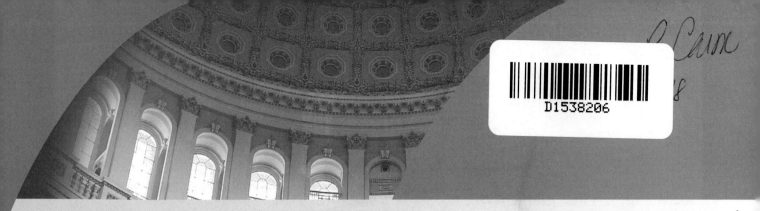

Essential Readings in Health Policy and Law

Joel B. Teitelbaum, JD, LLM

The George Washington University
School of Public Health and Health Services
Department of Health Policy
Washington, DC

Sara E. Wilensky, JD, MPP

The George Washington University
School of Public Health and Health Services
Department of Health Policy
Washington, DC

JONES AND BARTLETT PUBLISHERS
Sudbury, Massachusetts
BOSTON   TORONTO   LONDON   SINGAPORE

World Headquarters

Jones and Bartlett Publishers
40 Tall Pine Drive
Sudbury, MA 01776
978-443-5000
info@jbpub.com
www.jbpub.com

Jones and Bartlett Publishers Canada
6339 Ormindale Way
Mississauga, Ontario L5V 1J2
Canada

Jones and Bartlett Publishers
International
Barb House, Barb Mews
London W6 7PA
United Kingdom

Jones and Bartlett's books and products are available through most bookstores and online booksellers. To contact Jones and Bartlett Publishers directly, call 800-832-0034, fax 978-443-8000, or visit our website www.jbpub.com.

Substantial discounts on bulk quantities of Jones and Bartlett's publications are available to corporations, professional associations, and other qualified organizations. For details and specific discount information, contact the special sales department at Jones and Bartlett via the above contact information or send an email to specialsales@jbpub.com.

This publication is designed to provide accurate and authoritative information in regard to the Subject Matter covered. It is sold with the understanding that the publisher is not engaged in rendering legal, accounting, or other professional service. If legal advice or other expert assistance is required, the service of a competent professional person should be sought.

Production Credits
Publisher: Michael Brown
Production Director: Amy Rose
Associate Editor: Katey Birtcher
Production Editor: Tracey Chapman
Production Assistant: Roya Millard
Marketing Manager: Sophie Fleck
Manufacturing and Inventory Control Supervisor: Amy Bacus
Composition: Auburn Associates, Inc.
Cover Design: Kristin E. Ohlin
Cover Image: © Steve Maehl/ShutterStock, Inc.
Printing and Binding: Courier Stoughton
Cover Printing: John P. Pow Company

Library of Congress Cataloging-in-Publication Data
Essential readings of health policy and law / [edited by] Joel B. Teitelbaum, Sara E. Wilensky.
    p. ; cm. — (Essential public health)
  Includes bibliographical references and index.
  ISBN-13: 978-0-7637-3851-8 (pbk.)
  ISBN-10: 0-7637-3851-4 (pbk.)
  1. Medical policy—United States. 2. Medical care—United States. 3. Public health laws—United States. I. Teitelbaum, Joel Bern. II. Wilensky, Sara E. III. Series.
  [DNLM: 1. Health Policy—legislation & jurisprudence—United States—Collected Works. 2. Health Policy—legislation & jurisprudence—United States—Legal Cases. 3. Bioethical Issues—legislation & jurisprudence—United States—Collected Works. 4. Bioethical Issues—legislation & jurisprudence—United States—Legal Cases. 5. Delivery of Health Care—legislation & jurisprudence—United States—Collected Works. 6. Delivery of Health Care—legislation & jurisprudence—United States—Legal Cases. 7. Public Health—legislation & jurisprudence—United States—Collected Works. 8. Public Health—legislation & jurisprudence—United States—Legal Cases. 9. Quality of Health Care—legislation & jurisprudence—United States—Collected Works. 10. Quality of Health Care—legislation & jurisprudence—United States—Legal Cases. WA 33 AA1 E78 2009]
  RA395.A3E845 2009
  362.1—dc22
                            2008006665

6048
Printed in the United States of America
12 11 10 09 08   10 9 8 7 6 5 4 3 2 1

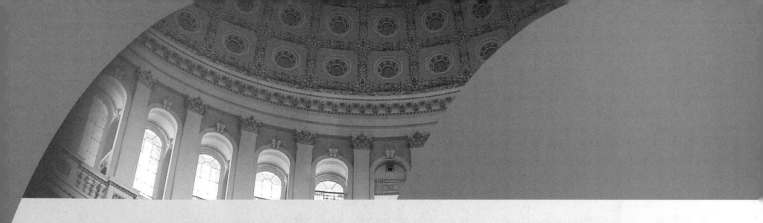

Contents

Part IV   Rethinking the Public Health and Health Care Systems   285

Part V   Tools for Health Policy Analysis   383

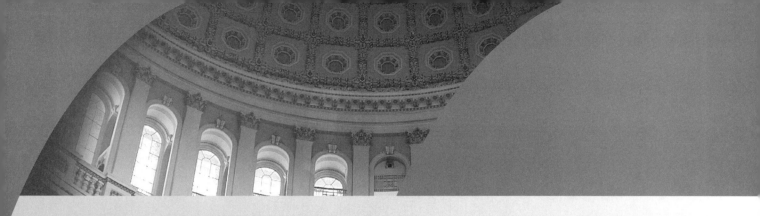

Series Page

See **www.jbpub.com/essentialpublichealth** for the latest information on the series.

ABOUT THE EDITOR:

Richard Riegalman, MD, MPH, PhD, is professor of Epidemiology-Biostatistics, Medicine, and Health Policy and founding dean at George Washington University School of Public Health and Health Services in Washington, DC.

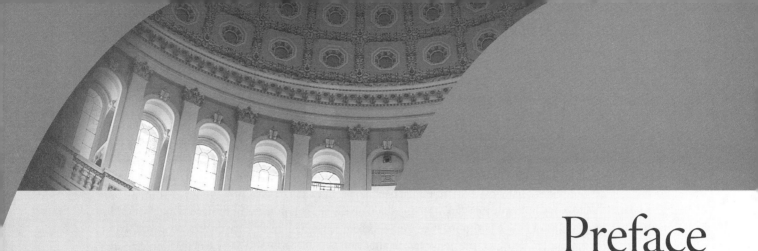

Preface

Essential Readings in Health Policy and Law is a companion to the *Essentials of Health Policy and Law* textbook. In the textbook, we explain how health policies and laws are influenced and formulated, describe a series of critical issues encountered in the study of health policy and law, and offer various frameworks for thinking about how to approach the issues going forward. The textbook is intentionally introductory and concise; it aims to provide the reader with a foundation in the seminal issues in American health policy and law and with a starting point for further reflection, research, and analysis.

As a companion to the textbook, *Essential Readings* is meant to assist introductory health policy and law students with their pursuit of more advanced study and discussion. It is a compilation of carefully selected readings—book chapters and articles, case law, statutes and regulations, and public policy "tools" such as health budget proposals—meant to allow for deeper analysis of topics covered in the textbook, as well as the study of a few topics not covered in the textbook due to space constraints.

Although this book is, in terms of its content, closely linked to its companion textbook, this is not the case in terms of its structure. Unlike the chapter structure of the textbook, this book is divided into five broad parts. We adopted this approach because of the flexibility it affords professors and students, given that the study of introductory health policy and law takes place across a spectrum: At some universities, introductory health policy might be taught, whereas health law is not; some institutions teach both health policy and law but do so as distinct courses (if not distinct disciplines), and some students study both health policy and law in the same course. Furthermore, many academic institutions are undertaking efforts to introduce basic health policy and/or law courses into their curriculum. It is our hope that the structure of the *Essentials of Health Policy and Law* textbook and this companion provide the requisite flexibility to be useful across this pedagogical spectrum.

Although the readings included herein can be fairly said to represent the perspectives of individual authors, policymakers, and judges that span the spectrum of political and social thought, this is true only generally, rather than with respect to each topic covered. This reflects our desire to reproduce a series of writings meant not to divide readers into specific camps—"I agree with that argument" or "I align myself most closely with this policy position"—but to offer thought-provoking readings intended to stimulate discussion, group reflection, and reassessment of one's own preexisting thoughts or beliefs. In other words, we hope to not only provide in-depth information on critical health policy and law issues facing the country but to create a classroom environment where free-flowing thought and discussion is more the norm than are preconceived positions seeking affirmation.

In somewhat the same vein, in most instances, we have reproduced the resources completely, rather than as edited versions. (One important exception to this is in the case of some judicial opinions, which can sometimes span dozens and dozens of pages when all related opinions—concurrences and dissents, in addition to the court majority's opinion—

are included.) We opted for this approach (rather than shortening documents in the hope of being able to include additional items) to maintain the authenticity and full context of the writings, thus allowing students to perhaps more easily form their views about a particular reading.

As mentioned, this book is divided into five parts, with each part including a brief introduction to the reading selections included. Part I provides a basic overview of public health. It is intended to be read by students with little or no background in the field or by those students looking to brush up on the key components of the field of public health, including the legal foundations of public health practice. Part II is concerned with healthcare quality, an area of critical policy and legal importance and one that has received great attention over the last few years, particularly as it relates to information technology. It is an area that deserves more attention among introductory students than we were able to provide in the companion textbook. Part III centers on the intersection of policy and law with medicine and ethics, including the evolution of public health ethics, which has long lingered in the shadow of medical ethics. In Part IV, we offer several resources on the topic of health system reform, which if nothing else is heralded for its ability to utterly defy consensus. The included articles are sure to spawn discussion about whether and how to reform the public health and healthcare systems. Finally, in Part V, we include a series of resources collectively called "Tools for Health Policy Analysis." These include practical articles describing the methods—and potential pitfalls—of policy analysis, as well as examples of the administrative regulations, informal government memoranda, and budget proposals that serve as important instruments in a policymaker's toolbox.

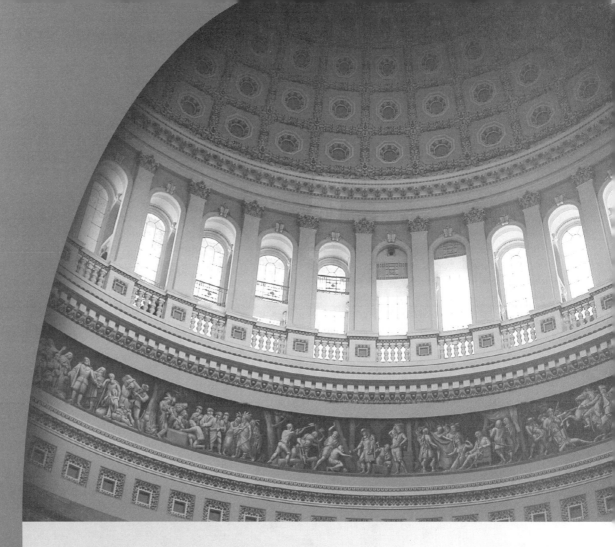

PART I

Overview of Public Health

The first Part in this series of readings provides foundational information about public health in the United States.[1] The selections included are intended to ensure that each reader has access to basic information about public health and public health policy and law, and they are also intended to spur debate about the proper role of public health in society.

As promised in *Essentials of Health Policy and Law,* Part I opens with a general description of public health. In "What is Public Health?" from the *Essentials of Public Health* textbook, Bernard Turnock defines public health, provides a brief history of U.S. public health efforts, reviews the features of the public health system, and discusses values associated with public health. (We recommend that readers review the subsequent chapters in Turnock's textbook for further information about the inner workings of public health.)

Following Turnock's overview is "The Law and the Public's Health: The Foundations," by Lawrence Gostin, Jeffrey Koplan, and Frank Grad. In it, the authors detail the role law plays in the field of public health and explain the underpinnings of public health law. The article also provides in-depth discussions of a number of topics touched upon in *Essentials of Health Policy and Law,* including state police powers. This discussion prepares readers for their first (of many) legal opinions reproduced in this book; in *Jacobson v. Massachusetts,* the United States Supreme Court ruled on the validity of a state mandatory vaccine law, whereas in *DeShaney v.*

Winnebago County Social Services Department and *Town of Castle Rock, Colorado v. Gonzales,* the Court discussed public health and welfare in the context of a "negative Constitution."

Part I ends with an overview of public health reform recommendations made by the Institute of Medicine in *The Future of the Public's Health in the 21st Century.* These recommendations illustrate the breadth of public health's influence on society by touching on areas as diverse as governmental public health infrastructure, community health, the health care delivery system, and the roles of business, employers, the media, and academia in public health reform efforts.

IN THIS SECTION

Bernard Turnock, "What Is Public Health?" from *Essentials of Public Health*
Larry Gostin et al., "The Law and the Public's Health: The Foundations" from *Law in Public Health Practice*
Case law: *Jacobson v. Massachusetts* (validity of state mandatory vaccine law)
Case law: *DeShaney v. Winnebago County Social Services Department* (public welfare and the "negative Constitution")
Case law: *Town of Castle Rock, Colorado v. Gonzales* (public welfare and the "negative Constitution")
Executive Summary from *The Future of the Public's Health in the 21st Century*

---

[1]The focus of this section is on public health, because many basic principles pertaining to the healthcare system were described at length in *Essentials of Health Policy and Law,* the companion to this book.

What Is Public Health?

Bernard J. Turnock

By permission of Jones and Bartlett Publishers, LLC. Reprinted from Turnock, BJ. *Essentials of Public Health*. Sudbury: Jones and Bartlett Publishers, 2001: 1–19.

LEARNING OBJECTIVES

After completing Chapter 1, learners will be proficient in describing what public health is, including its unique and important features, to general audiences. Key aspects of this competency expectation include:

- Articulating several different definitions of public health
- Describing the origins and content of public health responses over history
- Tracing the development of the public health system in the United States
- Broadly characterizing the contributions and value of public health
- Identifying three or more distinguishing features of public health
- Describing public health as a system with inputs, processes, outputs, and results, including the role of core functions and essential public health services and identifying five or more Internet Web sites that provide useful information on the U.S. public health system

The passing of one century and the arrival of another afford a rare opportunity to look back at where public health has been and forward to the challenges that lie ahead. Imagine a world 100 years from now where life expectancy is 30 years more and infant mortality rates are 95% lower than they are today. The average human life span would be more than 107 years, and less than one of every 2,000 infants would die before their first birthday. These seem like unrealistic expectations and unlikely achievements; yet, they are no greater than the gains realized during the 20th century in the United States. In 1900, few envisioned the century of progress in public health that lay ahead.

Yet by 1925 public health leaders such as C.E.A. Winslow were noting a nearly 50% increase in life expectancy (from 36 years to 53 years) for residents of New York City between the years 1880 and 1920.[1] Accomplishments such as these caused Winslow to speculate what might be possible through widespread application of scientific knowledge. With the even more spectacular achievements over the rest of the 20th century, we all should wonder what is possible in the century that has just begun.

The year 2006 will be remembered for many things, but it is unlikely that many people will remember it as a spectacular year for public health in the United States. No major discoveries, innovations, or triumphs set the year 2006 apart from other years in recent memory. Yet, on closer examination, maybe there were! Like the story of the wise man who invented the game of chess for his king and asked for payment by having the king place one grain of wheat on the first square of the chessboard, two on the second, four on the third, eight on the fourth, and so on, the small victories of public health over the past century have resulted in cumulative gains so vast in scope that they are difficult to comprehend.

In the year 2006, there were nearly 900,000 fewer cases of measles reported than in 1941, 200,000 fewer cases of diphtheria than in 1921, more than 250,000 fewer cases of whooping cough than in 1934, and 21,000 fewer cases of polio than in 1951.[2] The early years of the new century witnessed 50 million fewer smokers than would have been expected, given trends in tobacco use through 1965. More than 2 million Americans were alive that otherwise would have died from heart disease and stroke, and nearly 100,000 Americans were alive as a result of automobile seat belt use. Protection of the

U.S. blood supply had prevented more than 1.5 million hepatitis B and hepatitis C infections and more than 50,000 human immunodeficiency virus (HIV) infections, as well as more than $5 billion in medical costs associated with these three diseases.[3] Today, average blood lead levels in children are less than one third of what they were a quarter century ago. This catalog of accomplishments could be expanded many times over. Figure 1-1 summarizes this progress, as reflected in two of the most widely followed measures of a population's health status—life expectancy and infant mortality.

These results did not occur by themselves. They came about through decisions and actions that represent the essence of what public health is. It is the story of public health and its immense value and importance in our lives that is the focus of this text. With this impressive litany of accomplishments, it would seem that public health's story would be easily told. For many reasons, however, it is not. As a result, public health remains poorly understood by its prime beneficiary—the public—as well as many of its dedicated practitioners. Although public health's results, as measured in terms of improved health status, diseases prevented, scarce resources saved, and improved quality of life, are more apparent today than ever before, society seldom links the activities of public health with its results. This suggests that the public health community must more ef-

fectively communicate what public health is and what it does, so that its results can be readily traced to their source.

This chapter is an introduction to public health that links basic concepts to practice. It considers three questions:

- What is public health?
- Where did it come from?
- Why is it important in the United States today?

To address these questions, this chapter begins with a sketch of the historical development of public health activities in the United States. It then examines several definitions and characterizations of what public health is and explores some of its unique features. Finally, it offers insights into the value of public health in biologic, economic, and human terms.

Taken together, the topics in this chapter provide a foundation for understanding what public health is and why it is important. A conceptual framework that approaches public health from a systems perspective is introduced to identify the dimensions of the public health system and facilitate an understanding of the various images of public health that coexist in the United States today. We will see that, as in the story of the blind men examining the elephant, various sectors of our society have mistaken separate components of public health for the entire system. Later chapters will more thoroughly exam-

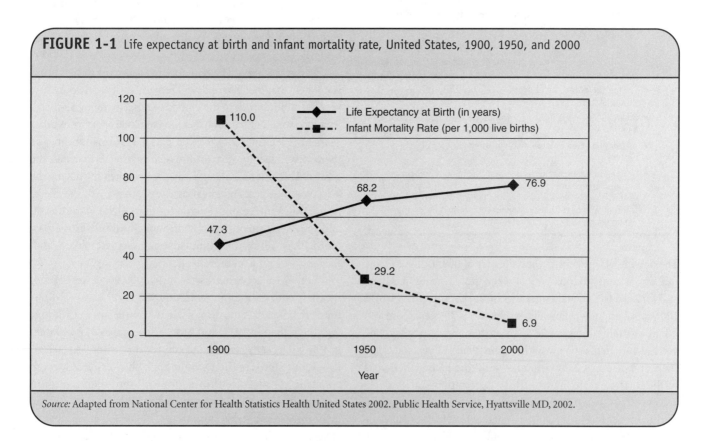

FIGURE 1-1 Life expectancy at birth and infant mortality rate, United States, 1900, 1950, and 2000

Source: Adapted from National Center for Health Statistics Health United States 2002. Public Health Service, Hyattsville MD, 2002.

ine and discuss the various components and dimensions of the public health system.

A BRIEF HISTORY OF PUBLIC HEALTH IN THE UNITED STATES

Early Influences on American Public Health

Although the complete history of public health is a fascinating saga in its own right, this section presents only selected highlights. Suffice it to say that when ancient cultures perceived illness as the manifestation of supernatural forces, they also felt that little in the way of either personal or collective action was possible. For many centuries, disease was synonymous with epidemic. Diseases, including horrific epidemics of infectious diseases such as the Black Death (plague), leprosy, and cholera, were phenomena to be accepted. It was not until the so-called Age of Reason and the Enlightenment that scholarly inquiry began to challenge the "givens" or accepted realities of society. Eventually, the expansion of the science and knowledge base would reap substantial rewards.

With the advent of industrialism and imperialism, the stage was set for epidemic diseases to increase their terrible toll. As populations shifted to urban centers for purpose of commerce and industry, public health conditions worsened. The mixing of dense populations living in unsanitary conditions and working long hours in unsafe and exploitative industries with wave-after-wave of cholera, smallpox, typhoid, tuberculosis, yellow fever, and other diseases was a formula for disaster. Such disaster struck again and again across the globe, but most seriously and most often at the industrialized seaport cities that provided the portal of entry for diseases transported as stowaways alongside commercial cargo. The experience, and subsequent susceptibility, of different cultures to these diseases partly explains how relatively small bands of Europeans were able to overcome and subjugate vast Native American cultures. Seeing the Europeans unaffected by scourges such as smallpox served to reinforce beliefs that these light-skinned visitors were supernatural figures, unaffected by natural forces.[4]

The British colonies in North America and the fledgling United States certainly bore their share of the burden. American diaries of the 17th and 18th centuries chronicle one infectious disease onslaught after another. These epidemics left their mark on families, communities, and even history. For example, the national capital had to be moved out of Philadelphia due to a devastating yellow fever epidemic in 1793. This epidemic also prompted the city to develop its first board of health in that same year.

The formation of local boards of distinguished citizens, the first boards of health, was one of the earliest organized responses to epidemics. This response was revealing in that it represented an attempt to confront disease collectively. Because science had not yet determined that specific microorganisms were the causes of epidemics, avoidance had long been the primary tactic used. Avoidance meant evacuating the general location of the epidemic until it subsided or isolating diseased individuals or those recently exposed to diseases on the basis of a mix of fear, tradition, and scientific speculation. Several developments, however, were swinging the pendulum ever closer to more effective counteractions.

The work of public health pioneers such as Edward Jenner, John Snow, and Edwin Chadwick illustrates the value of public health, even when its methods are applied amidst scientific uncertainty. Well before Koch's postulates established scientific methods for linking bacteria with specific diseases and before Pasteur's experiments helped to establish the germ theory, both Jenner and Snow used deductive logic and common sense to do battle with smallpox and cholera, respectively. In 1796, Jenner successfully used vaccination for a disease that ran rampant through communities across the globe. This was the initial shot in a long and arduous campaign that, by the year 1977, had totally eradicated smallpox from all of its human hiding places in every country in the world. The potential for its reemergence through the actions of terrorists is a topic left to a later chapter of this text.

Snow's accomplishments even further advanced the art and science of public health. In 1854, Snow traced an outbreak of cholera to the well water drawn from the pump at Broad Street and helped to prevent hundreds, perhaps thousands, of cholera cases. In that same year, he demonstrated that another large outbreak could be traced to one particular water company that drew its water from the Thames River, downstream from London, and that another company that drew its water upstream from London was not linked with cholera cases. In both efforts, Snow's ability to collect and analyze data allowed him to determine causation, which, in turn, allowed him to implement corrective actions that prevented additional cases. All of this occurred without benefit of the knowledge that there was an odd-shaped little bacterium that was carried in water and spread from person to person by hand-to-mouth contact!

England's General Board of Health conducted its own investigations of these outbreaks and concluded that air, rather than contaminated water, was the cause.[5] Its approach, however, was one of collecting a vast amount of information and accepting only that which supported its view of disease causation. Snow, on the other hand, systematically tested his hypothesis by exploring evidence that ran contrary to his initial expectations.

Chadwick was a more official leader of what has become known as the sanitary movement of the latter half of the 19th century. In a variety of official capacities, he played a major part in structuring government's role and responsibilities for protecting the public's health. Due to the growing concern over the social and sanitary conditions in England, a National Vaccination Board was established in 1837. Shortly thereafter, Chadwick's *Report on an Inquiry into the Sanitary Conditions of the Laboring Population of Great Britain* articulated a framework for broad public actions that served as a blueprint for the growing sanitary movement. One result was the establishment in 1848 of a General Board of Health. Interestingly, Chadwick's interest in public health had its roots in Jeremy Bentham's utilitarian movement. For Chadwick, disease was viewed as causing poverty, and poverty was responsible for the great social ills of the time, including societal disorder and high taxation to provide for the general welfare.[6] Public health efforts were necessary to reduce poverty and its wider social effects. This view recognizes a link between poverty and health that differs somewhat from current views. Today, it is more common to consider poor health as a result of poverty, rather than as its cause.

Chadwick was also a key participant in the partly scientific, partly political debate that took place in British government as to whether deaths should be attributed to clinical conditions or to their underlying factors, such as hunger and poverty. It was Chadwick's view that pathologic, as opposed to less proximal social and behavioral, factors should be the basis for classifying deaths.[6] Chadwick's arguments prevailed, although aspects of this debate continue to the present day. William Farr, sometimes called the *father of modern vital statistics*, championed the opposing view.

In the latter half of the 19th century, as sanitation and environmental engineering methods evolved, more effective interventions became available against epidemic diseases. Further, the scientific advances of this period paved the way for modern disease control efforts targeting specific microorganisms.

Growth of Local and State Public Health Activities in the United States

In the United States, Lemuel Shattuck's *Report of the Sanitary Commission of Massachusetts* in 1850 outlined existing and future public health needs for that state and became America's blueprint for development of a public health system. Shattuck called for the establishment of state and local health departments to organize public efforts aimed at sanitary inspections, communicable disease control, food sanitation, vital statistics, and services for infants and children. Although Shattuck's report closely paralleled Chadwick's efforts in Great Britain, ac-

ceptance of his recommendations did not occur for several decades. In the latter part of the century, his farsighted and far-reaching recommendations came to be widely implemented. With greater understanding of the value of environmental controls for water and sewage and of the role of specific control measures for specific diseases (including quarantine, isolation, and vaccination), the creation of local health agencies to carry out these activities supplemented—and, in some cases, supplanted—local boards of health. These local health departments developed rapidly in the seaports and other industrial urban centers, beginning with a health department in Baltimore in 1798, because these were the settings where the problems were reaching unacceptable levels.

Because infectious and environmental hazards are no respecters of local jurisdictional boundaries, states began to develop their own boards and agencies after 1870. These agencies often had very broad powers to protect the health and lives of state residents, although the clear intent at the time was that these powers be used to battle epidemics of infectious diseases. In later chapters, we will revisit these powers and duties because they serve as both a stimulus and a limitation for what can be done to address many contemporary public health issues and problems.

Federal Public Health Activities in the United States

This sketch of the development of public health in the United States would be incomplete without a brief introduction to the roles and powers of the federal government. Federal health powers, at least as enumerated in the U.S. Constitution, are minimal. It is surprising to some to learn that the word health does not even appear in the Constitution. As a result of not being a power granted to the federal government (such as defense, foreign diplomacy, international and interstate commerce, or printing money), health became a power to be exercised by states or reserved to the people themselves.

Two sections of the Constitution have been interpreted over time to allow for federal roles in health, in concert with the concept of the so-called implied powers necessary to carry out explicit powers. These are the ability to tax in order to provide for the "general welfare" (a phrase appearing in both the preamble and body of the Constitution) and the specific power to regulate commerce, both international and interstate. These opportunities allowed the federal government to establish a beachhead in health, initially through the Marine Hospital Service (eventually to become the Public Health Service). After the ratification of the 16th Amendment in 1916, authorizing a national income tax, the federal government acquired the ability to raise vast sums of money, which could then be directed toward promoting the general welfare. The specific means to this end were a variety of grants-in-aid to state and local governments. Beginning in the 1960s, federal grant-in-aid programs designed to fill gaps in the medical care system nudged state and local governments further and further into the business of medical service provision. Federal grant programs for other social, substance abuse, mental health, and community prevention services soon followed. The expansion of federal involvement into these areas, however, was not accomplished by these means alone.

Prior to 1900, and perhaps not until the Great Depression, Americans did not believe that the federal government should intervene in their social circumstances. Social values shifted dramatically during the Depression, a period of such great social insecurity and need that the federal government was now permitted—indeed, expected—to intervene. Later chapters will expand on the growth of the federal government's influence on public health activities and its impact on the activities of state and local governments.

To explain more easily the broad trends of public health in the United States, it is useful to delineate distinct eras in its history. One simple scheme, illustrated in Table 1-1, uses the years 1850, 1950, and 2000 as approximate dividers. Prior to 1850, the system was characterized by recurrent epidemics of infectious diseases, with little in the way of collective response possible. During the sanitary movement in the second half of the 19th and first half of the 20th century, science-based control measures were organized and deployed through a public health infrastructure that was developing in the form of local and state health departments. After 1950, gaps in the medical care system and federal grant dollars acted together to increase public provision of a wide range of health services. That increase set the stage for the current reexamination of the links between medical and public health practice. Some retrenchment from the direct service provision role has occurred since about 1990. As we will examine in subsequent chapters, a new era for public health that seeks to balance community-driven

TABLE 1-1 Major Eras in Public Health History in the United States

Before 1850	Battling epidemics
1850 to 1949	Building state and local infrastructure
1950 to 1999	Filling gaps in medical care delivery
After 1999	Preparing for and responding to community health threats

public health practice with preparedness and response for public health emergencies lies ahead.

IMAGES AND DEFINITIONS OF PUBLIC HEALTH

The historical development of public health activities in the United States provides a basis for understanding what public health is today. Nonetheless, the term *public health* evokes several different images among the general public and those dedicated to its improvement. To some, the term describes a broad social enterprise or system.

To others, the term describes the professionals and workforce whose job it is to solve certain important health problems. At a meeting in the early 1980s to plan a community-wide education and outreach campaign to encourage early prenatal care in order to reduce infant mortality, a community relations director of a large television station made some comments that reflected this view. When asked whether his station had been involved in infant mortality reduction efforts in the past, he responded, "Yes, but that's not our job. If you people in public health had been doing your job properly, we wouldn't be called on to bail you out!" Obviously, this man viewed public health as an effort of which he was not a part.

Still another image of public health is that of a body of knowledge and techniques that can be applied to health-related problems. Here, public health is seen as what public health does. Snow's investigations exemplify this perspective.

Similarly, many people perceive public health primarily as the activities ascribed to governmental public health agencies. For the majority of the public, this latter image represents public health in the United States, resulting in the common view that public health primarily involves the provision of medical care to indigent populations. Since 2001, however, public health has also emerged as a front line defense against bioterrorism and other threats to personal security and safety.

A final image of public health is that of the intended results of these endeavors. In this image, public health is literally the health of the public, as measured in terms of health and illness in a population.

This chapter will focus primarily on the first of these images, public health as a social enterprise or system. Later chapters will examine each of the other images of public health. It is important to understand what people mean when they speak of public health. As presented in Table 1-2, the profession, the methods, the governmental services, the ultimate outcomes, and even the broad social enterprise itself are all commonly encountered images of what public health is today.

With varying images of what public health is, we would expect no shortage of definitions. There have been many, and it serves little purpose to try to catalog all of them here. Three

TABLE 1-2 Images of Public Health

- Public health: the system and social enterprise
- Public health: the profession
- Public health: the methods (knowledge and techniques)
- Public health: governmental services (especially medical care for the poor)
- Public health: the health of the public

definitions, each separated by a generation, provide important insights into what public health is; these are summarized in Table 1-3.

In 1988 the prestigious Institute of Medicine (IOM) provided a useful definition in its landmark study of public health in the United States, *The Future of Public Health*. The IOM report characterized public health's mission as "fulfilling society's interest in assuring conditions in which people can be healthy."[7] This definition directs our attention to the many conditions that influence health and wellness, underscoring the broad scope of public health and legitimizing its interest in social, economic, political, and medical care factors that affect health and illness. The definition's premise that society has an interest in the health of its members implies that improving conditions and health status for others is acting in our own self-interest. The assertion that improving the health status of others provides benefits to all is a core value of public health.

Another core value of public health is reflected in the IOM definition's use of the term *assuring*. Assuring conditions in

TABLE 1-3 Selected Definitions of Public Health

- "The science and art of preventing disease, prolonging life and promoting health and efficiency through organized community effort"
- "Successive re-definings of the unacceptable"
- "Fulfilling society's interest in assuring conditions in which people can be healthy"

Source: Data are from the following: Institute of Medicine, National Academy of Sciences. *The Future of Public Health*. Washington, DC: National Academy Press: 1988; Winslow CEA. The untilled field of public health. *Mod Med*. 1920;2:183-191; and Vickers G. What sets the goals of public health? *Lancet*. 1958;1:599–604.

which people can be healthy means vigilantly promoting and protecting everyone's interests in health and well-being. This value echoes the wisdom in the often-quoted African aphorism that "it takes a village to raise a child." Former Surgeon General David Satcher, the first African-American to head this country's most respected federal public health agency, the Centers for Disease Control and Prevention (CDC), once described a visit to Africa in which he met with African teenagers to learn first hand of their personal health attitudes and behaviors. Satcher was struck by their concerns over the rapid urbanization of the various African nations and the changes that were affecting their culture and sense of community. These young people felt lost and abandoned; they questioned Satcher as to what CDC, the U.S. government, and the world community were willing to do to help them survive these changes. As one young man put it, "Where will we find our village?" Public health's role is one of serving us all as our village, whether we are teens in Africa or adults in the United States. The IOM report's characterization of public health advocated for just such a social enterprise and stands as a bold philosophical statement of mission and purpose.

The IOM report also sought to define the boundaries of public health by identifying three core functions of public health: assessment, policy development, and assurance. In one sense, these functions are comparable to those generally ascribed to the medical care system involving diagnosis and treatment. Assessment is the analogue of diagnosis, except that the diagnosis, or problem identification, is made for a group or population of individuals. Similarly, assurance is analogous to treatment and implies that the necessary remedies or interventions are put into place. Finally, policy development is an intermediate role of collectively deciding which remedies or interventions are most appropriate for the problems identified (the formulation of a treatment plan is the medical system's analogue). These core functions broadly describe what public health does (as opposed to what it is) and will be examined more thoroughly in later chapters.

The concepts embedded in the IOM definition are also reflected in Winslow's definition, developed more than 80 years ago. His definition describes both what public health does and how this gets done. It is a comprehensive definition that has stood the test of time in characterizing public health as

> . . . the science and art of preventing disease, prolonging life, and promoting health and efficiency through organized community effort for the sanitation of the environment, the control of communicable infections, the education of the individual in personal hygiene, the organization

of medical and nursing services for the early diagnosis and preventive treatment of disease, and
for the development of the social machinery to
insure everyone a standard of living adequate for
the maintenance of health, so organizing these
benefits as to enable every citizen to realize his
birthright of health and longevity.[8]

There is much to consider in Winslow's definition. The
phrases, "science and art," "organized community effort," and
"birthright of health and longevity" capture the substance and
aims of public health. Winslow's catalog of methods illumi-
nates the scope of the endeavor, embracing public health's initial targeting of infectious and environmental risks, as well as
current activities related to the organization, financing, and accountability of medical care services. His allusion to the "social
machinery necessary to insure everyone a standard of living
adequate for the maintenance of health" speaks to the relationship between social conditions and health in all societies.

There have been many other attempts to define public
health, although these have received less attention than either
the Winslow or IOM definitions. Several build on the observation that, over time, public health activities reflect the
interaction of disease with two other phenomena that can be
roughly characterized as science and social values: (1) what
do we know, and (2) what do we choose to do with that
knowledge?

A prominent British industrialist, Geoffrey Vickers, provided an interesting addition to this mix a half century ago
while serving as Secretary of the Medical Research Council.
In identifying the forces that set the agenda for public health,
Vickers noted, "The landmarks of political, economic, and
social history are the moments when some condition passed
from the category of the given into the category of the intolerable. I believe that the history of public health might well
be written as a record of successive re-definings of the
unacceptable."[9]

The usefulness of Vickers' formulation lies in its focus on
the delicate and shifting interface between science and social
values. Through this lens, we can view a tracing of public
health over history, facilitating an understanding of why and
how different societies have reacted to health risks differently
at various points in time and space. In this light, the history
of public health is one of blending knowledge with social values to shape responses to problems that require collective action after they have crossed the boundary from the acceptable
to the unacceptable.

Each of these definitions offers important insights into
what public health is and what it does. Individually and collec-

tively, they describe a social enterprise that is both important
and unique, as we will see in the section that follows.

PUBLIC HEALTH AS A SYSTEM

So what is public health? Maybe no single answer will satisfy
everyone. There are, in fact, several views of public health that
must be considered. One or more of them may be apparent to
the inquirer. The public health described in this chapter is a
broad social enterprise, more akin to a movement, that seeks to
extend the benefits of current knowledge in ways that will have
the maximum impact on the health status of a population. It
does so by identifying problems that call for collective action to
protect, promote, and improve health, primarily through preventive strategies. This public health is unique in its interdisciplinary approach and methods, its emphasis on preventive
strategies, its linkage with government and political decision
making, and its dynamic adaptation to new problems placed on
its agenda. Above all else, it is a collective effort to identify and
address the unacceptable realities that result in preventable and
avoidable health and quality of life outcomes, and it is the composite of efforts and activities that are carried out by people
and organizations committed to these ends.

With this broad view of public health as a social enterprise, the question shifts from what public health is to what
these other images of public health represent and how they relate to each other. To understand these separate images of public health, a conceptual model would be useful. Surprisingly, an
understandable and useful framework to tie these pieces together has been lacking. Other enterprises have found ways to
describe their complex systems, and, from what appears to be
an industrial production model, we can begin to look at the
various components of our public health system.

This framework brings together the mission and functions of public health in relation to the inputs, processes, outputs, and outcomes of the system. Table 1-4 provides general
descriptions for the terms used in this framework. It is sometimes easier to appreciate this model when a more familiar
industry, such as the automobile industry, is used as an example. The mission or purpose might be expressed as meeting the personal transportation needs of the population. This
industry carries out its mission by providing passenger cars to
its customers; this characterizes its function. In this light, we
can now examine the inputs, processes, outputs, and outcomes
of the system set up to carry out this function. Inputs would
include steel, rubber, plastic, and so forth, as well as the workers, know-how, technology, facilities, machinery, and support
services necessary to allow the raw materials to become automobiles. The key processes necessary to carry out the primary
function might be characterized as designing cars, making or

TABLE 1-4 Dimensions of the Public Health System

Capacity (Inputs):

- The resources and relationships necessary to carry out the core functions and essential services of public health (e.g., human resources, information resources, fiscal and physical resources, and appropriate relationships among the system components).

Process (Practices and Outputs):

- Those collective practices or processes that are necessary and sufficient to assure that the core functions and essential services of public health are being carried out effectively, including the key processes that iden-

tify and address health problems and their causative factors and the interventions intended to prevent death, disease, and disability and to promote quality of life.

Outcomes (Results):

- Indicators of health status, risk reduction, and quality-of-life enhancement outcomes are long-term objectives that define optimal, measurable future levels of health status; maximum acceptable levels of disease, injury, or dysfunction; or prevalence of risk factors.

Source: Adapted from Centers for Disease Control and Prevention, Public Health Program Office, 1990.

acquiring parts, assembling parts into automobiles, moving cars to dealers, and selling and servicing cars after purchase. No doubt this is an incomplete listing of this industry's processes; it is oversimplified here to make the point. In any event, these processes translate the abstract concept of getting cars to people into the operational steps necessary to carry out this basic function. The outputs of these processes are cars located where people can purchase them. The outcomes include satisfied customers and company profits.

Applying this same general framework to the public health system is also possible but may not be so obvious to the general public. The mission and functions of public health are well described in the IOM report's framework. The core functions of assessment, policy development, and assurance are considerably more abstract functions than making cars but still can be made operational through descriptions of their key steps or practices.[10,11] The inputs of the public health system include its human, organizational, informational, fiscal, and other resources. These resources and relationships are structured to carry out public health's core functions through a variety of processes that can also be termed *essential public health practices or services.* These processes include a variety of interventions that result from some of the more basic processes of assessing health needs and planning effective strategies.[12] These outputs or interventions are intended to produce the desired results, which, with public health, might well be characterized as health or quality-of-life outcomes. Figure 1-2 illustrates these relationships.

In this model, not all components are as readily understandable and measurable as others. Several of the inputs are

easily counted or measured, including human, fiscal, and organizational resources. Outputs are also generally easy to recognize and count (e.g., prenatal care programs, number of immunizations provided, health messages on the dangers of tobacco). Health outcomes are also readily understood in terms of mortality, morbidity, functional disability, time lost from work or school, and even more sophisticated measures, such as years of potential life lost and quality-of-life years lost. The elements that are most difficult to understand and visualize are the processes or essential services of the public health system. Although this is an evolving field, there have been efforts to characterize these operational aspects of public health. By such efforts, we are better able to understand public health practice, to measure it, and to relate it to its outputs and outcomes. A national work group was assembled by the U.S. Public Health Service in 1994 in an attempt to develop a consensus statement of what public health is and does in language understandable to those both inside and outside the field of public health. Table 1-5 presents the result of that process in a statement entitled "Public Health in America."[13] The conceptual framework identified in Figure 1-2 and the narrative representation in the "Public Health in America" statement are useful models for understanding the public health system and how it works, as we will see throughout this text.

This framework attempts to bridge the gap between what public health is, what it does (purpose/mission and functions, Figure 1-2), and how it does what it does (through its capacity, processes, and outcomes). It also allows us to examine the various components of the system so that we can better appreciate how the pieces fit together.

UNIQUE FEATURES OF PUBLIC HEALTH

Several unique features of public health individually and collectively serve to make understanding and appreciation of this enterprise difficult (Table 1-6). These include the underlying social justice philosophy of public health; its inherently political nature; its ever-expanding agenda, with new problems and issues being assigned over time; its link with government; its grounding in a broad base of biologic, physical, quantitative,

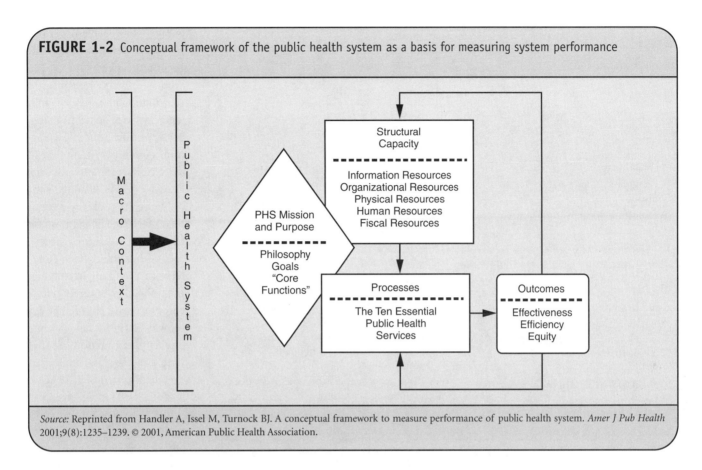

FIGURE 1-2 Conceptual framework of the public health system as a basis for measuring system performance

Source: Reprinted from Handler A, Issel M, Turnock BJ. A conceptual framework to measure performance of public health system. *Amer J Pub Health* 2001;9(8):1235–1239. © 2001, American Public Health Association.

social, and behavioral sciences; its focus on prevention as a prime intervention strategy; and the unique bond and sense of mission that links its proponents.

Social Justice Philosophy

It is vital to recognize the social justice orientation of public health and even more critical to understand the potential for conflict and confrontation that it generates. Social justice is said to be the foundation of public health. The concept first emerged around 1848, a time that might be considered the birth of modern public health. Social justice argues that public health is properly a public matter and that its results in terms of death, disease, health, and well-being reflect the decisions and actions that a society makes, for good or for ill.[14] Justice is an abstract concept that determines how each member of a society is allocated his or her fair share of collective burdens and benefits. Societal benefits to be distributed may include happiness, income, or social status. Burdens include restrictions of individual action and taxation. Justice dictates that there is fairness in the distribution of benefits and burdens; injustices occur when persons are denied some benefit to which they are entitled or when some burden is imposed unduly. If access to health services, or even health itself, is considered to

be a societal benefit (or if poor health is considered to be a burden), the links between the concepts of justice and public health become clear. Market justice and social justice represent two forms of modern justice.

Market justice emphasizes personal responsibility as the basis for distributing burdens and benefits. Other than respecting the basic rights of others, individuals are responsible primarily for their own actions and are free from collective obligations. Individual rights are highly valued, whereas collective responsibilities are minimized. In terms of health, individuals assume primary responsibility for their own health. There is little expectation that society should act to protect or promote the health of its members beyond addressing risks that cannot be controlled through individual action.

Social justice argues that significant factors within the society impede the fair distribution of benefits and burdens.[15] Examples of such impediments include social class distinctions, heredity, racism, and ethnism. Collective action, often leading to the assumption of additional burdens, is necessary to neutralize or overcome those impediments. In the case of public health, the goal of extending the potential benefits of the physical and behavioral sciences to all groups in the society, especially when the burden of disease and ill health within that

TABLE 1-5 Public Health in America

Vision:
Healthy People in Healthy Communities
Mission:
Promote Physical and Mental Health and Prevent Disease, Injury, and Disability

Public Health

- Prevents epidemics and the spread of disease
- Protects against environmental hazards
- Prevents injuries
- Promotes and encourages healthy behaviors
- Responds to disasters and assists communities in recovery
- Assures the quality and accessibility of health services

Essential Public Health Services

- Monitor health status to identify community health problems
- Diagnose and investigate health problems and health hazards in the community
- Inform, educate, and empower people about health issues

- Mobilize community partnerships to identify and solve health problems
- Develop policies and plans that support individual and community health efforts
- Enforce laws and regulations that protect health and ensure safety
- Link people with needed personal health services and assure the provision of health care when otherwise unavailable
- Assure a competent public health and personal health care workforce
- Evaluate effectiveness, accessibility, and quality of personal and population-based health services
- Research for new insights and innovative solutions to health problems

Source: Reprinted from Essential Public Health Services Working Group of the Core Public Health Functions Steering Committee, U.S. Public Health Service, 1994.

public policy problems remain unsolved, despite periodically becoming highly visible.[15] This scenario reflects responses to such intractable American problems as inadequate housing, poor public education systems, unemployment, racial discrimination, and poverty. However, it is also true for public health problems such as tobacco-related illnesses, infant mortality, substance abuse, mental health services, long-term care, and environmental pollution. The failure to effect comprehensive national health reform in 1994 is an example of this phenomenon. At that time, middle-class Americans deemed the modest price tag of health reform to be excessive, refusing to pay more out of their own pockets when they perceived that their own access and services were not likely to improve.

These and similar examples suggest that a critical challenge for public health as a social enterprise lies in overcoming the social and ethical barriers that prevent us from doing more with the tools already available to us.[15] Extending the frontiers of science and knowledge may not be as useful for improving public health as shifting the collective values of our society to act on what we already know. Recent public health successes, such as public attitudes toward smoking in both public and private locations and operating motor vehicles after alcohol consumption, provide evidence in support of this assertion. These advances came through changes in social norms, rather than through bigger and better science.

society is unequally distributed, is largely based on principles of social justice. It is clear that many modern public health (and other public policy) problems disproportionately affect some groups, usually a minority of the population, more than others. As a result, their resolution requires collective actions in which those less affected take on greater burdens, while not commensurately benefiting from those actions. When the necessary collective actions are not taken, even the most important

TABLE 1-6 Selected Unique Features of Public Health

- Basis in social justice philosophy
- Inherently political nature
- Dynamic, ever-expanding agenda
- Link with government
- Grounding in the sciences
- Use of prevention as a prime strategy
- Uncommon culture and bond

Inherently Political Nature

The social justice underpinnings of public health serve to stimulate political conflict. Public health is both public and political in nature. It serves populations, which are composites of many different communities, cultures, and values. Politics allows for issues to be considered, negotiated, and finally determined for populations. At the core of political processes are differing values and perspectives as to both the ends to be achieved and the means for achieving those ends. Advocating causes and agitating various segments of society to identify and address unacceptable conditions that adversely affect health status often lead to increased expectations and demands on society, generally through government. As a result, public health advocates appear at times as antigovernment and anti-institutional. Governmental public health agencies seeking to serve the interests of both government and public health are frequently caught in the middle. This creates tensions and conflict that can put these agencies at odds with governmental leaders on the one hand and external public health advocates on the other.

Expanding Agenda

A third unique feature of public health is its broad and ever-increasing scope. Traditional domains of public health interest include biology, environment, lifestyle, and health service organization. Within each of these domains are many factors that affect health status; in recent decades, many new public policy problems have been moved onto the public health agenda as their predisposing factors have been identified and found to fall into one or more of these domains.

The assignment of new problems to the public health agenda is an interesting phenomenon. For example, prior to 1900, the primary problems addressed by public health were infectious diseases and related environmental risks. After 1900, the focus expanded to include problems and needs of children and mothers to be addressed through health education and maternal and child health services as public sentiment over the health and safety of children increased. In the middle of the century, chronic disease prevention and medical care fell into public health's realm as an epidemiologic revolution began to identify causative agents for chronic diseases and links between use of health services and health outcomes. Later, substance abuse, mental illness, teen pregnancy, long-term care, and other issues fell to public health, as did several emerging problems, most notably the epidemics of violence and HIV infections, including acquired immune deficiency syndrome (AIDS). The public health agenda expanded even further as a result of the recent national dialogue over health reform and how health services will be organized and managed. Bioterrorism preparedness is an even more recent addition to this agenda amidst heightened concerns and expectations after the events of September 11, 2001, and the anthrax attacks the following month.

Link with Government

A fourth unique facet of public health is its link with government. Although public health is far more than the activities of federal, state, and local health departments, many people think only of governmental public health agencies when they think of public health. Government does play a unique role in seeing that the key elements are in place and that public health's mission gets addressed. Only government can exercise the enforcement provisions of our public policies that limit the personal and property rights of individuals and corporations in areas such as retail food establishments, sewage and water systems, occupational health and safety, consumer product safety, infectious disease control, and drug efficacy and safety. Government also can play the convener and facilitator role for identifying and prioritizing health problems that might be addressed through public resources and actions. These roles derive from the underlying principle of beneficence, in that government exists to improve the well-being of its members. Beneficence often involves a balance between maximizing benefits and minimizing harms on the one hand and doing no harm on the other.

Two general strategies are available for governmental efforts to influence public health. At the broadest level, governments can modify public policies that influence health through social and environmental conditions, such as policies for education, employment, housing, public safety, child welfare, pollution control, workplace safety, and family support. In line with the IOM report's definition of public health, these actions seek to ensure conditions in which people can be healthy. Another strategy of government is to directly provide programs and services that are designed to meet the health needs of the population. It is often easier to garner support for relatively small-scale programs directed toward a specific problem (such as tuberculosis or HIV infections) than to achieve consensus around broader health and social issues. This strategy is basically a "command-and-control" approach, in which government attempts to increase access to and utilization of services largely through deployment of its own resources rather than through working with others. A variation of this strategy for government is to ensure access to health care services through public financing approaches (Medicare and Medicaid are prime examples) or through specialized delivery systems (such as the Veterans Administration facilities, the Indian Health Service, and federally funded community health centers).

Whereas the United States has generally opted for the latter of these strategies, other countries have acted to place greater emphasis on broader social policies. Both the overall level of investment for and relative emphasis between these strategies contribute to the widely varying results achieved in terms of health status indicators among different nations (to be discussed in Chapter 2).

Many factors dictate the approaches used by a specific government at any point in time. These factors include history, culture, the structure of the government in question, and current social circumstances. There are also several underlying motivations that support government intervention. For paternalistic reasons, governments may act to control or restrict the liberties of individuals to benefit a group, whether or not that group seeks these benefits. For utilitarian reasons, governments intervene because of the perception that the state as a whole will benefit in some important way. For equality considerations, governments act to ensure that benefits and burdens are equally distributed among individuals. For equity considerations, governments justify interventions in order to distribute the benefits of society in proportion to need. These motivations reflect the views of each society as to whether health itself or merely access to health services is to be considered a right of individuals and populations within that society. Many societies, including the United States, act through government to ensure equal access to a broad array of preventive and treatment services. Equity in health status for all groups within the society may not be an explicit aspiration however, even where efforts are in place to ensure equality in access. Even more important for achieving equity in health status are concerted efforts to improve health status in population groups with the greatest disadvantage, mechanisms to monitor health status and contributing factors across all population groups, and participation of disadvantaged population groups in the key political decision-making processes within the society.[16] To the extent that equity in health status among all population groups does not guide actions of a society's government, these other elements will be only marginally effective.

As noted previously, the link between government and public health makes for a particularly precarious situation for governmental public health agencies. The conflicting value systems of public health and the wider community generally translate into public health agencies having to document their failure in order to make progress. It is said that only the squeaky wheel gets the grease; in public health, it often takes an outbreak, disaster, or other tragedy to demonstrate public health's value. Since 1985, increased funding for basic public health protection programs quickly followed outbreaks related to bacteria-contaminated milk in Illinois, tainted hamburgers in Washington state, and contaminated public water supplies in Milwaukee. Following concerns over preparedness of public health agencies to deal with bioterrorism and other public health threats, a massive infusion of federal funding occurred.

The assumption and delegation of public health responsibilities are quite complex in the United States, with different patterns in each of the 50 states (to be described in Chapter 4). Over recent decades, the concept of a governmental presence in health has emerged and gained widespread acceptance within the public health community. This concept characterizes the role of local government, often, but not necessarily always, operating through its official health agencies, which serve as the residual guarantors that needed services will actually be there when needed. In practice it means that, no matter how duties are assigned locally, there is a presence that ensures that health needs are identified and considered for collective action. We will return to this concept and how it is operationalized in Chapters 4 and 5.

Grounded in Science

One of the most unique aspects of public health—and one that continues to separate public health from many other social movements—is its grounding in science.[17] This relationship is clear for the medical and physical sciences that govern our understanding of the biologic aspects of humans, microorganisms, and vectors, as well as the risks present in our physical environments. However, it is also true for the social sciences of anthropology, sociology, and psychology that affect our understanding of human culture and behaviors influencing health and illness. The quantitative sciences of epidemiology and biostatistics remain essential tools and methods of public health practice. Often five basic sciences of public health are identified: epidemiology, biostatistics, environmental science, management sciences, and behavioral sciences. These constitute the core education of public health professionals.

The importance of a solid and diverse scientific base is both a strength and weakness of public health. Surely there is no substitute for science in the modern world. The public remains curiously attracted to scientific advances, at least in the physical and biologic sciences, and this base is important to market and promote public health interventions. For many years, epidemiology has been touted as the basic science of public health practice, suggesting that public health itself is applied epidemiology. Modern public health thinking views epidemiology less as the basic science of public health than as one of many contributors to a complex undertaking. In recent decades, knowledge from the social sciences has greatly enriched and supplemented the physical and biologic sciences. Yet these are areas less familiar to and perhaps less well appreciated by the public, making it difficult to garner public support for newer, more behaviorally mediated public health interventions. The old image of public health based on the scientific principles of environmental sanitation and communicable disease control is being superseded by a new image of public health approaches more grounded in what the public perceives to be "softer" science. This transition, at least temporarily, threatens public understanding and confidence in public health and its methods.

Focus on Prevention

If public health professionals were pressed to provide a one-word synonym for public health, the most frequent response would probably be prevention. In general, prevention characterizes actions that are taken to reduce the possibility that something will happen or in hopes of minimizing the damage that may occur if it does happen. Prevention is a widely appreciated and valued concept that is best understood when its object is identified. Although prevention is considered by many to be the purpose of public health, the specific intentions of prevention can vary greatly. Prevention can be aimed at deaths, hospital admissions, days lost from school, consumption of human and fiscal resources, and many other ends. There are as many targets for prevention as there are various health outcomes and effects to be avoided.

Prevention efforts often lack a clear constituency because success results in unseen consequences. Because these consequences are unseen, people are less likely to develop an attachment for or support the efforts preventing them. Advocates for such causes as mental health services, care for individuals with developmental disabilities, and organ transplants often make their presence felt. However, few state capitols have seen candlelight demonstrations by thousands of people who did not get diphtheria. This invisible constituency for prevention is partly a result of the interdisciplinary nature of public health. With no predominant discipline, it is even more difficult for people to understand and appreciate the work of public health.

From one perspective, the undervaluation of public health is understandable; the majority of the beneficiaries of recent and current public health prevention efforts have not yet been born! Despite its lack of recognition, prevention as a strategy has been remarkably successful and appears to offer great potential for future success, as well. Later chapters will explore this potential in greater depth.

Uncommon Culture

The final unique feature of public health to be discussed here appears to be both a strength and weakness. The tie that binds public health professionals is neither a common preparation through education and training nor a common set of work experiences and work settings. Public health is unique in that the common link is a set of intended outcomes toward which many different sciences, arts, and methods can contribute. As a result, public health professionals include anthropologists, sociologists, psychologists, physicians, nurses, nutritionists, lawyers, economists, political scientists, social workers, laboratorians, managers, sanitarians, engineers, epidemiologists, biostatisticians, gerontologists, disability specialists, and dozens of other professions and disciplines. All are bound to common ends, and all employ somewhat different perspectives from their diverse education, training, and work experiences. "Whatever it takes to get the job done" is the theme, suggesting that the basic task is one of problem solving around health issues. This aspect of public health is the foundation for strategies and methods that rely heavily on collaborations and partnerships.

This multidisciplinary and interdisciplinary approach is unique among professions, calling into question whether public health is really a profession at all. There are several strong arguments that public health is not a profession. There is no minimum credential or training that distinguishes public health professionals from either other professionals or nonprofessionals. Only a tiny proportion of those who work in organizations dedicated to improving the health of the public possess one of the academic public health degrees (the master's of public health degree and several other master's and doctoral degrees granted by schools of public health and other institutions). With the vast majority of public health workers not formally trained in public health, it is difficult to characterize its workforce as a profession. In many respects, it is more reasonable to view public health as a movement than as a profession.

VALUE OF PUBLIC HEALTH

How can we measure the value of public health efforts? This question is addressed both directly and indirectly throughout this text. Later chapters will examine the dimensions of public health's value in terms of lives saved and diseases prevented, as well as in dollars and cents. Nonetheless, some initial information will set the stage for greater detail later.

Public opinion polls conducted in recent years suggest that public health is highly valued in the United States.[18] The overwhelming majority of the public rated a variety of key public health services as "very important." Specifically,

- 91% of all adults believe that prevention of the spread of infectious diseases such as tuberculosis, measles, flu, and AIDS is very important
- 88% also believe that conducting research into the causes and prevention of disease is very important
- 87% believe that immunization to prevent diseases is very important
- 86% believe that ensuring that people are not exposed to unsafe water, air pollution, or toxic waste is very important
- 85% believe that it is very important to work to reduce death and injuries from violence
- 68% believe that it is important to encourage people to live healthier lifestyles, to eat well, and not to smoke
- 66% believe that it is important to work to reduce death and injuries from accidents at work, in the home, and on the streets

In a related poll conducted in 1999, the Pew Charitable Trusts found that 46% of all Americans thought that "public health/protecting populations from disease" was more important than "medicine/treating people who are sick." Almost 30% thought medicine was more important than public health; 22% said both were equally important, and 3% had no opinion. Public opinion surveys suggest that public health's contributions to health and quality of life have not gone unnoticed. Other assessments of the value of public health support this contention.

In 1965, McKeown concluded, "health has advanced significantly only since the late 18th century and until recently owed little to medical advances."[19] This conclusion is bolstered by more recent studies finding that public health's prevention efforts are responsible for 25 years of the nearly 30-year improvement in life expectancy at birth in the United States since 1900. This bold claim is based on evidence that only 5 years of the 30-year improvement are the result of medical care.[20] Of these 5 years, medical treatment accounts for 3.7 years, and clinical preventive services (such as immunizations and screening tests) account for 1.5 years. The remaining 25 years have resulted largely from prevention efforts in the form of social policies, community actions, and personal decisions. Many of these decisions and actions targeted infectious diseases affecting infants and children early in the 20th century. Later in that century, gains in life expectancy have also been achieved through reductions in chronic diseases affecting adults.

Many notable public health achievements occurred during the 20th century (Table 1-7). Several chapters of this text will highlight one or more of these achievements to illustrate the value of public health to American society in the 21st century by telling the story of its accomplishments in the preceding century. The first of these chronicles the prevention and control of infectious diseases in 20th-century America (see "Public Health Achievements in 20th-Century America: Prevention and Control of Infectious Disease," later in this chapter).

The value of public health in our society can be described in human terms as well as by public opinion, statistics of infections prevented, and values in dollars and cents. A poignant example dates from the 1950s, when the United States was in the midst of a terrorizing polio epidemic (Table 1-8). Few communities were spared during the periodic onslaughts of this serious disease during the first half of the 20th century in America. Public fear was so great that public libraries, community swimming pools, and other group activities were closed during the summers when the disease was most feared. Biomedical research had discovered a possible weapon against epidemic polio in the form of the Salk vaccine, however, which was developed in 1954 and licensed for use 1 year later. A massive and unprecedented campaign to immunize the public was quickly undertaken, setting the stage for a triumph of public health. The real triumph came in a way that might not have been expected, however, because soon into the campaign, isolated reports of vaccine-induced polio were identified in Chicago and California. Within 2 days of the initial case reports, action by governmental public health organizations at all levels resulted in the determination that these cases could be traced to one particular manufacturer. This determination was made only a few hours before the same vaccine was to be provided to hundreds of thousands of California children. The

---

TABLE 1-7 Ten Great Public Health Achievements—United States, 1900–1999

- Vaccination
- Motor-vehicle safety
- Safer workplaces
- Control of infectious diseases
- Decline in deaths from coronary heart disease and stroke
- Safer and healthier foods
- Healthier mothers and babies
- Family planning
- Fluoridation of drinking water
- Recognition of tobacco use as a health hazard

Source: Centers for Disease Control and Prevention. Ten great public health achievements—United States, 1900-1999. *MMWR Morb Mortal Wkly Rep.* 1999;48(12):241–243.

TABLE 1-8 The Value of Public Health: Fear of Polio, United States, 1950s

"I can remember no experience more horrifying than watching by the bedside of my five-year-old stricken with polio. The disease attacked his right leg, and we watched helplessly as his limb steadily weakened. On the third day, the doctor told us that he would survive and that paralysis was the worst he would suffer. I was grateful, although I continued to agonize about whether my wife and unborn child would be affected. What a blessing that no other parent will have to endure the terror that my wife and I and thousands of others shared that August."
—Morton Chapman, Sarasota, Florida

Source: Reprinted from U.S. Public Health Service. *For a Healthy Nation: Returns on Investments in Public Health.* Washington, DC: Public Health Service; 1994.

result was prevention of a disaster and rescue of the credibility of an immunization campaign that has virtually cut this disease off at its knees. The campaign proceeded on schedule and, five decades later, wild poliovirus has been eradicated from the western hemisphere.

Similar examples have occurred throughout history. The battle against diphtheria is a case in point. A major cause of death in 1900, diphtheria infections are virtually unheard of today. This achievement cannot be traced solely to advances in bacteriology and the antitoxins and immunizations that were deployed against this disease. Neither was it defeated by brilliant political and programmatic initiatives led by public health experts. It was the confluence of scientific advances and public perception of the disease itself that resulted in diphtheria's demise as a threat to entire populations. These forces shaped public health policies and the effectiveness of intervention strategies. In the end, diphtheria made some practices and politics possible, while it constrained others.[21] The story is one of science, social values, and public health.

CONCLUSION

Public health evokes different images for different people, and, even to the same people, it can mean different things in different contexts. The intent of this chapter has been to describe some of the common perceptions of public health in the United States. Is it a complex, dynamic, social enterprise, akin to a movement? Or is it best characterized as a goal of the improved health outcomes and health status that can be achieved by the work of all of us, individually and collectively? Or is public health some collection of activities that move us ever closer toward our aspirations? Or is it the profession that includes all of those dedicated to its cause? Or is public health merely what we see coming out of our official governmental health agencies— a strange mix of safety-net medical services for the poor and a variety of often-invisible community prevention services?

Public Health Achievements in 20th Century America: Prevention and Control of Infectious Diseases

Prior to 1900, infectious diseases represented the most serious threat to the health of populations across the globe. The 20th century witnessed a dramatic shift in the balance of power in the centuries-long battle between humans and microorganisms. Changes in both science and social values contributed to the assault on microbes, setting into motion the forces of organized community efforts to improve the health of the public. This approach served as a model for later public health initiatives targeting other major threats to health and well-being. Highlights of this achievement are captured in Figure 1-3 and Table 1-9. The rate of infectious diseases had been reduced to such low levels that the incidence of a few thousand cases of mumps in 2006 was regarded as a significant public health event (see Figure 1-4).

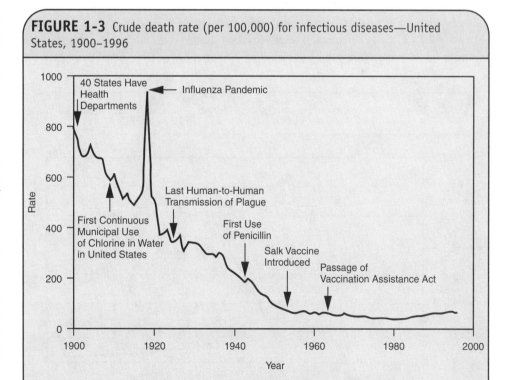

FIGURE 1-3 Crude death rate (per 100,000) for infectious diseases—United States, 1900–1996

Source: Repritned from Public Health Achievements, United States, 1900–1999; Control of Infectious Diseases, Morbidity and Mortality WeeklyReport, Vol. 48, No. 29, pp. 621–629, Centers for Disease Control and Prevention, 1999.

TABLE 1-9 Baseline 20th Century Annual Morbidity and 1998 Provisional Morbidity from Nine Diseases with Vaccines Recommended Before 1990 for Universal Use for Children, United States

	Baseline 20th Century Annual Morbidity	1998 Morbidity (Provisional)	Percentage Decrease
Smallpox	48,164	0	100
Diphtheria	175,885	1	100
Pertussis	147,271	6,279	95.7
Tetanus	1,314	34	97.4
Poliomyelitis (paralytic)	16,316	0	100
Measles	503,282	89	100
Mumps	152,209	606	99.6
Rubella	47,745	345	99.3
Congenital rubella syndrome	823	5	99.4
Haemophilus influenzae type b infection	20,000	54	99.7

Source: Reprinted from Centers for Disease Control and Prevention. Public health achievements, United States, 1900-1999: impact of vaccines universally recommended for children. *MMWR Morb Mortal Wkly Rep.* 1999;48:243–248.

Although it is tempting to consider expunging the term *public health* from our vocabularies because of the baggage associated with these various images, this would do little to address the obstacles to accomplishing our central task, because public health encompasses all of these images and perhaps more!

Based on principles of social justice, inherently political in its processes, addressing a constantly expanding agenda of problems, inextricably linked with government, grounded in science, emphasizing preventive strategies, and with a workforce bound by common aspirations, public health is unique in many ways. Its value, however, transcends its uniqueness. Public health efforts have been major contributors to recent improvements in health status and can contribute even more as we approach a new century with new challenges.

By carefully examining the various dimensions of the public health system in terms of its inputs, practices, outputs, and outcomes, we can gain insights into what it does, how it works, and how it can be improved. Better results do not come from setting new goals; they come from understanding and improving the processes that will then produce better outputs, in turn leading to better outcomes. This theme of understanding the public health system and public health practice as a necessary step toward its improvement will recur throughout this text.

FIGURE 1-4 Number of reported mumps cases by year, United States, 1980–2006

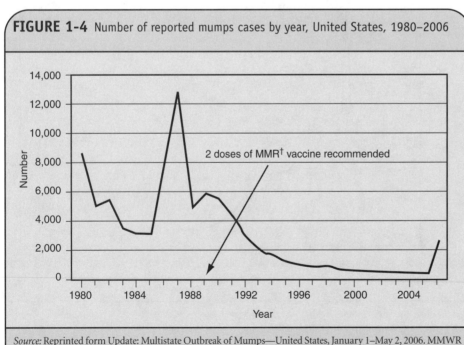

Source: Reprinted form Update: Multistate Outbreak of Mumps—United States, January 1–May 2, 2006. MMWR May 26, 2006, Vol. 55, No. 20, pp. 559–563. Centers for Disease Control and Prevention.

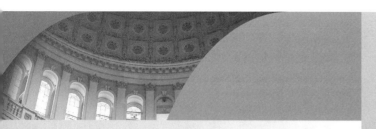

Discussion Questions and Exercises

1. What definition of public health best describes public health in the 21st century?

2. To what extent has public health contributed to improvement in health status and quality of life over history?

3. What historical phenomena are most responsible for the development of public health responses?

4. Which features of public health make it different from other fields? Which features are most unique and distinctive? Which is most important?

5. Because of your interest in a public health career, a producer working at a local television station has asked you to provide input into the development of a video explaining public health to the general public. What themes or messages would you suggest for this video? How would you propose presenting or packaging these messages?

6. There is little written in history books about public health problems and responses, suggesting that these issues have had little impact on history. Consider the European colonization of the Americas, beginning in the 16th century. How was it possible for Cortez and other European figures to overcome immense Native American cultures with millions of people? What role, if any, did public health themes and issues play?

7. Choose a relatively recent (within the last 3 years) occurrence/event that has drawn significant media attention to a public health issue or problem (e.g., bioterrorism, contaminated meat products, tobacco settlement, hurricane, flooding). Have different understandings of what public health is influenced public, as well as governmental responses to this event? If so, in what ways?

8. Review the history of public health activities in your state or community and describe how public health strategies and interventions have changed over time in the United States. What influences were most responsible for these changes? Does this suggest that public health functions have changed over time, as well?

9. Access the National Library of Medicine Web site (http://www.nlm.nih.gov) and conduct an online literature search of key words related to the definition, development, and current status of public health. Indicate the parameters used in this search and the general contents of the most useful article that you found.

10. Examine each of the Web sites listed here and become familiar with their general contents. Which ones are most useful for providing information and insights related to the question, "What is public health?" Why? Are there other Web sites you would suggest adding to this list?

    American Public Health Association (http://www.apha.org)

    Association of State and Territorial Health Officials (http://www.astho.org)

    National Association of County and City Health Officials (http://www.naccho.org)

    Public Health Foundation (http://www.phf.org)

    U.S. Department of Health and Human Services (http://www.dhhs/gov) and its various Public Service Agencies (e.g., Centers for Disease Control Prevention [http://www.cdc.org], Food and Drug Administration [http://www.fda.gov], Health Resources and Services Administration [http://www.hrsa.dhhs.gov], National Institutes of Health [http://www.nih.gov], Agency for Healthcare Research and Quality [http://www.ahrq.gov])

    U.S. Environmental Protection Agency (http://www.epa/gov)

    State health departments, available through the ASTHO Web site

    Local health departments, available through the Web sites of state health departments, NACCHO, and other national public health organizations

    Association of Schools of Public Health (http://www.asph.org) and individual schools, available through the Association of Schools of Public Health Web site

REFERENCES

1. Winslow CEA. Public health at the crossroads. *Am J Public Health*. 1926;16:1075–1085.

2. Hinman A. Eradication of vaccine-preventable diseases. *Ann Rev Public Health*. 1999;20:211–229.

3. U.S. Public Health Service. *For a Healthy Nation: Returns on Investment in Public Health*. Washington, DC: PHS; 1994.

4. McNeil WH. *Plagues and Peoples*. New York: Doubleday; 1977.

5. Paneth N, Vinten-Johansen P, Brody H. A rivalry of foulness: official and unofficial investigations of the London cholera epidemic of 1854. *Am J Public Health*. 1998;88:1545–1553.

6. Hamlin C. Could you starve to death in England in 1839? The Chadwick-Farr controversy and the loss of the "social" in public health. *Am J Public Health*. 1995;85:856–866.

7. Institute of Medicine, National Academy of Sciences. *The Future of Public Health*. Washington, DC: National Academy Press; 1988.

8. Winslow CEA. The untilled field of public health. *Mod Med*. 1920; 2:183–191.

9. Vickers G. What sets the goals of public health? *Lancet*. 1958; 1:599–604.

10. Baker EL, Melton RJ, Stange PV, et al. Health reform and the health of the public. *JAMA*. 1994;272:1276–1282.

11. Harrell JA, Baker EL. The essential services of public health. *Leadership Public Health*. 1994;3:27–30.

12. Handler A, Issel LM, Turnock BJ. A conceptual framework to measure performance of the public health system. *Am J Public Health*. 2001; 91:1235–1239.

13. Public Health Functions Steering Committee. *Public Health in America*. Washington, DC: U.S. Public Health Service; 1995.

14. Krieger N, Brin AE. A vision of social justice as the foundation of public health: commemorating 150 years of the spirit of 1848. *Am J Public Health*. 1998;88:1603–1606.

15. Beauchamp DE. Public health as social justice. *Inquiry*. 1976;13:3–14.

16. Susser M. Health as a human right: an epidemiologist's perspective on public health. *Am J Public Health*. 1993;83:418–426.

17. Afifi AA, Breslow L. The maturing paradigm of public health. *Ann Rev Public Health*. 1994;15:223–235.

18. Harris Polls. *Public Opinion about Public Health, United States. 1999*.

19. McKeown T. *Medicine in Modern Society*. London, England: Allen & Unwin; 1965.

20. Bunker JP, Frazier HS, Mosteller F. Improving health: measuring effects of medical care. *Milbank Q*. 1994;72:225–258.

21. Hammonds EM. *Childhood's Deadly Scourge: The Campaign to Control Diphtheria in New York City, 1880–1930*. Baltimore, MD: Johns Hopkins University Press; 1999.

The Law and the Public's Health: The Foundations from *Law in Public Health Practice*

Lawrence O. Gostin, Jeffrey P. Koplan, and Frank P. Grad

By permission of Oxford University Press, Inc. Reprinted from Gostin, LO, Koplan, JP, Grad, FP. The Law and the Public's Health: The Foundations. In: Goodman, RA, Hoffman, RE, Lopez, W, Mathews, GW, Rothstein, MA, Foster, KL, eds. *Law in Public Health Practice*. New York: Oxford University Press, Inc; 2003.

The law has played a vital role in public health since the founding of the Republic when the principal threats to health and safety were epidemic diseases. Law creates public health agencies, designates their mission, provides their authority, and limits their actions to protect a sphere of freedom outlined by the Constitution. The law, therefore, has always been vital to public health. The field of public health law, however, has never been more important than after the catastrophic threats to health that occurred after the events of September 11, 2001, particularly the dangers from anthrax. Just as these threats, old and new, teach us about the importance of a strong public health infrastructure, they also remind us of the need for appropriate public health powers. Public health law, of course, is about not only power, but also restraint. Public health officials, to be effective, need to act with strong scientific evidence and with fairness and tolerance.

In this chapter, we present the foundations of public health law—its definition, infrastructure, constitutional underpinnings, and powers. For more in-depth examinations of selected foundational topics, we refer readers to additional texts and resources.[1-3] Before turning to a careful exploration of the legal basis of public health, we examine fundamental aspects of the field of public health.

THE POPULATION BASIS FOR PUBLIC HEALTH

Defining Public Health

The effort to capture the entire spectrum of public health activity in one definition is bound to be complex and challenging. The field of public health is broad, and the mix of disciplines makes justice difficult to bestow on all of them. The Institute of Medicine's 1988 report, *The Future of Public Health*, offers a good starting point by describing public health's mis-sion as "fulfill[ing] society's interest in assuring the conditions in which people can be healthy."[4]

Several important and distinctive concepts are packed into this phrase: public health's collective action on society's behalf ("fulfill *society's interest*" and "*assuring* the conditions"), a broad view of the determinants of health ("the *conditions in which* people can be healthy"), and an emphasis on populations rather than on individuals ("in which *people* can be healthy"). In addition to these characteristics, public health is unique among health-related fields for the value and emphasis it places on prevention, protection, community health, education, and partnerships with varied organizations.

The mandate to "fulfill society's interests" and "assure" healthy conditions and quality services puts public health in frequent and compelling contact with the legal system. Likewise, "the conditions in which people can be healthy" recognizes the salience of the root causes or determinants of health—particularly those that may not be obvious, immediate, or perceived to be within the purview of other parts of the health system. In practice, this requires attention to the prevention of disease (not just to its detection and treatment) and to a view of disease that acknowledges the health implications of income, education, employment, and community.

Although the public health system often works in close partnership with the medical-care system to protect the public's health, many aspects of public health are not only essential but also unique. Different approaches to tobacco are a good example of these complementary approaches. Tobacco—the underlying cause of one of every five deaths in the United States—is a serious public health threat and causes a variety of diseases in smokers and others exposed to tobacco. The medical-care system focuses on treating the emphysema, lung cancer, and heart disease that result from tobacco use and provides individual counseling and perhaps assistance with smoking cessation (e.g., prescribing a nicotine patch for a smoker who wants to quit). The public health approach, on the other hand, seeks to change social norms about smoking (e.g., through media campaigns and by advocating smoke-free workplaces and public places) and has the goal of preventing tobacco addiction in the first place, especially among children.

Both approaches are needed, but their emphasis is at different points on the disease continuum (from prevention to treatment), and thus the two parts of the system employ different tools. In the medical-care system, health-care providers focus on diagnosing and treating an individual patient. In the public health system, the "patient" is the community or an entire population. The diagnosis focuses on identifying risk factors and preventing disease or its consequences, and the treatment might involve policy changes, media campaigns, environmental changes, or enforcement of regulations. Medical care usually is offered according to a medical model in selected settings—such as physicians' offices, hospitals, and clinics—while public health involves numerous disciplines (medicine, epidemiology, economics, political science), settings (such as schools and workplaces), and tools (including the media, regulatory authority, and changes to policies, the environment, and individual behavior).

Public health also is unique in its status as a common good. National disease surveillance systems that track the health status of populations, laboratory tests and techniques that track strains of disease, and teams of epidemiologists and other scientists that can be deployed when outbreaks occur are all examples of functions that no single private or non-profit entity could support and for which few, if any, market-based financial incentives exist. In this sense, the results of public health activities are truly common goods that benefit all of us, whether we are wealthy or poor, insured or uninsured, urban or rural, healthy or sick.

Public Health's Infrastructure

The 1988 Institute of Medicine report diagnosed a public health system in disarray and suggested three core functions for public health as a new framework to return public health to its roots: assessment, policy development, and assurance. The law is important in establishing each of these three vital roles within public health agencies. The three overlapping functions encompass the entire spectrum of public health activity, from surveillance functions that detect and monitor disease and injury patterns, to developing policies that promote health and prevent disease and disability, to ensuring

that data-driven interventions address the health issues identified through assessment activities. The cycle is continuously renewed as assessment activities detect whether progress has been made, leading to a subsequent set of policy actions, interventions, and reassessment (Figure 2-1). These core functions, in turn, were further delineated into more specific "essential services" of public health,[5] which have since formed the basis for planning documents (such as *Healthy People 2010*) and ongoing research on the status of public health practice.

Another way to describe public health is to consider its key components, or infrastructure. In a recent report to Congress,[6] The Centers for Disease Control and Prevention (CDC) identified three main components of the system's infrastructure, all of which work together to ensure that the public health system is fully prepared to carry out the core functions and essential services needed to protect communities across the country from both routine and acute health events. These elements are (1) workforce capacity and competency, (2) information and data systems, and (3) organizational capacity.

Like the Institute of Medicine report that preceded it, the CDC status report on public health's infrastructure found many areas for concern. The report concluded that despite recent efforts and some improvements, the system's infrastructure "is still structurally weak in nearly every area." The Institute of Medicine's new report, *Assuring the Health of the Public in the 21st Century*, similarly draws attention to the inadequacy of the public health infrastructure to detect and respond effectively to disease threats.[7]

Although the public health system has indeed been underfunded for decades, its contributions have been impressive. As British physician Geoffrey Rose[8] has observed,

> Measures to improve public health, relating as they do to such obvious and mundane matters as housing, smoking, and food, may lack the glamour of high-technology medicine, but what they lack in excitement they gain in their potential impact on health, precisely because they deal with the major causes of common disease and disabilities.

Public health's most dramatic accomplishment is the extension of the average life span, from 45 years at the turn of the twentieth century to nearly 80 years in 2002. Of these 35 years of "extra" longevity, only 5 or so can be attributed to advances in clinical medicine. Public health can take the credit for the other 30 years, thanks to improvements in sanitation, health education, the development of effective vaccines, and other advances (Table 2-1). U.S. census forms now include three digits for recording a respondent's age—a tribute to the growing

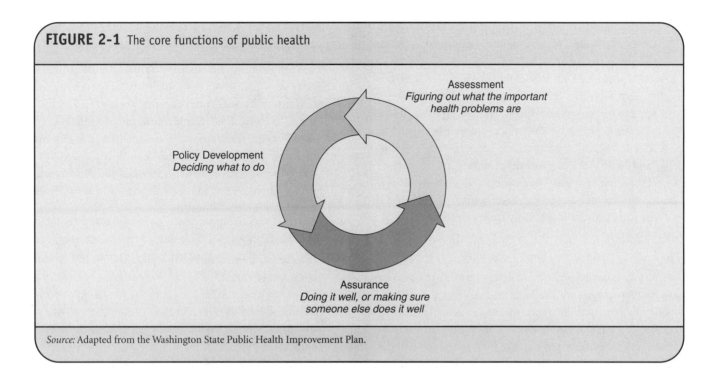

FIGURE 2-1 The core functions of public health

Assessment
Figuring out what the important health problems are

Policy Development
Deciding what to do

Assurance
Doing it well, or making sure someone else does it well

Source: Adapted from the Washington State Public Health Improvement Plan.

number of centenarians among us, now estimated to be approximately 70,000 Americans. Notice that for most of these achievements, law has played a vital role in relation to, for example, compulsory vaccinations, food and drug safety, regulation of the water supply, personal-control measures for contagious diseases, tobacco regulation (taxation, labeling and advertising, and tort actions), and regulation of car design and seatbelt use. Overall, these achievements highlight public health's protective role—the constant struggle to identify and minimize risk, whether it emanates from our own behaviors or those of others, the environments in which we live and work, our genetic legacy, or, as is often the case, some interplay among these.

Future Challenges

Of course, "fulfilling society's interest" is a task as immense as protecting the public's health (not only in the United States, but around the globe), and much remains undone. In the decades ahead, we are bound to face both known and unanticipated challenges. In the known category, challenges[10] include

- Achieving meaningful *changes in health-care systems,* including instituting a rational health-care system that balances equity, cost, and quality; and eliminating health disparities among racial and ethnic groups
- Focusing on the chronologic milestones of *childhood and old age* by investing in children's emotional and intellectual development and working to achieve not only a longer life span but also a longer "health span," one that offers a better quality of life, mobility, and independence for the growing population of seniors
- Addressing the *risks posed by our lifestyles and the environment,* such as incorporating healthy eating and physical activity into daily life (to combat the twin epidemics of obesity and diabetes, among many other adverse health outcomes); responding to emerging infectious diseases (including new pathogens spread by travel, migration, and commerce, as well as microbial

TABLE 2-1 A Century of Public Health Accomplishment—United States, 1900–1999

30 years of increased longevity
Vaccinations
Healthier mothers and babies
Family planning
Safer and healthier foods
Fluoridation of drinking water
Control of infectious diseases
Decline in deaths from heart disease and stroke
Recognition of tobacco use as a health hazard
Motor vehicle safety
Safer workplaces

Source: Adapted from the CDC.[9]

adaptation sped along by inappropriate use of antibiotics); and balancing economic growth with protection of our environment

- Applying what we already know and unlocking persistent mysteries about *the brain and human behavior* by recognizing and addressing the contributions of mental health to overall health and well-being and reducing the toll of violence (including homicide, suicide, and other types of violence) in society
- Exploring *new scientific frontiers* and applying *new scientific knowledge* (e.g., the mapping of the human genome) equitably, ethically, and responsibly

In many of these areas—including, for example, child development, mental health, obesity and physical activity, the environment, bioterrorism, and aging—promising science-based interventions are available and deserve support and broader implementation. In other areas, particularly the needs to delineate a rational health-care system, eliminate health disparities, curb violence, and manage new genetic knowledge, the course of action is less clear or even potentially divisive.

Like the public health achievements of the past, these future challenges will demand a blend of scientific innovation, technical and managerial expertise (especially regarding implementing health programs at the community level), persuasion, courage, and (last but not least) the skillful application of legal principles and tools. Public health's unique perspective can alter how these policy debates are framed and interpreted. By understanding and applying legal tools and principles that have already helped secure public health's achievements in the past century, the public health field can accelerate improvements in the public's health for decades to come.

CONCEPTUAL FOUNDATIONS OF PUBLIC HEALTH LAW

Public health law plays a unique role in ensuring the population's health. To demonstrate its importance, defining public health law and the public health law infrastructure are helpful.

Defining Public Health Law

A recent textbook defines public health law as "The study of the legal powers and duties of the state to assure the conditions for people to be healthy (e.g., to identify, prevent, and ameliorate risks to health in the population), and the limitations on the power of the state to constrain the autonomy, privacy, liberty, proprietary, or other legally protected interests of individuals for protection or promotion of community health."[1] This definition suggests five essential characteristics

of public health law, which correspond with the characteristics of public health itself described in the previous section:

- *Government:* Public health activities are the primary (but not exclusive) responsibility of government. Government creates policy and enacts laws and regulations designed to safeguard community health.
- *Populations:* Public health focuses on the health of populations. Certainly, public health authorities are concerned with access and quality in medical care, but their principal concern is to create the conditions in which communities can be healthy.
- *Relationships:* Public health contemplates the relationship between the state and the population (or between the state and individuals who place themselves or the community at risk).
- *Services:* Public health deals with the provision of population-based services grounded on the scientific methodologies of public health (e.g., biostatistics and epidemiology).
- *Coercion:* Public health authorities possess the power to coerce individuals and businesses for the protection of the community rather than relying on a near universal ethic of voluntarism.

The Public Health Law Infrastructure

The public health law infrastructure includes public health laws (statutes principally at the state level that establish the mission, functions, powers, and structures of public health agencies) and laws about the public's health (laws and regulations that offer a variety of tools to prevent injury and disease and promote the public's health). The Institute of Medicine[2] and the Department of Health and Human Services[11] recommended reform of state public health laws. Public health laws are scattered across countless statutes and regulations at the state and local levels. Problems of antiquity, inconsistency, redundancy, and ambiguity render these laws ineffective, or even counterproductive, in advancing the population's health. In particular, health codes frequently are outdated, constructed in layers over different periods of time, and highly fragmented among the 50 states and the territories.[12]

Problem of Antiquity

The most striking characteristic of state public health law—and the one that underlies many of its defects—is its overall antiquity. Certainly, some statutes are relatively recent in origin. However, much of public health law was framed in the late nineteenth and early to mid-twentieth centuries and contains elements that are 40 to 100 years old. Old public health statutes are often outmoded in ways that directly reduce their effectiveness and conformity with modern standards. These laws often do not reflect contemporary scientific understandings of injury and disease (e.g., surveillance, prevention, and response) or legal norms for protection of individual rights. Rather, public health laws use scientific and legal standards that prevailed when they were enacted. Society faces different sorts of risks today and deploys different methods of assessment and intervention. When many of these statutes were written, public health (e.g., epidemiology and biostatistics) and behavioral (e.g., client-centered counseling) sciences were in their infancy. Modern prevention and treatment methods did not exist.

Problem of Multiple Layers of Law

Related to the problem of antiquity is the problem of multiple layers of law. The law in most states consists of successive layers of statutes and amendments, constructed in some cases over 100 years or more in response to existing or perceived health threats. This is particularly troublesome in the area of infectious diseases, which forms a substantial part of state health codes. Because communicable disease laws have been enacted piecemeal, in response to specific epidemics, (e.g., smallpox, yellow fever, cholera, tuberculosis, venereal diseases, polio, and acquired immunodeficiency syndrome [AIDS]), they tell the story of the history of disease control in the United States. The disparate legal structures of state public health laws can significantly undermine their effectiveness. Laws enacted piecemeal over time are inconsistent, redundant, and ambiguous.

Problem of Inconsistency

Public health laws remain fragmented not only within states but also among them. Health codes within the states and territories have evolved independently, leading to profound variation in the structure, substance, and procedures for detecting, controlling, and preventing injury and disease. In fact, statutes and regulations among U.S. jurisdictions vary so significantly in definitions, methods, age, and scope that they defy orderly categorization. There is good reason for greater uniformity among the states in matters of public health. Health threats are rarely confined to single jurisdictions but pose risks within whole regions or the nation itself (e.g., air or water pollution, disposal of toxic waste, and the spread of infectious diseases, either naturally or through bioterrorist events).

One approach to rectifying inconsistencies in public health law is to reform laws so that they conform with modern scientific and legal standards, are more consistent within and among states, and more uniformly address different health threats. A single set of standards and procedures would add needed clarity and coherence to legal regulation and would reduce the opportunity for politically motivated disputes about how to classify newly emergent health threats.

Law as a Tool to Safeguard the Public's Health

Public health laws constitute the foundations for public health practice while providing tools for public health authorities. At least six models exist for legal intervention designed to prevent injury and disease and to promote the public's health. Although legal interventions can be effective, they often raise social, ethical, or constitutional concerns that warrant careful study.

Model 1 is the power to tax and spend. This power, given in federal and state constitutions, provides government with an important regulatory technique. The power to spend enables government to set conditions for the receipt of public funds. For example, the federal government grants highway funds to states on condition that they set the legal drinking age at 21 years.[13] The power to tax provides strong inducements to engage in beneficial behavior or refrain from risk behavior. For example, taxes on cigarettes significantly reduce smoking, particularly among young people.

Model 2 is the power to alter the informational environment. Government can add its voice to the marketplace of ideas through health promotion activities such as health communication campaigns; by providing relevant consumer information through labeling requirements; and by limiting harmful or misleading information through regulation of commercial advertising of unsafe products (e.g., cigarettes and alcoholic beverages).

Model 3 is direct regulation of individuals (e.g., seatbelt and motorcycle helmet laws), professionals (e.g., licenses), or businesses (e.g., inspections and occupational safety standards). Public health authorities regulate pervasively to reduce risks to the population.

Model 4 is indirect regulation through the tort system. Tort litigation can provide strong incentives for businesses to engage in less risky activities. Litigation has been used as a tool of public health to influence manufacturers of automobiles, cigarettes, and firearms. Litigation resulted in safer automobiles; reduced advertising and promotion of cigarettes to young people; and encouraged at least one manufacturer (Smith & Wesson) to develop safer firearms.

Model 5 is deregulation. The impact of laws may sometimes be detrimental to public health and may be an impediment to effective action. For example, criminal laws proscribe the possession and distribution of sterile syringes and needles. These laws, therefore, make engagement in human immunodeficiency virus (HIV) prevention activities more difficult for public health authorities.

The government, then, has many legal "levers" designed to prevent injury and disease and to promote the public's health. Legal interventions can be highly effective and need to be part of the public health officer's arsenal. At the same time, legal interventions can be controversial, raising important ethical, social, constitutional, and political issues. These conflicts are complex, important, and fascinating for students of public health law.

THE CONSTITUTIONAL UNDERPINNINGS OF PUBLIC HEALTH LAW

No inquiry is more important to public health law than understanding the role of government in the constitutional design. If, as we have suggested, public health law principally addresses government's assurance of the conditions for the population's health, then what activities must government undertake? The question is complex, requiring an assessment of duty (what government must do), authority (what government is empowered, but not obligated, to do), and limits (what government is prohibited from doing). In addition, this query raises a corollary question: Which government is to act? Some of the most divisive disputes in public health are among the federal government, the states, and the localities about which government has the power to intervene.

Government Duties to Ensure the Public's Health

Given the importance of government in maintaining public health (and many other communal benefits), one might expect the U.S. Constitution to create affirmative obligations for government to act. Yet, by standard accounts, the Constitution is cast purely in negative terms. The Supreme Court remains faithful to this negative conception of the Constitution, even in the face of dire personal consequences. In *DeShaney v. Winnebago County Department of Social Services*,[14] the Supreme Court held that government has no affirmative duty to protect citizens. In that case, a 1-year-old child, Joshua DeShaney, was beaten so badly by his father that he was left profoundly retarded and institutionalized. The social services department was aware of the abuse but took no steps to prevent further injuries to Joshua.

The Supreme Court has applied this line of reasoning in cases that bitterly divided the Court. In *Webster v. Reproductive Health Services*,[15] the majority saw no government obligation to provide services—in this case, medical services—to the poor[16] when a Missouri statute barred state employees from performing abortions and banned the use of public facilities for such. Referring to *DeShaney,* the Court rejected a positive

claim for basic government services: "[O]ur cases have recognized that the Due Process Clauses generally confer no affirmative right to governmental aid, even where such aid may be necessary to secure life, liberty, or property interests of which the government itself may not deprive the individual."[15] This negative theory of constitutional design, although well accepted, is highly simplified and, in the words of Justice Blackmun, represents "a sad commentary upon American life and constitutional principles."[14]

Federal Powers to Ensure the Conditions for Public Health

In theory, the United States is a government of limited powers, but the reality is quite different. The federal government possesses considerable authority to act and exerts extensive control in the realm of public health and safety. The Supreme Court, through an expansive interpretation of Congress's enumerated powers, has enabled the federal government to maintain a vast presence in public health—in matters ranging from biomedical research and the provision of health care to the control of infectious diseases, occupational health and safety, pure food and drugs, and environmental protection. The main constitutional powers for federal action in the realm of public health are the powers to tax and spend and to regulate interstate commerce.

At face value, the power to tax and spend has a single, overriding purpose: to raise revenue to provide for the good of the community. Without the ability to generate sufficient revenue, the legislature could not provide services such as transportation, education, medical services to the poor, sanitation, and environmental protection. The power to tax is also the power to regulate risk behavior and influence health-promoting activities. Broadly speaking, the tax code influences health-related behavior through tax relief and tax burdens. Tax relief encourages private health-promoting activity, and tax burdens discourage risk behavior.

Through various forms of tax relief, government provides incentives for private activities that it views as advantageous to community health. The tax code influences private health-related spending in many other ways: encouraging child care to enable parents to enter the work force; inducing investment in low-income housing; and stimulating charitable spending for research and care.

Taxation also regulates private behavior by economically penalizing risk-taking activities. Tax policy discourages a number of activities that government regards as unhealthy or dangerous. Consider excise or manufacturing taxes on tobacco, alcoholic beverages, or firearms. It is difficult to imagine a public health threat caused by human behavior or business activity that cannot be influenced by the taxing power. Similarly, the spending power does not simply grant Congress the authority to allocate resources; it is also an indirect regulatory device. Congress may prescribe the terms on which it disburses federal money to the states.

The Commerce Clause, more than any other enumerated power, affords Congress potent regulatory authority. The Commerce Clause gives Congress the power to regulate commerce "with foreign Nations, and among the several States, and with the Indian Tribes."[17] At face value, the Commerce Clause is limited to controlling the flow of goods and services across state lines. Yet, as interstate commerce has become ubiquitous; activities once considered purely local have come to have national effects and have accordingly come within Congress' commerce power. The Supreme Court's broad interpretation of the Commerce Clause has enabled national authorities to reach deeply into traditional realms of state public health power.

The Rehnquist Court, however, has begun to rethink the Commerce Clause as part of its agenda of gradually returning power from the federal government to the states. In the process, the Court has held that Congress lacks the power to engage in social and public health regulation primarily affecting intrastate activities. For example, the Court has held that Congress lacks the power to regulate firearms near schools[18] and to provide a remedy for victims of sexual violence.[19]

POLICE POWERS: STATE POWER TO REGULATE FOR THE PUBLIC'S HEALTH AND SAFETY

The "police power" is the most famous expression of the natural authority of sovereign governments to regulate private interests for the public good. One definition of the police power is

> the inherent authority of the state (and, through delegation, local government) to enact laws and promulgate regulations to protect, preserve and promote the health, safety, morals, and general welfare of the people. To achieve these communal benefits, the state retains the power to restrict, within federal and state constitutional limits, private interests—personal interests in autonomy, privacy, association, and liberty as well as economic interests in freedom to contract and uses of property.[1]

The linguistic and historical origins of the concept of "police" demonstrate a close association between government and civilization: *politia* (the state), *polis* (city), and *politeia* (citizenship).[20] "Police" was meant to describe those powers that

permitted sovereign government to control its citizens, particularly for promoting the general comfort, health, morals, safety, or prosperity of the public. The word had a secondary usage as well: "the cleansing or keeping clean." This use resonates with early twentieth century public health connotations of hygiene and sanitation.

States exercise police powers to ensure that communities live in safety and security, in conditions conducive to good health, with moral standards, and, generally speaking, without unreasonable interference with human well-being. Police powers legitimize state action to protect and promote broadly defined social goods.

Government, to achieve common goods, is empowered to enact legislation, regulate, and adjudicate in ways that necessarily limit, or even eliminate, private interests. Thus, government has inherent power to interfere with personal interests in autonomy, privacy, association, and liberty as well as economic interests in ownership, uses of private property, and freedom to contract. State power to restrict private rights is embodied in the common law maxim, *sic utere tuo ut alienum non laedas*, "use your own property in such a manner as not to injure that of another." The maxim supports the police power, giving government authority to determine safe uses of private property to diminish risks of injury and ill-health to others.[21] More generally, the police power affords government the authority to keep society free from noxious exercises of private rights. The state retains discretion to determine what is considered injurious or unhealthful and the manner in which to regulate, consistent with constitutional protections of personal interests.

The police powers have enabled states and their subsidiary municipal corporations to promote and preserve the public health in areas ranging from injury and disease prevention to sanitation, waste disposal, and water and air protections. Police powers exercised by the states include vaccination, isolation, and quarantine; inspection of commercial and residential premises; abatement of unsanitary conditions or other health nuisances; regulation of air and surface water contaminants; and restriction on the public's access to polluted areas, standards for pure food and drinking water, extermination of vermin, fluoridization of municipal water supplies, and licensure of physicians and other health-care professionals. These are the kinds of powers exercised daily by state and local public health agencies, as the following discussion demonstrates.

PUBLIC HEALTH POWERS: REGULATION OF PERSONS, PROFESSIONALS, AND BUSINESSES

The powers available to public health authorities in state statutes, as the previous discussion of police powers illustrates, are pervasive. Although systematically examining the full scope and complexity of the public health powers is not possible here, in this section we briefly outline selected principal authorities, many of which are detailed in subsequent chapters. These authorities group into the categories of the power to regulate persons, professionals, and businesses to safeguard the common good.

Regulation of Persons to Prevent Transmission of Communicable Disease: Autonomy, Privacy, and Liberty

Public health authorities have traditionally had a variety of powers to control personal behavior for preventing transmission of a communicable disease. These powers are essential to ensure effective surveillance and response to epidemics. The exercise of compulsory powers, however, also can interfere with autonomy, privacy, and liberty. As a society, we face hard trade-offs between the common good and the rights of individuals to a sphere of freedom. This section offers three illustrations of communicable disease powers: medical examination or testing, vaccination, and isolation or quarantine.

Medical Examination and Testing

State laws often provide public health authorities with the power to compel individuals to submit to testing or medical examination. Generally, testing and clinical examinations are not regarded as harsh legal requirements when the person may benefit. Some states require testing or examinations for sexually transmitted disease before marriage on the assumption that such testing can help prevent the spread of infection. Persons who engage in certain occupations, such as food handlers, nurses, and teachers, are required to submit to testing and examinations to be permitted to practice their occupation. Again, the rationale is that these examinations are useful in preventing disease (e.g., food handlers tested for typhoid or salmonellosis).

Compelling a person to undergo compulsory testing or examination is an invasion of autonomy and privacy and, therefore, requires a clear justification. Consider a recent Supreme Court decision that found compulsory drug testing of pregnant women to be a violation of the Fourth Amendment's proscription against unreasonable searches and seizures. Because the test information was shared with the police, the Court found that it lacked sufficient justification.[22] By analogy, a public health officer could not order a woman to undergo an examination for a sexually transmitted disease because there was no reason to believe she was infected.[23]

Compulsory Vaccination

Compulsory vaccination has become a major tool of public health practice, even though its constitutionality was not upheld by the U.S. Supreme Court until the seminal case of *Jacobson v. Massachusetts* in 1905.[24] The principle established in upholding required smallpox vaccination has been applied in other compulsory vaccination requirements, with particular applicability to childhood diseases such as measles, rubella, and mumps.

Virtually all states permit religious exemptions from compulsory vaccination. State Supreme Courts (with the exception of Mississippi)[25] have permitted legislatures to create exemptions for religious beliefs.[26,27] Even so, courts sometimes strictly construe religious exemptions, insisting that the belief against compulsory vaccination must be "genuine," "sincere," and an integral part of the religious doctrine.[28] A minority of states also permit exemptions based on conscientious objections.

Isolation and Quarantine

Public health authorities have the power to isolate or quarantine persons who are infected or exposed and who pose a danger to the public's health. It is a drastic remedy to prevent the spread of disease, and it is not used with any frequency today.

One tool for preventing the spread of infection is the exclusion of cases and contacts from populations that have not been exposed such as in schools or workplaces; sometimes isolation or quarantine requires a complete separation of the person from contact with others. As late as 1966, it was held that the health officer may make an isolation or quarantine order whenever he or she shall determine in a particular case that quarantine or isolation is necessary to protect the public health.[29] Still, the modern courts have required rigorous procedural due process before persons can be isolated or quarantined. In *Greene v. Edwards* (1980), the West Virginia Supreme Court reasoned that there is little difference between loss of liberty for mental health reasons and the loss of liberty for public health rationales.[30] Persons with an infectious disease, therefore, are entitled to similar procedural protections as persons with mental illness facing civil commitment. These procedural safeguards include the right to counsel, a hearing, and an appeal. Such rigorous procedural protections are justified by the fundamental invasion of liberty occasioned by long-term detention; the serious implications of erroneously finding a person dangerous; and the value of procedures in accurately determining the complex facts that are important to predicting future dangerous behavior.

Regulation of Professions and Businesses: Economic Liberty

Public health authorities have powers to regulate professions and businesses to safeguard the public's health and safety. These powers are important to ensure that professionals and businesses act in reasonably competent and safe ways. Professionals and businesses, however, also sometimes contest the validity of these powers because they interfere with economic freedoms to use property, enter into contracts, and pursue a profession. This section discusses several important regulatory powers: licensure, inspections, and nuisance abatement.

Licensure as a Tool of Public Health

When a person is born, his or her birth certificate is likely to be signed by a licensed physician. When a person dies, he or she is buried by a mortician, also licensed by a state agency. Between birth and death, many other agencies with health responsibilities are regulated through the device of professional, occupational, or institutional licensure. A discussion of licensure therefore follows logically the subject of restrictions of the person because licensure is a restriction, an imposition of conditions limiting the person's freedom to carry on an activity, profession, occupation, or business of choice. The license requirement thus limits both the person's liberty and the use of the person's property. The imposition of such a restraint is justified because it protects the public health, safety, and welfare. Public health law, as an early field of administrative law, has used licensure effectively for many generations. The occupations and callings in the general area of public health are among the earliest of licensed occupations.

Licensure, like other police powers, is an authority afforded by the legislature. It authorizes a licensing agency, either a board of health, a board of regents, or a special professional or occupational board, to promulgate rules relating to license applications and to control the licensed activity. The licensing law that delegates powers to the licensing agency may prescribe narrow or broad powers, granting it limited ministerial scope, such as collection of fees, or it may delegate broad regulatory powers to set rules for the exercise of the activity and giving the agency broad regulatory powers. The task does not end with granting licenses. The licensing agency generally has the continuing obligation to supervise the particular licensed activity. The obligation includes both the formulation of policy and standard setting in the light of what may be rapidly changing technology in the field and what may be changing needs of the people for protection.

Three major uses of licensure exist in areas related to public health. The first two are primarily matters of public health control or regulation. The first involves the licensing of people engaged in public health professions or occupations, such as physicians, dentists, nurses, physiotherapists, occupational therapists, psychologists, X-ray technologists, nutritionists, and many other allied health professionals. The second category is institutional licensure, such as state licensure of hospitals, intermediate-care facilities, nursing homes, clinics and ambulatory-care centers, and other places where patient health services are delivered, such as clinical and X-ray laboratories, including pharmacies and other businesses directly involved in rendering services. The third category is business that is not directly involved in providing health care and goods related to health care. Many businesses affect public health, including milk pasteurizing, food, energy, and public waste treatment.

Because licenses involve limits on a person's freedom to engage in particular activities, and because licensure grants a particular group of persons and businesses something of a monopoly, broad licensing powers can be justified only to protect the public health, safety, and welfare. Thus, all of the constitutional limitations that apply to the police power generally clearly apply to the grant of licenses and to the scope and fairness of licensing regulations. Licensure, in particular, should not be used as a device for economic control. Occupational licensure that restricts access to the field may be used by the "ins" to entrench themselves and to keep out the "outs." Licensure is used by some occupational groups to restrict competition, and it ought not to be misused for this purpose.

Licenses are now generally regarded as protected property rights. A license to carry on a business or engage in an occupation or profession has great value to the person or business that holds it. The question whether the government can revoke a license at any time because it was considered a mere privilege is no longer valid. A license, particularly in the field of institutional and occupational license in public health, incorporates valuable rights. Such a license is protected by due process and cannot be revoked or suspended without proper notice and hearing.

Searches and Inspections

Inspections are a common tool in public health designed to protect the population's health and safety. They are used to determine whether conditions exist that are deleterious to health and that violate public health standards or rules designed to bring about proper healthful performance of particular businesses, trades, and industries. Administrative inspections, unlike criminal law searches, are not primarily intended to uncover evidence to be used in the prosecution of a crime.

Although searches and inspections have a different emphasis, for constitutional purposes courts have generally regarded inspections as a lesser species of searches that must be conducted with constitutional safeguards. Inspections may uncover violations of health standards, for which violators may be prosecuted and penalties imposed. Inspections span the entire field of public health-related law. Inspections may be conducted to ensure health and safety in health care (e.g., hospitals and pharmacies), agriculture, nuclear power, food and drugs (Food and Drug Administration law), workplaces (Occupational Safety and Health Administration law), restaurants, housing, plumbing, and child care.

Sometimes inspections are referred to as administrative searches, but this term may sometimes be confusing in light of the use of the term *search*, which usually applies to criminal prosecutions. However, both searches and inspections are subject to review under the Fourth Amendment, which proscribes "unreasonable" searches and seizures. Before 1967, health and housing inspections were generally treated as reasonable searches, causing few constitutional problems. In *Camara v. Municipal Court of San Francisco* (1967), the U.S. Supreme Court held that the Fourth Amendment also applied to administrative searches and inspections.[31] Mr. Justice White, writing for the Court, held that a housing inspection was an intrusion on the privacy and security of individuals protected by the Fourth Amendment. Consequently, the public health authority must usually obtain a judicial warrant for an inspection. Inspection warrants, however, would normally be granted if the inspection is based on either the knowledge of an existing violation or a clear standard for routine inspections.

Although the Supreme Court has significantly changed the law of inspections, both before and after the decision in 1967 most inspections are carried out without a warrant because owners or occupants of premises generally will consent to inspections. Moreover, some exceptions exist to the inspection warrant requirement. For example, there is an exception for "pervasively regulated" businesses (e.g., firearms or alcoholic beverages). Pervasively regulated businesses are businesses so long and thoroughly regulated that persons who engage in the business have given up any "justifiable expectation of privacy."[32]

The Control of Nuisances and Dangerous Conditions

The vast field of tort law includes intentional or negligent injuries to persons and harm to property. It includes, for instance, medical malpractice and products liability affecting the manufacture of, *inter alia*, drugs and vaccines. The vastness and complexity of the broad area of torts prevents its general inclusion in this section, which focuses predominantly on public rather than private remedies.

The term *nuisance* covers both public and private nuisances. In the public health context, the primary concern is with public nuisances, a term that covers a variety of conditions that violate requirements of health and safety. A nuisance is a condition that constitutes an interference with the public right to pursue the normal conduct of life without the threat to health, comfort, and repose, ranging variously from matters of significant annoyance to conditions that impose significant risks to health and safety, for example, excessive noise, stenches, filth that attracts insects or rodents, and chemical wastes that contaminate the water supply. Facilities that generate smoke, soot, chemical odors, or other substances regarded as air pollutants may also be public nuisances. All these examples share interference with the rights of the public, and all are prohibited by law. Although any number of these examples would be treated in earlier days as common law nuisances, public nuisances are today defined by statute or ordinance[33,34] and are considered public offenses subject to criminal prosecution. Depending on the specific legislation, nuisances may also result in injunctive relief requiring "abatement."

The abatement of a public nuisance often involves the invasion of private property, so it must be clearly justified. If a health officer abates a nondangerous condition or acts excessively in light of the danger posed, then the purported abatement may constitute a "taking" or damaging of private property without due process of law, in violation of the Fourteenth Amendment. In such cases, the property owner may recover appropriate damages for the loss.[35]

The exercise of compulsory power clearly is a staple of public health law. Control over persons or property is necessary to promote the common good in a well-regulated society. At the same time, coercive measures infringe individual rights—autonomy, privacy, liberty, and property. Public health law, therefore, requires a careful examination of the tradeoffs between collective goods and personal freedoms.

THE FUTURE OF PUBLIC HEALTH LAW

Public health law is experiencing a renaissance in the United States. For example, the CDC has developed a public health law program (PHLP) designed to improve scientific understanding of the interaction between law and public health and to strengthen the legal foundation for public health practice. The PHLP has established a CDC Collaborating Center for Law and the Public's Health at Georgetown and Johns Hopkins universities; awarded a series of grants to investigate the connections between law and the public's health; and hosted the first national conference on public health law. At the same time, scholarship in public health law is blossoming, and new links are being formed between public health practitioners and attorneys.

National and state authorities are awakening to the possibilities of law reform to improve the public's health. The Robert Wood Johnson "Turning Point" Program is supporting the "Public Health Statute Modernization National Collaborative," a consortium of states and national public health organizations.[36] The Collaborative is conducting a comprehensive analysis of the structure and appropriateness of state public health statutes and developing a model state public health statute.

The events of September 11, 2001, provoked a national debate about the adequacy of the public health law infrastructure, and both federal and state governments began to examine the need for emergency health powers legislation. The CDC asked the Center for Law and the Public's Health at Georgetown and Johns Hopkins Universities to draft the Model Emergency Health Powers Act, which has now been adopted in whole or in part by a number of states.[37] Policy makers are realizing that the law relating to public health must be clear and consistent and afford strong and effective powers to public health authorities. At the same time, the law must respect personal freedoms and treat groups with fairness and tolerance.

The law, of course, cannot guarantee better public health. However, by crafting a consistent and uniform approach, carefully delineating the mission and functions of public health agencies, designating a range of flexible powers, specifying the criteria and procedures for using those powers, and protecting against discrimination and invasion of privacy, the law can become a catalyst, rather than an impediment, to reinvigorating the public health system.

REFERENCES

1. Gostin LO. *Public Health Law: Power, Duty, Restraint.* Berkeley: University of California Press, 2000.

2. Gostin LO. *Public Health Law and Ethics: A Reader.* Berkeley: University of California Press, 2002.

3. Grad F. *Public Health Law Manual,* 2nd ed. Washington, DC: American Public Health Association, 1990.

4. Institute of Medicine. *The Future of Public Health.* Washington, DC: National Academy Press, 1988.

5. Baker EL, Melton RJ, Stange PV, et al. Health reform and the health of the public. *JAMA.* 1994;272:1276–82.

6. U.S. Department of Health and Human Services, Centers for Disease Control and Prevention. *Public Health's Infrastructure: A Status Report.* Submitted to the Appropriations Committee of the U.S. Senate, 2001.

7. Institute of Medicine. *Assuring the Health of the Public in the 21st Century.* Washington, DC: National Academy Press, 2002.

8. Rose G. *The Strategy of Preventive Medicine.* Oxford: Oxford University Press, 1992: pp. 101.

9. CDC. Ten great public health achievements—United States, 1900–1999. *MMWR.* 1999;48:241–3.

10. Koplan JP, Fleming DW. Current and future public health challenges. *JAMA.* 2000;284:1696–8.

11. U.S. Department of Health and Human Services. *Healthy People 2010.* Washington, DC: U.S. Department of Health and Human Services, 2000.

12. Goslin LO. Public health law reform. *Am J Public Health.* 2001; 91:1365–8.

13. *South Dakota v. Dole,* 483 U.S. 203 (1987).

14. *DeShaney v. Winnebago County Department of Social Services,* 489 U.S. 189, 213 (1989).

15. *Webster v. Reproductive Health Services,* 492 U.S. 490, 507 (1989).

16. Tribe LH. The abortion funding conundrum: inalienable rights, affirmative duties, and the dilemma of dependence. *Harvard Law Rev.* 1985; 99:330–40.

17. U.S. Constitution, Article I, Section 8.

18. *United States v. Lopez,* 115 S. Ct. 1624 (1995).

19. *United States v. Morrison,* 120 S. Ct 1740 (2000).

20. *Webster's Third New International Dictionary, Unabridged.* Springfield, MA: Merriam-Webster, 1986: pp. 1753.

21. *Commonwealth v. Alger, 7 Cush.* 53, 96 (Mass. 1851).

22. *Ferguson v. City of Charleston,* 121 S. Ct. 1281 (2001).

23. *Irwin v. Arrendale,* 17 Ga. App. 1, 5–6, 159 S.E.2d 719, 724 (1967).

24. *Jacobson v. Massachusetts,* 197 U.S. 11 (1905).

25. *Brown v. Stone,* 378 So.2d 218,223 (Miss. 1979).

26. *Mason v. General Brown Cent. School Dist,* 851 F.2d 47 (2d Cir. 1988).

27. *Berg v. Glen Cove City Sch. Dist,* 853 F.Supp. 651 (E.D.N.Y. 1994).

28. *Brown v. City School Dist,* 429 N.Y.S.2d 355 (1980).

29. Application of Halko, 246 Cal. App.2d 553 (1966).

30. *Greene v. Edwards,* 263 S.E.2d 661, 663 (1980).

31. *Camara v. Municipal Court of San Francisco,* 381 U.S. 523 (1967).

32. *Colonnade Catering v. United States,* 397 U.S. 72 (1970).

33. *Lawton v. Steele,* 152 U.S. 133 (1894).

34. *State ex rel. Haas v. Dionne,* 42 Or. App. 851, 601 P.2d 894 (1979).

35. *Peters v. Township of Hopewell,* 534 F.Supp. 1324 (1982).

36. Turning Point. Available at http://www.turningpointprogram.org. Accessed December 18, 2001.

37. Model State Health Emergency Powers Act. Available at http://www. public healthlaw.net/MSEPHA/MSEPHA2.pdf. Accessed May 23, 2002.

Case Law: *Jacobson v. Massachusetts* (Validity of State Mandatory Vaccine Law)

JACOBSON v. COM. OF MASSACHUSETTS, **197 U.S. 11 (1905)**

HENNING JACOBSON, Plff. in Err.,

v.

COMMONWEALTH OF MASSACHUSETTS.

No. 70.

Argued December 6, 1904.

Decided February 20, 1905.

This case involves the validity, under the Constitution of the United States, of certain provisions in the statutes of Massachusetts relating to vaccination.

The revised laws of that commonwealth, chap 75, 137, provide that 'the board of health of a city or town, if, in its opinion, it is necessary for the public health or safety, shall require and enforce the vaccination and revaccination of all the inhabitants thereof, and shall provide them with the means of free vaccination. Whoever, being over twenty-one years of age and not under guardianship, refuses or neglects to comply with such requirement shall forfeit $5.'

An exception is made in favor of 'children who present a certificate, signed by a registered physician, that they are unfit subjects for vaccination.'139.

Proceeding under these statutes, the board of health of the city of Cambridge, Massachusetts, on the 27th day of February, 1902, adopted the following regulation: 'Whereas, smallpox has been prevalent to some extent in the city of Cambridge, and still continues to increase; and whereas, it is necessary for the speedy extermination of the disease that all

persons not protected by vaccination should be vaccinated; and whereas, in the opinion of the board, the public health and safety require the vaccination or revaccination of all the inhabitants of Cambridge; be it ordered, that all the inhabitants of the city who have not been successfully vaccinated since March 1st, 1897, be vaccinated or revaccinated.'

Subsequently, the board adopted an additional regulation empowering a named physician to enforce the vaccination of persons as directed by the board at its special meeting of February 27th.

These regulations being in force, the plaintiff in error, Jacobson, was proceeded against by a criminal complaint in one of the inferior courts of Massachusetts. The complaint charged that on the 17th day of July, 1902, the board of health of Cambridge, being of the opinion that it was necessary for the public health and safety, required the vaccination and revaccination of all the inhabitants thereof who had not been successfully vaccinated since the 1st day of March, 1897, and provided them with the means of free vaccination; and that the defendant, being over twenty-one years of age and not under guardianship, refused and neglected to comply with such requirement.

The defendant, having been arraigned, pleaded not guilty. The government put in evidence the previously mentioned regulations adopted by the board of health, and made proof tending to show that its chairman informed the defendant that, by refusing to be vaccinated, he would incur the penalty provided by the statute, and would be prosecuted therefor; that he offered to vaccinate the defendant without expense to him;

and that the offer was declined, and defendant refused to be vaccinated.

The prosecution having introduced no other evidence, the defendant made numerous offers of proof. But the trial court ruled that each and all of the facts offered to be proved by the defendant were immaterial, and excluded all proof of them.

The defendant, standing upon his offers of proof, and introducing no evidence, asked numerous instructions to the jury, among which were the following:

That 137 of chapter 75 of the Revised Laws of Massachusetts was in derogation of the rights secured to the defendant by the preamble to the Constitution of the United States, and tended to subvert and defeat the purposes of the Constitution as declared in its preamble;

That the section referred to was in derogation of the rights secured to the defendant by the 14th Amendment of the Constitution of the United States, and especially of the clauses of that amendment providing that no state shall make or enforce any law abridging the privileges or immunities of citizens of the United States, nor deprive any person of life, liberty, or property without due process of law, nor deny to any person within its jurisdiction the equal protection of the laws; and

That said section was opposed to the spirit of the Constitution.

Each of defendant's prayers for instructions was rejected, and he duly excepted. The defendant requested the court, but the court refused, to instruct the jury to return a verdict of not guilty. And the court instructed the jury, in substance, that, if they believed the evidence introduced by the commonwealth, and were satisfied beyond a reasonable doubt that the defendant was guilty of the offense charged in the complaint, they would be warranted in finding a verdict of guilty. A verdict of guilty was thereupon returned.

The case was then continued for the opinion of the supreme judicial court of Massachusetts. Santa Fe Pacific Railroad Company, the exceptions, sustained the action of the trial court, and thereafter, pursuant to the verdict of the jury, he was sentenced by the court to pay a fine of $5. And the court ordered that he stand committed until the fine was paid.

Messrs. Frederick H. Nash and Herbert Parker for defendant in error.

Mr. Justice Harlan delivered the opinion of the court:

We pass without extended discussion the suggestion that the particular section of the statute of Massachusetts now in question (137, chap. 75) is in derogation of rights secured by the preamble of the Constitution of the United States. Although that preamble indicates the general purposes for which the people ordained and established the Constitution, it has never been regarded as the source of any substantive power conferred on the government of the United States, or on any of its departments. Such powers embrace only those expressly granted in the body of the Constitution, and such as may be implied from those so granted. Although, therefore, one of the declared objects of the Constitution was to secure the blessings of liberty to all under the sovereign jurisdiction and authority of the United States, no power can be exerted to that end by the United States, unless, apart from the preamble, it be found in some express delegation of power, or in some power to be properly implied therefrom. 1 Story, Const. 462.

We also pass without discussion the suggestion that the above section of the statute is opposed to the spirit of the Constitution. Undoubtedly, as observed by Chief Justice Marshall, speaking for the court in *Sturges v. Crowninshield*, 4 Wheat. 122, 202, 4 L. ed. 529, 550, 'the spirit of an instrument, especially of a constitution, is to be respected not less than its letter; yet the spirit is to be collected chiefly from its words.' We have no need in this case to go beyond the plain, obvious meaning of the words in those provisions of the Constitution which, it is contended, must control our decision.

What, according to the judgment of the state court, are the scope and effect of the statute? What results were intended to be accomplished by it? These questions must be answered.

The supreme judicial court of Massachusetts said in the present case: 'Let us consider the offer of evidence which was made by the defendant Jacobson. The ninth of the propositions which he offered to prove, as to what vaccination consists of, is nothing more than a fact of common knowledge, upon which the statute is founded, and proof of it was unnecessary and immaterial. The thirteenth and fourteenth involved matters depending upon his personal opinion, which could not be taken as correct, or given effect, merely because he made it a ground of refusal to comply with the requirement. Moreover, his views could not affect the validity of the statute, nor entitle him to be excepted from its provisions. *Com. v. Connolly*, 163 Mass. 539, 40 N. E. 862; *Com. v. Has*, 122 Mass. 40; *Reynolds v. United States*, 98 U.S. 145, 25 L. ed. 244; *Reg. v. Downes*, 13 Cox, C. C. 111. The other eleven propositions all relate to alleged injurious or dangerous effects of vaccination. The defendant 'offered to prove and show be competent evidence' these socalled facts. Each of them, in its nature, is such that it cannot be stated as a truth, otherwise than as a matter of opinion. The only 'competent evidence' that could be presented to the court to prove these propositions was the testimony of experts, giving their opinions. It would not have been competent to introduce the medical history of individual cases. Assuming that medical experts could have been found who would have testified in support of these propositions, and that it had become the duty of the judge, in accordance with the law as stated in *Com. v. Anthes*, 5 Gray, 185, to instruct the jury as to whether or not the statute is constitutional, he would have been obliged to consider the evidence in connection with facts of common knowledge, which the court will always regard in passing upon the constitutionality of a statute. He would have considered this testimony of experts in connection with the facts that for nearly a century most of the members of the medical profession have regarded vaccination, repeated after intervals, as a preventive of smallpox; that, while they have recognized the possibility of injury to an individual from carelessness in the performance of it, or even in a conceivable case without carelessness, they generally have considered the risk of such an injury too small to be seriously weighed as against the benefits coming from the discreet and proper use of the preventive; and that not only the medical profession and the people generally have for a long time entertained these opinions, but legislatures and courts have acted upon them with general unanimity. If the defendant had been permitted to introduce such expert testimony as he had in support of these several propositions, it could not have changed the result. It would not have justified the court in holding that the legislature had transcended its power in enacting this statute on their judgment of what the welfare of the people demands.' *Com. v. Jacobson*, 183 Mass. 242, 66 N. E. 719.

While the mere rejection of defendant's offers of proof does not strictly present a Federal question, we may properly regard the exclusion of evidence upon the ground of its incompetency or immateriality under the statute as showing what, in the opinion of the state court, are the scope and meaning of the statute. Taking these observations of the state court as indicating the scope of the statute—and such is our duty. *Leffingwell v. Warren*, 2 Black, 599, 603, 17 L. ed. 261. 262; *Morley v. Lake Shore & M. S. R. Co.*, 146 U.S. 162, 167, 36 S. L. ed. 925, 928, 13 Sup. Ct. Rep. 54; *Tullis v. Lake Erie & W. R. Co.*, 175 U.S. 348, 44 L. ed. 192, 20 Sup. Ct. Rep. 136; *W. W. Cargill Co. v. Minnesota*, 180 U.S. 452, 466, 45 S. L. ed. 619, 625, 21 Sup. Ct. Rep. 423—we assume, for the purposes of the present inquiry, that its provisions require, at least as a general rule, that adults not under the guardianship and remaining within the limits of the city of Cambridge must submit to the regulation adopted by the board of health. Is the statute, so construed, therefore, inconsistent with the liberty which the Constitution of the United States secures to every person against deprivation by the state?

The authority of the state to enact this statute is to be referred to what is commonly called the police power—a power which the state did not surrender when becoming a member of the Union under the Constitution. Although this court has refrained from any attempt to define the limits of that power, yet it has distinctly recognized the authority of a state to enact quarantine laws and 'health laws of every description;' indeed, all laws that relate to matters completely within its territory and which do not by their necessary operation affect the people of other states. According to settled principles, the police power of a state must be held to embrace, at least, such reasonable regulations established directly by legislative enactment as will protect the public health and the public safety. *Gibbons v. Ogden*, 9 Wheat. 1, 203, 6 L. ed. 23, 71; *Hannibal & St. J. R. Co. v. Husen*, 95 U.S. 465, 470, 24 S. L. ed. 527, 530; *Boston Beer Co. v. Massachusetts*, 97 U.S. 25, 24 L. ed. 989; *New Orleans Gaslight Co. v. Louisiana Light & H. P. & Mfg. Co.*, 115 U.S. 650, 661, 29 S. L. ed. 516, 520, 6 Sup. Ct. Rep. 252; *Lawson v. Stecle*, 152 U.S. 133, 38 L. ed. 385, 14 Sup. Ct. Rep. 499. It is equally true that the state may invest local bodies called into existence for purposes of local administration with authority in some appropriate way to safeguard the public health and the public safety. The mode or manner in which those results are to be accomplished is within the discretion of the state, subject, of course, so far as Federal power is concerned, only to the condition that no rule prescribed by a state, nor any regulation adopted by a local governmental agency acting under the sanction of state legislation, shall contravene the Constitution of the United States, nor infringe any right granted or secured by that instrument. A local enactment or regulation, even if based on the acknowledged police powers of a state, must always yield in case of conflict with the exercise by the general government of any power it possesses under the Constitution, or with any right which that instrument gives or secures. *Gibbons v. Ogden*, 9 Wheat. 1, 210, 6 L. ed. 23, 73; *Sinnot v. Davenport*, 22 How. 227, 243, 16 L. ed. 243, 247; *Missouri, K. & T. R. Co. v. Haber*, 169 U.S. 613, 626, 42 S. L. ed. 878, 882, 18 Sup. Ct. Rep. 488.

We come, then, to inquire whether any right given or secured by the Constitution is invaded by the statute as interpreted by the state court. The defendant insists that his liberty is invaded when the state subjects him to fine or imprisonment for neglecting or refusing to submit to vaccination; that a compulsory vaccination law is unreasonable, arbitrary, and oppressive, and, therefore, hostile to the inherent right of every freeman to care for his own body and health in such way as to him seems best; and that the execution of such a law against one who objects to vaccination, no matter for what reason, is nothing short of an assault upon his person. But the liberty secured by the Constitution of the United States to every person within its jurisdiction does not import an absolute right in each person to be, at all times and in all circumstances, wholly freed from restraint. There are manifold restraints to which every person is necessarily subject for the common good. On any other basis organized society could not exist with safety to its members. Society based on the rule that each one is a law unto himself would soon be confronted with disorder and anarchy. Real liberty for all could not exist under the operation of a principle which recognizes the right of each individual person to use his own, whether in respect of his person or his property, regardless of the injury that may be done to others. This court has more than once recognized it as a fundamental principle that 'persons and property are subjected to all kinds of restraints and burdens in order to secure the general comfort, health, and prosperity of the state; of the perfect right of the legislature to do which no question ever was, or upon acknowledged general principles ever can be, made, so far as natural persons are concerned.' *Hannibal & St. J. R. Co. v. Husen*, 95 U.S. 465, 471, 24 S. L. ed. 527, 530; *Missouri, K. & T. R. Co. v. Haber*, 169 U.S. 613, 628, 629 S., 42 L. ed. 878–883, 18 Sup. Ct. Rep. 488; *Thorpe v. Rutland & B. R. Co.*, 27 Vt. 148, 62 Am. Dec. 625. In *Crowley v. Christensen*, 137 U.S. 86, 89, 34 S. L. ed. 620, 621, 11 Sup. Ct. Rep. 13, we said: 'The possession and enjoyment of all rights are subject to such reasonable conditions as may be deemed by the governing authority of the country essential to the safety, health, peace, good order, and morals of the community. Even liberty itself, the greatest of all rights, is not unrestricted license to act according to one's own will. It is only freedom from restraint under conditions essential to the equal enjoyment of the same right by others. It is, then, liberty regulated by law.' In the Constitution of Massachusetts adopted in 1780 it was laid down as a fundamental principle of the social compact that the whole people covenants with each citizen, and each citizen with the whole people, that all shall be governed by certain laws for 'the common good,' and that government is instituted 'for the common good, for the protection, safety, prosperity, and happiness of the people, and not for the profit, honor, or private interests of any one man, family, or class of men.' The good and welfare of the commonwealth, of which the legislature is primarily the judge, is the basis on which the police power rests in *Massachusetts. Com. v. Alger*, 7 Cush. 84.

Applying these principles to the present case, it is to be observed that the legislature of Massachusetts required the inhabitants of a city or town to be vaccinated only when, in the opinion of the board of health, that was necessary for the public health or the public safety. The authority to determine for all what ought to be done in such an emergency must have been lodged somewhere or in some body; and surely it was appropriate for the legislature to refer that question, in the first instance, to a board of health composed of persons residing in the locality affected, and appointed, presumably, because of their fitness to determine such questions. To invest such a body

with authority over such matters was not an unusual, nor an unreasonable or arbitrary, requirement. Upon the principle of self-defense, of paramount necessity, a community has the right to protect itself against an epidemic of disease which threatens the safety of its members. It is to be observed that when the regulation in question was adopted smallpox, according to the recitals in the regulation adopted by the board of health, was prevalent to some extent in the city of Cambridge, and the disease was increasing. If such was the situation—and nothing is asserted or appears in the record to the contrary—if we are to attach, any value whatever to the knowledge which, it is safe to affirm, in common to all civilized peoples touching smallpox and the methods most usually employed to eradicate that disease, it cannot be adjudged that the present regulation of the board of health was not necessary in order to protect the public health and secure the public safety. Smallpox being prevalent and increasing at Cambridge, the court would usurp the functions of another branch of government if it adjudged, as matter of law, that the mode adopted under the sanction of the state, to protect the people at large was arbitrary, and not justified by the necessities of the case. We say necessities of the case, because it might be that an acknowledged power of a local community to protect itself against an epidemic threatening the safety of all might be exercised in particular circumstances and in reference to particular persons in such an arbitrary, unreasonable manner, or might go so far beyond what was reasonably required for the safety of the public, as to authorize or compel the courts to interfere for the protection of such persons. *Wisconsin, M. & P. R. Co. v. Jacobson*, 179 U.S. 287, 301, 45 S. L. ed. 194, 201, 21 Sup. Ct. Rep. 115; 1 Dill. Mun. Corp. 4th ed. 319–325, and authorities in notes; Freurid, Police Power, 63 et seq. In *Hannibal & St. J. R. Co. v. Husen*, 95 U.S. 465, 471–473, 24 L. ed. 527, 530, 531, this court recognized the right of a state to pass sanitary laws, laws for the protection of life, liberty, health, or property within its limits, laws to prevent persons and animals suffering under contagious or infectious diseases, or convicts, from coming within its borders. But, as the laws there involved went beyond the necessity of the case, and, under the guise of exerting a police power, invaded the domain of Federal authority, and violated rights secured by the Constitution, this court deemed it to be its duty to hold such laws invalid. If the mode adopted by the commonwealth of Massachusetts for the protection of its local communities against smallpox proved to be distressing, inconvenient, or objectionable to some—if nothing more could be reasonably affirmed of the statute in question—the answer is that it was the duty of the constituted authorities primarily to keep in view the welfare, comfort, and safety of the many, and not permit the interests of the many to be subordinated to the wishes or convenience of the few. There is, of course, a sphere within which the individual may assert the supremacy of his own will, and rightfully dispute the authority of any human government—especially of any free government existing under a written constitution, to interfere with the exercise of that will. But it is equally true that in every well-ordered society charged with the duty of conserving the safety of its members the rights of the individual in respect of his liberty may at times, under the pressure of great dangers, be subjected to such restraint, to be enforced by reasonable regulations, as the safety of the general public may demand. An American citizen arriving at an American port on a vessel in which, during the voyage, there had been cases of yellow fever or Asiatic cholera, he, although apparently free from disease himself, may yet, in some circumstances, be held in quarantine against his will on board of such vessel or in a quarantine station, until it be ascertained by inspection, conducted with due diligence, that the danger of the spread of the disease among the community at large has disappeared. The liberty secured by the 14th Amendment, this court has said, consists, in part, in the right of a person 'to live and work where he will' (*Allgeyer v. Louisiana*, 165 U.S. 578, 41 L. ed. 832, 17 Sup. Ct. Rep. 427); and yet he may be compelled, by force if need be, against his will and without regard to his personal wishes or his pecuniary interests, or even his religious or political convictions, to take his place in the ranks of the army of his country, and risk the chance of being shot down in its defense. It is not, therefore, true that the power of the public to guard itself against imminent danger depends in every case involving the control of one's body upon his willingness to submit to reasonable regulations established by the constituted authorities, under the sanction of the state, for the purpose of protecting the public collectively against such danger.

It is said, however, that the statute, as interpreted by the state court, although making an exception in favor of children certified by a registered physician to be unfit subjects for vaccination, makes no exception in case of adults in like condition. But this cannot be deemed a denial of the equal protection of the laws to adults; for the statute is applicable equally to all in like condition, and there are obviously reasons why regulations may be appropriate for adults which could not be safely applied to persons of tender years.

Looking at the propositions embodied in the defendant's rejected offers of proof, it is clear that they are more formidable by their number than by their inherent value. Those offers in the main seem to have had no purpose except to state the general theory of those of the medical profession who attach little or no value to vaccination as a means of preventing the spread of smallpox, or who think that vaccination causes other diseases of the body. What everybody knows the court must know, and therefore the state court judicially knew, as this court knows, that an opposite theory accords with the common belief, and is maintained by high medical authority. We must assume that, when the statute in question was passed, the legislature of Massachusetts was not unaware of these opposing theories, and was compelled, of necessity, to choose between them. It was not compelled to commit a matter involving the public health and safety to the final decision of a court or jury. It is no part of the function of a court or a jury to determine which one of two modes was likely to be the most effective for the protection of the public against disease. That was for the legislative department to determine in the light of all the information it had or could obtain. It could not properly abdicate its function to guard the public health and safety. The state legislature proceeded upon the theory which recognized vaccination as at least an effective, if not the best-known, way in which to meet and suppress the evils of a smallpox epidemic that imperiled an entire population. Upon what sound principles as to the relations existing between the different departments of government can the court review this action of the legislature? If there is any such power in the judiciary to review legislative action in respect of a matter affecting the general welfare, it can only be when that which the legislature has done comes within the rule that, if a statute purporting to have been enacted to protect the public health, the public morals, or the public safety, has no real or substantial relation to those objects, or is, beyond all question, a plain, palpable invasion of rights secured by the fundamental law, it is the duty of the courts to so adjudge, and thereby give effect to the Constitution. *Mugler v. Kansas*, 123 U.S. 623, 661, 31 S. L. ed. 205, 210, 8 Sup. Ct. Rep. 273; *Minnesota v. Barber*, 136 U.S. 313, 320, 34 S. L. ed. 455, 458, 3 Inters. Com. Rep. 185, 10 Sup. Ct. Rep. 862; *Atkin v. Kansas*, 191 U.S. 207, 223, 48 S. L. ed. 148, 158, 24 Sup. Ct. Rep. 124.

Whatever may be thought of the expediency of this statute, it cannot be affirmed to be, beyond question, in palpable conflict with the Constitution. Nor, in view of the methods employed to stamp out the disease of smallpox, can anyone confidently assert that the means prescribed by the state to that end has no real or substantial relation to the protection of the public health and the public safety. Such an assertion would not be consistent with the experience of this and other countries whose authorities have dealt with the disease of smallpox. And the principle of vaccination as a means to prevent the spread of smallpox has been enforced in many states by statutes making the vaccination of children a condition of their right to enter or remain in public schools. *Blue v. Beach*, 155 Ind. 121, 50 L. R. A. 64, 80 Am. St. Rep. 195, 56 N. E. 89; *Morris v. Columbus*, 102 Ga. 792, 42 L. R. A. 175, 66 Am. St. Rep. 243, 30

S. E. 850; *State v. Hay*, 126 N. C. 999, 49 L. R. A. 588, 78 Am. St. Rep. 691, 35 S. E. 459; *Abeel v. Clark*, 84 Cal. 226, 24 Pac. 383; *Bissell v. Davison*, 65 Conn. 183, 29 L. R. A. 251, 32 Atl. 348; *Hazen v. Strong*, 2 Vt. 427; *Duffield v. Williamsport School District*, 162 Pa. 476, 25 L. R. A. 152, 29 Atl. 742.

The latest case upon the subject of which we are aware is *Viemester v. White*, decided very recently by the court of appeals of New York. That case involved the validity of a statute excluding from the public schools all children who had not been vaccinated. One contention was that the statute and the regulation adopted in exercise of its provisions was inconsistent with the rights, privileges, and liberties of the citizen. The contention was overruled, the court saying, among other things:

'Smallpox is known of all to be a dangerous and contagious disease. If vaccination strongly tends to prevent the transmission or spread of this disease, it logically follows that children may be refused admission to the public schools until they have been vaccinated. The appellant claims that vaccination does not tend to prevent smallpox, but tends to bring about other diseases, and that it does much harm, with no good. It must be conceded that some laymen, both learned and unlearned, and some physicians of great skill and repute, do not believe that vaccination is a preventive of smallpox. The common belief, however, is that it has a decided tendency to prevent the spread of this fearful disease, and to render it less dangerous to those who contract it. While not accepted by all, it is accepted by the mass of the people, as well as by most members of the medical profession. It has been general in our state, and in most civilized nations for generations. It is generally accepted in theory, and generally applied in practice, both by the voluntary action of the people, and in obedience to the command of law. Nearly every state in the Union has statutes to encourage, or directly or indirectly to require, vaccination; and this is true of most nations of Europe. . . . A common belief, like common knowledge, does not require evidence to establish its existence, but may be acted upon without proof by the legislature and the courts. . . . The fact that the belief is not universal is not controlling, for there is scarcely any belief that is accepted by everyone. The possibility that the belief may be wrong, and that science may yet show it to be wrong, is not conclusive; for the

legislature has the right to pass laws which, according to the common belief of the people, are adapted to prevent the spread of contagious diseases. In a free country, where the government is by the people, through their chosen representatives, practical legislation admits of no other standard of action, for what the people believe is for the common welfare must be accepted as tending to promote the common welfare, whether it does in fact or not. Any other basis would conflict with the spirit of the Constitution, and would sanction measures opposed to a Republican form of government. While we do not decide, and cannot decide, that vaccination is a preventive of smallpox, we take judicial notice of the fact that this is the common belief of the people of the state, and, with this fact as a foundation, we hold that the statute in question is a health law, enacted in a reasonable and proper exercise of the police power.' 179 N. Y. 235, 72 N. E. 97.

Since, then, vaccination, as a means of protecting a community against smallpox, finds strong support in the experience of this and other countries, no court, much less a jury, is justified in disregarding the action of the legislature simply because in its or their opinion that particular method was—perhaps, or possibly—not the best either for children or adults.

Did the offers of proof made by the defendant present a case which entitled him, while remaining in Cambridge, to claim exemption from the operation of the statute and of the regulation adopted by the board of health? We have already said that his rejected offers, in the main, only set forth the theory of those who had no faith in vaccination as a means of preventing the spread of smallpox, or who thought that vaccination, without benefiting the public, put in peril the health of the person vaccinated. But there were some offers which it is contended embodied distinct facts that might properly have been considered. Let us see how this is.

The defendant offered to prove that vaccination 'quite often' caused serious and permanent injury to the health of the person vaccinated; that the operation 'occasionally' resulted in death; that it was 'impossible' to tell 'in any particular case' what the results of vaccination would be, or whether it would injure the health or result in death; that 'quite often' one's blood is in a certain condition of impurity when it is not prudent or safe to vaccinate him; that there is no practical test by which to determine 'with any degree of certainty' whether one's blood is in such condition of impurity as to render vaccination necessarily unsafe or dangerous; that vaccine matter is 'quite often' impure and dangerous to be used, but whether impure or not cannot be ascertained by any known practical test; that the defendant refused to submit to vaccination for the reason that he had, 'when a child,' been caused great and extreme suffering for a long period by a disease produced by vaccination; and that he had witnessed a similar result of vaccination, not only in the case of his son, but in the cases of others.

These offers, in effect, invited the court and jury to go over the whole ground gone over by the legislature when it enacted the statute in question. The legislature assumed that some children, by reason of their condition at the time, might not be fit subjects of vaccination; and it is suggested—and we will not say without reason—that such is the case with some adults. But the defendant did not offer to prove that, by reason of his then condition, he was in fact not a fit subject of vaccination at the time he was informed of the requirement of the regulation adopted by the board of health. It is entirely consistent with his offer of proof that, after reaching full age, he had become, so far as medical skill could discover, and when informed of the regulation of the board of health was, a fit subject of vaccination, and that the vaccine matter to be used in his case was such as any medical practitioner of good standing would regard as proper to be used. The matured opinions of medical men everywhere, and the experience of mankind, as all must know, negative the suggestion that it is not possible in any case to determine whether vaccination is safe. Was defendant exempted from the operation of the statute simply because of his dread of the same evil results experienced by him when a child, and which he had observed in the cases of his son and other children? Could he reasonably claim such an exemption because 'quite often,' or 'occasionally,' injury had resulted from vaccination, or because it was impossible, in the opinion of some, by any practical test, to determine with absolute certainty whether a particular person could be safely vaccinated?

It seems to the court that an affirmative answer to these questions would practically strip the legislative department of its function to care for the public health and the public safety when endangered by epidemics of disease. Such an answer would mean that compulsory vaccination could not, in any conceivable case, be legally enforced in a community, even at the command of the legislature, however widespread the epidemic of smallpox, and however deep and universal was the belief of the community and of its medical advisers that a system of general vaccination was vital to the safety of all.

We are not prepared to hold that a minority, residing or remaining in any city or town where smallpox is prevalent, and enjoying the general protection afforded by an organized local government, may thus defy the will of its constituted authorities, acting in good faith for all, under the legislative sanction of the state. If such be the privilege of a minority, then a like privilege would belong to each individual of the community, and the spectacle would be presented of the welfare and safety of an entire population being subordinated to the notions of a single individual who chooses to remain a part of that population. We are unwilling to hold it to be an element in the liberty secured by the Constitution of the United States that one person, or a minority of persons, residing in any community and enjoying the benefits of its local government, should have the power thus to dominate the majority when supported in their action by the authority of the state. While this court should guard with firmness every right appertaining to life, liberty, or property as secured to the individual by the supreme law of the land, it is of the last importance that it should not invade the domain of local authority except when it is plainly necessary to do so in order to enforce that law. The safety and the health of the people of Massachusetts are, in the first instance, for that commonwealth to guard and protect. They are matters that do not ordinarily concern the national government. So far as they can be reached by any government, they depend, primarily, upon such action as the state, in its wisdom, may take; and we do not perceive that this legislation has invaded any right secured by the Federal Constitution.

Before closing this opinion we deem it appropriate, in order to prevent misapprehension as to our views, to observe—perhaps to repeat a thought already sufficiently expressed, namely—that the police power of a state, whether exercised directly by the legislature, or by a local body acting under its authority, may be exerted in such circumstances, or by regulations so arbitrary and oppressive in particular cases, as to justify the interference of the courts to prevent wrong and oppression. Extreme cases can be readily suggested. Ordinarily such cases are not safe guides in the administration of the law. It is easy, for instance, to suppose the case of an adult who is embraced by the mere words of the act, but yet to subject whom to vaccination in a particular condition of his health or body would be cruel and inhuman in the last degree. We are not to be understood as holding that the statute was intended to be applied to such a case, or, if it was so intended, that the judiciary would not be competent to interfere and protect the health and life of the individual concerned. 'All laws,' this court has said, 'should receive a sensible construction. General terms should be so limited in their application as not to lead to injustice, oppression, or an absurd consequence. It will always, therefore, be presumed that the legislature intended exceptions to its language which would avoid results of this character. The reason of the law in such cases should prevail over its letter.' *United States v. Kirby*, 7 Wall. 482, 19 L. ed. 278; *Lau Ow*

Bew v. United States, 144 U.S. 47, 58, 36 S. L. ed. 340, 344, 12 Sup. Ct. Rep. 517. Until otherwise informed by the highest court of Massachusetts, we are not inclined to hold that the statute establishes the absolute rule that an adult must be vaccinated if it be apparent or can be shown with reasonable certainty that he is not at the time a fit subject of vaccination, or that vaccination, by reason of his then condition, would seriously impair his health, or probably cause his death. No such case is here presented. It is the cause of an adult who, for aught that appears, was himself in perfect health and a fit subject of vaccination, and yet, while remaining in the community, refused to obey the statute and the regulation adopted in execution of its provisions for the protection of the public health and the public safety, confessedly endangered by the presence of a dangerous disease.

We now decide only that the statute covers the present case, and that nothing clearly appears that would justify this court in holding it to be unconstitutional and inoperative in its application to the plaintiff in error.

The judgment of the court below must be affirmed.

It is so ordered.

Mr. Justice Brewer and Mr. Justice Peckham dissent.

Footnotes

'State-supported facilities for vaccination began in England in 1808 with the National Vaccine Establishment. In 1840 vaccination fees were made payable out of the rates. The first compulsory act was passed in 1853, the guardians of the poor being intrusted with the carrying out of the law; in 1854 the public vacinations under one year of age were 408,824 as against an average of 180,960 for several years before. In 1867 a new act was passed, rather to remove some technical difficulties than to enlarge the scope of the former act; and in 1871 the act was passed which compelled the boards of guardians to appoint vaccination officers. The guardians also appoint a public vaccinator, who must be duly qualified to practise medicine, and whose duty it is to vaccinate (for a fee of one shilling and sixpence) any child resident within his district brought to him for that purpose, to examine the same a week after, to give a certificate, and to certify to the vaccination officer the fact of vaccination or of insusceptibility. . . .

Vaccination was made compulsory in Bavarla in 1807, and subsequently in the following countries: Denmark (1810), Sweden (1814), Wurttemberg, Hesse, and other German states (1818), Prussia (1835), Roumania (1874), Hungary (1876), and Servia (1881). It is compulsory by cantonal law in 10 out of the 22 Swiss cantons; an attempt to pass a Federal compulsory law was defeated by a plebiscite in 1881. In the following countries there is no compulsory law, but governmental facilities and compulsion on various classes more or less directly

under governmental control, such as soldiers, state employees, apprentices, school pupils, etc.: France, Italy, Spain, Portugal, Belgium. Norway, Austria, Turkey. . . . Vaccination has been compulsory in South Australia since 1872, in Victoria since 1874, and in Western Australia since 1878. In Tasmania a compulsory act was passed in 1882. In New South Wales there is no compulsion, but free facilities for vaccination. Compulsion was adopted at Calcutta in 1880, and since then at 80 other towns of Bengal, at Madras in 1884, and at Bombay and elsewhere in the presidency a few years earlier. Revaccination was made compulsory in Denmark in 1871, and in Roumania in 1874; in Holland it was enacted for all school pupils in 1872. The various laws and administrative orders which had been for many years in force as to vaccination and revaccination in the several German states were consolidated in an imperial statute of 1874. ' 24 *Encyclopaedia Britannica* (1894), Vaccination.

'In 1857 the British Parliament received answers from 552 physicians to questions which were asked them in reference to the utility of vaccination, and only two of these spoke against it. Nothing proves this utility more clearly than the statistics obtained. Especially instructive are those which Flinzer compiled respecting the epidemic in Chemnitz which prevailed in 1870–71. At this time in the town there were 64,255 inhabitants, of whom 53,891, or 83.87 per cent, were vaccinated, 5,712, or 8.89 per cent were unvaccinated, and 4,652, or 7.24 per cent, had had the smallpox before. Of those vaccinated 953, or 1.77 per cent, became affected with smallpox, and of the uninocculated 2,643, or 46.3 per cent, had the disease. In the vaccinated the mortality from the disease was 0.73 per cent, and in the unprotected it was 9.16 per cent. In general, the danger of infection is six times as great, and the mortality 68 times as great, in the unvaccinated, as in the vaccinated. Statistics derived from the civil population are in general not so instructive as those derived from armies, where vaccination is usually more carefully performed, and where statistics can be more accurately collected. During the Franco-German war (1870–71) there was in France a widespread epidemic of smallpox, but the German army lost during the campaign only 450 cases, or 58 men to the 100,000; in the French army, however, where vaccination was not carefully carried out, the number of deaths from smallpox was 23,400, *Johnson's Universal Cyclopaedia* (1897), Vaccination.

'The degree of protection afforded by vaccination thus became a question of great interest. Its extreme value was easily demonstrated by statistical researches. In England, in the last half of the eighteenth century, out of every 1,000 deaths, 96 occurred from smallpox; in the first half of the present century, out of every 1,000 deaths, but 35 were caused by that disease.

The amount of mortality in a country by smallpox seems to bear a fixed relation to the extent to which vaccination is carried out In all England and Wales, for some years previous to 1853, the proportional mortality by smallpox was 21.9 to 1,000 deaths from all causes; in London it was but 16 to 1,000; in Ireland, where vaccination was much less general, it was 49 to 1,000, while in Connaught it was 60 to 1,000. On the other hand, in a number of European countries where vaccination was more or less compulsory, the proportionate number of deaths from smallpox about the same time varied from 2 per 1,000 of all causes in Bohemia, Lombardy, Venice, and Sweden, to 8.33 per 1,000 in Saxony. Although in many instances persons who had been vaccinated were attacked with smallpox in a more or less modified form, it was noticed that the persons so attacked had been commonly vaccinated many years previously.' 16 *American Cyclopedia*, Vaccination (1883).

'Dr Buchanan, the medical officer of the London Government Board, reported as the result of statistics that the smallpox death rate among adult persons vaccinated was 90 to a million; whereas among those unvaccinated it was 3,350 to a million; whereas among vaccinated children under five years of age, 42 ½ per million; whereas among unvaccinated children of the same age it was 5,950 per million.' Hardway, *Essentials of Vaccination* (1882). The same author reports that, among

other conclusions reached by the Academie de Medicine of France, was one that, 'without vaccination, hygienic measures (isolation, disinfection, etc.) are of themselves insufficient for preservation from smallpox.' Ibid.

'The Belgian Academy of Medicine appointed a committee to make an exhaustive examination of the whole subject, and among the conclusions reported by them were: 1. 'Without vaccination, hygienic measures and means, whether public or private, are powerless in preserving mankind from smallpox. . . . 3. Vaccination is always an inoffensive operation when practised with proper care on healthy subjects. . . . 4. It is highly desirable, in the interests of the health and lives of our countrymen, that vaccination should be rendered compulsory.' Edwards, *Vaccination* (1882).

The English Royal Commission, appointed with Lord Herschell, the Lord Chancellor of England, at its head, to inquire, among other things, as to the effect of vaccination in reducing the prevalence of, and mortality from, smallpox, reported, after several years of investigation: 'We think that it diminishes the liability to be attacked by the disease; that it modifies the character of the disease and renders it less fatal,—of a milder and less severe type; that the protection it affords against attacks of the disease is greatest during the years immediately succeeding the operation of vaccination.'

Case Law: *DeShaney v. Winnebago County Social Services Department* (Public Welfare and the "Negative Constitution")

DESHANEY v. WINNEBAGO CTY. SOC. SERVS. DEPT., 489 U.S. 189 (1989)

DESHANEY, A MINOR, BY HIS GUARDIAN AD LITEM, ET AL. v. WINNEBAGO COUNTY DEPARTMENT OF SOCIAL SERVICES ET AL.

CERTIORARI TO THE UNITED STATES COURT OF APPEALS FOR THE SEVENTH CIRCUIT

No. 87-154.

Argued November 2, 1988

Decided February 22, 1989

REHNQUIST, C. J., delivered the opinion of the Court, in which WHITE, STEVENS, O'CONNOR, SCALIA, and KENNEDY, JJ., joined. BRENNAN, J., filed a dissenting opinion, in which MARSHALL and BLACKMUN, JJ., joined, post, p. 203. BLACKMUN, J., filed a dissenting opinion, post, p. 212.

CHIEF JUSTICE REHNQUIST delivered the opinion of the Court.

Petitioner is a boy who was beaten and permanently injured by his father, with whom he lived. Respondents are social workers and other local officials who received complaints that petitioner was being abused by his father and had reason to believe that this was the case, but nonetheless did not act to remove petitioner from his father's custody. Petitioner sued respondents claiming that their failure to act deprived him of his liberty in violation of the Due Process Clause of the Fourteenth Amendment to the United States Constitution. We hold that it did not.

I

The facts of this case are undeniably tragic. Petitioner Joshua DeShaney was born in 1979. In 1980, a Wyoming court granted his parents a divorce and awarded custody of Joshua to his father, Randy DeShaney. The father shortly thereafter moved to Neenah, a city located in Winnebago County, Wisconsin, taking the infant Joshua with him. There he entered into a second marriage, which also ended in divorce.

The Winnebago County authorities first learned that Joshua DeShaney might be a victim of child abuse in January 1982, when his father's second wife complained to the police, at the time of their divorce, that he had previously "hit the boy causing marks and [was] a prime case for child abuse." App. 152–153. The Winnebago County Department of Social Services (DSS) interviewed the father, but he denied the accusations, and DSS did not pursue them further. In January 1983, Joshua was admitted to a local hospital with multiple bruises and abrasions. The examining physician suspected child abuse and notified DSS, which immediately obtained an order from a Wisconsin juvenile court placing Joshua in the temporary custody of the hospital. Three days later, the county convened an ad hoc "child protection team"—consisting of a pediatrician, a psychologist, a police detective, the county's lawyer, several DSS case workers, and various hospital personnel—to consider Joshua's situation. At this meeting, the Team decided that there was insufficient evidence of child abuse to retain Joshua in the custody of the court. The Team did, however, decide to recommend several measures to protect Joshua, including enrolling him in a preschool program, providing his father with certain counseling services, and encouraging his father's girlfriend to move out of the home. Randy DeShaney entered into a voluntary agreement with DSS in which he promised to cooperate with them in accomplishing these goals.

Based on the recommendation of the child protection team, the juvenile court dismissed the child protection case and returned Joshua to the custody of his father. A month later, emergency room personnel called the DSS caseworker handling Joshua's case to report that he had once again been treated for suspicious injuries. The caseworker concluded that there was no basis for action. For the next six months, the caseworker made monthly visits to the DeShaney home, during which she observed a number of suspicious injuries on Joshua's head; she also noticed that he had not been enrolled in school, and that the girlfriend had not moved out. The caseworker dutifully recorded these incidents in her files, along with her continuing suspicions that someone in the DeShaney household was physically abusing Joshua, but she did nothing more. In November 1983, the emergency room notified DSS that Joshua had been treated once again for injuries that they believed to be caused by child abuse. On the caseworker's next two visits to the DeShaney home, she was told that Joshua was too ill to see her. Still DSS took no action.

In March 1984, Randy DeShaney beat 4-year-old Joshua so severely that he fell into a life-threatening coma. Emergency brain surgery revealed a series of hemorrhages caused by traumatic injuries to the head inflicted over a long period of time. Joshua did not die, but he suffered brain damage so severe that he is expected to spend the rest of his life confined to an institution for the profoundly retarded. Randy DeShaney was subsequently tried and convicted of child abuse.

Joshua and his mother brought this action under 42 U.S.C. 1983 in the United States District Court for the Eastern District of Wisconsin against respondents Winnebago County, DSS, and various individual employees of DSS. The complaint alleged that respondents had deprived Joshua of his liberty without due process of law, in violation of his rights under the Fourteenth Amendment, by failing to intervene to protect him against a risk of violence at his father's hands of which they knew or should have known. The district court granted summary judgment for respondents.

The Court of Appeals for the Seventh Circuit affirmed, 812 F.2d 298 (1987), holding that petitioners had not made out an actionable 1983 claim for two alternative reasons. First, the court held that the Due Process Clause of the Fourteenth Amendment does not require a state or local governmental entity to protect its citizens from "private violence, or other mishaps not attributable to the conduct of its employees." *Id.*, at 301. In so holding, the court specifically rejected the posi-

tion endorsed by a divided panel of the Third Circuit in *Estate of Bailey by Oare v. County of York*, 768 F.2d 503, 510–511 (1985), and by dicta in *Jensen v. Conrad*, 747 F.2d 185, 190–194 (CA4 1984), cert. denied, 470 U.S. 1052 (1985), that once the State learns that a particular child is in danger of abuse from third parties and actually undertakes to protect him from that danger, a "special relationship" arises between it and the child which imposes an affirmative constitutional duty to provide adequate protection. 812 F.2d, at 303–304. Second, the court held, in reliance on our decision in *Martinez v. California*, 444 U.S. 277, 285 (1980), that the casual connection between respondents' conduct and Joshua's injuries was too attenuated to establish a deprivation of constitutional rights actionable under 1983. 812 F.2d, at 301–303. The court therefore found it unnecessary to reach the question whether respondents' conduct evinced the "state of mind" necessary to make out a due process claim after *Daniels v. Williams*, 474 U.S. 327 (1986), and *Davidson v. Cannon*, 474 U.S. 344 (1986). 812 F.2d, at 302.

Because of the inconsistent approaches taken by the lower courts in determining when, if ever, the failure of a state or local governmental entity or its agents to provide an individual with adequate protective services constitutes a violation of the individual's due process rights, see *Archie v. Racine*, 847 F.2d 1211, 1220–1223, and n. 10 (CA7 1988) (en banc) (collecting cases), cert. pending, No. 88-576, and the importance of the issue to the administration of state and local governments, we granted certiorari. 485 U.S. 958 (1988). We now affirm.

II

The Due Process Clause of the Fourteenth Amendment provides that "[n]o State shall . . . deprive any person of life, liberty, or property, without due process of law." Petitioners contend that the State[1] deprived Joshua of his liberty interest in "free[dom] from . . . unjustified intrusions on personal security," see *Ingraham v. Wright*, 430 U.S. 651, 673 (1977), by failing to provide him with adequate protection against his father's violence. The claim is one invoking the substantive rather than the procedural component of the Due Process Clause; petitioners do not claim that the State denied Joshua protection without according him appropriate procedural safeguards, see *Morrissey v. Brewer*, 408 U.S. 471, 481 (1972), but that it was categorically obligated to protect him in these circumstances, see *Youngberg v. Romeo*, 457 U.S. 307, 309 (1982).[2]

---

[1] As used here, the term "State" refers generically to state and local governmental entities and their agents.

[2] Petitioners also argue that the Wisconsin child protection statutes gave Joshua an "entitlement" to receive protective services in accordance with the terms of the statute, an entitlement which would enjoy due process protection against state deprivation under our decision in *Board of Regents of State Colleges v.*

But nothing in the language of the Due Process Clause itself requires the State to protect the life, liberty, and property of its citizens against invasion by private actors. The Clause is phrased as a limitation on the State's power to act, not as a guarantee of certain minimal levels of safety and security. It forbids the State itself to deprive individuals of life, liberty, or property without "due process of law," but its language cannot fairly be extended to impose an affirmative obligation on the State to ensure that those interests do not come to harm through other means. Nor does history support such an expansive reading of the constitutional text. Like its counterpart in the Fifth Amendment, the Due Process Clause of the Fourteenth Amendment was intended to prevent government "from abusing [its] power, or employing it as an instrument of oppression," *Davidson v. Cannon, supra,* at 348; see also *Daniels v. Williams, supra,* at 331 ("to secure the individual from the arbitrary exercise of the powers of government," and "to prevent governmental power from being used for purposes of oppression") (internal citations omitted); *Parratt v. Taylor,* 451 U.S. 527, 549 (1981) (Powell, J., concurring in result) (to prevent the "affirmative abuse of power"). Its purpose was to protect the people from the State, not to ensure that the State protected them from each other. The Framers were content to leave the extent of governmental obligation in the latter area to the democratic political processes.

Consistent with these principles, our cases have recognized that the Due Process Clauses generally confer no affirmative right to governmental aid, even where such aid may be necessary to secure life, liberty, or property interests of which the government itself may not deprive the individual. See, e. g., *Harris v. McRae,* 448 U.S. 297, 317–318 (1980) (no obligation to fund abortions or other medical services) (discussing Due Process Clause of Fifth Amendment); *Lindsey v. Normet,* 405 U.S. 56, 74 (1972) (no obligation to provide adequate housing) (discussing Due Process Clause of Fourteenth Amendment); see also *Youngberg v. Romeo, supra,* at 317 ("As a general matter, a State is under no constitutional duty to provide substantive services for those within its border"). As we said in *Harris v. McRae*: "Although the liberty protected by the Due Process Clause affords protection against unwarranted government interference . . ., it does not confer an entitlement to such [governmen-

tal aid] as may be necessary to realize all the advantages of that freedom." 448 U.S., at 317–318 (emphasis added). If the Due Process Clause does not require the State to provide its citizens with particular protective services, it follows that the State cannot be held liable under the Clause for injuries that could have been averted had it chosen to provide them.[3] As a general matter, then, we conclude that a State's failure to protect an individual against private violence simply does not constitute a violation of the Due Process Clause.

Petitioners contend, however, that even if the Due Process Clause imposes no affirmative obligation on the State to provide the general public with adequate protective services, such a duty may arise out of certain "special relationships" created or assumed by the State with respect to particular individuals. Brief for Petitioners 13–18. Petitioners argue that such a "special relationship" existed here because the State knew that Joshua faced a special danger of abuse at his father's hands, and specifically proclaimed, by word and by deed, its intention to protect him against that danger. Id., at 18–20. Having actually undertaken to protect Joshua from this danger—which petitioners concede the state played no part in creating—the state acquired an affirmative "duty," enforceable through the Due Process Clause, to do so in a reasonably competent fashion. Its failure to discharge that duty, so the argument goes, was an abuse of governmental power that so "shocks the conscience," *Rochin v. California,* 342 U.S. 165, 172 (1952), as to constitute a substantive due process violation. Brief for Petitioners 20.[4]

We reject this argument. It is true that in certain limited circumstances the Constitution imposes upon the State affirmative duties of care and protection with respect to particular individuals. In *Estelle v. Gamble,* 429 U.S. 97 (1976), we recognized that the Eighth Amendment's prohibition against cruel and unusual punishment, made applicable to the States through the Fourteenth Amendment's Due Process Clause, *Robinson v. California,* 370 U.S. 660 (1962), requires the State to provide adequate medical care to incarcerated prisoners.

Roth, 408 U.S. 564 (1972). Brief for Petitioners 24–29. But this argument is made for the first time in petitioners' brief to this Court: it was not pleaded in the complaint, argued to the Court of Appeals as a ground for reversing the District Court, or raised in the petition for certiorari. We therefore decline to consider it here. See *Youngberg v. Romeo,* 457 U.S., at 316, n. 19; *Dothard v. Rawlinson,* 433 U.S. 321, 323, n. 1 (1977); *Duignan v. United States,* 274 U.S. 195, 200 (1927); *Old Jordan Mining & Milling Co. v. Societe Anonyme des Mines,* 164 U.S. 261, 264–265 (1896).

---

[3]The State may not, of course, selectively deny its protective services to certain disfavored minorities without violating the Equal Protection Clause. See *Yick Wo v. Hopkins,* 118 U.S. 356 (1886). But no such argument has been made here.

[4]The genesis of this notion appears to lie in a statement in our opinion in *Martinez v. California,* 444 U.S. 277 (1980). In that case, we were asked to decide, inter alia, whether state officials could be held liable under the Due Process Clause of the Fourteenth Amendment for the death of a private citizen at the hands of a parolee. Rather than squarely confronting the question presented here—whether the Due Process Clause imposed upon the State an affirmative duty to protect—we affirmed the dismissal of the claim on the narrower ground that the causal connection between the state officials' decision to release the parolee from prison and the murder was too attenuated to establish a "deprivation" of constitutional rights within the meaning of 1983.

429 U.S., at 103–104.[5] We reasoned that because the prisoner is unable "by reason of the deprivation of his liberty [to] care for himself," it is only "just" that the State be required to care for him. Ibid., quoting *Spicer v. Williamson,* 191 N.C. 487, 490, 132 S. E. 291, 293 (1926).

In *Youngberg v. Romeo,* 457 U.S. 307 (1982), we extended this analysis beyond the Eighth Amendment setting,[6] holding that the substantive component of the Fourteenth Amendment's Due Process Clause requires the State to provide involuntarily committed mental patients with such services as are necessary to ensure their "reasonable safety" from themselves and others. *Id.,* at 314–325; see *id.,* at 315, 324 (dicta indicating that the State is also obligated to provide such individuals with "adequate food, shelter, clothing, and medical care"). As we explained: "If it is cruel and unusual punishment to hold convicted criminals in unsafe conditions, it must be unconstitutional [under the Due Process Clause] to confine the involuntarily committed—who may not be punished at all—in unsafe conditions." *Id.,* at 315–316; see also *Revere v. Massachusetts General Hospital,* 463 U.S. 239, 244 (1983) (hold-

---

Id., at 284–285. But we went on to say:

> [T]he parole board was not aware that appellants' decedent, as distinguished from the public at large, faced any special danger. We need not and do not decide that a parole officer could never be deemed to "deprive" someone of life by action taken in connection with the release of a prisoner on parole. But we do hold that at least under the particular circumstances of this parole decision, appellants' decedent's death is too remote a consequence of the parole officers' action to hold them responsible under the federal civil rights law. *Id.,* at 285 (footnote omitted).

Several of the Courts of Appeals have read this language as implying that once the State learns that a third party poses a special danger to an identified victim, and indicates its willingness to protect the victim against that danger, a "special relationship" arises between State and victim, giving rise to an affirmative duty, enforceable through the Due Process Clause, to render adequate protection. See *Estate of Bailey by Oare v. County of York,* 768 F.2d 503, 510–511 (CA3 1985); *Jensen v. Conrad,* 747 F.2d 185, 190–194, and n. 11 (CA4 1984) (dicta), cert. denied, 470 U.S. 1052 (1985)); *Balistreri v. Pacifica Police Dept.,* 855 F.2d 1421, 1425–1426 (CA9 1988). But see, in addition to the opinion of the Seventh Circuit below, *Estate of Gilmore v. Buckley,* 787 F.2d 714, 720–723 (CA1), cert. denied, 479 U.S. 882 (1986); *Harpole v. Arkansas Dept. of Human Services,* 820 F.2d 923, 926–927 (CA8 1987); *Wideman v. Shallowford Community Hospital Inc.,* 826 F.2d 1030, 1034–1037 (CA11 1987).

[5]To make out an Eighth Amendment claim based on the failure to provide adequate medical care, a prisoner must show that the state defendants exhibited "deliberate indifference" to his "serious" medical needs; the mere negligent or inadvertent failure to provide adequate care is not enough. *Estelle v. Gamble,* 429 U.S., at 105–106. In *Whitley v. Albers,* 475 U.S. 312 (1986), we suggested that a similar state of mind is required to make out a substantive due process claim in the prison setting. *Id.,* at 326–327.

[6]The Eighth Amendment applies "only after the State has complied with the constitutional guarantees traditionally associated with criminal prosecutions. . . . [T]he State does not acquire the power to punish with which the Eighth Amendment is concerned until after it has secured a formal adjudication of guilt in accordance with due process of law." *Ingraham v. Wright,* 430 U.S. 651, 671–672, n. 40 (1977); see also *Revere v. Massachusetts General Hospital,* 463 U.S. 239, 244 (1983); *Bell v. Wolfish,* 441 U.S. 520, 535, n. 16 (1979).

---

ing that the Due Process Clause requires the responsible government or governmental agency to provide medical care to suspects in police custody who have been injured while being apprehended by the police).

But these cases afford petitioners no help. Taken together, they stand only for the proposition that when the State takes a person into its custody and holds him there against his will, the Constitution imposes upon it a corresponding duty to assume some responsibility for his safety and general well-being. See *Youngberg v. Romeo, supra,* at 317 ("When a person is institutionalized—and wholly dependent on the State[,] . . . a duty to provide certain services and care does exist").[7] The rationale for this principle is simple enough: when the State by the affirmative exercise of its power so restrains an individual's liberty that it renders him unable to care for himself, and at the same time fails to provide for his basic human needs—e. g., food, clothing, shelter, medical care, and reasonable safety—it transgresses the substantive limits on state action set by the Eighth Amendment and the Due Process Clause. See *Estelle v. Gamble, supra,* at 103–104; *Youngberg v. Romeo, supra,* at 315–316. The affirmative duty to protect arises not from the State's knowledge of the individual's predicament or from its expressions of intent to help him, but from the limitation which it has imposed on his freedom to act on his own behalf. See *Estelle v. Gamble, supra,* at 103 ("An inmate must rely on prison authorities to treat his medical needs; if the authorities fail to do so, those needs will not be met"). In the substantive due process analysis, it is the State's affirmative act of restraining the individual's freedom to act on his own behalf—through incarceration, institutionalization, or other similar restraint of personal liberty—which is the "deprivation of liberty" triggering the protections of the Due Process Clause, not its failure to act to protect his liberty interests against harms inflicted by other means.[8]

The Estelle-Youngberg analysis simply has no applicability in the present case. Petitioners concede that the harms Joshua suffered occurred not while he was in the State's custody, but while he was in the custody of his natural father, who

---

[7]Even in this situation, we have recognized that the State "has considerable discretion in determining the nature and scope of its responsibilities." *Youngberg v. Romeo,* 457 U.S., at 317.

[8]Of course, the protections of the Due Process Clause, both substantive and procedural, may be triggered when the State, by the affirmative acts of its agents, subjects an involuntarily confined individual to deprivations of liberty which are not among those generally authorized by his confinement. See, e. g., *Whitley v. Albers, supra,* at 326–327 (shooting inmate); *Youngberg v. Romeo, supra,* at 316 (shackling involuntarily committed mental patient); *Hughes v. Rowe,* 449 U.S. 5, 11 (1980) (removing inmate from general prison population and confining him to administrative segregation); *Vitek v. Jones,* 445 U.S. 480, 491–494 (1980) (transferring inmate to mental health facility).

was in no sense a state actor.[9] While the State may have been aware of the dangers that Joshua faced in the free world, it played no part in their creation, nor did it do anything to render him any more vulnerable to them. That the State once took temporary custody of Joshua does not alter the analysis, for when it returned him to his father's custody, it placed him in no worse position than that in which he would have been had it not acted at all; the State does not become the permanent guarantor of an individual's safety by having once offered him shelter. Under these circumstances, the State had no constitutional duty to protect Joshua.

It may well be that, by voluntarily undertaking to protect Joshua against a danger it concededly played no part in creating, the State acquired a duty under state tort law to provide him with adequate protection against that danger. See Restatement (Second) of Torts 323 (1965) (one who undertakes to render services to another may in some circumstances be held liable for doing so in a negligent fashion); see generally W. Keeton, D. Dobbs, R. Keeton, & D. Owen, Prosser and Keeton on the Law of Torts 56 (5th ed. 1984) (discussing "special relationships" which may give rise to affirmative duties to act under the common law of tort). But the claim here is based on the Due Process Clause of the Fourteenth Amendment, which, as we have said many times, does not transform every tort committed by a state actor into a constitutional violation. See *Daniels v. Williams*, 474 U.S., at 335–336; *Parratt v. Taylor*, 451 U.S., at 544; *Martinez v. California*, 444 U.S. 277, 285 (1980); *Baker v. McCollan*, 443 U.S. 137, 146 (1979); *Paul v. Davis*, 424 U.S. 693, 701 (1976). A State may, through its courts and legislatures, impose such affirmative duties of care and protection upon its agents as it wishes. But not "all common-law duties owed by government actors were . . . constitutionalized by the Fourteenth Amendment." *Daniels v. Williams*, supra, at 335. Because, as explained previously here, the State had no constitutional duty to protect Joshua against his father's violence, its failure to do so—though calamitous in hind-

sight—simply does not constitute a violation of the Due Process Clause.[10]

Judges and lawyers, like other humans, are moved by natural sympathy in a case like this to find a way for Joshua and his mother to receive adequate compensation for the grievous harm inflicted upon them. But before yielding to that impulse, it is well to remember once again that the harm was inflicted not by the State of Wisconsin, but by Joshua's father. The most that can be said of the state functionaries in this case is that they stood by and did nothing when suspicious circumstances dictated a more active role for them. In defense of them it must also be said that had they moved too soon to take custody of the son away from the father, they would likely have been met with charges of improperly intruding into the parent–child relationship, charges based on the same Due Process Clause that forms the basis for the present charge of failure to provide adequate protection.

The people of Wisconsin may well prefer a system of liability which would place upon the State and its officials the responsibility for failure to act in situations such as the present one. They may create such a system, if they do not have it already, by changing the tort law of the State in accordance with the regular lawmaking process. But they should not have it thrust upon them by this Court's expansion of the Due Process Clause of the Fourteenth Amendment.

Affirmed.

JUSTICE BRENNAN, with whom JUSTICE MARSHALL and JUSTICE BLACKMUN join, dissenting.

"The most that can be said of the state functionaries in this case," the Court today concludes, "is that they stood by and did nothing when suspicious circumstances dictated a more active role for them." *Ante* this page. Because I believe that this description of respondents' conduct tells only part of the story and that, accordingly, the Constitution itself "dictated a more active role" for respondents in the circumstances presented here, I cannot agree that respondents had no constitutional duty to help Joshua DeShaney.

It may well be, as the Court decides, *ante*, at 194–197, that the Due Process Clause as construed by our prior cases creates

---

[9]Complaint 16, App. 6 ("At relevant times to and until March 8, 1984, [the date of the final beating,] Joshua DeShaney was in the custody and control of Defendant Randy DeShaney"). Had the State by the affirmative exercise of its power removed Joshua from free society and placed him in a foster home operated by its agents, we might have a situation sufficiently analogous to incarceration or institutionalization to give rise to an affirmative duty to protect. Indeed, several Courts of Appeals have held, by analogy to *Estelle* and *Youngberg*, that the State may be held liable under the Due Process Clause for failing to protect children in foster homes from mistreatment at the hands of their foster parents. See *Doe v. New York City Dept. of Social Services*, 649 F.2d 134, 141–142 (CA2 1981), *after remand*, 709 F.2d 782, *cert. denied sub nom. Catholic Home Bureau v. Doe*, 464 U.S. 864 (1983); *Taylor ex rel. Walker v. Ledbetter*, 818 F.2d 791, 794–797 (CA11 1987) (en banc), *cert. pending Ledbetter v. Taylor*, No. 87–521. We express no view on the validity of this analogy, however, as it is not before us in the present case.

[10]Because we conclude that the Due Process Clause did not require the State to protect Joshua from his father, we need not address respondents' alternative argument that the individual state actors lacked the requisite "state of mind" to make out a due process violation. See *Daniels v. Williams*, 474 U.S., at 334, n. 3. Similarly, we have no occasion to consider whether the individual respondents might be entitled to a qualified immunity defense, see *Anderson v. Creighton*, 483 U.S. 635 (1987), or whether the allegations in the complaint are sufficient to support a 1983 claim against the county and DSS under *Monell v. New York City Dept. of Social Services*, 436 U.S. 658 (1978), and its progeny.

no general right to basic governmental services. That, however, is not the question presented here; indeed, that question was not raised in the complaint, urged on appeal, presented in the petition for certiorari, or addressed in the briefs on the merits. No one, in short, has asked the Court to proclaim that, as a general matter, the Constitution safeguards positive as well as negative liberties.

This is more than a quibble over dicta; it is a point about perspective, having substantive ramifications. In a constitutional setting that distinguishes sharply between action and inaction, one's characterization of the misconduct alleged under 1983 may effectively decide the case. Thus, by leading off with a discussion (and rejection) of the idea that the Constitution imposes on the States an affirmative duty to take basic care of their citizens, the Court foreshadows—perhaps even preordains—its conclusion that no duty existed even on the specific facts before us. This initial discussion establishes the baseline from which the Court assesses the DeShaneys' claim that, when a State has—"by word and by deed," *ante*, at 197—announced an intention to protect a certain class of citizens and has before it facts that would trigger that protection under the applicable state law, the Constitution imposes upon the State an affirmative duty of protection.

The Court's baseline is the absence of positive rights in the Constitution and a concomitant suspicion of any claim that seems to depend on such rights. From this perspective, the DeShaneys' claim is first and foremost about inaction (the failure, here, of respondents to take steps to protect Joshua), and only tangentially about action (the establishment of a state program specifically designed to help children like Joshua). And from this perspective, holding these Wisconsin officials liable—where the only difference between this case and one involving a general claim to protective services is Wisconsin's establishment and operation of a program to protect children—would seem to punish an effort that we should seek to promote.

I would begin from the opposite direction. I would focus first on the action that Wisconsin has taken with respect to Joshua and children like him, rather than on the actions that the State failed to take. Such a method is not new to this Court. Both *Estelle v. Gamble*, 429 U.S. 97 (1976), and *Youngberg v. Romeo*, 457 U.S. 307 (1982), began by emphasizing that the States had confined J. W. Gamble to prison and Nicholas Romeo to a psychiatric hospital. This initial action rendered these people helpless to help themselves or to seek help from persons unconnected to the government. See *Estelle, supra*, at 104 ("[I]t is but just that the public be required to care for the prisoner, who cannot by reason of the deprivation of his liberty, care for himself"); *Youngberg, supra*, at 317 ("When a person is institutionalized—and wholly dependent on the

State—it is conceded by petitioners that a duty to provide certain services and care does exist"). Cases from the lower courts also recognize that a State's actions can be decisive in assessing the constitutional significance of subsequent inaction. For these purposes, moreover, actual physical restraint is not the only state action that has been considered relevant. See, e. g., *White v. Rochford*, 592 F.2d 381 (CA7 1979) (police officers violated due process when, after arresting the guardian of three young children, they abandoned the children on a busy stretch of highway at night).

Because of the Court's initial fixation on the general principle that the Constitution does not establish positive rights, it is unable to appreciate our recognition in *Estelle* and *Youngberg* that this principle does not hold true in all circumstances. Thus, in the Court's view, *Youngberg* can be explained (and dismissed) in the following way: "In the substantive due process analysis, it is the State's affirmative act of restraining the individual's freedom to act on his own behalf—through incarceration, institutionalization, or other similar restraint of personal liberty—which is the 'deprivation of liberty' triggering the protections of the Due Process Clause, not its failure to act to protect his liberty interests against harms inflicted by other means." *Ante*, at 200. This restatement of *Youngberg*'s holding should come as a surprise when one recalls our explicit observation in that case that Romeo did not challenge his commitment to the hospital, but instead "argue[d] that he ha[d] a constitutionally protected liberty interest in safety, freedom of movement, and training within the institution; and that petitioners infringed these rights by failing to provide constitutionally required conditions of confinement." 457 U.S., at 315 (emphasis added). I do not mean to suggest that "the State's affirmative act of restraining the individual's freedom to act on his own behalf," *ante*, at 200, was irrelevant in *Youngberg*; rather, I emphasize that this conduct would have led to no injury, and consequently no cause of action under 1983, unless the State then had failed to take steps to protect Romeo from himself and from others. In addition, the Court's exclusive attention to state-imposed restraints of "the individual's freedom to act on his own behalf," *ante*, at 200, suggests that it was the State that rendered Romeo unable to care for himself, whereas in fact—with an I. Q. of between 8 and 10, and the mental capacity of an 18-month-old child, 457 U.S., at 309—he had been quite incapable of taking care of himself long before the State stepped into his life. Thus, the fact of hospitalization was critical in *Youngberg* not because it rendered Romeo helpless to help himself, but because it separated him from other sources of aid that, we held, the State was obligated to replace. Unlike the Court, therefore, I am unable to see in *Youngberg* a neat and decisive divide between action and inaction.

Moreover, to the Court, the only fact that seems to count as an "affirmative act of restraining the individual's freedom to act on his own behalf" is direct physical control. *Ante*, at 200 (listing only "incarceration, institutionalization, [and] other similar restraint of personal liberty" in describing relevant "affirmative acts"). I would not, however, give *Youngberg* and *Estelle* such a stingy scope. I would recognize, as the Court apparently cannot, that "the State's knowledge of [an] individual's predicament [and] its expressions of intent to help him" can amount to a "limitation . . . on his freedom to act on his own behalf" or to obtain help from others. *Ante*, at 200. Thus, I would read *Youngberg* and *Estelle* to stand for the much more generous proposition that, if a State cuts off private sources of aid and then refuses aid itself, it cannot wash its hands of the harm that results from its inaction.

Youngberg and *Estelle* are not alone in sounding this theme. In striking down a filing fee as applied to divorce cases brought by indigents, see *Boddie v. Connecticut*, 401 U.S. 371 (1971), and in deciding that a local government could not entirely foreclose the opportunity to speak in a public forum, see, e. g., *Schneider v. State*, 308 U.S. 147 (1939); *Hague v. Committee for Industrial Organization*, 307 U.S. 496 (1939); *United States v. Grace*, 461 U.S. 171 (1983), we have acknowledged that a State's actions—such as the monopolization of a particular path of relief—may impose upon the State certain positive duties. Similarly, *Shelley v. Kraemer*, 334 U.S. 1 (1948), and *Burton v. Wilmington Parking Authority*, 365 U.S. 715 (1961), suggest that a State may be found complicit in an injury even if it did not create the situation that caused the harm.

Arising as they do from constitutional contexts different from the one involved here, cases like *Boddie* and *Burton* are instructive rather than decisive in the case before us. But they set a tone equally well established in precedent as, and contradictory to, the one the Court sets by situating the DeShaneys' complaint within the class of cases epitomized by the Court's decision in *Harris v. McRae*, 448 U.S. 297 (1980). The cases that I have cited tell us that *Goldberg v. Kelly*, 397 U.S. 254 (1970) (recognizing entitlement to welfare under state law), can stand side by side with *Dandridge v. Williams*, 397 U.S. 471, 484 (1970) (implicitly rejecting idea that welfare is a fundamental right), and that *Goss v. Lopez*, 419 U.S. 565, 573 (1975) (entitlement to public education under state law), is perfectly consistent with *San Antonio Independent School Dist. v. Rodriguez*, 411 U.S. 1, 29–39 (1973) (no fundamental right to education). To put the point more directly, these cases signal that a State's prior actions may be decisive in analyzing the constitutional significance of its inaction. I thus would locate the DeShaneys' claims within the framework of cases like *Youngberg* and *Estelle* and more generally, *Boddie* and

Schneider, by considering the actions that Wisconsin took with respect to Joshua.

Wisconsin has established a child-welfare system specifically designed to help children like Joshua. Wisconsin law places upon the local departments of social services such as respondent (DSS or Department) a duty to investigate reported instances of child abuse. See Wis. Stat. 48.981(3) (1987–1988). While other governmental bodies and private persons are largely responsible for the reporting of possible cases of child abuse, see 48.981(2), Wisconsin law channels all such reports to the local departments of social services for evaluation and, if necessary, further action. 48.981(3). Even when it is the sheriff's office or police department that receives a report of suspected child abuse, that report is referred to local social services departments for action, see 48.981(3)(a); the only exception to this occurs when the reporter fears for the child's immediate safety. 48.981(3)(b). In this way, Wisconsin law invites—indeed, directs—citizens and other governmental entities to depend on local departments of social services such as respondent to protect children from abuse.

The specific facts before us bear out this view of Wisconsin's system of protecting children. Each time someone voiced a suspicion that Joshua was being abused, that information was relayed to the Department for investigation and possible action. When Randy DeShaney's second wife told the police that he had "hit the boy causing marks and [was] a prime case for child abuse," the police referred her complaint to DSS. *Ante*, at 192. When, on three separate occasions, emergency room personnel noticed suspicious injuries on Joshua's body, they went to DSS with this information. *Ante*, at 192–193. When neighbors informed the police that they had seen or heard Joshua's father or his father's lover beating or otherwise abusing Joshua, the police brought these reports to the attention of DSS. App. 144–145. And when respondent Kemmeter, through these reports and through her own observations in the course of nearly 20 visits to the DeShaney home, *id.*, at 104, compiled growing evidence that Joshua was being abused, that information stayed within the Department—chronicled by the social worker in detail that seems almost eerie in light of her failure to act upon it. (As to the extent of the social worker's involvement in, and knowledge of, Joshua's predicament, her reaction to the news of Joshua's last and most devastating injuries is illuminating: "I just knew the phone would ring some day and Joshua would be dead." 812 F.2d 298, 300 (CA7 1987).)

Even more telling than these examples is the Department's control over the decision whether to take steps to protect a particular child from suspected abuse. While many different people contributed information and advice to this decision, it was up to the people at DSS to make the ultimate decision (subject to the approval of the local government's corporation counsel) whether to disturb the family's current arrangements. App. 41, 58. When Joshua first appeared at a local hospital with injuries signaling physical abuse, for example, it was DSS that made the decision to take him into temporary custody for the purpose of studying his situation—and it was DSS, acting in conjunction with the corporation counsel, that returned him to his father. *Ante*, at 192. Unfortunately for Joshua DeShaney, the buck effectively stopped with the Department.

In these circumstances, a private citizen, or even a person working in a government agency other than DSS, would doubtless feel that her job was done as soon as she had reported her suspicions of child abuse to DSS. Through its child-welfare program, in other words, the State of Wisconsin has relieved ordinary citizens and governmental bodies other than the Department of any sense of obligation to do anything more than report their suspicions of child abuse to DSS. If DSS ignores or dismisses these suspicions, no one will step in to fill the gap. Wisconsin's child-protection program thus effectively confined Joshua DeShaney within the walls of Randy DeShaney's violent home until such time as DSS took action to remove him. Conceivably, then, children like Joshua are made worse off by the existence of this program when the persons and entities charged with carrying it out fail to do their jobs.

It simply belies reality, therefore, to contend that the State "stood by and did nothing" with respect to Joshua. *Ante*, at 203. Through its child-protection program, the State actively intervened in Joshua's life and, by virtue of this intervention, acquired ever more certain knowledge that Joshua was in grave danger. These circumstances, in my view, plant this case solidly within the tradition of cases like *Youngberg* and *Estelle*.

It will be meager comfort to Joshua and his mother to know that, if the State had "selectively den[ied] its protective services" to them because they were "disfavored minorities," *ante*, at 197, n. 3, their 1983 suit might have stood on sturdier ground. Because of the posture of this case, we do not know why respondents did not take steps to protect Joshua; the Court, however, tells us that their reason is irrelevant so long as their inaction was not the product of invidious discrimination. Presumably, then, if respondents decided not to help Joshua because his name began with a "J" or because he was born in the spring, or because they did not care enough about him even to formulate an intent to discriminate against him based on an arbitrary reason, respondents would not be liable to the DeShaneys because they were not the ones who dealt the blows that destroyed Joshua's life.

I do not suggest that such irrationality was at work in this case; I emphasize only that we do not know whether or not it was. I would allow Joshua and his mother the opportunity to show that respondents' failure to help him arose, not out of the sound exercise of professional judgment that we recognized in *Youngberg* as sufficient to preclude liability, see 457 U.S., at 322–323, but from the kind of arbitrariness that we have in the past condemned. See, e. g., *Daniels v. Williams*, 474 U.S. 327, 331 (1986) (purpose of Due Process Clause was "to secure the individual from the arbitrary exercise of the powers of government" (citations omitted)); *West Coast Hotel Co. v. Parrish*, 300 U.S. 379, 399 (1937) (to sustain state action, the Court need only decide that it is not "arbitrary or capricious"); *Euclid v. Ambler Realty Co.*, 272 U.S. 365, 389 (1926) (state action invalid where it "passes the bounds of reason and assumes the character of a merely arbitrary fiat," quoting *Purity Extract & Tonic Co. v. Lynch*, 226 U.S. 192, 204 (1912)).

Youngberg's deference to a decisionmaker's professional judgment ensures that once a caseworker has decided, on the basis of her professional training and experience, that one course of protection is preferable for a given child, or even that no special protection is required, she will not be found liable for the harm that follows. (In this way, *Youngberg*'s vision of substantive due process serves a purpose similar to that served by adherence to procedural norms, namely, requiring that a state actor stop and think before she acts in a way that may lead to a loss of liberty.) Moreover, that the Due Process Clause is not violated by merely negligent conduct, see *Daniels*, *supra*, and *Davidson v. Cannon*, 474 U.S. 344 (1986), means that a social worker who simply makes a mistake of judgment under what are admittedly complex and difficult conditions will not find herself liable in damages under 1983.

As the Court today reminds us, "the Due Process Clause of the Fourteenth Amendment was intended to prevent government 'from abusing [its] power, or employing it as an instrument of oppression.'" *Ante*, at 196, quoting *Davidson*, *supra*, U.S., at 348. My disagreement with the Court arises from its failure to see that inaction can be every bit as abusive of power as action, that oppression can result when a State undertakes a vital duty and then ignores it. Today's opinion construes the Due Process Clause to permit a State to displace private sources of protection and then, at the critical moment, to shrug its shoulders and turn away from the harm that it has promised to try to prevent. Because I cannot agree that our Constitution is indifferent to such indifference, I respectfully dissent.

JUSTICE BLACKMUN, dissenting.

Today, the Court purports to be the dispassionate oracle of the law, unmoved by "natural sympathy." *Ante*, at 202. But, in this pretense, the Court itself retreats into a sterile formalism which prevents it from recognizing either the facts of the case before it or the legal norms that should apply to those facts. As JUSTICE BRENNAN demonstrates, the facts here involve not mere passivity, but active state intervention in the life of Joshua DeShaney—intervention that triggered a fundamental duty to aid the boy once the State learned of the severe danger to which he was exposed.

The Court fails to recognize this duty because it attempts to draw a sharp and rigid line between action and inaction. But such formalistic reasoning has no place in the interpretation of the broad and stirring Clauses of the Fourteenth Amendment. Indeed, I submit that these Clauses were designed, at least in part, to undo the formalistic legal reasoning that infected antebellum jurisprudence, which the late Professor Robert Cover analyzed so effectively in his significant work entitled *Justice Accused* (1975).

Like the antebellum judges who denied relief to fugitive slaves, see *id.*, at 119–121, the Court today claims that its decision, however harsh, is compelled by existing legal doctrine. On the contrary, the question presented by this case is an open one, and our Fourteenth Amendment precedents may be read more broadly or narrowly depending upon how one chooses to read them. Faced with the choice, I would adopt a "sympathetic" reading, one which comports with dictates of fundamental justice and recognizes that compassion need not be exiled from the province of judging. Cf. A. Stone, Law, Psychiatry, and Morality 262 (1984) ("We will make mistakes if we go forward, but doing nothing can be the worst mistake. What is required of us is moral ambition. Until our composite sketch becomes a true portrait of humanity we must live with our uncertainty; we will grope, we will struggle, and our compassion may be our only guide and comfort").

Poor Joshua! Victim of repeated attacks by an irresponsible, bullying, cowardly, and intemperate father, and abandoned by respondents who placed him in a dangerous predicament and who knew or learned what was going on, and yet did essentially nothing except, as the Court revealingly observes, *ante*, at 193, "dutifully recorded these incidents in [their] files." It is a sad commentary upon American life, and constitutional principles—so full of late of patriotic fervor and proud proclamations about "liberty and justice for all"—that this child, Joshua DeShaney, now is assigned to live out the remainder of his life profoundly retarded. Joshua and his mother, as petitioners here, deserve—but now are denied by this Court—the opportunity to have the facts of their case considered in the light of the constitutional protection that 42 U.S.C. 1983 is meant to provide.

Case Law: *Town of Castle Rock, Colorado v. Gonzales* (Public Welfare and the "Negative Constitution")

TOWN OF CASTLE ROCK, COLORADO v. GONZALES, *individually and a next best friend of her deceased minor children,* **GONZALES et al.**

CERTIORARI TO THE UNITED STATES COURT OF APPEALS FOR THE TENTH CIRCUIT

No. 04-278. Argued March 21, 2005—Decided June 27, 2005

Scalia, J., delivered the opinion of the Court, in which *Rehnquist*, C. J., and *O'Connor, Kennedy, Souter, Thomas*, and *Breyer*, JJ., joined. *Souter*, J., filed a concurring opinion, in which *Breyer*, J., joined. *Stevens*, J., filed a dissenting opinion, in which *Ginsburg*, J., joined.

On writ of certiorari to the United States Court of appeals for the tenth circuit.

[June 27, 2005]

Justice Scalia delivered the opinion of the Court.

We decide in this case whether an individual who has obtained a state-law restraining order has a constitutionally protected property interest in having the police enforce the restraining order when they have probable cause to believe it has been violated.

I

The horrible facts of this case are contained in the complaint that respondent Jessica Gonzales filed in Federal District Court. (Because the case comes to us on appeal from a dismissal of the complaint, we assume its allegations are true. See *Swierkiewicz v. Sorema N. A.*, 534 U. S. 506, 508, n. 1 (2002).) Respondent alleges that petitioner, the town of Castle Rock, Colorado, violated the Due Process Clause of the Fourteenth Amendment to the United States Constitution when its police officers, act-

ing pursuant to official policy or custom, failed to respond properly to her repeated reports that her estranged husband was violating the terms of a restraining order.[1]

The restraining order had been issued by a state trial court several weeks earlier in conjunction with respondent's divorce proceedings. The original form order, issued on May 21, 1999, and served on respondent's husband on June 4, 1999, commanded him not to "molest or disturb the peace of [respondent] or of any child" and to remain at least 100 yards from the family home at all times. 366 F. 3d 1093, 1143 (CA10 2004) (en banc) (appendix to dissenting opinion of O'Brien, J.). The bottom of the pre-printed form noted that the reverse side contained "Important notices for restrained parties and law enforcement officials." *Ibid.* (emphasis deleted). The preprinted text on the back of the form included the following "Warning":

"A knowing violation of a restraining order is a crime.... A violation will also constitute contempt of court. You may be arrested without notice if a law enforcement officer has probable cause to believe that you have knowingly violated this order." *Id.*, at 1144.

The preprinted text on the back of the form also included a "Notice to Law Enforcement Officials," which read in part:

---

[1]Petitioner claims that respondent's complaint "did not allege ... that she ever notified the police of her contention that [her husband] was actually in violation of the restraining order." Brief for Petitioner 7, n. 2. The complaint does allege, however, that respondent "showed [the police] a copy of the [temporary restraining order (TRO)] and requested that it be enforced." App. to Pet. for Cert. 126a. At this stage in the litigation, we may assume that this reasonably implied the order was being violated. See *Steel Co. v. Citizens for Better Environment*, 523 U. S. 83, 104 (1998).

"You shall use every reasonable means to enforce this restraining order. You shall arrest, or, if an arrest would be impractical under the circumstances, seek a warrant for the arrest of the restrained person when you have information amounting to probable cause that the restrained person has violated or attempted to violate any provision of this order and the restrained person has been properly served with a copy of this order or has received actual notice of the existence of this order." *Ibid.*

On June 4, 1999, the state trial court modified the terms of the restraining order and made it permanent. The modified order gave respondent's husband the right to spend time with his three daughters (ages 10, 9, and 7) on alternate weekends, for two weeks during the summer, and, "'upon reasonable notice,'" for a mid-week dinner visit "'arranged by the parties'"; the modified order also allowed him to visit the home to collect the children for such "parenting time." *Id.*, at 1097 (majority opinion).

According to the complaint, at about 5 or 5:30 p.m. on Tuesday, June 22, 1999, respondent's husband took the three daughters while they were playing outside the family home. No advance arrangements had been made for him to see the daughters that evening. When respondent noticed the children were missing, she suspected her husband had taken them. At about 7:30 p.m., she called the Castle Rock Police Department, which dispatched two officers. The complaint continues: "When [the officers] arrived. . . , she showed them a copy of the TRO and requested that it be enforced and the three children be returned to her immediately. [The officers] stated that there was nothing they could do about the TRO and suggested that [respondent] call the police department again if the three children did not return home by 10:00 p.m." App. to Pet. for Cert. 126a.[2]

At approximately 8:30 p.m., respondent talked to her husband on his cellular telephone. He told her "he had the three children [at an] amusement park in Denver." *Ibid.* She called the police again and asked them to "have someone check for" her husband or his vehicle at the amusement park and "put out an [all points bulletin]" for her husband, but the officer with whom she spoke "refused to do so," again telling her to "wait until 10:00 p.m. and see if" her husband returned the girls. *Id.*, at 126a–127a.

At approximately 10:10 p.m., respondent called the police and said her children were still missing, but she was now told to wait until midnight. She called at midnight and told

the dispatcher her children were still missing. She went to her husband's apartment and, finding nobody there, called the police at 12:10 a.m.; she was told to wait for an officer to arrive. When none came, she went to the police station at 12:50 a.m. and submitted an incident report. The officer who took the report "made no reasonable effort to enforce the TRO or locate the three children. Instead, he went to dinner." *Id.*, at 127a.

At approximately 3:20 a.m., respondent's husband arrived at the police station and opened fire with a semiautomatic handgun he had purchased earlier that evening. Police shot back, killing him. Inside the cab of his pickup truck, they found the bodies of all three daughters, whom he had already murdered. *Ibid.*

On the basis of the foregoing factual allegations, respondent brought an action under Rev. Stat. §1979, 42 U. S. C. §1983, claiming that the town violated the Due Process Clause because its police department had "an official policy or custom of failing to respond properly to complaints of restraining order violations" and "tolerate[d] the non-enforcement of restraining orders by its police officers." App. to Pet. for Cert. 129a.[3] The complaint also alleged that the town's actions "were taken either willfully, recklessly or with such gross negligence as to indicate wanton disregard and deliberate indifference to" respondent's civil rights. *Ibid.*

Before answering the complaint, the defendants filed a motion to dismiss under Federal Rule of Civil Procedure 12(b)(6). The District Court granted the motion, concluding that, whether construed as making a substantive due process or procedural due process claim, respondent's complaint failed to state a claim upon which relief could be granted.

A panel of the Court of Appeals affirmed the rejection of a substantive due process claim, but found that respondent had alleged a cognizable procedural due process claim. 307 F. 3d 1258 (CA10 2002). On rehearing en banc, a divided court reached the same disposition, concluding that respondent had a "protected property interest in the enforcement of the terms of her restraining order" and that the town had deprived her of due process because "the police never 'heard' nor seriously entertained her request to enforce and protect her interests in the restraining order." 366 F. 3d, at 1101, 1117. We granted certiorari. 543 U. S. ___ (2004).

II

The Fourteenth Amendment to the United States Constitution provides that a State shall not "deprive any person of life, lib-

---

[2]It is unclear from the complaint, but immaterial to our decision, whether respondent showed the police only the original "TRO" or also the permanent, modified restraining order that had superseded it on June 4.

[3]Three police officers were also named as defendants in the complaint, but the Court of Appeals concluded that they were entitled to qualified immunity, 366 F. 3d 1093, 1118 (CA10 2004) (en banc). Respondent did not file a cross-petition challenging that aspect of the judgment.

erty, or property, without due process of law." Amdt. 14, §1. In 42 U. S. C. §1983, Congress has created a federal cause of action for "the deprivation of any rights, privileges, or immunities secured by the Constitution and laws." Respondent claims the benefit of this provision on the ground that she had a property interest in police enforcement of the restraining order against her husband; and that the town deprived her of this property without due process by having a policy that tolerated nonenforcement of restraining orders.

As the Court of Appeals recognized, we left a similar question unanswered in *DeShaney v. Winnebago County Dept. of Social Servs.*, 489 U. S. 189 (1989), another case with "undeniably tragic" facts: Local child protection officials had failed to protect a young boy from beatings by his father that left him severely brain damaged. *Id.*, at 191–193. We held that the so-called substantive component of the Due Process Clause does not "requir[e] the State to protect the life, liberty, and property of its citizens against invasion by private actors." *Id.*, at 195. We noted, however, that the petitioner had not properly preserved the argument that—and we thus "decline[d] to consider" whether—state "child protection statutes gave [him] an 'entitlement' to receive protective services in accordance with the terms of the statute, an entitlement which would enjoy due process protection." *Id.*, at 195, n. 2.

The procedural component of the Due Process Clause does not protect everything that might be described as a "benefit": "To have a property interest in a benefit, a person clearly must have more than an abstract need or desire" and "more than a unilateral expectation of it. He must, instead, have a legitimate claim of entitlement to it." *Board of Regents of State Colleges v. Roth*, 408 U. S. 564, 577 (1972). Such entitlements are " 'of course . . . , not created by the Constitution. Rather, they are created and their dimensions are defined by existing rules or understandings that stem from an independent source such as state law.' " *Paul v. Davis*, 424 U. S. 693, 709 (1976) (quoting *Roth*, *supra*, at 577); see also *Phillips v. Washington Legal Foundation*, 524 U. S. 156, 164 (1998).

A

Our cases recognize that a benefit is not a protected entitlement if government officials may grant or deny it in their discretion. See, *e.g.*, *Kentucky Dept. of Corrections v. Thompson*, 490 U. S. 454, 462–463 (1989). The Court of Appeals in this case determined that Colorado law created an entitlement to enforcement of the restraining order because the "court-issued restraining order . . . specifically dictated that its terms must be enforced" and a "state statute command[ed]" enforcement of the order when certain objective conditions were met (probable cause to believe that the order had been violated and that

the object of the order had received notice of its existence). 366 F. 3d, at 1101, n. 5; see also *id.*, at 1100, n. 4; *id.*, at 1104–1105, and n. 9. Respondent contends that we are obliged "to give deference to the Tenth Circuit's analysis of Colorado law on" whether she had an entitlement to enforcement of the restraining order. Tr. of Oral Arg. 52.

We will not, of course, defer to the Tenth Circuit on the ultimate issue: whether what Colorado law has given respondent constitutes a property interest for purposes of the Fourteenth Amendment. That determination, despite its state-law underpinnings, is ultimately one of federal constitutional law. "Although the underlying substantive interest is created by 'an independent source such as state law,' *federal constitutional law* determines whether that interest rises to the level of a 'legitimate claim of entitlement' protected by the Due Process Clause." *Memphis Light, Gas & Water Div. v. Craft*, 436 U. S. 1, 9 (1978) (emphasis added) (quoting *Roth*, *supra*, at 577); cf. *United States ex rel. TVA v. Powelson*, 319 U. S. 266, 279 (1943). Resolution of the federal issue begins, however, with a determination of what it is that state law provides. In the context of the present case, the central state-law question is whether Colorado law gave respondent a right to police enforcement of the restraining order. It is on this point that respondent's call for deference to the Tenth Circuit is relevant.

We have said that a "presumption of deference [is] given the views of a federal court as to the law of a State within its jurisdiction." *Phillips*, *supra*, at 167. That presumption can be overcome, however, see *Leavitt v. Jane L.*, 518 U. S. 137, 145 (1996) (*per curiam*), and we think deference inappropriate here. The Tenth Circuit's opinion, which reversed the Colorado District Judge, did not draw upon a deep well of state-specific expertise, but consisted primarily of quoting language from the restraining order, the statutory text, and a state-legislative-hearing transcript. See 366 F. 3d, at 1103–1109. These texts, moreover, say nothing distinctive to Colorado, but use mandatory language that (as we shall discuss) appears in many state and federal statutes. As for case law: the only state-law cases about restraining orders that the Court of Appeals relied upon were decisions of Federal District Courts in Ohio and Pennsylvania and state courts in New Jersey, Oregon, and Tennessee. *Id.*, at 1104–1105, n. 9, 1109.[4] Moreover, if we were simply to

---

[4]Most of the Colorado-law cases cited by the Court of Appeals appeared in footnotes declaring them to be irrelevant because they involved only substantive due process (366 F. 3d, at 1100–1101, nn. 4–5), only statutes without restraining orders (*id.*, at 1101, n. 5), or Colorado's Government Immunity Act, which the Court of Appeals concluded applies "only to . . . state tort law claims" (*id.*, at 1108–1109, n. 12). Our analysis is likewise unaffected by the Immunity Act or by the way that Colorado has dealt with substantive due process or cases that do not involve restraining orders.

accept the Court of Appeals' conclusion, we would necessarily have to decide conclusively a federal constitutional question (i.e., whether such an entitlement constituted property under the Due Process Clause and, if so, whether petitioner's customs or policies provided too little process to protect it). We proceed, then, to our own analysis of whether Colorado law gave respondent a right to enforcement of the restraining order.[5]

B

The critical language in the restraining order came not from any part of the order itself (which was signed by the state-court trial judge and directed to the restrained party, respondent's husband), but from the preprinted notice to law-enforcement personnel that appeared on the back of the order. See *supra,* at 2–3. That notice effectively restated the statutory provision describing "peace officers' duties" related to the crime of violation of a restraining order. At the time of the conduct at issue in this case, that provision read as follows:

"(a) Whenever a restraining order is issued, the protected person shall be provided with a copy of such order. *A peace officer shall use every reasonable means to enforce a restraining order.*

"(b) *A peace officer shall arrest, or, if an arrest would be impractical under the circumstances, seek a warrant for the arrest of a restrained person* when the peace officer has information amounting to probable cause that:

"(I) The restrained person has violated or attempted to violate any provision of a restraining order; and

"(II) The restrained person has been properly served with a copy of the restraining order or the restrained person has received actual notice of the existence and substance of such order.

"(c) In making the probable cause determination described in paragraph (b) of this subsection (3), a peace officer shall assume that the information received from the registry is accurate. *A peace officer shall enforce a valid restraining order whether or not there is a record of the restraining order in the registry.*" Colo. Rev. Stat. §18-6-803.5(3) (Lexis 1999) (emphases added)."

The Court of Appeals concluded that this statutory provision—especially taken in conjunction with a statement

from its legislative history,[6] and with another statute restricting criminal and civil liability for officers making arrests[7]—established the Colorado Legislature's clear intent "to alter the fact that the police were not enforcing domestic abuse restraining orders" and thus its intent "that the recipient of a domestic abuse restraining order have an entitlement to its enforcement." 366 F. 3d, at 1108. Any other result, it said, "would render domestic abuse restraining orders utterly valueless." *Id.,* at 1109.

This last statement is sheer hyperbole. Whether or not respondent had a right to enforce the restraining order, it rendered certain otherwise lawful conduct by her husband both criminal and in contempt of court. See §§18-6-803.5(2)(a), (7). The creation of grounds on which he could be arrested, criminally prosecuted, and held in contempt was hardly "valueless"—even if the prospect of those sanctions ultimately failed to prevent him from committing three murders and a suicide.

We do not believe that these provisions of Colorado law truly made enforcement of restraining orders *mandatory.* A well established tradition of police discretion has long coexisted with apparently mandatory arrest statutes.

"In each and every state there are long-standing statutes that, by their terms, seem to preclude nonenforcement by the police. . . . However, for a number of reasons, including their legislative history, insufficient resources, and sheer physical impossibility, it has been recognized that such statutes cannot be interpreted literally. . . . [T]hey clearly do not mean that a police officer may not lawfully decline to make an arrest. As to third parties in these states, the full-enforcement statutes simply have no effect, and their significance is further diminished." 1 ABA Standards for Criminal Justice 1–4.5, commentary, pp. 1–124 to 1–125 (2d ed. 1980) (footnotes omitted).

The deep-rooted nature of law-enforcement discretion, even in the presence of seemingly mandatory legislative commands, is illustrated by *Chicago v. Morales,* 527 U. S. 41 (1999),

---

[5]In something of an anyone-but-us approach, the dissent simultaneously (and thus unpersuasively) contends not only that this Court should certify a question to the Colorado Supreme Court, *post,* at 5–7 (opinion of *Stevens,* J.), but also that it should defer to the Tenth Circuit (which itself did not certify any such question), *post,* at 3–4. No party in this case has requested certification, even as an alternative disposition. See Tr. of Oral Arg. 56 (petitioner's counsel "disfavor[ing]" certification); *id.,* at 25–26 (counsel for the United States arguing against certification). At oral argument, in fact, respondent's counsel declined *Justice Stevens'* invitation to request it. *Id.,* at 53.

[6]The Court of Appeals quoted one lawmaker's description of how the bill " 'would really attack the domestic violence problems' ":

" '[T]he entire criminal justice system must act in a consistent manner, which does not now occur. The police must make probable cause arrests. The prosecutors must prosecute every case. Judges must apply appropriate sentences, and probation officers must monitor their probationers closely. And the offender needs to be sentenced to offender-specific therapy. [T]he entire system must send the same message . . . [that] violence is criminal. And so we hope that House Bill 1253 starts us down this road.' " 366 F. 3d, at 1107 (quoting Tr. of Colorado House Judiciary Hearings on House Bill 1253, Feb. 15, 1994) (emphases omitted).

[7]Under Colo. Rev. Stat. §18-6-803.5(5) (Lexis 1999), "[a] peace officer arresting a person for violating a restraining order or otherwise enforcing a restraining order" was not to be held civilly or criminally liable unless he acted "in bad faith and with malice" or violated "rules adopted by the Colorado supreme court."

which involved an ordinance that said a police officer "'shall order'" persons to disperse in certain circumstances, *id.*, at 47, n. 2. This Court rejected out of hand the possibility that "the mandatory language of the ordinance . . . afford[ed] the police *no* discretion." *Id.*, at 62, n. 32. It is, the Court proclaimed, simply "common sense that *all* police officers must use some discretion in deciding when and where to enforce city ordinances." *Ibid.* (emphasis added).

Against that backdrop, a true mandate of police action would require some stronger indication from the Colorado Legislature than "shall use every reasonable means to enforce a restraining order" (or even "shall arrest . . . or . . . seek a warrant"), §§18-6-803.5(3)(a), (b). That language is not perceptibly more mandatory than the Colorado statute which has long told municipal chiefs of police that they "shall pursue and arrest any person fleeing from justice in any part of the state" and that they "shall apprehend any person in the act of committing any offense . . . and, forthwith and without any warrant, bring such person before a . . . competent authority for examination and trial." Colo. Rev. Stat. §31-4-112 (Lexis 2004). It is hard to imagine that a Colorado peace officer would not have some discretion to determine that—despite probable cause to believe a restraining order has been violated—the circumstances of the violation or the competing duties of that officer or his agency counsel decisively against enforcement in a particular instance.[8] The practical necessity for discretion is particularly apparent in a case such as this one, where the suspected violator is not actually present and his whereabouts are unknown. Cf. *Donaldson v. Seattle*, 65 Wash. App. 661, 671–672, 831 P. 2d 1098, 1104 (1992) ("There is a vast difference between a mandatory duty to arrest [a violator who is on the scene] and a mandatory duty to conduct a follow up investigation [to locate an absent violator]. . . . A mandatory duty to investigate would be completely open-ended as to priority, duration and intensity").

The dissent correctly points out that, in the specific context of domestic violence, mandatory-arrest statutes have been found in some States to be more mandatory than traditional mandatory-arrest statutes. *Post*, at 7–13 (opinion of *Stevens*, J.). The Colorado statute mandating arrest for a domestic-violence offense is different from but related to the one at issue here, and it includes similar though not identical phrasing. See

Colo. Rev. Stat. §18-6-803.6(1) (Lexis 1999) ("When a peace officer determines that there is probable cause to believe that a crime or offense involving domestic violence . . . has been committed, the officer shall, without undue delay, arrest the person suspected of its commission. . ."). Even in the domestic-violence context, however, it is unclear how the mandatory-arrest paradigm applies to cases in which the offender is not present to be arrested. As the dissent explains, *post*, at 9–10, and n. 8, much of the impetus for mandatory-arrest statutes and policies derived from the idea that it is better for police officers to arrest the aggressor in a domestic-violence incident than to attempt to mediate the dispute or merely to ask the offender to leave the scene. Those other options are only available, of course, when the offender is present at the scene. See Hanna, No Right to Choose: Mandated Victim Participation in Domestic Violence Prosecutions, 109 Harv. L. Rev. 1849, 1860 (1996) ("[T]he clear trend in police practice is to arrest the batterer *at the scene* . . . " (emphasis added)).

As one of the cases cited by the dissent, *post*, at 12, recognized, "there will be situations when no arrest is possible, *such as when the alleged abuser is not in the home.*" *Donaldson*, 65 Wash. App., at 674, 831 P. 2d, at 1105 (emphasis added). That case held that Washington's mandatory arrest statute required an arrest only in "cases where the offender is on the scene" and that it "d[id] not create an on-going mandatory duty to conduct an investigation" to locate the offender. *Id.*, at 675, 831 P. 2d, at 1105. Colorado's restraining-order statute appears to contemplate a similar distinction, providing that when arrest is "impractical," which was likely the case when the whereabouts of respondent's husband were unknown—the officers' statutory duty is to "seek a warrant" rather than "arrest." §18-6-803.5(3)(b).

Respondent does not specify the precise means of enforcement that the Colorado restraining-order statute assertedly mandated—whether her interest lay in having police arrest her husband, having them seek a warrant for his arrest, or having them "use every reasonable means, up to and including arrest, to enforce the order's terms," Brief for Respondent 29–30.[9] Such indeterminacy is not the hallmark of a duty that is mandatory. Nor can someone be safely deemed "entitled" to something when the identity of the alleged entitlement is vague. See *Roth*, 408 U. S., at 577 (considering whether "certain

---

[8]Respondent in fact concedes that an officer may "properly" decide not to enforce a restraining order when the officer deems "a technical violation" too "immaterial" to justify arrest. Respondent explains this as a determination that there is no probable cause. Brief for Respondent 28. We think, however, that a determination of no probable cause to believe a violation has occurred is quite different from a determination that the violation is too insignificant to pursue.

[9]Respondent characterizes her entitlement in various ways. See Brief for Respondent 12 ("'entitlement' to receive protective services"); *id.*, at 13 ("interest in police enforcement action"); *id.*, at 14 ("specific government benefit" consisting of "the government service of enforcing the objective terms of the court order protecting her and her children against her abusive husband"); *id.*, at 32 ("[T]he restraining order here mandated the arrest of Mr. Gonzales under specified circumstances, or at a minimum required the use of reasonable means to enforce the order").

benefits" were "secure[d]" by rule or understandings); cf. *Natale v. Ridgefield*, 170 F. 3d 258, 263 (CA2 1999) ("There is no reason . . . to restrict the 'uncertainty' that will preclude existence of a federally protectable property interest to the uncertainty that inheres in the exercise of discretion"). The dissent, after suggesting various formulations of the entitlement in question,[10] ultimately contends that the obligations under the statute were quite precise: either make an arrest or (if that is impractical) seek an arrest warrant, *post*, at 14. The problem with this is that the seeking of an arrest warrant would be an entitlement to nothing but procedure—which we have held inadequate even to support standing, see *Lujan v. Defenders of Wildlife*, 504 U. S. 555 (1992); much less can it be the basis for a property interest. See *post*, at 3–4 (*Souter*, J., concurring). After the warrant is sought, it remains within the discretion of a judge whether to grant it, and after it is granted, it remains within the discretion of the police whether and when to execute it.[11] Respondent would have been assured nothing but the seeking of a warrant. This is not the sort of "entitlement" out of which a property interest is created.

Even if the statute could be said to have made enforcement of restraining orders "mandatory" because of the domestic-violence context of the underlying statute, that would not necessarily mean that state law gave *respondent* an entitlement to *enforcement* of the mandate. Making the actions of government employees obligatory can serve various legitimate ends other than the conferral of a benefit on a specific class of people. See, *e.g., Sandin v. Conner*, 515 U. S. 472, 482 (1995) (finding no constitutionally protected liberty interest in prison regulations phrased in mandatory terms, in part because "[s]uch guidelines are not set forth solely to benefit the prisoner"). The serving of public rather than private ends is the normal course of the criminal law because criminal acts, "besides the injury [they do] to individuals, ... strike at the very being of society; which cannot possibly subsist, where actions of this sort are suffered to escape with impunity." 4 W. Blackstone, Commentaries on the Laws of England 5 (1769); see also *Huntington v. Attrill*, 146 U. S. 657, 668 (1892). This

principle underlies, for example, a Colorado district attorney's discretion to prosecute a domestic assault, even though the victim withdraws her charge. See *People v. Cunefare*, 102 P. 3d 302, 311–312 (Colo. 2004) (Bender, J., concurring in part, dissenting in part, and dissenting in part to the judgment).

Respondent's alleged interest stems only from a State's *statutory* scheme—from a restraining order that was authorized by and tracked precisely the statute on which the Court of Appeals relied. She does not assert that she has any common-law or contractual entitlement to enforcement. If she was given a statutory entitlement, we would expect to see some indication of that in the statute itself. Although Colorado's statute spoke of "protected person[s]" such as respondent, it did so in connection with matters other than a right to enforcement. It said that a "protected person shall be provided with a copy of [a restraining] order" when it is issued, §18-6-803.5(3)(a); that a law enforcement agency "shall make all reasonable efforts to contact the protected party upon the arrest of the restrained person," §18-6-803.5(3)(d); and that the agency "shall give [to the protected person] a copy" of the report it submits to the court that issued the order, §18-6-803.5(3)(e). Perhaps most importantly, the statute spoke directly to the protected person's power to "initiate contempt proceedings against the restrained person if the order [was] issued in a civil action or request the prosecuting attorney to initiate contempt proceedings if the order [was] issued in a criminal action." §18-6-803.5(7). The protected person's express power to "initiate" civil contempt proceedings contrasts tellingly with the mere ability to "request" initiation of criminal contempt proceedings—and even more dramatically with the complete silence about any power to "request" (much less demand) that an arrest be made.

The creation of a personal entitlement to something as vague and novel as enforcement of restraining orders cannot "simply g[o] without saying." *Post*, at 17, n. 16 (*Stevens*, J., dissenting). We conclude that Colorado has not created such an entitlement.

C

Even if we were to think otherwise concerning the creation of an entitlement by Colorado, it is by no means clear that an individual entitlement to enforcement of a restraining order could constitute a "property" interest for purposes of the Due Process Clause. Such a right would not, of course, resemble any traditional conception of property. Although that alone does not disqualify it from due process protection, as *Roth* and its progeny show, the right to have a restraining order enforced does not "have some ascertainable monetary value," as even our "*Roth*-type property-as-entitlement" cases have implicitly

---

[10]See *post*, at 1 ("entitlement to police protection"); *post*, at 2 ("entitlement to mandatory individual protection by the local police force"); *ibid.* ("a right to police assistance"); *post*, at 8 ("a citizen's interest in the government's commitment to provide police enforcement in certain defined circumstances"); *post*, at 18 ("respondent's property interest in the enforcement of her restraining order"); *post*, at 20 (the "service" of "protection from her husband"); *post*, at 21–22 ("interest in the enforcement of the restraining order").

[11]The dissent asserts that the police would lack discretion in the execution of this warrant, *post*, at 13–14, n. 12, but cites no statute mandating immediate execution. The general Colorado statute governing arrest provides that police "may arrest" when they possess a warrant "commanding" arrest. Colo. Rev. Stat. §16-3-102(1) (Lexis 1999).

required. Merrill, The Landscape of Constitutional Property, 86 Va. L. Rev. 885, 964 (2000).[12] Perhaps most radically, the alleged property interest here arises *incidentally*, not out of some new species of government benefit or service, but out of a function that government actors have always performed—to wit, arresting people who they have probable cause to believe have committed a criminal offense.[13]

The indirect nature of a benefit was fatal to the due process claim of the nursing-home residents in *O'Bannon v. Town Court Nursing Center*, 447 U. S. 773 (1980). We held that, while the withdrawal of "direct benefits" (financial payments under Medicaid for certain medical services) triggered due process protections, *id.*, at 786–787, the same was not true for the "indirect benefit[s]" conferred on Medicaid patients when the Government enforced "minimum standards of care" for nursing-home facilities, *id.*, at 787. "[A]n indirect and incidental result of the Government's enforcement action . . . does not amount to a deprivation of any interest in life, liberty, or property." *Ibid.* In this case, as in *O'Bannon*, "[t]he simple distinction between government action that directly affects a citizen's legal rights . . . and action that is directed against a third party and affects the citizen only indirectly or incidentally, provides a sufficient answer to" respondent's reliance on cases that found government-provided services to be entitlements. *Id.*, at 788. The *O'Bannon* Court expressly noted, *ibid.*, that the distinction between direct and indirect benefits distinguished *Memphis Light, Gas & Water Div. v. Craft*, 436 U. S. 1 (1978), one of the government-services cases on which the dissent relies, *post*, at 19.

III

We conclude, therefore, that respondent did not, for purposes of the Due Process Clause, have a property interest in police enforcement of the restraining order against her husband. It is accordingly unnecessary to address the Court of Appeals' determination (366 F. 3d, at 1110–1117) that the town's custom or policy prevented the police from giving her due process when they deprived her of that alleged interest. See *American Mfrs. Mut. Ins. Co. v. Sullivan*, 526 U. S. 40, 61 (1999).[14]

In light of today's decision and that in *DeShaney*, the benefit that a third party may receive from having someone else arrested for a crime generally does not trigger protections under the Due Process Clause, neither in its procedural nor in its "substantive" manifestations. This result reflects our continuing reluctance to treat the Fourteenth Amendment as "'a font of tort law,'" *Parratt v. Taylor*, 451 U. S. 527, 544 (1981) (quoting *Paul v. Davis*, 424 U. S., at 701), but it does not mean States are powerless to provide victims with personally enforceable remedies. Although the framers of the Fourteenth Amendment and the Civil Rights Act of 1871, 17 Stat. 13 (the original source of §1983), did not create a system by which police departments are generally held financially accountable for crimes that better policing might have prevented, the people of Colorado are free to craft such a system under state law. Cf. *DeShaney*, 489 U. S., at 203.[15]

The judgment of the Court of Appeals is Reversed.

---

[12] The dissent suggests that the interest in having a restraining order enforced does have an ascertainable monetary value because one may "contract with a private security firm . . . to provide protection" for one's family. *Post*, at 2, 20, and n. 18. That is, of course, not as precise as the analogy between public and private schooling that the dissent invokes. *Post*, at 20, n. 18. Respondent probably could have hired a private firm to guard her house, to prevent her husband from coming onto the property, and perhaps even to search for her husband after she discovered that her children were missing. Her alleged entitlement here, however, does not consist in an abstract right to "protection," but (according to the dissent) in enforcement of her restraining order through the arrest of her husband, or the seeking of a warrant for his arrest, after she gave the police probable cause to believe the restraining order had been violated. A private person would not have the power to arrest under those circumstances because the crime would not have occurred in his presence. Colo. Rev. Stat. §16-3-201 (Lexis 1999). And, needless to say, a private person would not have the power to obtain an arrest warrant.

[13] In other contexts, we have explained that "a private citizen lacks a judicially cognizable interest in the prosecution or nonprosecution of another." *Linda R. S. v. Richard D.*, 410 U. S. 614, 619 (1973).

[14] Because we simply do not address whether the process would have been adequate if respondent had had a property interest, the dissent is correct to note that we do not "contest" the point, *post*, at 2. Of course, we do not *accept* it either.

[15] In Colorado, the general statutory immunity for government employees does not apply when "the act or omission causing . . . injury was willful and wanton." Colo. Rev. Stat. §24-10-118(2)(a) (Lexis 1999). Respondent's complaint does allege that the police officers' actions "were taken either willfully, recklessly or with such gross negligence as to indicate wanton disregard and deliberate indifference to" her civil rights. App. to Pet. for Cert. 128a. The state cases cited by the dissent that afford a cause of action for police failure to enforce restraining orders, *post*, at 11–12, 14–15, n. 13, vindicate state common-law or statutory tort claims—not procedural due process claims under the Federal Constitution. See *Donaldson v. Seattle*, 65 Wash. App. 661, 881 P. 2d 1098 (1992) (city could be liable under some circumstances for *per se* negligence in failing to meet statutory duty to arrest); *Matthews v. Pickett County*, 996 S. W. 2d 162 (Tenn. 1999) (county could be liable under Tennessee's Governmental Tort Liability Act where restraining order created a special duty); *Campbell v. Campbell*, 294 N. J. Super. 18, 682 A. 2d 272 (1996) (rejecting four specific defenses under the New Jersey Tort Claims Act in negligence action against individual officers); *Sorichetti v. New York*, 65 N. Y. 2d 461, 482 N. E. 2d 70 (1985) (city breached duty of care arising from special relationship between police and victim); *Nearing v. Weaver*, 295 Ore. 702, 670 P. 2d 137 (1983) (statutory duty to individual plaintiffs arising independently of tort-law duty of care).

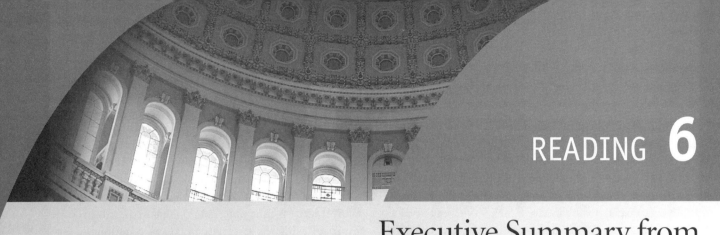

Executive Summary from *The Future of the Public's Health in the 21st Century*

The Future of the Public's Health in the 21st Century

Committee on Assuring the Health of the Public in the 21st Century

Board on Health Promotion and Disease Prevention

Institute of Medicine of the National Academies, 2002

The beginning of the twenty-first century provided an early preview of the health challenges that the United States will face in the coming decades. The systems and entities that protect and promote the public's health, already challenged by problems like obesity, toxic environments, a large uninsured population, and health disparities, must also confront emerging threats, such as antimicrobial resistance and bioterrorism. The social, cultural, and global contexts of the nation's health are also undergoing rapid and dramatic change. Scientific and technological advances, such as genomics and informatics, extend the limits of knowledge and human potential more rapidly than their implications can be absorbed and acted upon. At the same time, people, products, and germs migrate and the nation's demographics are shifting in ways that challenge public and private resources. Against this background, the Committee on Assuring the Health of the Public in the 21st Century was charged with describing a framework for assuring the public's health in the new century.

The report reviews national health achievements in recent decades, but also examines the hidden vulnerabilities that undercut current health potential, and that, if not addressed, could produce a decline in the future health status of the American people. The concept of health as a public good is discussed, as is the fundamental duty of government to promote and protect the health of the public. The report describes the rationale for multisectoral engagement in partnership with government and the roles that different actors can play to support a healthy future for the American people. Finally, it describes major trends that are likely to influence the nation's health in the coming decades.

The committee's work began with a vision—*healthy people in healthy communities.* This is not a new idea, but it is the guiding vision of *Healthy People 2010,* the health agenda for the nation. The committee embraced that vision and began discussing who should be responsible for assuring America's health at the beginning of the twenty-first century—a duty historically assigned to governmental public health agencies, through the work of national, state, tribal, and local departments of health. Current realities indicate that this is no longer sufficient. On the one hand, government has a unique responsibility to promote and protect the health of the people built on a constitutional, theoretical, and practical foundation. However, governmental public health agencies alone cannot assure the nation's health. First, public resources are finite, and the public's health is just one of many priorities. Second, democratic societies define and limit the types of actions that can be undertaken only by government and reserve other social choices for private institutions. Third, the determinants that interact to create good or ill health derive from various sources and sectors. Among other factors, health is shaped by laws and policies, employment and income, and social norms and influences (McGinnis et al., 2002). Fourth, there is a growing recognition that individuals, communities, and various social institutions can form powerful collaborative relationships to improve health that government alone cannot replicate.

Health is a primary public good because many aspects of human potential such as employment, social relationships, and political participation are contingent on it. In view of the value of health to employers, business, communities, and society in general, creating the conditions for people to be healthy should also be a shared social goal. The special role of government must be allied with the contributions of other sectors of society. This report builds on the foundation of the *Future of Public Health* report, which asserted that public health is "what we as a society do collectively to assure the conditions in which people can be healthy" (IOM, 1988). In addition to assessing the state and needs of the governmental public health infrastructure—the backbone of the public health system—this report also focuses on the roles and actions of other entities that could be potential partners within such a system.

The emphasis on an intersectoral public health system does not supersede the special duty of the governmental public health agencies but, rather, complements it with a call for the contributions of other sectors of society that have enormous power to influence health. A public health system would include the governmental public health agencies, the health care delivery system, and the public health and health sciences academia, sectors that are heavily engaged and more clearly identified with health activities. The committee has also identified communities and their many entities (e.g., schools, organizations, and religious congregations), businesses and employers, and the media as potential actors in the public health system. Businesses play important, often dual, roles in shaping population health. In the occupational setting, through environmental impacts, as members of communities, and as purveyors of products available for mass consumption, businesses may undermine health by polluting, spreading environmental toxicants, and producing or marketing products detrimental to health. However, businesses can and often do take steps to contribute to population health through efforts such as facilitating economic development and regional employment and workplace-specific contributions such as health promotion and the provision of health care benefits. The media is also featured because of its deeply influential role as a conduit for information and as a shaper of public opinion about health and related matters.

The events of the autumn of 2001 placed the governmental public health infrastructure under unprecedented public and political scrutiny. Although motivated by concern about its preparedness to respond to a potential crisis, this scrutiny offered an opportunity to assess the overall adequacy of the governmental public health infrastructure to promote and protect the public's health in the new century. This status check revealed facts that were well known to the public health community but that surprised many policy makers and much of the public. The governmental public health infrastructure has suffered from political neglect and from the pressure of political agendas and public opinion that frequently override empirical evidence. Under the glare of a national crisis, policy makers and the public became aware of vulnerable and outdated health information systems and technologies, an insufficient and inadequately trained public health workforce, antiquated laboratory capacity, a lack of real-time surveillance and epidemiological systems, ineffective and fragmented communications networks, incomplete domestic preparedness and emergency response capabilities, and communities without access to essential public health services. These problems leave the nation's health vulnerable—and not only to exotic germs and bioterrorism. The health of the public is also at risk when social and other environmental conditions undermine health, including toxic water, air, and housing; inaccurate and confusing health information; poverty; a lack of health care; and unequal opportunities for health. Government's partners, potential actors in the public health system, can contribute to assuring population health by helping to change the conditions for health in communities, at work, and through the media.

AREAS OF ACTION AND CHANGE

To address the present and future challenges faced by the nation's public health system—including potential actors in the private and nonprofit sectors—this report proposes six areas of action and change to be undertaken by all who work to assure population health. These areas include

1. Adopting a population health approach that considers the multiple determinants of health;
2. Strengthening the governmental public health infrastructure, which forms the backbone of the public health system;
3. Building a new generation of intersectoral partnerships that also draw on the perspectives and resources of diverse communities and actively engage them in health action;
4. Developing systems of accountability to assure the quality and availability of public health services;
5. Making evidence the foundation of decision making and the measure of success; and
6. Enhancing and facilitating communication within the public health system (e.g., among all levels of the governmental public health infrastructure and between public health professionals and community members).

FINDINGS AND RECOMMENDATIONS
Governmental Public Health Infrastructure

Finding: Public health law at the federal, state, and local levels is often outdated and internally inconsistent. This leads to inefficiency and a lack of coordination and may even pose a danger in a crisis requiring an immediate and effective public health response. Pioneering work at the national level has gone into developing models and guidance to assist states in reforming their public health laws as appropriate for their unique legal structures and public health preparedness needs, but a more comprehensive effort is needed.

1. The Secretary of the Department of Health and Human Services (DHHS), in consultation with states, should appoint a national commission to develop a framework and recommendations for state public health law reform. In particular, the national commission would review all existing public health law as well as the Turning Point[1] Model State Public Health Act and the Model State Emergency Health Powers Act[2]; provide guidance and technical assistance to help states reform their laws to meet modern scientific and legal standards; and help foster greater consistency within and among states, especially in their approach to different health threats (Chapter 3).

Finding: The public health workforce must have appropriate education and training to perform its role. Today, a majority of governmental public health workers have little or no training in public health. Enhancing the knowledge and skills of governmental public health workers and nongovernmental workers who perform public health functions is necessary to ensure that essential public health services are competently delivered. Assessing and strengthening competence will help to ensure workforce preparedness, nurture leadership, and assure the quality of public health services.

2. All federal, state, and local governmental public health agencies should develop strategies to ensure that public health workers who are involved in the provision of essential public health services demonstrate mastery of the core public health competencies appropriate to their jobs. The Council on Linkages between Academia

and Public Health Practice[3] should also encourage the competency development of public health professionals working in public health system roles in for-profit and nongovernmental entities (Chapter 3).

3. Congress should designate funds for the Centers for Disease Control and Prevention (CDC) and the Health Resources and Services Administration (HRSA) to periodically assess the preparedness of the public health workforce, to document the training necessary to meet basic competency expectations, and to advise on the funding necessary to provide such training (Chapter 3).

4. Leadership training, support, and development should be a high priority for governmental public health agencies and other organizations in the public health system and for schools of public health that supply the public health infrastructure with its professionals and leaders (Chapter 3).

5. A formal national dialogue should be initiated to address the issue of public health workforce credentialing. The Secretary of DHHS should appoint a national commission on public health workforce credentialing to lead this dialogue. The commission should be charged to determine if a credentialing system would further the goal of creating a competent workforce and, if applicable, the manner and time frame for implementation by governmental public health agencies at all levels. The dialogue should include representatives from federal, state, and local public health agencies, academia, and public health professional organizations who can represent and discuss the various perspectives on the workforce credentialing debate (Chapter 3).

Finding: Developments in communication and information technologies present both opportunities and challenges to attaining the vision of healthy people in healthy communities. Harnessing the potential of these technologies will enable public health officials to collect and disseminate information more efficiently, improve the effectiveness of public health interventions, and enable the public to understand what services should be provided, and thus what they have the right to expect from their public officials.

---

[1]Turning Point, a program funded by the Robert Wood Johnson and the W. K. Kellogg foundations, works to strengthen the public health infrastructure at the local and state levels across the United States and spearheads the Turning Point National Collaborative on Public Health Statute Modernization.

[2]The Model State Emergency Health Powers Act (MSEHPA) provides states with the powers needed "to detect and contain bioterrorism or a naturally occurring disease outbreak. Legislative bills based on the MSEHPA have been introduced in 34 states" (Gostin et al., 2002).

[3]The Council on Linkages between Academia and Public Health Practice is comprised of leaders from national organizations representing the public health practice and academic communities. The Council grew out of the Public Health Faculty/Agency Forum, which developed recommendations for improving the relevance of public health education to the demands of public health in the practice sector. The Council and its partners have focused attention on the need for a public health practice research agenda.

6. All partners within the public health system should place special emphasis on communication as a critical core competency of public health practice. Governmental public health agencies at all levels should use existing and emerging tools (including information technologies) for effective management of public health information and for internal and external communication. To be effective, such communication must be culturally appropriate and suitable to the literacy levels of the individuals in the communities they serve (Chapter 3).

Finding: Existing information networks make it difficult, and sometimes impossible, for governmental public health agencies to exchange information and communicate effectively with the health care delivery system for the purposes of surveillance, reporting, and appropriately responding to threats to the public's health. Clear communication and enhanced information gathering, processing, and dissemination mechanisms will increase the accountability and effectiveness of governmental public health agencies and other public health system actors. Individuals and communities may also benefit by being able to contribute and collect information directly relevant to them.

7. The Secretary of DHHS should provide leadership to facilitate the development and implementation of the National Health Information Infrastructure (NHII). Implementation of NHII should take into account, where possible, the findings and recommendations of the National Committee on Vital and Health Statistics (NCVHS) working group on NHII. Congress should consider options for funding the development and deployment of NHII (e.g., in support of clinical care, health information for the public, and public health practice and research) through payment changes, tax credits, subsidized loans, or grants (Chapter 3).

Finding: At this time, DHHS lacks a system for conducting regular assessments of the adequacy and capacity of the governmental public health infrastructure. Such assessments are urgently needed to keep Congress and the public informed and would play an important role in supporting a regular process of assessment and evaluation at state and local public health agency levels.

8. DHHS should be accountable for assessing the state of the nation's governmental public health infrastructure and its capacity to provide the essential public health services to every community and for reporting that assessment annually to Congress and the nation.

The assessment should include a thorough evaluation of federal, state, and local funding for the nation's governmental public health infrastructure and should be conducted in collaboration with state and local officials. The assessment should identify strengths and gaps and serve as the basis for plans to develop a funding and technical assistance plan to assure sustainability. The public availability of these reports will enable state and local public health agencies to use them for continual self-assessment and evaluation (Chapter 3).

Finding: The capacity of the nation's public health laboratories should be assessed. Every state has at least one state public health laboratory to support infectious disease surveillance and other public health activities. About 60 percent of the 3,000 local health departments provide some laboratory services. Enhanced funding has been provided to prepare states and some urban areas for bioterrorism and other emergencies. The adequacy of these funds and how effectively they are being used to address laboratory capacity problems are unknown. The appropriate funding levels to sustain current capacity and enable the laboratories to integrate new technologies as they emerge have not been determined and require investigation.

9. DHHS should evaluate the status of the nation's public health laboratory system, including an assessment of the impact of recent increased funding. The evaluation should identify remaining gaps, and funding should be allocated to close them. Working with the states, DHHS should agree on a base funding level that will maintain the enhanced laboratory system and allow the rapid deployment of newly developed technologies (Chapter 3).

Finding: After adequate funding levels are determined for the governmental public health infrastructure, the appropriate investment level is needed to assure that every community has access to the essential public health services.

10. DHHS should develop a comprehensive investment plan for a strong national governmental public health infrastructure with a timetable, clear performance measures, and regular progress reports to the public. State and local governments should also provide adequate, consistent, and sustainable funding for the governmental public health infrastructure (Chapter 3).

Finding: Current funding structures frequently burden the work of state and local public health jurisdictions with administrative requirements. "Stove-pipe" (i.e., categorical) funding is often inflexible, at times discouraging evidence-based planning and use of funds or the blending of resources in special circumstances.

11. The federal government and states should renew efforts to experiment with clustering or consolidation of categorical grants for the purpose of increasing local flexibility to address priority health concerns and enhance the efficient use of limited resources (Chapter 3).

Finding: Although the health care delivery system has several mechanisms for accreditation and quality assurance, the committee found that there are no such structures for the governmental public health infrastructure. Accreditation mechanisms may help to ensure the robustness and efficiency of the governmental public health infrastructure, assure the quality of public health services, and transparently provide information to the public about the quality of the services delivered.

12. The Secretary of DHHS should appoint a national commission to consider if an accreditation system would be useful for improving and building state and local public health agency capacities. If such a system is deemed useful, the commission should make recommendations on how it would be governed and develop mechanisms (e.g., incentives) to gain state and local government participation in the accreditation effort. Membership on this commission should include representatives from CDC, the Association of State and Territorial Health Officials, the National Association of County and City Health Officials, and nongovernmental organizations (Chapter 3).

Finding: Research is needed to guide policy decisions that shape public health practice. The committee had hoped to provide specific guidance elaborating on the types and levels of workforce, infrastructure, related resources, and financial investments necessary to ensure the availability of essential public health services to all of the nation's communities. However, such evidence is limited, and there is no agenda or support for this type of research, despite the critical need for such data to promote and protect the nation's health.

13. CDC, in collaboration with the Council on Linkages between Academia and Public Health Practice and other public health system partners, should develop a research agenda and estimate the funding needed to build the evidence base that will guide policy making for public health practice (Chapter 3).

Finding: Effective interagency collaboration on health issues at the federal level is crucial but difficult because of the specialized nature of agency structures and responsibilities. Furthermore, many agencies not traditionally associated with health issues make policy and manage programs with potential implications for health. More effective coordinating structures are needed to reduce obstacles to the effective use of federal regulatory and standard-setting powers in health. Mechanisms are needed to develop collaborative relationships and to harmonize regulations within DHHS, across federal agencies, and among federal state and local governments to assure effective action for protecting the population's health.

14. The Secretary of DHHS should review the regulatory authorities of DHHS agencies with health-related responsibilities to reduce overlap and inconsistencies, ensure that the department's management structure is best suited to coordinate among agencies within DHHS with health-related responsibilities, and, to the extent possible, simplify relationships with state and local governmental public health agencies. Similar efforts should be made to improve coordination with other federal cabinet agencies performing important public health services, such as the Department of Agriculture and the Environmental Protection Agency (Chapter 3).

Finding: The success of the public health system depends in part on collaboration among all levels of government. Although noting the importance of preserving state autonomy and the ability to address local circumstances, the National Governors' Association (1997) acknowledged a need for a federal role in certain domestic issues—where issues are national in scope and where the national interest is at risk—and to help states meet the needs of special populations. Collaboration on such issues would also improve the alignment of policy across federal agencies. The committee believes that a more formal entity could facilitate the link between the Secretary of DHHS and state health officers for the purpose of improving communication, coordination, and collaborative action on a national health agenda.

15. Congress should mandate the establishment of a National Public Health Council. This National Public Health Council would bring together the Secretary of DHHS and state health commissioners at least annually to
     • Provide a forum for communication and collaboration on action to achieve national health goals as articulated in *Healthy People 2010*;
     • Advise the Secretary of DHHS on public health issues

- Advise the Secretary of DHHS on financing and regulations that affect governmental public health capacity at the state and local levels;
- Provide a forum for overseeing the development of an incentive-based federal-state-funded system to sustain a governmental public health infrastructure that can assure the availability of essential public health services to every American community and can monitor progress toward this goal (e.g., through report cards);
- Review and evaluate the domestic policies of other cabinet agencies for their impact on national health outcomes (e.g., through health impact reports) and on the reduction and elimination of health disparities; and
- Submit an annual report on their deliberations and recommendations to Congress.

The Council should be chaired by the Secretary of DHHS and cochaired by a state health director on a rotating basis. An appropriately resourced secretariat should be established in the Office of the Secretary to ensure that the Council has access to the information and expertise of all DHHS agencies during its deliberations (Chapter 3).

Community

Finding: Community organizations are close to the populations they serve and are therefore a crucial part of the public health system for identifying needs and responses and evaluating results. Communication and collaboration between community organizations and health departments are often limited, leading to the duplication of effort and an inefficient use of resources. Moreover, foundation and governmental funding mechanisms are often not structured in ways that encourage broad community engagement and leadership at all stages. Communities are sometimes brought into the effort late, after planning has begun, or they are simply used as informants or subjects of research. The goal of achieving lasting change for health improvement should guide community groups and public and private funders.

16. Local governmental public health agencies should support community-led efforts to inventory resources, assess needs, formulate collaborative responses, and evaluate outcomes for community health improvement and the elimination of health disparities. Governmental public health agencies should provide community organizations and coalitions with technical assistance and support in identifying and securing resources as needed and at all phases of the process (Chapter 4).

17. Governmental and private-sector funders of community health initiatives should plan their investments with a focus on long-lasting change. Such a focus would include realistic time lines, an emphasis on ongoing community engagement and leadership, and a final goal of institutionalizing effective project components in the local community or public health system as appropriate (Chapter 4).

Health Care Delivery System

Finding: Health care is an important determinant of population and individual health. Although most Americans receive the health care services that they require, the approximately 41 million people who have no health insurance experience difficulty in accessing care and are often unable to obtain needed services. Furthermore, the services that they do receive may not be timely, appropriate, or well coordinated. Recent Institute of Medicine (IOM) reports have found that health insurance coverage is associated with better health outcomes for children and adults. It is also associated with having a regular source of care and with the greater and more appropriate use of health services. These factors, in turn, improve the likelihood of disease screening and early detection, the management of chronic illnesses, and the effective treatment of acute conditions. The ultimate result is better health for children, adults, and families. Increased health insurance coverage would likely reduce racial and ethnic disparities in the use of appropriate health care services and may also reduce disparities in morbidity and mortality among ethnic groups.

18. Adequate population health cannot be achieved without making comprehensive and affordable health care available to every person residing in the United States. It is the responsibility of the federal government to lead a national effort to examine the options available to achieve stable health care coverage of individuals and families and to assure the implementation of plans to achieve that result (Chapter 5).

Finding: In addition to a lack of health care coverage, many people are covered by health insurance plans that do not include coverage for preventive health care, mental health, substance abuse treatment, and dental health services or require copayments that lessen access (Allukian, 1999; King, 2000; Solanki et al., 2000). This causes many individuals to live with undiagnosed mental illness and others to go without treatment (DHHS, 1999). Many children and adults suffer from oral health conditions that may affect their overall health status (DHHS, 2000). These often-neglected services constitute gaps in efforts to assure the health of the population.

19. All public and privately funded insurance plans should include age-appropriate preventive services as recommended by the U.S. Preventive Services Task Force and provide evidence-based coverage of oral health, mental health, and substance abuse treatment services (Chapter 5).

Finding: As the public health system strains to meet the challenges posed by increasing costs, an aging population, and a range of threats to health, it will need a meaningful partnership with the health care delivery sector to attain their shared population health goals.

20. Bold, large-scale demonstrations should be funded by the federal government and other major investors in health care to test radical new approaches to increase the efficiency and effectiveness of health care financing and delivery systems. The experiments should effectively link delivery systems with other components of the public health system and focus on improving population health while eliminating disparities. The demonstrations should be supported by adequate resources to enable innovative ideas to be fairly tested (Chapter 5).

Businesses and Employers

Finding: Employers play a major role in the health of their employees and the population at large through their impacts on natural and built environments, through workplace conditions, and through their relationship with communities. For example, employers may be an important part of a region's economic development, which, in turn, may support health improvement. In addition, low unemployment rates and vibrant businesses are likely to mean better housing, higher incomes, and improved overall quality of life within communities. Furthermore, employers facilitate access to health care services by purchasing health care for their employees.

21. The federal government should develop programs to assist small employers and employers with low-wage workers to purchase health insurance at reasonable rates (Chapter 6).

22. The corporate community and public health agencies should initiate and enhance joint efforts to strengthen health promotion and disease and injury prevention programs for employees and their communities. As an early step, the corporate and governmental public health community should:
    a. Strengthen partnership and collaboration by
       • Developing direct linkages between local public health agencies and business leaders to forge a common language and understanding of employee and community health problems and to participate in setting community health goals and strategies for achieving them, and
       • Developing innovative ways for the corporate and governmental public health communities to gather, interpret, and exchange mutually meaningful data and information, such as the translation of health information to support corporate health promotion and health care purchasing activities.
    b. Enhance communication by
       • Developing effective employer and community communication and education programs focused on the benefits of and options for health promotion and disease and injury prevention; and
       • Using proven marketing and social marketing techniques to promote individual behavioral and community change.
    c. Develop the evidence base for workplace and community interventions through greater public, private, and philanthropic investments in research to extend the science and improve the effectiveness of workplace and community interventions to promote health and prevent disease and injury.
    d. Recognize business leadership in employee and community health by elevating the level of recognition given to corporate investment in employee and community health. The Secretaries of DHHS and the Department of Commerce, along with business leaders (e.g., chambers of commerce and business roundtables), should jointly sponsor a Corporate Investment in Health Award. The award would recognize private-sector entities that have demonstrated exemplary civic and social responsibility for improving the health of their workers and the community (Chapter 6).

Media

Finding: Both the news and entertainment media shape public opinion and influence decision making, with potentially critical effects on population health. Moreover, public health efforts and especially the activities of governmental public health agencies often receive and attract little media attention, explaining in part the widespread lack of understanding about the concepts and content of public health activities (i.e., population-level health promotion and protection, as well as disease prevention). Editors and journalists and medical and public health officials generally do not understand each other's perspectives, methods, and objectives. This lack of understanding frequently leads to the provision of inaccurate or inadequate health information and missed opportunities to communicate effectively to the public. The journalism and public health communities have identified a clear need for training, research, and dialogue to improve their ability to accurately inform and communicate with the public, communities, and other actors in the public health system.

23. An ongoing dialogue should be maintained between medical and public health officials and editors and journalists at the local level and their representative associations nationally. Furthermore, foundations and governmental health agencies should provide opportunities to develop and evaluate educational and training programs that provide journalists with experiences that will deepen their knowledge of public health subject matter and provide public health workers with a foundation in communication theory, messaging, and application (Chapter 7).

24. The television networks, television stations, and cable providers should increase the amount of time they donate to public service announcements (PSAs) as partial fulfillment of the public service requirement in their Federal Communications Commission (FCC) licensing agreements (Chapter 7).

25. The FCC should review its regulations for PSA broadcasting on television and radio to ensure a more balanced broadcasting schedule that will reach a greater proportion of the viewing and listening audiences (Chapter 7).

26. Public health officials and local and national entertainment media should work together to facilitate the communication of accurate information about disease and about medical and health issues in the entertainment media (Chapter 7).

27. Public health and communication researchers should develop an evidence base on media influences on health knowledge and behavior, as well as on the promotion of healthy public policy (Chapter 7).

Academia

Finding: Academia provides degree and continuing education to a significant proportion of the public health workforce. Consistent with the previous recommendations to assess workforce competency and develop strategies to overcome deficits, changes are needed in both academic settings and curricula and in the financial support available to students training for careers in public health.

28. Academic institutions should increase integrated interdisciplinary learning opportunities for students in public health and other related health science professions. Such efforts should include not only multidisciplinary education but also interdisciplinary education and appropriate incentives for faculty to undertake such activities (Chapter 8).

29. Congress should increase funding for HRSA programs that provide financial support for students enrolled in public health degree programs through mechanisms such as training grants, loan repayments, and service obligation grants. Funding should also be provided to strengthen the Public Health Training Center program to effectively meet the educational needs of the existing public health workforce and to facilitate public health worker access to the centers. Support for leadership training of state and local health department directors and local community leaders should continue through funding of the National and Regional Public Health Leadership Institutes and distance-learning materials developed by HRSA and CDC (Chapter 8).

Finding: The committee finds that health-related research is disproportionately biomedical, focused on the health and health problems of individuals. Funding and incentives for population-level research and community-based prevention research are low, as these are not priority areas within academia or the governmental public health infrastructure.

30. Federal funders of research and academic institutions should recognize and reward faculty scholarship related to public health practice research (Chapter 8).

31. The committee recommends that Congress provide funds for CDC to enhance its investigator-initiated program for prevention research while maintaining a strong Centers, Institutes, and Offices (CIO)-generated research program. CDC should take steps that include
   • Expanding the external peer review mechanism for review of investigator-initiated research;
   • Allowing research to be conducted over the more generous time lines often required by prevention research; and
   • Establishing a central mechanism for coordination of investigator-initiated proposal submissions (Chapter 8).

32. CDC should authorize an analysis of the funding levels necessary for effective Prevention Research Center functioning, taking into account the levels authorized

by P.L. 98-551 as well as the amount of prevention research occurring in other institutions and organizations (Chapter 8).

33. NIH should increase the portion of its budget allocated to population- and community-based prevention research that
    - Addresses population-level health problems;
    - Involves a definable population and operates at the level of the whole person;
    - Evaluates the application and impacts of new discoveries on the actual health of the population; and
    - Focuses on the behavioral and environmental (social, economic, cultural, physical) factors associated with primary and secondary prevention of disease and disability in populations.

Furthermore, the committee recommends that the Director of NIH report annually to the Secretary of DHHS on the scope of population- and community-based prevention research activities undertaken by the NIH centers and institutes (Chapter 8).

34. Academic institutions should develop criteria for recognizing and rewarding faculty scholarship related to service activities that strengthen public health practice (Chapter 8).

The findings and recommendations outlined above illustrate the areas of action and change that the committee believes should be emphasized by all potential actors in the public health system. Recommendations are directed to many parties, because in a society as diverse and decentralized as that of the United States, achieving population health requires contributions from all levels of government, the private business sector, and the variety of institutions and organizations that shape opportunities, attitudes, behaviors, and resources affecting health. Governmental public health agencies have the responsibility to facilitate and nurture the conditions conducive to good health. Without the active collaboration of other important institutions, however, they cannot produce the healthy people in healthy communities envisioned in *Healthy People 2010*.

REFERENCES

Allukian M. 1999. Dental insurance is essential, but not enough. In Closing the Gap, a newsletter. Office of Minority Health, Department of Health and Human Services, July, Washington, DC.

DHHS (Department of Health and Human Services). 1999. Mental Health: A Report of the Surgeon General. Rockville, MD: Substance Abuse and Mental Health Administration, National Institute of Mental Health, National Institutes of Health, DHHS.

DHHS. 2000. Oral Health in America: A Report of the Surgeon General. Rockville, MD: National Institute of Dental and Craniofacial Research, National Institutes of Health, DHHS.

Gostin LO, Sapsin JW, Teret SP, Burris S, Mair JS, Hodge JG Jr, Vernick JS. 2002. The Model State Emergency Health Powers Act: planning for and response to bioterrorism and naturally occurring infectious diseases. Journal of the American Medical Association 288(5):622–628.

IOM (Institute of Medicine). 1988. The Future of Public Health, p. 1. Washington, DC: National Academy Press.

King JS. 2000. Grant Results Report: Assessing insurance coverage of preventive services by private employers. Robert Wood Johnson Foundation. Available online at www.rwjf.org/app/rw_grant_results_reports/rw_grr/029975s.htm. Accessed April 19, 2002.

McGinnis MJ, Williams-Russo P, Knickman JR. 2002. The case for more active policy attention to health promotion. To succeed, we need leadership that informs and motivates, economic incentives that encourage change, and science that moves the frontiers. Health Affairs 21(2):78–93.

NGA (National Governors Association). 1997. Policy positions. Washington, DC: National Governors Association.

Solanki G, Schauffler HH, Miller LS. 2000. The direct and indirect effects of cost-sharing on the use of preventive services. Health Services Research 34(6):1331–1350.

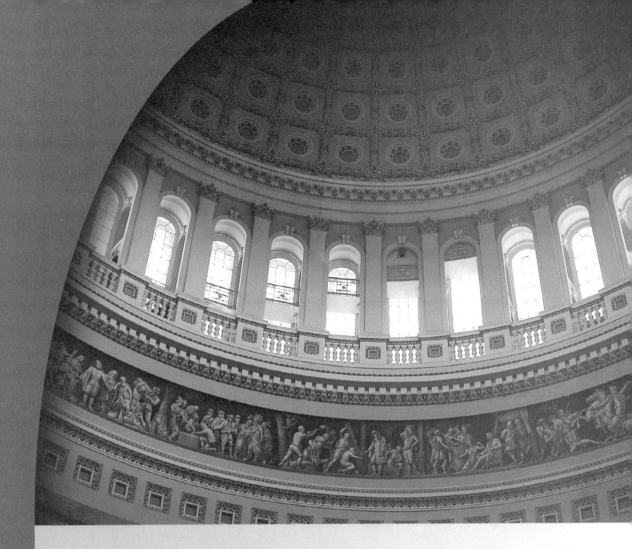

PART II

Health Care Quality

This Part includes five readings on the topic of health care quality, viewed from the perspectives of policy, health services research, and law. The opening reading is the Executive Summary from the Institute of Medicine's (IOM) influential report, "Crossing the Quality Chasm." In it, the IOM addresses one of the most pressing issues in today's health care delivery system: whether the care actually being delivered to people in this country is, in fact, the care they should be receiving. The IOM report studies this question in the context of preventive, acute, chronic, and end-of-life care.

In the article "The Quality of Health Care Delivered to Adults in the United States," Elizabeth McGlynn and her colleagues analyze the extent to which standard processes involved in health care are consistently applied across a range of patients and medical conditions. The results of their study indicated that delivery of recommended, standard processes for basic care—an important dimension of health care quality—was lacking often enough to pose "serious threats" to the health of the population.

The third reading in this series, the Summary from the IOM's landmark study on health disparities ("Unequal Treatment: Confronting Racial and Ethnic Disparities in Health Care"), revealed the scope and depth of a critical health care quality problem. This IOM report clearly showed that even after controlling for insurance status, income, and other health care access-related factors, racial and ethnic minorities receive lower quality care than nonminorities. "Unequal Treatment" placed health disparities atop the policy agenda and should be required reading for all health policy students.

The final two readings are legal opinions meant to exemplify the role that law in general and courts in particular play in the shaping of health care quality policy. In the case of *Canterbury v. Spence*, a federal appellate court issued an historic opinion shifting the standard of health care informed consent from one that was universally perceived and applied as being physician-oriented to one that relied on what a reasonable patient would view as amounting to an adequate disclosure of critical information when making health care decisions. In *Jones v. Chicago*, the Supreme Court of Illinois ruled that health maintenance organizations can properly be held accountable for negligence stemming from their actions as an arranger and provider of health care services.

IN THIS SECTION

Executive Summary from
Crossing the Quality Chasm

Crossing the Quality Chasm: A New Health System for the 21st Century
Committee on Quality of Health Care in America
Institute of Medicine, 2001

The American health care delivery system is in need of fundamental change. Many patients, doctors, nurses, and health care leaders are concerned that the care delivered is not, essentially, the care we should receive (Donelan et al., 1999; Reed and St. Peter, 1997; Shindul-Rothschild et al., 1996; Taylor, 2001). The frustration levels of both patients and clinicians have probably never been higher. Yet the problems remain. Health care today harms too frequently and routinely fails to deliver its potential benefits.

Americans should be able to count on receiving care that meets their needs and is based on the best scientific knowledge. Yet there is strong evidence that this frequently is not the case.[1] Crucial reports from disciplined review bodies document the scale and gravity of the problems (Chassin et al., 1998; Institute of Medicine, 1999; Advisory Commission on Consumer Protection and Quality in the Health Care Industry, 1998). Quality problems are everywhere, affecting many patients. Between the health care we have and the care we could have lays not just a gap, but a chasm.

The Committee on the Quality of Health Care in America was formed in June 1998 and charged with developing a strategy that would result in a substantial improvement in the qual-

ity of health care over the next 10 years. In carrying out this charge, the committee commissioned a detailed review of the literature on the quality of care; convened a communications workshop to identify strategies for raising the awareness of the general public and key stakeholders of quality concerns; identified environmental forces that encourage or impede efforts to improve quality; developed strategies for fostering greater accountability for quality; and identified important areas of research that should be pursued to facilitate improvements in quality. The committee has focused on the personal health care delivery system, specifically, the provision of preventive, acute, chronic, and end-of-life health care for individuals. Although the committee recognizes the critical role of the public health system in protecting and improving the health of our communities, this issue lies beyond the purview of the present study.

The committee has already spoken to one urgent quality problem—patient safety. In our first report, *To Err Is Human: Building a Safer Health System*, we concluded that tens of thousands of Americans die each year from errors in their care, and hundreds of thousands suffer or barely escape from nonfatal injuries that a truly high-quality care system would largely prevent (Institute of Medicine, 2000b).

As disturbing as the committee's report on safety is, it reflects only a small part of the unfolding story of quality in American health care. Other defects are even more widespread and, taken together, detract still further from the health, functioning, dignity, comfort, satisfaction, and resources of Americans. This report addresses these additional quality problems. As the patient safety report was a call for action to make

[1]See [Appendix A] of this report for a review of the literature on the quality of care.

care safer, this report is a call for action to improve the American health care delivery system as a whole, in all its quality dimensions, for all Americans.

WHY ACTION IS NEEDED NOW

At no time in the history of medicine has the growth in knowledge and technologies been so profound. Since the first contemporary randomized controlled trial was conducted more than 50 years ago, the number of trials conducted has grown to nearly 10,000 annually (Chassin, 1998). Between 1993 and 1999, the budget of the National Institutes of Health increased from $10.9 to $15.6 billion, while investments by pharmaceutical firms in research and development increased from $12 to $24 billion (National Institutes of Health, 2000; Pharmaceutical Research and Manufacturers of America, 2000). Genomics and other new technologies on the horizon offer the promise of further increasing longevity, improving health and functioning, and alleviating pain and suffering. Advances in rehabilitation, cell restoration, and prosthetic devices hold potential for improving the health and functioning of many with disabilities. Americans are justifiably proud of the great strides that have been made in the health and medical sciences.

As medical science and technology have advanced at a rapid pace, however, the health care delivery system has floundered in its ability to provide consistently high-quality care to all Americans. Research on the quality of care reveals a health care system that frequently falls short in its ability to translate knowledge into practice, and to apply new technology safely and appropriately. During the last decade alone, more than 70 publications in leading peer-reviewed journals have documented serious quality shortcomings [***]. The performance of the health care system varies considerably. It may be exemplary, but often is not, and millions of Americans fail to receive effective care. If the health care system cannot consistently deliver today's science and technology, we may conclude that it is even less prepared to respond to the extraordinary scientific advances that will surely emerge during the first half of the 21st century. And finally, more than 40 million Americans remain without health insurance, deprived of critically important access to basic care (U.S. Census Bureau, 2000).

The health care system as currently structured does not, as a whole, make the best use of its resources. There is little doubt that the aging population and increased patient demand for new services, technologies, and drugs are contributing to the steady increase in health care expenditures, but so, too, is waste. Many types of medical errors result in the subsequent need for additional health care services to treat patients who have been harmed (Institute of Medicine, 2000b). A highly fragmented delivery system that largely lacks even rudimen-

tary clinical information capabilities results in poorly designed care processes characterized by unnecessary duplication of services and long waiting times and delays. And there is substantial evidence documenting overuse of many services—services for which the potential risk of harm outweighs the potential benefits (Chassin et al., 1998; Schuster et al., 1998).

What is perhaps most disturbing is the absence of real progress toward restructuring health care systems to address both quality and cost concerns, or toward applying advances in information technology to improve administrative and clinical processes. Despite the efforts of many talented leaders and dedicated professionals, the last quarter of the 20th century might best be described as the "era of Brownian motion in health care." Mergers, acquisitions, and affiliations have been commonplace within the health plan, hospital, and physician practice sectors (Colby, 1997). Yet all this organizational turmoil has resulted in little change in the way health care is delivered. Some of the new arrangements have failed following disappointing results. Leaders of health care institutions are under extraordinary pressure, trying on the one hand to strategically reposition their organizations for the future, and on the other to respond to today's challenges, such as reductions in third-party payments (Guterman, 1998), shortfalls in nurse staffing (Egger, 2000), and growing numbers of uninsured patients seeking uncompensated care (Institute of Medicine, 2000a).

For several decades, the needs of the American public have been shifting from predominantly acute, episodic care to care for chronic conditions. Chronic conditions are now the leading cause of illness, disability, and death; they affect almost half of the U.S. population and account for the majority of health care expenditures (Hoffman et al., 1996; The Robert Wood Johnson Foundation, 1996). As the need for community-based acute and long-term care services has grown, the portion of health care resources devoted to hospital care has declined, while that expended on pharmaceuticals has risen dramatically (Copeland, 1999). Yet there remains a dearth of clinical programs with the infrastructure required to provide the full complement of services needed by people with heart disease, diabetes, asthma, and other common chronic conditions (Wagner et al., 1996). The fact that more than 40 percent of people with chronic conditions have more than one such condition argues strongly for more sophisticated mechanisms to communicate and coordinate care (The Robert Wood Johnson Foundation, 1996). Yet physician groups, hospitals, and other health care organizations operate as silos, often providing care without the benefit of complete information about the patient's condition, medical history, services provided in other settings, or medications prescribed by other clinicians. For those without insurance, care is often unobtainable except in emergencies. It is not surprising, then, that studies of patient experience document that the health system for some is a "nightmare to navigate" (Picker Institute and American Hospital Association, 1996).

QUALITY AS A SYSTEM PROPERTY

The committee is confident that Americans can have a health care system of the quality they need, want, and deserve. But we are also confident that this higher level of quality cannot be achieved by further stressing current systems of care. The current care systems cannot do the job. Trying harder will not work. Changing systems of care will.

The committee's report on patient safety offers a similar conclusion in its narrower realm. Safety flaws are unacceptably common, but the effective remedy is not to browbeat the health care workforce by asking them to try harder to give safe care. Members of the health care workforce are already trying hard to do their jobs well. In fact, the courage, hard work, and commitment of doctors, nurses, and others in health care are today the only real means we have of stemming the flood of errors that are latent in our health care systems.

Health care has safety and quality problems because it relies on outmoded systems of work. Poor designs set the workforce up to fail, regardless of how hard they try. If we want safer, higher-quality care, we will need to have redesigned systems of care, including the use of information technology to support clinical and administrative processes.

Throughout this report, the committee offers a strategy and action plan for building a stronger health system over the coming decade, one that is capable of delivering on the promise of state-of-the-art health care to all Americans. In some areas, achieving this ideal will require crossing a large chasm between today's system and the possibilities of tomorrow.

AN AGENDA FOR CROSSING THE CHASM

The need for leadership in health care has never been greater. Transforming the health care system will not be an easy process. But the potential benefits are large as well. Narrowing the quality chasm will make it possible to bring the benefits of medical science and technology to all Americans in every community, and this in turn will mean less pain and suffering, less disability, greater longevity, and a more productive workforce. To this end, the committee proposes the following agenda for redesigning the 21st-century health care system:

- That all health care constituencies, including policymakers, purchasers, regulators, health professionals, health care trustees and management, and consumers, commit to a national statement of purpose for the health care system as a whole and to a shared agenda of six

aims for improvement that can raise the quality of care to unprecedented levels.
- That clinicians and patients, and the health care organizations that support care delivery, adopt a new set of principles to guide the redesign of care processes.
- That the Department of Health and Human Services identify a set of priority conditions upon which to focus initial efforts, provide resources to stimulate innovation, and initiate the change process.
- That health care organizations design and implement more effective organizational support processes to make change in the delivery of care possible.
- That purchasers, regulators, health professions, educational institutions, and the Department of Health and Human Services create an environment that fosters and rewards improvement by (1) creating an infrastructure to support evidence-based practice, (2) facilitating the use of information technology, (3) aligning payment incentives, and (4) preparing the workforce to better serve patients in a world of expanding knowledge and rapid change.

The committee recognizes that implementing this agenda will be a complex process and that it will be important to periodically evaluate progress and reassess strategies for overcoming barriers.

Establishing Aims for the 21st-Century Health Care System

The committee proposes six aims for improvement to address key dimensions in which today's health care system functions at far lower levels than it can and should. Health care should be:

- *Safe*—avoiding injuries to patients from the care that is intended to help them.
- *Effective*—providing services based on scientific knowledge to all who could benefit and refraining from providing services to those not likely to benefit (avoiding underuse and overuse, respectively).
- *Patient-centered*—providing care that is respectful of and responsive to individual patient preferences, needs, and values and ensuring that patient values guide all clinical decisions.
- *Timely*—reducing waits and sometimes harmful delays for both those who receive and those who give care.
- *Efficient*—avoiding waste, including waste of equipment, supplies, ideas, and energy.
- *Equitable*—providing care that does not vary in quality because of personal characteristics such as gender, ethnicity, geographic location, and socioeconomic status.

A health care system that achieved major gains in these six dimensions would be far better at meeting patient needs. Patients would experience care that was safer, more reliable, more responsive, more integrated, and more available. Patients could count on receiving the full array of preventive, acute, and chronic services from which they are likely to benefit. Such a system would also be better for clinicians and others who would experience the satisfaction of providing care that was more reliable, more responsive to patients, and more coordinated than is the case today.

The entire enterprise of care would ideally be united across these aims by a single, overarching purpose for the American health care system as a whole. For this crucial statement of purpose, the committee endorses and adopts the phrasing of the Advisory Commission on Consumer Protection and Quality in the Health Care Industry (1998).

> Recommendation 1: All health care organizations, professional groups, and private and public purchasers should adopt as their explicit purpose to continually reduce the burden of illness, injury, and disability, and to improve the health and functioning of the people of the United States.

> Recommendation 2: All health care organizations, professional groups, and private and public purchasers should pursue six major aims; specifically, health care should be safe, effective, patient-centered, timely, efficient, and equitable.

Additionally, without ongoing tracking to assess progress in meeting the six aims, policy makers, leaders within the health professions and health organizations, purchasers, and consumers will be unable to determine progress or understand where improvement efforts have succeeded and where further work is most needed. The National Quality Report has the potential to play an important role in continuing to raise the awareness of the American public about the quality-of-care challenges facing the health care system. Public awareness of shortcomings in quality is critical to securing public support for the steps that must be taken to address these concerns.

> Recommendation 3: Congress should continue to authorize and appropriate funds for, and the Department of Health and Human Services should move forward expeditiously with the establishment of, monitoring and tracking processes for use in evaluating the progress of the health system in pursuit of the above-cited

aims of safety, effectiveness, patient-centeredness, timeliness, efficiency, and equity. The Secretary of the Department of Health and Human Services should report annually to Congress and the President on the quality of care provided to the American people.

The committee applauds Congress and the Administration for their current efforts to establish a National Quality Report for tracking the quality of care. Ongoing input from the many public- and private-sector associations, professional groups, and others involved in quality measurement and improvement will contribute to the success of these efforts. The establishment of specific goals for each of the six aims could further enhance the usefulness of this monitoring and tracking system as a stimulus for performance improvement. Continued funding for this activity should be ensured, as well as regular reports that communicate progress to all concerned. It should be noted that although this report focuses only on health care for individuals, the previous overarching statement of purpose and six aims for improvement are sufficiently robust that they can be applied equally to decisions and evaluations at the population-health level.

Formulating New Rules to Redesign and Improve Care

As discussed earlier, improved performance will depend on new system designs. The committee believes it would be neither useful nor possible for us to specify in detail the design of 21st-century health care delivery systems. Imagination and valuable pluralism abound at the local level in the nation's health care enterprise. At the same time, we believe local efforts to implement innovation and achieve improvement can benefit from a set of simple rules to guide the redesign of the health care system.

In formulating these rules, the committee has been guided by the belief that care must be delivered by systems that are carefully and consciously designed to provide care that is safe, effective, patient-centered, timely, efficient, and equitable. Such systems must be designed to serve the needs of patients, and to ensure that they are fully informed, retain control and participate in care delivery whenever possible, and receive care that is respectful of their values and preferences. Such systems must facilitate the application of scientific knowledge to practice, and provide clinicians with the tools and supports necessary to deliver evidence-based care consistently and safely.

> Recommendation 4: Private and public purchasers, health care organizations, clinicians, and

patients should work together to redesign health care processes in accordance with the following rules:

1. *Care based on continuous healing relationships.* Patients should receive care whenever they need it and in many forms, not just face-to-face visits. This rule implies that the health care system should be responsive at all times (24 hours a day, every day) and that access to care should be provided over the Internet, by telephone, and by other means in addition to face-to-face visits.

2. *Customization based on patient needs and values.* The system of care should be designed to meet the most common types of needs, but have the capability to respond to individual patient choices and preferences.

3. *The patient as the source of control.* Patients should be given the necessary information and the opportunity to exercise the degree of control they choose over health care decisions that affect them. The health system should be able to accommodate differences in patient preferences and encourage shared decision making.

4. *Shared knowledge and the free flow of information.* Patients should have unfettered access to their own medical information and to clinical knowledge. Clinicians and patients should communicate effectively and share information.

5. *Evidence-based decision making.* Patients should receive care based on the best available scientific knowledge. Care should not vary illogically from clinician to clinician or from place to place.

6. *Safety as a system property.* Patients should be safe from injury caused by the care system. Reducing risk and ensuring safety require greater attention to systems that help prevent and mitigate errors.

7. *The need for transparency.* The health care system should make information available to patients and their families that allows them to make informed decisions when selecting a health plan, hospital, or clinical practice, or choosing among alternative treatments. This should include information

describing the system's performance on safety, evidence-based practice, and patient satisfaction.

8. *Anticipation of needs.* The health system should anticipate patient needs, rather than simply reacting to events.

9. *Continuous decrease in waste.* The health system should not waste resources or patient time.

10. *Cooperation among clinicians.* Clinicians and institutions should actively collaborate and communicate to ensure an appropriate exchange of information and coordination of care.

These rules will lead the redesign effort in the right direction, guiding the innovation required to achieve the aims for improvement outlined earlier. Widespread application of these ten rules, each grounded in both logic and varying degrees of evidence, will represent a new paradigm for health care delivery. As the redesign effort moves forward, it will be important to assess not only progress toward meeting the aims, but also the specific effects attributable to the new rules and to adapt the rules as appropriate.

Design ideas are not enough, however. To initiate the process of change, both an action agenda and resources are needed.

Taking the First Steps

The committee recognizes the enormity of the change that will be required to achieve a substantial improvement in the nation's health care system. Although steps can be taken immediately to apply the ten rules set forth previously to the redesign of health care, widespread application will require commitment to the provision of evidence-based care that is responsive to individual patients' needs and preferences. Well-designed and well-run systems of care will be required as well. These changes will occur most rapidly in an environment in which public policy and market forces are aligned and in which the change process is supported by an appropriate information technology infrastructure.

To initiate the process of change, the committee believes the health care system must focus greater attention on the development of care processes for the common conditions that afflict many people. A limited number of such conditions, about 15 to 25, account for the majority of health care services (Centers for Disease Control and Prevention, 1999; Medical Expenditure Panel Survey, 2000; Ray et al., 2000). Nearly all of these conditions are chronic. By focusing attention on a limited number of common conditions, the committee believes it will be possible to make sizable improvements in the quality of care received by many individuals within the coming decade.

Health care for chronic conditions is very different from care for acute episodic illnesses. Care for the chronically ill needs to be a collaborative, multidisciplinary process. Effective methods of communication, both among caregivers and between caregivers and patients, are critical to providing high-quality care. Personal health information must accompany patients as they transition from home to clinical office setting to hospital to nursing home and back.

Carefully designed, evidence-based care processes, supported by automated clinical information and decision support systems, offer the greatest promise of achieving the best outcomes from care for chronic conditions. Some efforts are now under way to synthesize the clinical evidence pertaining to common chronic conditions and to make this information available to consumers and clinicians on the Web and by other means (Lindberg and Humphreys, 1999). In addition, evidence-based practice guidelines have been developed for many chronic conditions (Eisenberg, 2000). Yet studies of the quality of care document tremendous variability in practice for many such conditions. Given these variations and the prevalence of chronic conditions, these conditions represent an excellent starting point for efforts to better define optimum care or best practices, and to design care processes to meet patient needs. Moreover, such efforts to improve quality must be supported by payment methods that remove barriers to integrated care and provide strong incentives and rewards for improvement.

To facilitate this process, the Agency for Healthcare Research and Quality should identify a limited number of priority conditions that affect many people and account for a sizable portion of the national health burden and associated expenditures. In identifying these priority conditions, the agency should consider using the list of conditions identified through the Medical Expenditure Panel Survey (2000). According to the most recent survey data, the top 15 priority conditions are cancer, diabetes, emphysema, high cholesterol, HIV/AIDS, hypertension, ischemic heart disease, stroke, arthritis, asthma, gall bladder disease, stomach ulcers, back problems, Alzheimer's disease and other dementias, and depression and anxiety disorders. Health care organizations, clinicians, purchasers, and other stakeholders should then work together to (1) organize evidence-based care processes consistent with best practices, (2) organize major prevention programs to target key health risk behaviors associated with the onset or progression of these conditions, (3) develop the information infrastructure needed to support the provision of care and the ongoing measurement of care processes and patient outcomes, and (4) align the incentives inherent in payment and accountability processes with the goal of quality improvement.

> Recommendation 5: The Agency for Healthcare Research and Quality should identify not fewer than 15 priority conditions, taking into account frequency of occurrence, health burden, and resource use. In collaboration with the National Quality Forum, the agency should convene stakeholders, including purchasers, consumers, health care organizations, professional groups, and others, to develop strategies, goals, and action plans for achieving substantial improvements in quality in the next 5 years for each of the priority conditions.

Redirecting the health care industry toward the implementation of well-designed care processes for priority conditions will require significant resources. Capital will be required to invest in enhancing organizational capacity, building an information infrastructure, and training multidisciplinary care teams, among other things. The committee believes it is appropriate for the public sector to take the lead in establishing an innovation fund to seed promising projects, but not to shoulder the full burden of the transition. Private-sector organizations, including foundations, purchasers, health care organizations, and others, should also make investments. High priority should be given to projects that are likely to result in making available in the public domain new programs, tools, and technologies that are broadly applicable throughout the health care sector.

> Recommendation 6: Congress should establish a Health Care Quality Innovation Fund to support projects targeted at (1) achieving the six aims of safety, effectiveness, patient-centeredness, timeliness, efficiency, and equity; and/or (2) producing substantial improvements in quality for the priority conditions. The fund's resources should be invested in projects that will produce a public-domain portfolio of programs, tools, and technologies of widespread applicability.

Americans now invest annually $1.1 trillion, or 13.5 percent, of the nation's gross domestic product (GDP) in the health care sector (Health Care Financing Administration, 1999). This figure is expected to grow to more than $2 trillion, or 16 percent of GDP, by 2007 (Smith et al., 1998). The committee believes a sizable commitment, on the order of $1 billion over 3 to 5 years, is needed to strongly communicate the need for rapid and significant change in the health care system and to help initiate the transition. Just as a vigorous public commitment has led to the mapping of human DNA, a similar commitment is needed to help the nation's health care system achieve the aims for improvement outlined previously.

Building Organizational Supports for Change

Supporting front-line teams that deliver care are many types of health care organizations. Today, these are hospitals, physician practices, clinics, integrated delivery systems, and health plans, but new forms will unquestionably emerge. Whatever those forms, care that is responsive to patient needs and makes consistent use of the best evidence requires far more conscious and careful organization than we find today.

Organizations will need to negotiate successfully six major challenges. The first is to redesign care processes to serve more effectively the needs of the chronically ill for coordinated, seamless care across settings and clinicians and over time. The use of tools to organize and deliver care has lagged far behind biomedical and clinical knowledge. A number of well-understood design principles, drawn from other industries as well as some of today's health care organizations, could help greatly in improving the care that is provided to patients.

A second challenge is making effective use of information technologies to automate clinical information and make it readily accessible to patients and all members of the care team. An improved information infrastructure is needed to establish effective and timely communication among clinicians and between patients and clinicians.

A third challenge is to manage the growing knowledge base and ensure that all those in the health care workforce have the skills they need. Making use of new knowledge requires that health professionals develop new skills or assume new roles. It requires that they use new tools to access and apply the expanding knowledge base. It also requires that training and ongoing licensure and certification reflect the need for lifelong learning and evaluation of competencies.

A fourth challenge for organizations is coordination of care across patient conditions, services, and settings over time. Excellent information technologies and well-thought-out and -implemented modes of ongoing communication can reduce the need to craft laborious, case-by-case strategies for coordinating patient care.

A fifth challenge is to continually advance the effectiveness of teams. Team practice is common, but the training of health professionals is typically isolated by discipline. Making the necessary changes in roles to improve the work of teams is often slowed or stymied by institutional, labor, and financial structures, and by law and custom.

Finally, all organizations—whether or not health care related—can improve their performance only by incorporating care process and outcome measures into their daily work. Use of such measures makes it possible to understand the degree to which performance is consistent with best practices, and the extent to which patients are being helped.

> Recommendation 7: The Agency for Healthcare Research and Quality and private foundations should convene a series of workshops involving representatives from health care and other industries and the research community to identify, adapt, and implement state-of-the-art approaches to addressing the following challenges:

> - Redesign of care processes based on best practices
> - Use of information technologies to improve access to clinical information and support clinical decision making
> - Knowledge and skills management
> - Development of effective teams
> - Coordination of care across patient conditions, services, and settings over time
> - Incorporation of performance and outcome measurements for improvement and accountability

Establishing a New Environment for Care

To enable the profound changes in health care recommended in this report, the *environment* of care must also change. The committee believes the current environment often inhibits the changes needed to achieve quality improvement. Two types of environmental change are needed:

- *Focus and align the environment toward the six aims for improvement.* To effect this set of changes, purchasers and health plans, for example, should eliminate or modify payment practices that fragment the care system, and should establish incentives designed to encourage and reward innovations aimed at improving quality. Purchasers and regulators should also create precise streams of accountability and measurement reflecting achievements in the six aims. Moreover, efforts should be made to help health care consumers understand the aims, why they are important, and how to interpret the levels of performance of various health care systems.

- *Provide, where possible, assets and encouragement for positive change.* For example, national funding agencies could promote research on new designs for the care of priority conditions, state and national activities could be undertaken to facilitate the exchange of best practices and shared learning among health care delivery systems, and a national system for monitoring progress toward the six aims for improvement could help improvement efforts remain on track.

Such environmental changes need to occur in four major areas: the infrastructure that supports the dissemination and application of new clinical knowledge and technologies, the information technology infrastructure, payment policies, and preparation of the health care workforce.

Changes will also be needed in the quality oversight and accountability processes of public and private purchasers. This issue is not addressed here. The IOM will be issuing a separate report on federal quality measurement and improvement programs in Fall 2002. In addition, the National Quality Forum has an extensive effort under way to develop a national framework for quality measurement and accountability and will be issuing a report in Summer 2001.

Applying Evidence to Health Care Delivery

In the current health care system, scientific knowledge about best care is not applied systematically or expeditiously to clinical practice. An average of about 17 years is required for new knowledge generated by randomized controlled trials to be incorporated into practice, and even then application is highly uneven (Balas and Boren, 2000). The extreme variability in practice in clinical areas in which there is strong scientific evidence and a high degree of expert consensus about best practices indicates that current dissemination efforts fail to reach many clinicians and patients, and that there are insufficient tools and incentives to promote rapid adoption of best practices. The time has come to invest in the creation of a more effective infrastructure for the application of knowledge to health care delivery:

> Recommendation 8: The Secretary of the Department of Health and Human Services should be given the responsibility and necessary resources to establish and maintain a comprehensive program aimed at making scientific evidence more useful and accessible to clinicians and patients. In developing this program, the Secretary should work with federal agencies and in collaboration with professional and health care associations, the academic and research

communities, and the National Quality Forum and other organizations involved in quality measurement and accountability.

It is critical that leadership from the private sector, both professional and other health care leaders and consumer representatives, be involved in all aspects of this effort to ensure its applicability and acceptability to clinicians and patients. The infrastructure developed through this public- and private-sector partnership should focus initially on priority conditions and include:

- Ongoing analysis and synthesis of the medical evidence
- Delineation of specific practice guidelines
- Identification of best practices in the design of care processes
- Enhanced dissemination efforts to communicate evidence and guidelines to the general public and professional communities
- Development of decision support tools to assist clinicians and patients in applying the evidence
- Establishment of goals for improvement in care processes and outcomes
- Development of quality measures for priority conditions

More systematic approaches are needed to analyze and synthesize medical evidence for both clinicians and patients. Far more sophisticated clinical decision support systems will be required to assist clinicians and patients in selecting the best treatment options and delivering safe and effective care. Many promising private- and public-sector activities now under way can serve as excellent models and building blocks for a more expanded effort. In particular, the Cochrane Collaboration and the Agency for Healthcare Research and Quality's Evidence-Based Practice Centers represent important efforts to synthesize medical evidence. The growth of the Internet has also opened up many new opportunities to make evidence more accessible to clinicians and consumers. The efforts of the National Library of Medicine to facilitate access to the medical literature by both consumers and health care professionals and to design Web sites that organize large amounts of information on particular health needs are particularly promising.

The development of a more effective infrastructure to synthesize and organize evidence around priority conditions would also offer new opportunities to enhance quality measurement and reporting. A stronger and more organized evidence base should facilitate the adoption of best practices, as well as the development of valid and reliable quality measures for priority conditions that could be used for both internal quality improvement and external accountability.

Using Information Technology

Health care delivery has been relatively untouched by the revolution in information technology that has been transforming nearly every other aspect of society. The majority of patient and clinician encounters take place for purposes of exchanging clinical information: patients share information with clinicians about their general health, symptoms, and concerns, and clinicians use their knowledge and skills to respond with pertinent medical information, and in many cases reassurance. Yet it is estimated that only a small fraction of physicians offer email interaction, a simple and convenient tool for efficient communication, to their patients (Hoffman, 1997).

The meticulous collection of personal health information throughout a patient's life can be one of the most important inputs to the provision of proper care. Yet for most individuals, that health information is dispersed in a collection of paper records that are poorly organized and often illegible, and frequently cannot be retrieved in a timely fashion, making it nearly impossible to manage many forms of chronic illness that require frequent monitoring and ongoing patient support.

Although growth in clinical knowledge and technology has been profound, many health care settings lack basic computer systems to provide clinical information or support clinical decision making. The development and application of more sophisticated information systems is essential to enhance quality and improve efficiency.

The Internet has enormous potential to transform health care through information technology applications in such areas as consumer health, clinical care, administrative and financial transactions, public health, professional education, and biomedical and health services research (National Research Council, 2000). Many of these applications are currently within reach, including remote medical consultation with patients in their homes or offices; consumer and clinician access to the medical literature; creation of "communities" of patients and clinicians with shared interests; consumer access to information on health plans, participating providers, eligibility for procedures, and covered drugs in a formulary; and videoconferencing among public health officials during emergency situations. Other applications are more experimental, such as simulation of surgical procedures; consultation among providers involving manipulation of digital images; and control of experimental equipment, such as electron microscopes.

The Internet also supports rising interest among consumers in information and convenience in all areas of commerce, including health care. The number of Americans who use the Internet to retrieve health-related information is estimated to be about 70 million (Cain et al., 2000). Consumers access health-related Web sites to research an illness or disease; seek information on nutrition and fitness; research drugs and their interactions; and search for doctors, hospitals, and online medical support groups.

The committee believes information technology must play a central role in the redesign of the health care system if a substantial improvement in quality is to be achieved over the coming decade. Automation of clinical, financial, and administrative transactions is essential to improving quality, preventing errors, enhancing consumer confidence in the health system, and improving efficiency.

Central to many information technology applications is the automation of patient-specific clinical information. A fully electronic medical record, including all types of patient information, is not needed to achieve many, if not most, of the benefits of automated clinical data. Sizable benefits can be derived in the near future from automating certain types of data, such as medication orders. Efforts to automate clinical information date back several decades, but progress has been slow (Institute of Medicine, 1991), in part because of the barriers and risks involved. An important constraint is that consumers and policy makers share concerns about the privacy and confidentiality of these data (Cain et al., 2000; Goldman, 1998). The United States also lacks national standards for the capture, storage, communication, processing, and presentation of health information (Work Group on Computerization of Patient Records, 2000).

The challenges of applying information technology to health care should not be underestimated. Health care is undoubtedly one of the most, if not the most, complex sector of the economy. The number of different types of transactions (i.e., patient needs, interactions, and services) is very large. Sizable capital investments and multiyear commitments to building systems will be required. Widespread adoption of many information technology applications will require behavioral adaptations on the part of large numbers of patients, clinicians, and organizations. Yet, the Internet is rapidly transforming many aspects of society, and many health-related processes stand to be reshaped as well.

In the absence of a national commitment and financial support to build a national health information infrastructure, the committee believes that progress on quality improvement will be painfully slow. The automation of clinical, financial, and administrative information and the electronic sharing of such information among clinicians, patients, and appropriate others within a secure environment are critical if the 21st-century health care system envisioned by the committee is to be realized.

> Recommendation 9: Congress, the executive
> branch, leaders of health care organizations,

public and private purchasers, and health informatics associations and vendors should make a renewed national commitment to building an information infrastructure to support health care delivery, consumer health, quality measurement and improvement, public accountability, clinical and health services research, and clinical education. This commitment should lead to the elimination of most handwritten clinical data by the end of the decade.

Aligning Payment Policies with Quality Improvement

Current payment methods do not adequately encourage or support the provision of quality health care. Although payment is not the only factor that influences provider and patient behavior, it is an important one.

All payment methods affect behavior and quality. For example, fee-for-service payment methods for physicians and hospitals raise concerns about potential overuse of services—the provision of services that may not be necessary or may expose the patient to greater potential harm than benefit. On the other hand, capitation and per case payment methods for physicians and hospitals raise questions about potential underuse—the failure to provide services from which the patient would likely benefit. Indeed, no payment method perfectly aligns financial incentives with the goal of quality improvement for all health care decision makers, including clinicians, hospitals, and patients. This is one reason for the widespread interest in blended methods of payment designed to counter the disadvantages of one payment method with the advantages of another.

Too little attention has been paid to the careful analysis and alignment of payment incentives with quality improvement. The current health care environment is replete with examples of payment policies that work against the efforts of clinicians, health care administrators, and others to improve quality. The following example, presented at an Institute of Medicine workshop on payment and quality held on April 24, 2000,[2] illustrates how payment policies can work against the efforts of clinicians, health care administrators, and others to improve quality:

A physician group paid primarily on a fee-for-service basis instituted a new program to im-

prove blood sugar control for diabetic patients. Specifically, pilot studies suggested that tighter diabetic management could decrease hemoglobin Alc levels by 2 percentage points for about 40 percent of all diabetic patients managed by the physician group. Data from two randomized controlled trials demonstrated that better sugar controls should translate into lower rates of retinopathy, nephropathy, peripheral neurological damage, and heart disease. The savings in direct health care costs (i.e., reduced visits and hospital episodes) from avoided complications have been estimated to generate a net savings of about $2,000 per patient per year, on average, over 15 years. Across the more than 13,000 diabetic patients managed by the physician group, the project had the potential to generate over $10 million in net savings each year. The project was costly to the medical group in two ways. First, expenses to conduct the project, including extra clinical time for tighter management, fell to the physician group. Second, over time, as diabetic complication rates fell, the project would reduce patient visits and, thus, revenues as well. But the savings from avoided complications would accrue to the insurer or a self-funded purchaser.

The committee believes that all purchasers, both public and private, should carefully reexamine their payment policies.

> Recommendation 10: Private and public purchasers should examine their current payment methods to remove barriers that currently impede quality improvement, and to build in stronger incentives for quality enhancement.

Payment methods should:

- Provide fair payment for good clinical management of the types of patients seen. Clinicians should be adequately compensated for taking good care of all types of patients, neither gaining nor losing financially for caring for sicker patients or those with more complicated conditions. The risk of random incidence of disease in the population should reside with a larger risk pool, whether that be large groups of providers, health plans, or insurance companies.
- Provide an opportunity for providers to share in the benefits of quality improvement. Rewards should be located close to the level at which the reengineering and

---

[2]This case study has been excerpted from a paper prepared by and presented at the IOM workshop by Brent James, Intermountain Health Care, Salt Lake City, Utah, April 2000.

process redesign needed to improve quality are likely to take place.

- Provide the opportunity for consumers and purchasers to recognize quality differences in health care and direct their decisions accordingly. In particular, consumers need to have good information on quality and the ability to use that information as they see fit to meet their needs.
- Align financial incentives with the implementation of care processes based on best practices and the achievement of better patient outcomes. Substantial improvements in quality are most likely to be obtained when providers are highly motivated and rewarded for carefully designing and fine-tuning care processes to achieve increasingly higher levels of safety, effectiveness, patient-centeredness, timeliness, efficiency, and equity.
- Reduce fragmentation of care. Payment methods should not pose a barrier to providers' ability to coordinate care for patients across settings and over time.

To assist purchasers in the redesign of payment policy based on these fundamental principles, a vigorous program of pilot testing and evaluating alternative design options should be pursued.

> Recommendation 11: The Health Care Financing Administration and the Agency for Healthcare Research and Quality, with input from private payers, health care organizations, and clinicians, should develop a research agenda to identify, pilot test, and evaluate various options for better aligning current payment methods with quality improvement goals.

Examples of possible means of achieving this end include blended methods of payment for providers, multiyear contracts, payment modifications to encourage use of electronic interaction among clinicians and between clinicians and patients, risk adjustment, bundled payments for priority conditions, and alternative approaches for addressing the capital investments needed to improve quality.

Preparing the Workforce

A major challenge in transitioning to the health care system of the 21st century envisioned by the committee is preparing the workforce to acquire new skills and adopt new ways of relating to patients and each other. At least three approaches can be taken to support the workforce in this transition. One is to redesign the way health professionals are trained to emphasize the aims for improvement set forth earlier, including teaching evidence-based practice and using multidisciplinary approaches. Second is to modify the ways in which health pro-

fessionals are regulated to facilitate the needed changes in care delivery. Scope-of-practice acts and other workforce regulations need to allow for innovation in the use of all types of clinicians to meet patient needs in the most effective and efficient way possible. Third is to examine how the liability system can constructively support changes in care delivery while remaining part of an overall approach to accountability for health care professionals and organizations. All three approaches are important and require additional study.

> Recommendation 12: A multidisciplinary summit of leaders within the health professions should be held to discuss and develop strategies for (1) restructuring clinical education to be consistent with the principles of the 21st-century health system throughout the continuum of undergraduate, graduate, and continuing education for medical, nursing, and other professional training programs; and (2) assessing the implications of these changes for provider credentialing programs, funding, and sponsorship of education programs for health professionals.

> Recommendation 13: The Agency for Healthcare Research and Quality should fund research to evaluate how the current regulatory and legal systems (1) facilitate or inhibit the changes needed for the 21st-century health care delivery system, and (2) can be modified to support health care professionals and organizations that seek to accomplish the six aims set forth in Chapter 2.

SUMMARY

The changes needed to realize a substantial improvement in health care involve the health care system as a whole. The new rules set forth in this report will affect the role, self-image, and work of front-line doctors, nurses, and all other staff. The needed new infrastructures will challenge today's health care leaders—both clinical leaders and management. The necessary environmental changes will require the interest and commitment of payers, health plans, government officials, and regulatory and accrediting bodies. New skills will require new approaches by professional educators. The 21st-century health care system envisioned by the committee—providing care that is evidence-based, patient-centered, and systems-oriented—also implies new roles and responsibilities for patients and their families, who must become more aware, more participative, and more demanding in a care system that should be meeting their needs. And all involved must be united by the overarching purpose of reducing the burden of illness, injury, and disability in our nation.

American health care is beset by serious problems, but they are not intractable. Perfect care may be a long way off, but much better care is within our grasp. The committee envisions a system that uses the best knowledge, that is focused intensely on patients, and that works across health care providers and settings. Taking advantage of new information technologies will be an important catalyst to moving us beyond where we are today. The committee believes that achieving such a system is both possible and necessary.

REFERENCES

Advisory Commission on Consumer Protection and Quality in the Health Care Industry. 1998. "Quality First: Better Health Care for All Americans." Online. Available at http://www.hcqualitycommission.gov/final/ [accessed Sept. 9, 2000].

Balas, E. Andrew and Suzanne A. Boren. Managing Clinical Knowledge for Health Care Improvement. *Yearbook of Medical Informatics.* National Library of Medicine, Bethesda, MD:65–70, 2000.

Cain, Mary M., Robert Mittman, Jane Sarasohn-Kahn, and Jennifer C. Wayne. *Health e-People: The Online Consumer Experience.* Oakland, CA: Institute for the Future, California Health Care Foundation, 2000.

Centers for Disease Control and Prevention. 1999. "Chronic Diseases and Their Risk Factors: The Nation's Leading Causes of Death." Online. Available at http://www.cdc.gov/nccdphp/statbookl statbook.htm [accessed Dec. 7, 2000].

Chassin, Mark R. Is Health Care Ready for Six Sigma Quality? *Milbank Quarterly* 76(4):575–91, 1998.

Chassin, Mark R., Robert W. Galvin, and the National Roundtable on Health Care Quality. The Urgent Need to Improve Health Care Quality. *JAMA* 280(11):1000–5, 1998.

Colby, David C. Doctors and their Discontents. *Health Affairs* 16(6):112–4, 1997.

Copeland, C. Prescription Drugs: Issues of Cost, Coverage and Quality. *EBRI Issue Brief* April(208):1–21, 1999.

Donelan, Karen, Robert J. Blendon, Cathy Schoen, et al. The Cost of Health System Change: Public Discontent in Five Nations. *Health Affairs* 18(3):206–16, 1999.

Egger, Ed. Nurse Shortage Worse Than You Think, But Sensitivity May Help Retain Nurses. *Health Care Strategic Management* 18(5):16–8, 2000.

Eisenberg, John M. Quality Research for Quality Healthcare: The Data Connection. *Health Services Research* 35:xii–xvii, 2000.

Goldman, Janlori. Protecting Privacy to Improve Health Care. *Health Affairs* 17(6):47–60, 1998.

Guterman, Stuart. The Balanced Budget Act of 1997: Will Hospitals Take a Hit on Their PPS Margins? *Health Affairs* 17(1):159–66, 1998.

Health Care Financing Administration. 1999. "1998 National Health Expenditures. Department of Health and Human Services. Washington, DC." Online. Available at http://www.hcfa.gov/stats/nhe-oact/hilites.htm [accessed Jan. 10, 2000].

Hoffman, A. Take 2 and E-mail me in the Morning: Doctors Consult Patients Electronically. *New York Times.* June 3, 1997.

Hoffman, Catherine, Dorothy P. Rice, and Hai-Yen Sung. Persons with Chronic Conditions. Their Prevalence and Costs. *JAMA* 276(18):1473–9, 1996.

Institute of Medicine *The Computer-Based Patient Record: An Essential Technology for Health Care.* Richard S. Dick and Elaine B. Steen, eds. Washington, D.C.: National Academy Press, 1991.

—— *Ensuring Quality Cancer Care.* Maria Hewitt and Joseph V. Simone, eds. Washington, D.C.: National Academy Press, 1999.

—— *America's Health Care Safety Net. Intact but Endangered.* Marion E. Lewin and Stuart Altman, eds. Washington, D.C.: National Academy Press, 2000a.

—— *To Err Is Human: Building a Safer Health System.* Linda T. Kohn, Janet M. Corrigan, and Molla S. Donaldson, eds. Washington, D.C: National Academy Press, 2000b.

Lindberg, Donald A. B. and Betsy L. Humphreys. A Time of Change for Medical Informatics in the USA. *Yearbook of Medical Informatics* National Library of Medicine, Bethesda, MD:53–7, 1999.

Medical Expenditure Panel Survey. 2000. "MEPS HC-006R: 1996 Medical Conditions." Online. Available at http://www.meps.ahrq.gov/catlist.htm [accessed Dec. 7, 2000].

National Institutes of Health. 2000. "An Overview." Online. Available at http://www.nih.gov/about/NIHoverview.html [accessed Aug. 11, 2000].

National Research Council. *Networking Health: Prescriptions for the Internet.* Washington, DC: National Academy Press, 2000.

Pharmaceutical Research and Manufacturers of America. 2000. "PhRMA Annual Report, 2000–2001." Online. Available at http://www.phrma.org/ publications/publications/annual2000/ [accessed Nov. 11, 2000].

Picker Institute and American Hospital Association. *Eye on Patients Report.* 1996.

Ray, G. Thomas, Tracy Lieu, Bruce Fireman, et al. The Cost of Health Conditions in a Health Maintenance Organization. *Medical Care Research and Review* 57(1):92–109, 2000.

Reed, Marie C. and Robert F. St. Peter *Satisfaction and Quality: Patient and Physician Perspectives.* Washington, D.C.: Center for Studying Health System Change, 1997.

Schuster, Mark A., Elizabeth A. McGlynn, and Robert H Brook. How Good is the Quality of Health Care in the United States? *The Milbank Quarterly* 76(4):517–63, 1998.

Shindul-Rothschild, Judith, Diane Berry, and Ellen Long-Middleton. Where Have All the Nurses Gone? Final Results of Our Patient Care Survey. *American Journal of Nursing* 96(11):25–39, 1996.

Smith, Sheila, Mark Freeland, Stephen Heffler, et al. The Next Ten Years of Health Spending: What Does the Future Hold? *Health Affairs* 17(3):128–40, 1998.

Taylor, Humphrey. 2001. "Harris Poll #3, Most People Continue to Think Well of Their Health Plans." Online. Available at http://www.harrisblackintl. com/ harris_poll/index.asp [accessed Jan. 11, 2001].

The Robert Wood Johnson Foundation. *Chronic Care in America: A 21st Century Challenge.* Princeton, NJ: The Robert Wood Johnson Foundation, 1996. Online. Available at http://www.rwjf.org/library/chrcare/ [accessed Sept. 19, 2000].

U.S. Census Bureau. Health Insurance Coverage: 1999. *Current Population Survey.* by Robert J. Mills. Washington, D.C.: U.S. Census Bureau. September, 2000. Online. Available at: *http://* www.census.gov/hhes/www/hlthin99.html [accessed Jan. 22, 2001].

Wagner, Edward H., Brian T. Austin, and Michael Von Korff. Organizing Care for Patients with Chronic Illness. *Milbank Quarterly* 74(4):511–42, 1996.

Work Group on Computerization of Patient Records. *Toward a National Health Information Infrastructure: Report of the Work Group on Computerization of Patient Records.* Washington, D.C.: U.S. Department of Health and Human Services, 2000.

The Quality of Health Care Delivered to Adults in the United States

Elizabeth A. McGlynn, Steven M. Asch, John Adams, Joan Keesey, Jennifer Hicks, Alison DeCristofaro, and Eve A. Kerr

Source: Copyright © 2003 Massachusetts Medical Society. All Rights Reserved. The Quality of Health Care Delivered to Adults in the United States. Elizabeth A. McGlynn, PhD, Steven M. Asch, MD, MPH, John Adams, PhD, Joan Keesey, BA, Jennifer Hicks, MPH, PhD, Alison DeCristofaro, MPH, and Eve A. Kerr, MD, MPH. The New England Journal of Medicine, 348, 26:2635 (June 26, 2003).

ABSTRACT

Background

We have little systematic information about the extent to which standard processes involved in health care—a key element of quality—are delivered in the United States.

Methods

We telephoned a random sample of adults living in 12 metropolitan areas in the United States and asked them about selected health care experiences. We also received written consent to copy their medical records for the most recent two-year period and used this information to evaluate performance on 439 indicators of quality of care for 30 acute and chronic conditions as well as preventive care. We then constructed aggregate scores.

Results

Participants received 54.9 percent (95 percent confidence interval, 54.3 to 55.5) of recommended care. We found little difference among the proportion of recommended preventive care provided (54.9 percent), the proportion of recommended acute care provided (53.5 percent), and the proportion of rec-ommended care provided for chronic conditions (56.1 percent). Among different medical functions, adherence to the processes involved in care ranged from 52.2 percent for screening to 58.5 percent for follow-up care. Quality varied substantially according to the particular medical condition, ranging from 78.7 percent of recommended care (95 percent confidence interval, 73.3 to 84.2) for senile cataract to 10.5 percent of recommended care (95 percent confidence interval, 6.8 to 14.6) for alcohol dependence.

Conclusions

The deficits we have identified in adherence to recommended processes for basic care pose serious threats to the health of the American public. Strategies to reduce these deficits in care are warranted.

The degree to which health care in the United States is consistent with basic quality standards is largely unknown.[1,2] Although previous studies have documented serious quality deficits, they provide a limited perspective on the issue.[3–5] Most have assessed a single condition,[6,7] a small number of indicators of quality,[8,9] persons with a single type of insurance coverage,[10] or persons receiving care in a small geographic area.[11,12] The few national studies have been limited to specific segments of the population, such as Medicare beneficiaries[13–15] or enrollees in managed-care plans[16]; have focused on a limited set of topics, such as preventive care,[17] diabetes,[18] or human immunodeficiency virus[19]; or have assessed health outcomes without a link to specific processes involved in care.[20] As a result, we have no comprehensive view of the level of quality of care given to the average person in the United States. This information gap contributes to a persistent belief that quality is not a serious national problem.[1]

In this article, we report results from the Community Quality Index (CQI) study, a collateral study of the Community Tracking Study (CTS).[21] The CTS, conducted by the Center for Studying Health System Change (CSHSC), monitors changes in health care markets in the United States. The CTS obtains self-reported information from a random sample of the U.S. population on their insurance coverage, patterns of utilization of health care services, and health status. The CSHSC has reported on trends in health care costs,[22] factors affecting the choice of employer-sponsored or public insurance,[23] and changes in the structure of managed-care plans.[24] However, the CTS lacks detailed information about the implications of these variations in health care markets for the quality of health care. By collaborating with the CSHSC, we were able to assess the extent to which the recommended processes of medical care—one critical dimension of quality—are delivered to a representative sample of the U.S. population for a broad spectrum of conditions.

METHODS

Recruitment of Participants

In 12 metropolitan areas (Boston; Cleveland; Greenville, S.C.; Indianapolis; Lansing, Mich.; Little Rock, Ark; Miami; Newark, N.J.; Orange County, Calif.; Phoenix, Ariz.; Seattle; and Syracuse, N.Y.), using random-digit-dial telephone surveys, the CTS deliberately recruited enough participants to assess how structural characteristics in each market (e.g., the penetration of managed care) affect patterns of access to and utilization of health care services. Between October 1998 and August 2000, we recontacted by telephone households that had participated in the CTS interviews. Participants were asked to complete a telephone interview regarding their health history and to provide a listing of all individual or institutional health care providers whom they had seen during the previous two years. Participants who orally agreed to provide access to their medical records were sent written consent forms to sign and return to RAND. Photocopies of the medical records of participants providing written consent were sent to RAND for central abstracting.

Response Rates

Because of the complex, multistage nature of the study design, several calculations of the response rate are provided. Among the 20,028 adults in the initial sample, 2091 (10 percent) were deemed ineligible, primarily because they had left the area. Among the 17,937 eligible adults, 13,275 (74 percent) participated in the telephone interview regarding their health history,

including 863 (7 percent) who had had no visits to a health care provider during the previous two years. Among the 12,412 participants who had had visits, 10,404 (84 percent) agreed orally to provide access to their medical records. We obtained written consent from 7528 (61 percent of those with visits to a provider). Participants reported having seen between 1 and 17 providers (mean, 2.6) during the study period. We obtained at least one record for 6712 (89 percent) of those who returned their consent forms. Overall, we received 84 percent of the records for which we had consent forms; we received all expected records for 4612 of the 6712 participants with consent forms and records (69 percent) and all but one record for 1547 of these participants (23 percent). Sensitivity analyses revealed few differences in results related to the completeness of records, so all participants for whom we obtained at least one record were included in the results we report (37 percent of the sample of eligible adults).

Development of Indicators of Quality

The indicators of quality used in the study were derived from RAND's Quality Assessment Tools system.[25] RAND staff members selected acute and chronic conditions that represented the leading causes of illness, death, and utilization of health care in each age group, as well as preventive care related to these causes. For each condition, staff physicians reviewed established national guidelines and the medical literature and proposed indicators of quality for all phases of care or medical functions (screening, diagnosis, treatment, and follow-up). We developed indicators to assess potential problems with the overuse and underuse of key processes. We primarily chose measures of processes as indicators, because they represent the activities that clinicians control most directly, because they do not generally require risk adjustment beyond the specification of eligibility, and because they are consistent with the structure of national guidelines.[5,26]

Four nine-member, multispecialty expert panels were convened to assess the validity of the indicators proposed by the staff, using the RAND-UCLA modified Delphi method.[27] The members of the panels, nominated by the appropriate specialty societies, were diverse with respect to geography, practice setting, and sex. Indicators were rated on a 9-point scale (with 1 denoting not valid and 9 very valid). Only indicators with a median validity score of 7 or higher were included in the Quality Assessment Tools system. This method of selecting indicators is reliable[28] and has been shown to have content, construct, and predictive validity in other applications.[29–32]

The criteria for the selection of conditions, reviews of the literature, the process followed by the panels, and the final indicators have been published elsewhere.[33–36] (Further information on all the quality indicators used in this study is available at http://www.rand.org/health/mcglynn_appa.pdf or from the National Auxiliary Publications Service.*) Table 8-1 provides a brief description and classifications for a sample of the indicators we used. The classifications enabled us to examine quality from the perspective of what is being done (type of care), why it is being done (function), how it is being delivered (mode), and the nature of the quality problem (underuse or overuse). Results are based on 439 indicators for 30 conditions and preventive care.

---

*See NAPS document no. 05610 for 50 pages of supplementary material. To order, contact NAPS, c/o Microfiche Publications, 248 Hempstead Tpke,. West Hempstead, NY 11552.

TABLE 8-1 Selected Quality-of-Care Indicators and Classifications Used in the Community Quality Index Study*

Condition†	Description of Selected Indicator	Classification for Aggregate Scores			
		Type of Care	Function	Mode	Problem With Quality
Alcohol dependence (5 indicators)					
Indicator 2	Assessment of alcohol dependence among regular or binge drinkers	For chronic condition	Diagnosis	History	Underuse
Indicator 4	Treatment referral for persons given a diagnosis of alcohol dependence	For chronic condition	Treatment	Encounter or other intervention	Underuse
Asthma (25 indicators)					
Indicator 4	Long-acting agents for patients with frequent use of short-acting beta-agonists	For chronic condition	Treatment	Medication	Underuse
Indicator 6	Inhaled corticosteroids for patients receiving long-term systemic corticosteroid therapy	For chronic condition	Treatment	Medication	Underuse
Breast cancer (9 indicators)					
Indicator 1	Appropriate follow-up of palpable mass	For chronic condition	Diagnosis	Laboratory testing or radiography	Underuse
Indicator 5	Choice of surgical treatments for stage I or II cancer	For chronic condition	Treatment	Surgery	Underuse
Cerebrovascular disease (10 indicators)					
Indicator 4	Antiplatelet therapy for noncardiac stroke or transient ischemic attack	For chronic condition	Treatment	Medication	Underuse
Indicator 5	Carotid imaging for patients with symptomatic cardiovascular disease or transient ischemic attack	For chronic condition	Diagnosis	Laboratory testing or radiography	Underuse
Colorectal cancer (12 indicators)					
Indicator 1	Screening for high-risk patients starting at 40 yr of age	Preventive	Screening	Laboratory testing or radiography	Underuse
Indicator 7	Appropriate surgical treatment	For chronic condition	Treatment	Surgery	Underuse
Congestive heart failure (36 indicators)					
Indicator 1	Ejection fraction assessed before medical therapy	For chronic condition	Diagnosis	Laboratory testing or radiography	Underuse
Indicator 32	ACE inhibitors for patients with congestive heart failure and an ejection fraction < 40%	For chronic condition	Treatment	Medication	Underuse
Coronary artery disease (37 indicators)					
Indicator 3	Counseling on smoking cessation	For chronic condition	Treatment	Counseling or education	Underuse
Indicator 11	Avoidance of nifedipine for patients with an acute myocardial infarction	For chronic condition	Treatment	Medication	Overuse

continues

TABLE 8-1 Selected Quality-of-Care Indicators and Classifications Used in the Community Quality Index Study (continued)

Condition[†]	Description of Selected Indicator	Type of Care	Function	Mode	Problem With Quality
			Classification for Aggregate Scores		
Diabetes (13 indicators)					
Indicator 9	Diet and exercise counseling	For chronic condition	Treatment	Counseling or education	Underuse
Indicator 12	Angiotensin-converting enzyme inhibitors for patients with proteinuria	For chronic condition	Treatment	Medication	Underuse
Headache (21 indicators)					
Indicator 11	CT or MRI for patients with new-onset headache and an abnormal neurologic examination	Acute	Diagnosis	Laboratory testing or radiography	Underuse
Indicator 15	Use of appropriate first-line agents for patients with acute migraine	Acute	Treatment	Medication	Overuse
Hip fracture (9 indicators)					
Indicator 6	Prophylactic antibiotics given on day of hip-repair surgery	Acute	Treatment	Medication	Underuse
Indicator 7	Prophylactic antithrombotic drugs given on admission for patients with hip fracture	Acute	Treatment	Medication	Underuse
Hyperlipidemia (7 indicators)					
Indicator 4	Treatment of high LDL cholesterol levels in patients with coronary artery disease	For chronic condition	Treatment	Medication	Underuse
Hypertension (27 indicators)					
Indicator 16	Lifestyle modification for patients with mild hypertension	For chronic condition	Treatment	Counseling or education	Underuse
Indicator 18	Pharmacotherapy for uncontrolled mild hypertension	For chronic condition	Treatment	Medication	Underuse
Indicator 27	Change in treatment when blood pressure is persistently uncontrolled	For chronic condition	Follow-up	Medication	Underuse
Acute low back pain (6 indicators)					
Indicator 1	Rule out cancer, fracture, infection, cauda equina syndrome, and neurologic causes	Acute	Diagnosis	History	Underuse
Indicator 6	Avoidance of prolonged bed rest	Acute	Treatment	Other	Overuse
Preventive care (38 indicators)					
Indicator 1	Screening for problem drinking	Preventive	Screening	History	Underuse
Indicator 2	Mammographic screening for breast cancer	Preventive	Screening	Laboratory testing or radiography	Underuse
Indicator 3	Screening for colorectal cancer in persons at average risk	Preventive	Screening	Laboratory testing or radiography	Underuse
Indicator 8	Influenza vaccine for persons ≥ yr of age	Preventive	Treatment	Immunization	Underuse
Indicator 21	HIV testing for those at risk	Preventive	Screening	Laboratory testing or radiography	Underuse
Indicator 25	Screening for cervical cancer	Preventive		Laboratory testing or radiography	Underuse

continues

TABLE 8-1 Selected Quality-of-Care Indicators and Classifications Used in the Community Quality Index Study (continued)

Condition[†]	Description of Selected Indicator	Classification for Aggregate Scores			
		Type of Care	Function	Mode	Problem With Quality
Indicator 29	Smoking status documented	Preventive	Screening	History	Underuse
Indicator 31	Annual advice for smokers to quit smoking	Preventive	Screening Treatment	Counseling or education	Underuse
Sexually transmitted diseases (26 indicators)					
Indicator 9	Chlamydia screening for high-risk women	Preventive	Screening	Laboratory testing or radiography	Underuse
Indicator 24	HIV screening in patients with sexually transmitted diseases	Acute		Laboratory testing or radiography	Underuse

* ACE denotes angiotensin-converting enzyme, CT computed tomography, MRI magnetic resonance imaging, LDL low-density lipoprotein, and HIV human immuno-deficiency virus.
† The number of indicators given in parentheses after each condition is the total number of indicators of quality of care for that condition; the indicators listed below each condition are examples.

Health History Interview

We obtained selective information directly from respondents to augment information in their medical records. The health history took an average of 13 minutes to complete. The data obtained in this interview were used to refine the analysis of a respondent's eligibility for inclusion in the analysis or to augment the scoring for 22 of the 439 indicators. For example, we used reports of symptoms from participants with asthma to classify those with moderate-to-severe disease. We augmented scores for influenza or pneumococcal immunizations and screening for cancer on the basis of self-reports.

Abstracting of Charts

We developed computer-assisted abstraction software on a Visual Basic platform (version 6.0, Microsoft). The software allowed the manual abstraction of charts to be tailored to the specific record being reviewed and provided interactive checks of the quality of the data (for consistency and range), calculations (e.g., the determination of the presence of high blood pressure), and classifications (e.g., the determination of drug class) during abstraction.

Data for the study were abstracted by 20 trained registered nurses who had successfully abstracted a complex standard chart after a two-week training program. Charts were abstracted separately for each health care provider of each participant (i.e., at the dyad level). The average time required to abstract a chart for a participant-provider dyad was 50 minutes.

To assess interrater reliability, we re-abstracted charts from a randomly selected 4 percent sample of participants. Average reliability, with the use of the kappa statistic, ranged from substantial to almost perfect[37] at three levels: the presence or absence of a given condition ($\kappa = 0.83$), the participant's eligibility for the process represented by a given indicator ($\kappa = 0.76$), and scoring of a given indicator ($\kappa = 0.80$).

Statistical Analysis

We specified the combination of variables necessary to determine whether each participant was or was not eligible for the process specified by each indicator and whether each participant did or did not receive each process or some proportion of it. Each indicator was scored at one of three levels—that of the individual participant, that of the participant–provider dyad, or that of the episode—depending on the nature of the process being evaluated. The level at which an indicator was scored affected the number of times a participant was eligible for the specified process; the resulting number served as the denominator in the calculation of the aggregate score. For participant-level indicators, we gave the participant a score of "pass" if at least one of his or her health care providers had delivered the indicated care (e.g., influenza vaccination). For indicators scored at the level of the participant-provider dyad (e.g., smoking status noted in the chart), we scored every dyad separately, so the number of times the participant was counted in the denominator depended on the number of providers who saw the participant and could have performed the specified process. For indicators scored at the episode level (e.g., follow-up after hospitalization for an exacerbation of asthma), we scored every event rendering the participant eligible for the specified process and involving any of the participant's providers, so the number of eligibility events depended on the number of episodes that occurred.

In order to produce aggregate scores, we divided all instances in which recommended care was delivered by the number of times participants were eligible for indicators in the category. For example, Table 8-1 presents information about seven of the indicators for acute care; the number of times participants were eligible for these indicators would constitute the denominator for the acute care score. The results are presented as proportions, theoretically ranging in value from 0 to 100 percent. We used the bootstrap method to estimate standard errors directly for all the aggregate scores.[38]

Because everyone in the initial sample for the CQI study had participated in the CTS, we had a rich set of variables for assessing nonresponse. We used logistic-regression analysis to estimate the relations between individual characteristics (age, sex, race, educational level, income, self-reported level of use of physicians and hospitals, insurance status, and health status) and participation in the study. In general, participants tended to be older than nonparticipants ($P < 0.001$) and were more likely than nonparticipants to be female ($P < 0.001$) and white ($P < 0.001$), with higher levels of education ($P < 0.001$) and income ($P < 0.001$). They were also more likely to have used health care services ($P < 0.001$) and to be in other than excellent health ($P = 0.03$). We used the coefficients from the regression equation to adjust the scores for nonresponse, and we weighted the data for the participants to be representative of the population from which they were drawn.

RESULTS

Characteristics of the Participants

Table 8-2 summarizes the characteristics of the participants; these characteristics differ from population averages but parallel the profile of persons receiving medical care. For example, the average age of patients in the National Ambulatory Medical Care Survey[39] is 44.7 years. Women have higher rates of visits than men (319.9 vs. 234.9 visits per 100 persons per year), and whites have higher rates of visits than blacks (293.2 vs. 210.7 visits per 100 persons per year).[39] Participants were well educated. Forty-three percent had one or more of the chronic conditions we assessed, and 34 percent had one or more of the acute conditions. Preventive care was assessed for all participants; in addition, participants' care was assessed for 1.5 chronic or acute conditions, on average, for a total of 2.5 (range, 1 to 13). Participants were included in the overall denominator an average of 16 times (range, 2 to 304).

Analysis of Care Delivered

Tables 8-3, 8-4, and 8-5 show the number of indicators included in the aggregate score, the number of persons eligible

TABLE 8-2 Characteristics of the 6,712 Participants*

Characteristic	Value
Age (yr)	
Mean	45.5 ± 0.2
Range	18–97
Female sex (%)	59.6 ± 0.006
Nonwhite race (%)	18.6 ± 0.005
Education (yr)	13.7 ± 0.03
≥ 1 Chronic conditions (%)	44.7 ± 0.006
≥ 1 Acute conditions (%)	36.3 ± 0.006
Number of conditions and preventive care for which participants were eligible	
Mean	2.5 ± 0.02
Range	1–13
Number of times participants eligible for indicators†	
Mean	15.8 ± 0.17
Range	2–304

* Plus–minus values are means or percentages ± SE.
† The number of times a participant is eligible for an indicator is a function of the level at which the indicator is scored (participant, participant–provider dyad, or episode), the number of participants eligible for the specified process, and the number of indicators in the aggregate-score category.

for one or more processes within the category, the number of times participants in the sample were eligible for indicators, and the weighted mean proportion (and 95 percent confidence interval) of recommended processes that were delivered.

Overall, participants received 54.9 percent of recommended care (95 percent confidence interval, 54.3 to 55.5) (Table 8-3). This level of performance was similar in the areas of preventive care, acute care, and care for chronic conditions. The level of performance according to the particular medical function ranged from 52.2 percent (95 percent confidence interval, 51.3 to 53.2) for screening to 58.5 percent (95 percent confidence interval, 56.6 to 60.4) for follow-up care.

"Mode" refers to the mechanism of care delivery required for the provision of the indicated process. Analysis of performance in terms of mode may identify areas in which system-wide interventions could offer solutions to problems of quality, such as improved methods for ordering, processing, and communicating laboratory results. We found greater variation among modes than among functions in adherence to the processes we studied (Table 8-4). Care requiring an encounter or other intervention (e.g., the annual visit recommended for patients with hypertension) had the highest rates of adherence (73.4 percent [95 percent confidence interval, 71.5 to 75.3]),

TABLE 8-3 Adherence to Quality Indicators, Overall and According to Type of Care and Function

Variable	Number of Indicators	Number of Participants Eligible	Total Number of Times Indicator Eligibility Was Met	Percentage of Recommended Care Received (95% CI)*
Overall care	439	6,712	98,649	54.9 (54.3–55.5)
Type of care				
Preventive	38	6,711	55,268	54.9 (54.2–55.6)
Acute	153	2,318	19,815	53.5 (52.0–55.0)
Chronic	248	3,387	23,566	56.1 (55.0–57.3)
Function				
Screening	41	6,711	39,486	52.2 (51.3–53.2)
Diagnosis	178	6,217	29,679	55.7 (54.5–56.8)
Treatment	173	6,707	23,019	57.5 (56.5–58.4)
Follow-up	47	2,413	6,465	58.5 (56.6–60.4)

* CI denotes confidence interval.

and processes involving counseling or education (e.g., advising smokers with chronic obstructive pulmonary disease to quit smoking) had the lowest rates of adherence (18.3 percent [95 percent confidence interval, 16.7 to 20.0]). All pairwise differences were statistically significant at $P < 0.001$ except those between the prescribing of medication and care requiring an encounter or other intervention ($P = 0.02$), physical examination and immunization ($P = 0.001$), surgery and immunization ($P = 0.004$), and surgery and physical examination ($P = 0.05$). The difference between surgery and laboratory testing or radiography was not significant ($P = 0.39$).

Problems With Quality of Care

We also classified indicators according to the problem with quality that was deemed most likely to occur, and we found greater problems with underuse (46.3 percent of participants did not receive recommended care [95 percent confidence interval, 45.8 to 46.8]) than with overuse (11.3 percent of participants received care that was not recommended and was potentially harmful [95 percent confidence interval, 10.2 to 12.4]).

Variations in Quality

Table 8-5 shows substantial variability in the quality-of-care scores for the 25 conditions for which at least 100 persons were eligible for analysis. Persons with senile cataracts received 78.7 percent of the recommended care (95 percent confidence interval, 73.3 to 84.2); persons with alcohol dependence received 10.5 percent of the recommended care (95 percent confidence interval, 6.8 to 14.6). The aggregate scores for individual con-

ditions were generally not sensitive to the presence or absence of any single indicator of quality.

DISCUSSION

Overall, participants received about half of the recommended processes involved in care. These deficits in care have important implications for the health of the American public. For example, only 24 percent of participants in our study who had diabetes received three or more glycosylated hemoglobin tests over a two-year period. This finding parallels the finding by Saaddine and colleagues that 29 percent of adults with diabetes who participated in the nationally representative Behavioral Risk Factor Surveillance System reported having their blood sugar tested during the previous year.[18] This routine monitoring is essential to the assessment of the effectiveness of treatment, to ensuring appropriate responses to poor glycemic control, and to the identification of complications of the disease at an early stage so that serious consequences may be prevented. In the United Kingdom Prospective Diabetes Study, tight blood glucose control and biannual monitoring decreased the risk of microvascular complications by 25 percent.[40]

In our study, persons with hypertension received 64.7 percent of the recommended care (95 percent confidence interval, 62.6 to 66.7). We have previously demonstrated a link between blood-pressure control and adherence to process-related measures of quality of care for hypertension.[41] Persons whose blood pressure is persistently above normal are at increased risk for heart disease, stroke, and death.[42] Poor blood-pressure control contributes to more than 68,000 preventable deaths annually.[43]

Overall, 68.0 percent (95 percent confidence interval, 64.2 to 71.8) of the recommended care for coronary artery disease was received, but only 45 percent of persons presenting with a myocardial infarction received beta-blockers, which reduce the risk of death by 13 percent during the first week of treatment and by 23 percent over the long term.[44] Only 61 percent of participants with a myocardial infarction who were appropriate candidates for aspirin therapy received aspirin, which has been shown in randomized trials to reduce the risk of death from vascular causes by 15 percent, to reduce the risk of nonfatal myocardial infarction by 30 percent, and to reduce the risk of nonfatal stroke by 40 percent.[45]

TABLE 8-4 Adherence to Quality Indicators, According to Mode

Mode	Number of Indicators	Number of Participants Eligible	Total Number of Times Indicator Eligibility Was Met	Percentage of Recommended Care Received (95% CI)*
Encounter or other intervention	30	2,843	4,329	73.4 (71.5–75.3)
Medication	95	2,964	8,389	68.6 (67.0–70.3)
Immunization	8	6,700	9,748	65.7 (64.3–67.0)
Physical examination	67	6,217	19,428	62.9 (61.8–64.0)
Laboratory testing or radiography	131	5,352	18,605	61.7 (60.4–63.0)
Surgery	21	244	312	56.9 (51.3–62.5)
History	64	6,711	36,032	43.4 (42.4–44.3)
Counseling or education	23	2,838	3,806	18.3 (16.7–20.0)

* CI denotes confidence interval. All pairwise differences were statistically significant at $P < 0.001$, except those between medication and encounter or other intervention ($P = 0.02$), physical examination and immunization ($P = 0.001$), surgery and immunization ($P = 0.004$), and surgery and physical examination ($P = 0.05$). The difference between surgery and laboratory testing or radiography was not significant ($P = 0.39$).

Deficits in processes involved in primary and secondary preventive care are also associated with preventable deaths. Among elderly participants, only 64 percent had received or been offered a pneumococcal vaccine; nearly 10,000 deaths from pneumonia could be prevented annually by appropriate vaccinations.[43] About 38 percent of participants had been screened for colorectal cancer; annual fecal occult-blood tests could prevent about 9600 deaths annually.[43]

Nonresponse bias is a potential limitation of the study. Because the sample we analyzed included 37 percent of the eligible adults, the results are likely to be biased, but the direction of that bias is not clear. For example, because our participants were more likely to use the health care system than were eligible persons who did not participate in the study, our results may be biased toward an underestimation of deficits in quality related to underuse.

The study relied primarily on the review of medical records to score indicators, which may lead some to conclude that we have identified problems with documentation rather than quality. This issue has been examined in studies that compared process-based quality scores using standardized patients, vignettes, and abstraction of medical records[46] and studies that compared standardized patients with audiotapes of encounters.[47] Overall, the process scores among the four conditions studied were 5 percentage points lower with the use of medical records than with the use of vignettes and 10 percentage points lower with the use of medical records than with the use of standardized patients. About two thirds of the disagreement between data from standardized patients and data from audiotapes was attributable to reports by standardized patients that they received care processes that were not confirmed by audiotape. A related study reported a false positive rate of 6.4 percent in medical-record documentation, with the highest false positive rates found for physical examination and elements of the diagnostic process.[48] Thus, our scores might have been as much as 10 percentage points higher if we had used a different method of obtaining data. We used the interview about the participant's health history to partially offset this effect. For example, among elderly participants, only 15 percent had a note in any chart indicating that an influenza vaccination had been received, but 85 percent reported having received one. In general, the inclusion of self-reported data improved scores.

Our results indicate that, on average, Americans receive about half of recommended medical care processes. Although this point estimate of the size of the quality problem may continue to be debated, the gap between what we know works and what is actually done is substantial enough to warrant attention. These deficits, which pose serious threats to the health and well-being of the U.S. public, persist despite initiatives by both the federal government and private health care delivery systems to improve care.

What can we do to break through this impasse? Given the complexity and diversity of the health care system, there will be no simple solution. A key component of any solution, however, is the routine availability of information on performance at all levels. Making such information available will require a

TABLE 8-5 Adherence to Quality Indicators, According to Condition*

Condition	Number of Indicators	Number of Participants Eligible	Total Number of Times Indicator Eligibility Was Met	Percentage of Recommended Care Received (95% CI)
Senile cataract	10	159	602	78.7 (73.3–84.2)
Breast cancer	9	192	202	75.7 (69.9–81.4)
Prenatal care	39	134	2,920	73.0 (69.5–76.6)
Low back pain	6	489	3,391	68.5 (66.4–70.5)
Coronary artery disease	37	410	2,083	68.0 (64.2–71.8)
Hypertension	27	1,973	6,643	64.7 (62.6–66.7)
Congestive heart failure	36	104	1,438	63.9 (55.4–72.4)
Cerebrovascular disease	10	101	210	59.1 (49.7–68.4)
Chronic obstructive pulmonary disease	20	169	1,340	58.0 (51.7–64.4)
Depression	14	770	3,011	57.7 (55.2–60.2)
Orthopedic conditions	10	302	590	57.2 (50.8–63.7)
Osteoarthritis	3	598	648	57.3 (53.9–60.7)
Colorectal cancer	12	231	329	53.9 (47.5–60.4)
Asthma	25	260	2,332	53.5 (50.0–57.0)
Benign prostatic hyperplasia	5	138	147	53.0 (43.6–62.5)
Hyperlipidemia	7	519	643	48.6 (44.1–53.2)
Diabetes mellitus	13	488	2,952	45.4 (42.7–48.3)
Headache	21	712	8,125	45.2 (43.1–47.2)
Urinary tract infection	13	459	1,216	40.7 (37.3–44.1)
Community-acquired pneumonia	5	144	291	39.0 (32.1–45.8)
Sexually transmitted diseases or vaginitis	26	410	2,146	36.7 (33.8–39.6)
Dyspepsia and peptic ulcer disease	8	278	287	32.7 (26.4–39.1)
Atrial fibrillation	10	100	407	24.7 (18.4–30.9)
Hip fracture	9	110	167	22.8 (6.2–39.5)
Alcohol dependence	5	280	1,036	10.5 (6.8–14.6)

* Condition-specific scores are not reported for management of pain due to cancer and its palliation, management of symptoms of menopause, hysterectomy, prostate cancer, and cesarean section, because fewer than 100 people were eligible for analysis of these categories. CI denotes confidence interval.

major overhaul of our current health information systems, with a focus on automating the entry and retrieval of key data for clinical decision making and for the measurement and reporting of quality.[49] Establishing a national base line for performance makes it possible to assess the effect of policy changes and to evaluate large-scale national, regional, state, or local efforts to improve quality.

ACKNOWLEDGMENTS

Supported by the Robert Wood Johnson Foundation and by career development awards (to Drs. Asch and Kerr) from the Veterans Affairs Health Services Research and Development program.

We are indebted to Maureen Michael, James Knickman, and Robert Hughes at the Robert Wood Johnson Foundation for their support; to Paul Ginsburg at the Center for Studying Health System Change for his support of this collaboration; to Richard Strauss at Mathematica Policy Research for developing systems for passing the initial sample from the Community Tracking Study household survey to RAND for this study; to RAND's Survey Research Group (Josephine Levy and Laural Hill) and the telephone interviewers for recruiting participants; to Peggy Wallace, Karen Ricci, and Belle Griffin for their assistance in the design of the data-collection tool, for hiring and training the nurse abstractors, and for overseeing the data-collection process; to Liisa Hiatt for serving as the project manager; and to Vector Research for developing the data-collection software.

REFERENCES

1. McGlynn EA, Brook RH. Keeping quality on the policy agenda. *Health Aff (Millwood)*. 2001;20(3):82–90.

2. Institute of Medicine. *Crossing the quality chasm: A new health system for the 21st century.* Washington, DC: National Academy Press; 2001.

3. Schuster MA, McGlynn EA, Brook RH. How good is the quality of health care in the United States? *Milbank Q.* 1998;76:517–63.

4. Miller RH, Luft HS. Managed care plan performance since 1980: a literature analysis. *JAMA.* 1994;271:1512–9.

5. Jencks SM, Cuerdon T, Burwen DR, et al. Quality of medical care delivered to Medicare beneficiaries: a profile at state and national levels. *JAMA.* 2000;284:1670–6.

6. Ellerbeck EF, Jencks SF, Radford MJ, et al. Quality of care for Medicare patients with acute myocardial infarction: a four-state pilot study from the Cooperative Cardiovascular Project. *JAMA.* 1995;273:1509–14.

7. Murata PJ, McGlynn EA, Siu AL, et al. Quality measures for prenatal care: a comparison of care in six health care plans. *Arch Fam Med.* 1994;3:41–9.

8. Krumholz HM, Radford MJ, Ellerbeck EF, et al. Aspirin in the treatment of acute myocardial infarction in elderly Medicare beneficiaries: patterns of use and outcomes. *Circulation.* 1995;92:2841–7.

9. Brechner RJ, Cowie CC, Howie LJ, Herman WH, Will JC, Harris MI. Ophthalmic examination among adults with diagnosed diabetes mellitus. *JAMA.* 1993;270:1714–8.

10. Starfield B, Powe NR, Weiner JR, et al. Costs vs quality in different types of primary care settings. *JAMA.* 1994;272:1903–8.

11. Payne SM, Donahue C, Rappo P, et al. Variations in pediatric pneumonia and bronchitis/asthma admission rates: is appropriateness a factor? *Arch Pediatr Adolesc Med.* 1995;149:162–9.

12. Udvarhelyi IS, Jennison K, Phillips RS, Epstein AM. Comparison of the quality of ambulatory care for fee-for-service and prepaid patients. *Ann Intern Med.* 1991;115:394–400.

13. Jencks SF, Huff ED, Cuerdon T. Change in the quality of care delivered to Medicare beneficiaries, 1998–1999 to 2000–2001. *JAMA.* 2003;289: 305–12.

14. Asch SM, Sloss EM, Hogan C, Brook RH, Kravitz RL. Measuring underuse of necessary care among elderly Medicare beneficiaries using inpatient and outpatient claims. *JAMA.* 2000;284:2325–33.

15. Kahn KL, Keeler EB, Sherwood MJ, et al. Comparing outcomes of care before and after implementation of the DRG-based prospective payment system. *JAMA.* 1990;264:1984–8.

16. *The state of health care quality, 2002.* Washington, DC: National Committee for Quality Assurance. (Accessed May 30,2003, at http://www.ncqa.org/sohc2002/.)

17. Nelson DE, Bland S, Powell-Griner E, et al. State trends in health risk factors and receipt of clinical preventive services among US adults during the 1990s. *JAMA.* 2002;287:2659–67.

18. Saaddine JB, Engelgau MM, Beckles GL, Gregg EW, Thompson TJ, Narayan KM. A diabetes report card for the United States: quality of care in the 1990s. *Ann Intern Med.* 2002;136:565–74.

19. Asch SM, Gifford AL, Bozzette SA, et al. Underuse of primary Mycobacterium avium complex and Pneumocystis carinii prophylaxis in the United States. *J Acquir Immune Defic Syndr.* 2001;28:340–4.

20. Hyman DJ, Pavlik VN. Characteristics of patients with uncontrolled hypertension in the United States. *N Engl J Med.* 2001;345:479–86. [Erratum, *N Engl J Med.* 2002;346:544.]

21. Kemper PD, Blumenthal D, Corrigan JM, et al. The design of the Community Tracking Study: a longitudinal study of health system change and its effects on people. *Inquiry.* 1996;33:195–206.

22. Strunk BC, Ginsburg PB, Gabel JR. Tracking health care costs: hospital care surpasses drugs as the key cost driver. Bethesda, MD: *Health Affairs,* September 2001. (Accessed May 30, 2003, at http://www.healthaffairs.org1110_web_exclusives.php.)

23. Cunningham PJ. Declining employer-sponsored coverage: the role of public programs and implications for access to care. *Med Care Res Rev.* 2002;59:79–98.

24. Draper DA, Hurley RE, Lesser CS, Strunk BC. The changing face of managed care. *Health Aff (Millwood).* 2002;21(1):11–23.

25. McGlynn EA, Kerr EA, Asch SM. New approach to assessing the clinical quality of care for women: the QA Tool system. *Womens Health Issues.* 1999;9:184–92.

26. McGlynn EA. Choosing and evaluating clinical performance measures. *Jt Comm J Qual Improv.* 1998;24:470–9.

27. Brook RH. The RAND/UCLA appropriateness method. In: McCormick KA, Moore SR, Siegel RA, eds. *Clinical practice guideline development: Methodology perspectives.* Rockville, MD: Agency for Health Care Policy and Research; November 1994:59–70. (AHCPR publication no. 95–0009).

28. Shekelle PG, Kahan JP, Bernstein SJ, Leape LL, Kamberg CJ, Park RE. The reproducibility of a method to identify the overuse and underuse of medical procedures. *N Engl J Med.* 1998;338:1888–95.

29. Shekelle PG, Chassin MR, Park RE. Assessing the predictive validity of the RANDI UCLA appropriateness method criteria for performing carotid endarterectomy. *Int J TechnolAssess Health Care.* 1998;14:707–27.

30. Kravitz RL, Park RE, Kahan JP. Measuring the clinical consistency of panelists' appropriateness ratings: the case of coronary artery bypass surgery. *Health Policy.* 1997;42:135–43.

31. Selby JV, Fireman BH, Lundstrom RJ, et al. Variation among hospitals in coronary-angiography practices and outcomes after myocardial infarction in a large health maintenance organization. *N Engl J Med.* 1996; 335:1888–96.

32. Hemingway H, Crook AM, Feder G, et al. Underuse of coronary revascularization procedures in patients considered appropriate candidates for revascularization. *N Engl J Med.* 2001;344:645–54.

33. McGlynn EA, Kerr EA, Damberg CL, Asch SM, eds. *Quality of care for women: A review of selected clinical conditions and quality indicators.* Santa Monica, CA: RAND; 2000.

34. Kerr EA, Asch SM, Hamilton EG, McGlynn EA, eds. *Quality of care for cardiopulmonary conditions: A review of the literature and quality indicators.* Santa Monica, CA: RAND; 2000.

35. Idem. *Quality of care for general medical conditions: A review of the literature and quality indicators.* Santa Monica, CA: RAND; 2000.

36. Asch SM, Kerr EA, Hamilton EG, Reifel JL, McGlynn EA, eds. *Quality of care for oncologic conditions and HIV: A review of the literature and quality indicators.* Santa Monica, CA: RAND; 2000.

37. Landis RJ, Koch GG. The measurement of observer agreement for categorical data. *Biometrics.* 1977;33:159–74.

38. Efron B, Tibshirani R. *An introduction to the bootstrap.* New York, NY: Chapman & Hall; 1993.

39. Cherry DK, Burt CW, Woodwell DA. National ambulatory medical care survey: 1999 summary: Advance data from vital and health statistics. No. 322. Hyattsville, MD: National Center for Health Statistics, July 2001. (DHHS publication no. (PHS) 2001-1250 01-0383.)

40. UK Prospective Diabetes Study (UKPDS) Group. Intensive blood-glucose control with sulphonylureas or insulin compared with conventional treatment and risk of complications in patients with type 2 diabetes (UKPDS 33). *Lancet.* 1998;352:837–853. [Erratum, *Lancet.* 1999;354:602.]

41. Asch SM, Kerr EA, Lapuerta P, Law A, McGlynn EA. A new approach for measuring quality of care for women with hypertension. *Arch Intern Med.* 2001;161:1329–35.

42. Collins R, Peto R, MacMahon S, et al. Blood pressure, stroke, and coronary heart disease. 2. Short-term reductions in blood pressure: overview of randomised drug trials in their epidemiological context. *Lancet.* 1990;335:827–38.

43. Woolf SH. The need for perspective in evidence-based medicine. *JAMA.* 1999;282:2358–65.

44. Hennekens CH, Albert CM, Godfried SL, Gaziano JM, Buring JE. Adjunctive drug therapy of acute myocardial infarction evidence from clinical trials. *N Engl J Med.* 1996;335:1660–7.

45. Antman EM, Lau J, Kupelnick B, Mosteller F, Chalmers TC. A comparison of results of meta-analyses of randomized control trials and recommendations of clinical experts: treatments for myocardial infarction. *JAMA.* 1992;268:240–8.

46. Peabody JW, Luck J, Glassman P, Dresselhaus TR, Lee M. Comparison of vignettes, standardized patients, and chart abstraction: a prospective validation study of 3 methods for measuring quality. *JAMA.* 2000;283:1715–22.

47. Luck J, Peabody LW. Using standardised patients to measure physicians' practice: validation study using audio recordings. *BMJ.* 2002; 325:679.

48. Dresselhaus TR, Luck J, Peabody JW. The ethical problem of false positives: a prospective evaluation of physician reporting in the medical record. *J Med Ethics.* 2002;28:291–4.

49. Berwick DM, James B, Coye MJ. Connections between quality measurement and reporting. *Med Care.* 2003;41:Suppl:I-30–I-38.

Summary From *Unequal Treatment*

Brian D. Smedley, Adrienne Y. Stith, and Alan R. Nelson, Editors

Source: Unequal Treatment: Confronting Racial and Ethnic Disparities in Health Care, Brian D. Smedley, Adrienne Y. Stith, and Alan R. Nelson, Editors. Committee on Understanding and Eliminating Racial and Ethnic Disparities in Health Care, Board on Health Sciences Policy, Institute of Medicine, The National Academies Press, Washington, DC, 2003.

SUMMARY

Abstract

Racial and ethnic minorities tend to receive a lower quality of healthcare than non-minorities, even when access-related factors, such as patients' insurance status and income, are controlled. The sources of these disparities are complex, are rooted in historic and contemporary inequities, and involve many participants at several levels, including health systems, their administrative and bureaucratic processes, utilization managers, healthcare professionals, and patients. Consistent with the charge, the study committee focused part of its analysis on the clinical encounter itself, and found evidence that stereotyping, biases, and uncertainty on the part of healthcare providers can all contribute to unequal treatment. The conditions in which many clinical encounters take place—characterized by high time pressure, cognitive complexity, and pressures for cost-containment—may enhance the likelihood that these processes will result in care poorly matched to minority patients' needs. Minorities may experience a range of other barriers to accessing care, even when insured at the same level as whites, including barriers of language, geography, and cultural familiarity. Further, financial and institutional arrangements of health systems, as well as the legal, regulatory, and policy environment in which they operate, may have disparate and negative effects on minorities' ability to attain quality care.

A comprehensive, multi-level strategy is needed to eliminate these disparities. Broad sectors—including healthcare providers, their patients, payors, health plan purchasers, and society at large—should be made aware of the healthcare gap between racial and ethnic groups in the United States. Health systems should base decisions about resource allocation on published clinical guidelines, insure that physician financial incentives do not disproportionately burden or restrict minority patients' access to care, and take other steps to improve access—including the provision of interpretation services, where community need exists. Economic incentives should be considered for practices that improve provider–patient communication and trust, and reward appropriate screening, preventive, and evidence-based clinical care. In addition, payment systems should avoid fragmentation of health plans along socioeconomic lines.

The healthcare workforce and its ability to deliver quality care for racial and ethnic minorities can be improved substantially by increasing the proportion of underrepresented U.S. racial and ethnic minorities among health professionals. In addition, both patients and providers can benefit from education. Patients can benefit from culturally appropriate education programs to improve their knowledge of how to access care and their ability to participate in clinical decision making. The greater burden of education, however, lies with providers. Cross-cultural curricula should be integrated early into the training of future healthcare providers, and practical, case-based, rigorously evaluated training should persist through practitioner continuing education programs. Finally, collection, reporting, and monitoring of patient care data by health plans and federal and state payors should be encouraged as a means to assess progress in eliminating disparities, to evaluate intervention efforts, and to assess potential civil rights violations.

Looking gaunt but determined, 59-year-old Robert Tools was introduced on August 21, 2001, as a medical miracle—the first surviving recipient of a fully implantable artificial heart. At a news conference, Tools spoke with emotion about his second chance at life and the quality of his care. His physicians looked on with obvious affection, grateful and honored to have extended Tools' life. Mr. Tools has since lost his battle for life, but will be remembered as a hero for undergoing an experimental technology and paving the way for other patients to undergo the procedure. Moreover, the fact that Tools was African American and his doctors were white seemed, for most Americans, to symbolize the irrelevance of race in 2001. According to two recent polls, a significant majority of Americans believe that blacks like Tools receive the same quality of healthcare as whites (Lillie-Blanton et al., 2000; Morin, 2001).

Behind these perceptions, however, lies a sharply contrasting reality. A large body of published research reveals that racial and ethnic minorities experience a lower quality of health services, and are less likely to receive even routine medical procedures than are white Americans. Relative to whites, African Americans—and in some cases, Hispanics—are less likely to receive appropriate cardiac medication (e.g., Herholz et al., 1996) or to undergo coronary artery bypass surgery (e.g., Ayanian et al., 1993; Hannan et al., 1999; Johnson et al., 1993; Petersen et al., 2002), are less likely to receive peritoneal dialysis and kidney transplantation (e.g., Epstein et al., 2000; Barker-Cummings et al., 1995; Gaylin et al., 1993), and are likely to receive a lower quality of basic clinical services (Ayanian et al., 1999) such as intensive care (Williams et al., 1995), even when variations in such factors as insurance status, income, age, co-morbid conditions, and symptom expression are taken into account. Significantly, these differences are associated with greater mortality among African-American patients (Peterson et al., 1997; Bach et al., 1999).

STUDY CHARGE AND COMMITTEE ASSUMPTIONS

These disparities prompted Congress to request an Institute of Medicine (IOM) study to assess differences in the kinds and quality of healthcare received by U.S. racial and ethnic minori-

ties and non-minorities. Specifically, Congress requested that the IOM:

- Assess the extent of racial and ethnic differences in healthcare that are not otherwise attributable to known factors such as access to care (e.g., ability to pay or insurance coverage);
- Evaluate potential sources of racial and ethnic disparities in healthcare, including the role of bias, discrimination, and stereotyping at the individual (provider and patient), institutional, and health system levels; and,
- Provide recommendations regarding interventions to eliminate healthcare disparities.

This Executive Summary presents only abbreviated versions of the study committee's findings and recommendations. For the full findings and recommendations, and a more extensive justification of each, the reader is referred to the committee report. Later here, findings and recommendations are preceded by text summarizing the evidence base from which they are drawn. For purposes of clarity, some findings and recommendations are presented in a different sequence than they appear in the full report; however, their numeric designation remains the same.

Defining Racial and Ethnic Healthcare Disparities

The study committee defines *disparities* in healthcare as racial or ethnic differences in the quality of healthcare that are not due to access-related factors or clinical needs, preferences,[1] and appropriateness of intervention (Figure 9-1). The committee's analysis is focused at two levels: 1) the operation of healthcare systems and the legal and regulatory climate in which health systems function; and 2) discrimination at the individual, patient-provider level. Discrimination, as the committee uses the term, refers to differences in care that result from biases, prejudices, stereotyping, and uncertainty in clinical communication and decision-making. It should be emphasized that these definitions are not legal definitions. Different sources of federal, state and international law define discrimination in varying ways, with some focusing on intent and others emphasizing disparate impact.

---

1. The committee defines patient *preferences* as patients' choices regarding healthcare that are based on a full and accurate understanding of treatment options. As discussed in Chapter 3 of this report, patients' understanding of treatment options is often shaped by the quality and content of provider–patient communication, which in turn may be influenced by factors correlated with patients and providers' race, ethnicity, and culture. Patient preferences that are not based on a full and accurate understanding of treatment options may therefore be a source of racial and ethnic disparities in care. The committee recognizes that patients' preferences and clinicians' presentation of clinical information and alternatives influence each other but found separation of the two to be analytically useful.

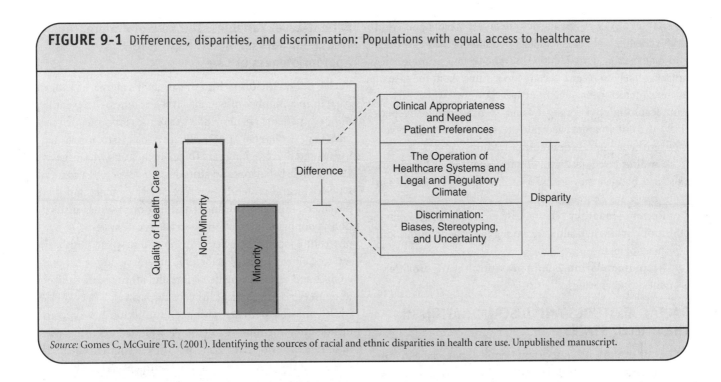

FIGURE 9-1 Differences, disparities, and discrimination: Populations with equal access to healthcare

Source: Gomes C, McGuire TG. (2001). Identifying the sources of racial and ethnic disparities in health care use. Unpublished manuscript.

EVIDENCE OF HEALTHCARE DISPARITIES

Evidence of racial and ethnic disparities in healthcare is, with few exceptions, remarkably consistent across a range of illnesses and healthcare services. These disparities are associated with socioeconomic differences and tend to diminish significantly, and in a few cases, disappear altogether when socioeconomic factors are controlled. The majority of studies, however, find that racial and ethnic disparities remain even after adjustment for socioeconomic differences and other healthcare access-related factors (for more extensive reviews of this literature, see Kressin and Petersen, 2001; Geiger, this volume; and Mayberry, Mili, and Ofili, 2000).

Studies of racial and ethnic differences in cardiovascular care provide some of the most convincing evidence of healthcare disparities. The most rigorous studies in this area assess both potential underuse and overuse of services and appropriateness of care by controlling for disease severity using well-established clinical and diagnostic criteria (e.g., Schneider et al., 2001; Ayanian et al., 1993; Allison et al., 1996; Weitzman et al., 1997) or matched patient controls (Giles et al., 1995). Several studies, for example, have assessed differences in treatment regimen following coronary angiography, a key diagnostic procedure. These studies have demonstrated that differences in treatment are not due to clinical factors such as racial differences in the severity of coronary disease or overuse of services by whites (e.g., Schneider et al., 2001; Laouri et al., 1997; Canto

et al., 2000; Peterson et al., 1997). Further, racial disparities in receipt of coronary revascularization procedures are associated with higher mortality among African Americans (Peterson et al., 1997).

Healthcare disparities are also found in other disease areas. Several studies demonstrate significant racial differences in the receipt of appropriate cancer diagnostic tests (e.g., McMahon et al., 1999), treatments (e.g., Imperato et al., 1996), and analgesics (e.g., Bernabei et al., 1998), while controlling for stage of cancer at diagnosis and other clinical factors. As is the case in studies of cardiovascular disease, evidence suggests that disparities in cancer care are associated with higher death rates among minorities (Bach et al., 1999). Similarly, African Americans with HIV infection are less likely than non-minorities to receive antiretroviral therapy (Moore et al., 1994), prophylaxis for pneumocystic pneumonia, and protease inhibitors (Shapiro et al., 1999). These disparities remain even after adjusting for age, gender, education, CD4 cell count, and insurance coverage (e.g., Shapiro et al., 1999). In addition, differences in the quality of HIV care are associated with poorer survival rates among minorities, even at equivalent levels of access to care (Bennett et al., 1995; Cunningham et al., 2000).

Racial and ethnic disparities are found in a range of other disease and health service categories, including diabetes care (e.g., Chin, Zhang, and Merrell, 1998), end-stage renal disease and kidney transplantation (e.g., Epstein et al., 2000; Kasiske, London, and Ellison, 1998; Barker-Cummings et al., 1995;

Ayanian et al., 1999), pediatric care and maternal and child health, mental health, rehabilitative and nursing home services, and many surgical procedures. In some instances, minorities are *more* likely to receive certain procedures. As in the case of bilateral orchiectomy and amputation, however (which African Americans undergo at rates 2.4 and 3.6 times greater, respectively, than their white Medicare peers; Gornick et al., 1996), these are generally less desirable procedures.

Finding 1-1: Racial and ethnic disparities in healthcare exist and, because they are associated with worse outcomes in many cases, are unacceptable.

Recommendation 2-1: Increase awareness of racial and ethnic disparities in healthcare among the general public and key stakeholders.

Recommendation 2-2: Increase healthcare providers' awareness of disparities.

RACIAL ATTITUDES AND DISCRIMINATION IN THE UNITED STATES

By way of context, it is important to note that racial and ethnic disparities are found in many sectors of American life. African Americans, Hispanics, American Indians, and Pacific Islanders, and some Asian-American subgroups are disproportionately represented in the lower socioeconomic ranks, in lower quality schools, and in poorer-paying jobs. These disparities can be traced to many factors, including historic patterns of legalized segregation and discrimination. Unfortunately, some discrimination remains. For example, audit studies of mortgage lending, housing, and employment practices using paired "testers" demonstrate persistent discrimination against African Americans and Hispanics. These studies illustrate that much of American social and economic life remains ordered by race and ethnicity, with minorities disadvantaged relative to whites. In addition, these findings suggest that minorities' experiences in the world outside of the healthcare practitioner's office are likely to affect their perceptions and responses in care settings.

Finding 2-1: Racial and ethnic disparities in healthcare occur in the context of broader historic and contemporary social and economic inequality, and evidence of persistent racial and ethnic discrimination in many sectors of American life.

ASSESSING POTENTIAL SOURCES OF DISPARITIES IN CARE

The studies cited above suggest that a range of patient-level, provider-level, and system-level factors may be involved in racial and ethnic healthcare disparities, beyond access-related factors.

Patient-Level Variables: The Role of Preferences, Treatment Refusal, and the Clinical Appropriateness of Care

Racial and ethnic disparities in care may emerge, at least in part, from a number of patient-level attributes. For example, minority patients are more likely to refuse recommended services (e.g., Sedlis et al., 1997), adhere poorly to treatment regimens, and delay seeking care (e.g., Mitchell and McCormack, 1997). These behaviors and attitudes can develop as a result of a poor cultural match between minority patients and their providers, mistrust, misunderstanding of provider instructions, poor prior interactions with healthcare systems, or simply from a lack of knowledge of how to best use healthcare services. However, racial and ethnic differences in patient preferences and care-seeking behaviors and attitudes are unlikely to be major sources of healthcare disparities. For example, while minority patients have been found to refuse recommended treatment more often than whites, differences in refusal rates are small and have not fully accounted for racial and ethnic disparities in receipt of treatments (Hannan et al., 1999; Ayanian et al., 1999). Overuse of some clinical services (i.e., use of services when not clinically indicated) may be more common among white than minority patients, and may contribute to racial and ethnic differences in discretionary procedures. Several recent studies, however, have assessed racial differences relative to established criteria (Hannan et al., 1999; Laouri et al., 1997; Canto et al., 2000; Peterson et al., 1997) or objective diagnostic information, and still find racial differences in receipt of care. Other studies find that overuse of cardiovascular services among whites does not explain racial differences in service use (Schneider et al., 2001).

Finally, some researchers have speculated that biologically based racial differences in clinical presentation or response to treatment may justify racial differences in the type and intensity of care provided. For example, racial and ethnic group differences are found in response to drug therapies such as enalapril, an angiotensin-converting-enzyme inhibitor used to reduce the risk of heart failure (Exner et al., 2001). These differences in response to drug therapy, however, are not due to "race" per se but can be traced to differences in the distribution of polymorphic traits between population groups (Wood, 2001), and are small in relation to the common benefits of most therapeutic interventions. Further, as noted above, the majority of studies document disparities in healthcare services and disease areas when interventions are equally effective across population groups—making the "racial differences" hypothesis an unlikely explanation for observed disparities in care.

Finding 4-2: A small number of studies suggest that racial and ethnic minority patients are more likely than white patients to refuse treatment. These studies find that differences in refusal rates are generally small and that minority patient refusal does not fully explain healthcare disparities.

Healthcare Systems-Level Factors

Aspects of health systems—such as the ways in which systems are organized and financed, and the availability of services—may exert different effects on patient care, particularly for racial and ethnic minorities. Language barriers, for example, pose a problem for many patients where health systems lack the resources, knowledge, or institutional priority to provide interpretation and translation services. Nearly 14 million Americans are not proficient in English, and as many as one in five Spanish-speaking Latinos reports not seeking medical care due to language barriers (The Robert Wood Johnson Foundation, 2001). Similarly, time pressures on physicians may hamper their ability to accurately assess presenting symptoms of minority patients, especially where cultural or linguistic barriers are present. Further, the geographic availability of healthcare institutions—while largely influenced by economic factors that are outside the charge of this study—may have a differential impact on racial and ethnic minorities, independent of insurance status (Kahn et al., 1994). A study of the availability of opioid supplies, for example, revealed that only one in four pharmacies located in predominantly non-white neighborhoods carried adequate supplies, compared with 72% of pharmacies in predominantly white neighborhoods (Morrison et al., 2000). Perhaps more significantly, changes in the financing and delivery of healthcare services—such as the shifts brought by cost-control efforts and the movement to managed care—may pose greater barriers to care for racial and ethnic minorities than for non-minorities (Rice, this volume). Increasing efforts by states to enroll Medicaid patients in managed care systems, for example, may disrupt traditional community-based care and displace providers who are familiar with the language, culture, and values of ethnic minority communities (Leigh, Lillie-Blanton, Martinez, and Collins, 1999). In addition, research indicates that minorities enrolled in publicly funded managed care plans are less likely to access services after mandatory enrollment in an HMO, compared with whites and other minorities enrolled in non-managed care plans (Tai-Seale et al., 2001).

Care Process-Level Variables: The Role of Bias, Stereotyping, Uncertainty

Three mechanisms might be operative in healthcare disparities from the provider's side of the exchange: bias (or prejudice) against minorities; greater clinical uncertainty when interacting with minority patients; and beliefs (or stereotypes) held by the provider about the behavior or health of minorities (Balsa and McGuire, 2001). Patients might also react to providers' behavior associated with these practices in a way that also contributes to disparities. Unfortunately, little research has been conducted to elucidate how patient race or ethnicity may influence physician decision-making and how these influences affect the quality of care provided. In the absence of such research, the study committee drew upon a mix of theory and relevant research to understand how clinical uncertainty, biases or stereotypes, and prejudice might operate in the clinical encounter.

Clinical Uncertainty

Any degree of uncertainty a physician may have relative to the condition of a patient can contribute to disparities in treatment. Doctors must depend on inferences about severity based on what they can see about the illness and on what else they observe about the patient (e.g., race). The doctor can therefore be viewed as operating with prior beliefs about the likelihood of patients' conditions, "priors" that will be different according to age, gender, socioeconomic status, and race or ethnicity. When these priors—which are taught as a cognitive heuristic to medical students are considered alongside the information gained in a clinical encounter, both influence medical decisions.

Doctors must balance new information gained from the patient (sometimes with varying levels of accuracy) and their prior expectations about the patient to determine the diagnosis and course of treatment. If the physician has difficulty accurately understanding the symptoms or is less sure of the "signal"—the set of clues and indications that physicians rely upon to make diagnostic decisions—then he or she is likely to place greater weight on the "priors." The consequence is that treatment decisions and patients' needs are potentially less well matched.

The Implicit Nature of Stereotypes

A large body of research in psychology has explored how stereotypes evolve, persist, shape expectations, and affect interpersonal interactions. Stereotyping can be defined as the process by which people use social categories (e.g., race, sex) in acquiring, processing, and recalling information about others. The beliefs (stereotypes) and general orientations (attitudes) that people bring to their interactions help to organize and simplify complex or uncertain situations and give perceivers greater confidence in their ability to understand a situation and respond in efficient and effective ways (Mackie, Hamilton, Susskind, and Rosselli, 1996).

Although functional, social stereotypes and attitudes also tend to be systematically biased. These biases may exist in overt, explicit forms, as represented by traditional bigotry. However, because their origins arise from virtually universal social categorization processes, they may also exist, often unconsciously, among people who strongly endorse egalitarian principles and truly believe that they are not prejudiced (Dovidio and Gaertner, 1998). In the United States, because of shared socialization influences, there is considerable empirical evidence that even well-meaning whites who are not overtly biased and who do not believe that they are prejudiced typically demonstrate unconscious implicit negative racial attitudes and stereotypes (Dovidio, Brigham, Johnson, and Gaertner, 1996). Both implicit and explicit stereotypes significantly shape interpersonal interactions, influencing how information is recalled and guiding expectations and inferences in systematic ways. They can also produce self-fulfilling prophecies in social interaction, in that the stereotypes of the perceiver influence the interaction with others in ways that conform to stereotypical expectations Jussim, 1991).

Healthcare Provider Prejudice or Bias

Prejudice is defined in psychology as an unjustified negative attitude based on a person's group membership (Dovidio et al., 1996). Survey research suggests that among white Americans, prejudicial attitudes toward minorities remain more common than not, as over half to three-quarters believe that relative to whites, minorities—particularly African Americans—are less intelligent, more prone to violence, and prefer to live off of welfare (Bobo, 2001). It is reasonable to assume, however, that the vast majority of healthcare providers find prejudice morally abhorrent and at odds with their professional values. But healthcare providers, like other members of society, may not recognize manifestations of prejudice in their own behavior.

While there is no direct evidence that provider biases affect the quality of care for minority patients, research suggests that healthcare providers' diagnostic and treatment decisions, as well as their feelings about patients, are influenced by patients' race or ethnicity. Schulman et al. (1999), for example, found that physicians referred white male, black male, and white female hypothetical "patients" (actually videotaped actors who displayed the same symptoms of cardiac disease) for cardiac catheterization at the same rates (approximately 90% for each group), but were significantly less likely to recommend catheterization procedures for black female patients exhibiting the same symptoms. Weisse et al. (2001), using a similar methodology as that of Schulman, found that male

physicians prescribed twice the level of analgesic medication for white "patients" than for black "patients." Female physicians, in contrast, prescribed higher doses of analgesics for black than for white "patients," suggesting that male and female physicians may respond differently to gender and/or racial cues. In another experimental design, Abreu (1999) found that mental health professionals subliminally "primed" with African American stereotype-laden words were more likely to evaluate the same hypothetical patient (whose race was not identified) more negatively than when primed with neutral words. And in a study based on actual clinical encounters, van Ryn and Burke (2000) found that doctors rated black patients as less intelligent, less educated, more likely to abuse drugs and alcohol, more likely to fail to comply with medical advice, more likely to lack social support, and less likely to participate in cardiac rehabilitation than white patients, even after patients' income, education, and personality characteristics were taken into account. These findings suggest that while the relationship between race or ethnicity and treatment decisions is complex and may also be influenced by gender, providers' perceptions and attitudes toward patients are influenced by patient race or ethnicity, often in subtle ways.

Medical Decisions Under Time Pressure With Limited Information

Studies suggest that several characteristics of the clinical encounter increase the likelihood that stereotypes, prejudice, or uncertainty may influence the quality of care for minorities (van Ryn, 2002). In the process of care, health professionals must come to judgments about patients' conditions and make decisions about treatment, often without complete and accurate information. In most cases, they must do so under severe time pressure and resource constraints. The assembly and use of these data are affected by many influences, including various "gestalts" or cognitive shortcuts. In fact, physicians are commonly trained to rely on clusters of information that functionally resemble the application of "prototypic" or stereotypic constellations. These conditions of time pressure, resource constraints, and the need to rely on gestalts map closely onto those factors identified by social psychologists as likely to produce negative outcomes due to lack of information, to stereotypes, and to biases (van Ryn, 2002).

Patient Response: Mistrust and Refusal

As noted above, the responses of racial and ethnic minority patients to healthcare providers are also a potential source of disparities. Little research has been conducted as to how patients may influence the clinical encounter. It is reasonable to speculate, however, that if patients convey mistrust, refuse treatment, or comply poorly with treatment, providers may become less engaged in the treatment process, and patients are less likely to be provided with more vigorous treatments and services. But these kinds of reactions from minority patients may be understandable as a response to negative racial experiences in other contexts, or to real or perceived mistreatment by providers. Survey research, for example, indicates that minority patients perceive higher levels of racial discrimination in healthcare than non-minorities (LaVeist, Nickerson, and Bowie, 2000; Lillie-Blanton et al., 2000). Patients' and providers' behavior and attitudes may therefore influence each other reciprocally, but reflect the attitudes, expectations, and perceptions that each has developed in a context where race and ethnicity are often more salient than these participants are even aware of. In addition, it is clear that the healthcare provider, rather than the patient, is the more powerful actor in clinical encounters. Providers' expectations, beliefs, attitudes, and behaviors are therefore likely to be a more important target for intervention efforts.

Finding 3-1: Many sources—including health systems, healthcare providers, patients, and utilization managers—may contribute to racial and ethnic disparities in healthcare.

Finding 4-1: Bias, stereotyping, prejudice, and clinical uncertainty on the part of healthcare providers may contribute to racial and ethnic disparities in healthcare. While indirect evidence from several lines of research supports this statement, a greater understanding of the prevalence and influence of these processes is needed and should be sought through research.

INTERVENTIONS TO ELIMINATE RACIAL AND ETHNIC DISPARITIES IN HEALTHCARE

Legal, Regulatory, and Policy Interventions

"De-Fragmentation" of Healthcare Financing and Delivery

Racial and ethnic minorities are more likely than whites to be enrolled in "lower-end" health plans, which are characterized by higher per capita resource constraints and stricter limits on covered services (Phillips et al., 2000). The disproportionate presence of racial and ethnic minorities in lower-end health plans is a potential source of healthcare disparities, given that efforts to control for insurance status in studies of healthcare disparities have not taken detailed account of variations among health plans. Such socioeconomic fragmentation of health plans engenders different clinical cultures, with different practice norms, tied to varying per capita resource constraints (Bloche, 2001).

Equalizing access to high-quality plans can limit such fragmentation. Public healthcare payors such as Medicaid should strive to help beneficiaries access the same health products as privately-insured patients. This recommendation is also reflected in the IOM Quality Chasm report's strategies for focusing health systems on quality, in its call to "eliminate or modify payment practices that fragment the care system" (IOM, 2001, p. 13).

Recommendation 5-1: Avoid fragmentation of health plans along socioeconomic lines.

Strengthening Doctor-Patient Relationships

Several lines of research suggest that the consistency and stability of the doctor-patient relationship is an important determinant of patient satisfaction and access to care. Having a usual source of care is associated, for example, with use of preventive care services (Agency for Healthcare Research and Quality, 2001). In addition, having a consistent relationship with a primary care provider may help to address minority patient mistrust of healthcare systems and providers, particularly if the relationship is with a provider who is able to bridge cultural and linguistic gaps (LaVeist, Nickerson, and Bowie, 2000). Minority patients, however, are less likely to enjoy a consistent relationship with a provider, even when insured at the same levels as white patients (Lillie-Blanton, Martinez, and Salganicoff, 2001). This is due in part to the types of health systems in which they are enrolled and the relative lack of providers located in minority communities.

Health systems should attempt to ensure that every patient, whether insured privately or publicly, has a sustained relationship with an attending physician able to help the patient effectively navigate the healthcare bureaucracy. Federal and state performance standards for Medicaid managed care plans, for example, should include guidelines to ensure the stability of patients' assignments to primary care providers (and these providers' accessibility), reasonable patient loads per primary care physician, and time allotments for patient visits.

Recommendation 5-2: Strengthen the stability of patient-provider relationships in publicly funded health plans.

Patient and provider relationships will also be strengthened by greater racial and ethnic diversity in the health professions. Racial concordance of patient and provider is associated with greater patient participation in care processes, higher patient satisfaction, and greater adherence to treatment (Cooper-Patrick et al., 1999). In addition, racial and ethnic minority providers are more likely than their non-minority colleagues to serve in minority and medically underserved communities (Komaromy et al., 1996). The benefits of diversity in health professions fields are significant, and illustrate that a continued commitment to affirmative action is necessary for graduate health professions education programs, residency recruitment, and other professional opportunities.

Recommendation 5-3: Increase the proportion of under-represented U.S. racial and ethnic minorities among health professionals.

Patient Protections

Much of the political focus on Capitol Hill in the summer of 2001 was devoted to managed care regulation. To one extent or another, the various bills debated would all extend protections to enrollees in private managed care organizations, providing avenues for appeal of care denial decisions, improving access to specialty care, requiring health plans to disclose information about coverage, banning physician "gag" clauses, and providing other legal remedies to resolve disputes. Publicly funded health plans, however, are not addressed in these legislative proposals. Given that many minorities are disproportionately represented among the publicly insured who receive care within managed care organizations, the same patient protections that apply to the privately insured should apply to those in publicly funded plans (Hashimoto, 2001).

Recommendation 5-4: Apply the same managed care protections to publicly funded HMO enrollees that apply to private HMO enrollees.

Civil Rights Enforcement

Enforcement of regulation and statute is also an important component of a comprehensive strategy to address healthcare disparities, but unfortunately has been too often relegated to low-priority status. The U.S. DHHS Office of Civil Rights (OCR) is charged with enforcing several relevant federal statutes and regulations that prohibit discrimination in healthcare (principally Title VI of the 1964 Civil Rights Act). The agency, however, has suffered from insufficient resources to investigate complaints of possible violations, and has long abandoned proactive, investigative strategies (Smith, 1999). Complaints to the agency declined in the early 1990s, but have increased in recent years, while funding has remained level in terms of appropriated dollars but lower in terms of spending power after adjusting for inflation (U.S. Commission on Civil Rights, 2001). The agency should be equipped with sufficient resources to better address these complaints and carry out its oversight responsibilities.

Recommendation 5-5: Provide greater resources to the U.S. DHHS Office for Civil Rights to enforce civil rights laws.

Health Systems Interventions

A variety of interventions applied at the level of health systems may be effective as a part of a comprehensive, multi-level strategy to address racial and ethnic disparities in healthcare.

Evidence-Based Cost Control

In the current era of continually escalating healthcare costs, cost containment is an important goal of all health systems. To the extent possible, however, medical limit setting by health plans should be based on evidence of effectiveness. The application of evidence to healthcare delivery, such as through the use of evidence-based guidelines, can help to address the problem of potential underuse of services resulting from capitation or per case payment methods, as noted in the IOM Quality Chasm report (IOM, 2001). Evidence-based guidelines offer the advantages of consistency, predictability, and objectivity that general, discretionary advisory statements do not. In addition, because evidence-based guidelines and standards directly promote accountability, they also indirectly affect equity of care.

In actual practice, however, a pragmatic balance must be sought between the advantages and limitations of guidelines, such as the tension between the goal of standardization versus the need for clinical flexibility. Disclosing health plans' clinical protocols offers one means of achieving this balance, as it would aid both private sector and public efforts in balancing the virtues of rules and discretion. To achieve this, private accrediting entities and state regulatory bodies could require that health plans publish their clinical practice protocols, along with supporting evidence, thereby opening these protocols to professional and consumer review (Bloche, 2001).

Recommendation 5-6: Promote the consistency and equity of care through the use of evidence-based guidelines.

Financial Incentives in Healthcare

Financial factors, such as capitation and health plan incentives to providers to practice frugally, can pose greater barriers to racial and ethnic minority patients than to white patients, even among patients insured at the same level. Low payment rates limit the supply of physician (and other healthcare provider) services to low-income groups, disproportionately affecting ethnic minorities (Rice, this volume). Inadequate supply takes the form of too few providers participating in plans serving the poor and provider unwillingness to spend adequate time with patients. This time pressure may contribute to poor information exchange between physicians and members of minority groups.

If appropriately crafted, however, financial incentives to physicians can serve a positive role in efforts to reduce disparities in care. Economic rewards for time spent engaging patients and their families can help physicians to overcome barriers of culture, communication, and empathy. In addition, incentives that encourage physicians to adhere to evidence-based protocols for frugal practice and to engage in age- and gender-appropriate disease screening can promote efficient, quality care and penalize deviations, regardless of race or ethnicity. Further, financial incentives linked to favorable clinical outcomes, where reasonably measurable (e.g., control of diabetes, asthma, and high blood pressure) can also promote equity of care (Bloche, 2001). Again, this recommendation is consistent with the IOM *Quality Chasm* report, which calls for healthcare organizations, clinicians, purchasers, and other stakeholders to "align the incentives inherent in payment and accountability processes with the goal of quality improvement" (IOM, 2001, p. 10).

Recommendation 5-7: Structure payment systems to ensure an adequate supply of services to minority patients and limit provider incentives that may promote disparities.

Recommendation 5-8: Enhance patient-provider communication and trust by providing financial incentives for practices that reduce barriers and encourage evidence-based practice.

Interpretation Services

As noted above, many racial and ethnic minorities find that language barriers pose a significant problem in their efforts to access healthcare. Language barriers may affect the delivery of adequate care through poor exchange of information, loss of important cultural information, misunderstanding of physician instruction, poor shared decision making, or ethical compromises (e.g., difficulty obtaining informed consent; Woloshin et al., 1995). Linguistic difficulties may also result in decreased adherence with medication regimes, poor appointment attendance (Manson, 1988), and decreased satisfaction with services (Carrasquillo et al., 1999; David and Rhee, 1998; Derose and Baker, 2000).

Broader use of professional interpretation services has been hampered by a number of logistical and resource constraints. For example, in some regions of the country, few trained professional interpreters are available, and reimbursement for interpretation services via publicly funded insurance such as Medicaid is often inadequate. Greater resources are needed to support professional interpretation services, and more research and innovation should identify effective means to harness new technologies (e.g., simultaneous telephone interpretation) to aid interpretation.

Recommendation 5-9: Support the use of interpretation services where community need exists.

Community Health Workers

Community health workers—often termed lay health advisors, neighborhood workers, indigenous health workers, health aides, *consejera,* or *promotora*—fulfill multiple functions in helping to improve access to healthcare. Community health workers can serve as liaisons between patients and providers, educate providers about community needs and the culture of the community, provide patient education, contribute to continuity and coordination of care, assist in appointment attendance and adherence to medication regimens, and help to increase the use of preventive and primary care services (Brownstein et al., 1992; Earp and Flax, 1999; Jackson and Parks, 1997). In addition, some evidence suggests that lay health workers can help improve the quality of care and reduce costs (Witmer et al., 1995), and improve general wellness by facilitating community access to and negotiation for services (Rodney et al., 1998).

Recommendation 5-10: Support the use of community health workers.

Multidisciplinary Teams

Research demonstrates that multidisciplinary team approaches—including physicians, nurses, dietitians, and social workers, among others—can effectively optimize patient care. This effect is found in randomized controlled studies of patients with coronary heart disease, hypertension, and other diseases, and has extended to strategies for reducing risk behaviors and conditions such as smoking, sedentary lifestyle and obesity (Hill and Miller, 1996). Multidisciplinary teams coordinate and streamline care, enhance patient adherence through follow-up techniques, and address the multiple behavioral and social risks faced by patients. These teams may save costs and improve the efficiency of care by reducing the need for face-to-face physician visits and improve patients' day-to-day care between visits. Further, such strategies have proven effective in improving health outcomes of minorities previously viewed as "difficult to serve" (Hill and Miller, 1996). Multidisciplinary team approaches should be more widely instituted as strategy for improving care delivery, implementing secondary prevention strategies, and enhancing risk reduction.

Recommendation 5-11: Implement multidisciplinary treatment and preventive care teams.

Patient Education and Empowerment

Increasingly, researchers are recognizing the important role of patients as active participants in clinical encounters (Korsch, 1984). Patient education efforts have taken many forms, including the use of books and pamphlets, in-person instruction, CD-ROM-based educational materials, and internet-based information. These materials guide patients through typical office visits and provide information about asking appropriate questions and having their questions answered, communicating with the provider when instructions are not understood or cannot be followed, and being an active participant in decision-making. While evaluation data are limited, particularly with respect to racial and ethnic minority patients, preliminary evidence suggests that patient education can improve patients' skills and knowledge of clinical encounters and improve their participation in care decisions.

Recommendation 5-12: Implement patient education programs to increase patients' knowledge of how to best access care and participate in treatment decisions.

Cross-Cultural Education in the Health Professions

Given the increasing racial and ethnic diversity of the U.S. population, the development and implementation of training programs for healthcare providers offers promise as a key intervention strategy in reducing healthcare disparities. As a result, cross-cultural education programs have been developed to enhance health professionals' awareness of how cultural and social factors influence healthcare, while providing methods to obtain, negotiate and manage this information clinically once it is obtained. Cross-cultural education can be divided into three conceptual approaches focusing on *attitudes* (cultural sensitivity/awareness approach), *knowledge* (multicultural/categorical approach), and *skills* (cross-cultural approach), and has been taught using a variety of interactive and experiential methodologies. Research to date demonstrates that training is effective in improving provider knowledge of cultural and behavioral aspects of healthcare and building effective communication strategies. Despite progress in the field, however, several challenges exist, including the need to define educational core competencies, reach consensus on approaches and methodologies, determine methods of integration into the medical and nursing curriculum, and develop and implement appropriate evaluation strategies. These challenges should be addressed to realize the potential of cross-cultural education strategies.

Recommendation 6-1: Integrate cross-cultural education into the training of all current and future health professionals.

DATA COLLECTION AND MONITORING

Standardized data collection is critically important in the effort to understand and eliminate racial and ethnic disparities in healthcare. Data on patient and provider race and ethnicity would allow researchers to better disentangle factors that are associated with healthcare disparities, help health plans to monitor performance, ensure accountability to enrolled members and payors, improve patient choice, allow for evaluation of intervention programs, and help identify discriminatory practices. Unfortunately, standardized data on racial and eth-

nic differences in care are generally unavailable. Federal and state-supported data collection efforts are scattered and unsystematic, and many health plans, with a few notable exceptions, do not collect data on enrollees' race, ethnicity, or primary language.

A number of ethical, logistical, and fiscal concerns present challenges to data collection and monitoring, including the need to protect patient privacy, the costs of data collection, and resistance from healthcare providers, institutions, plans and patients. In addition, health plans have raised significant concerns about how such data will be analyzed and reported. The challenges to data collection should be addressed, as the costs of failing to assess racial and ethnic disparities in care may outweigh new burdens imposed by data collection and analysis efforts.

Recommendation 7-1: Collect and report data on healthcare access and utilization by patients' race, ethnicity, socioeconomic status, and where possible, primary language.

Recommendation 7-2: Include measures of racial and ethnic disparities in performance measurement.

Recommendation 7-3: Monitor progress toward the elimination of healthcare disparities.

Recommendation 7-4: Report racial and ethnic data by federally defined categories, but use subpopulation groups where possible.

NEEDED RESEARCH

While the literature that the committee reviewed provides significant evidence of racial and ethnic disparities in care, the evidence base from which to better understand and eliminate disparities in care remains less than clear. Several broad areas of research are needed to clarify how race and ethnicity are associated with disparities in the process, structure, and outcomes of care. Research must provide a better understanding of the contribution of patient, provider, and institutional characteristics on the quality of care for minorities. Research has been notably absent in other areas. More research is needed, for example, to understand the extent of disparities in care faced by Asian-American, Pacific-Islander, American Indian and Alaska Native, and Hispanic populations, and to better understand and surmount barriers to research on healthcare disparities, including those related to ethical issues in data collection.

Recommendation 8-1: Conduct further research to identify sources of racial and ethnic disparities and assess promising intervention strategies.

Recommendation 8-2: Conduct research on ethical issues and other barriers to eliminating disparities.

REFERENCES

Abreu JM. (1999). Conscious and nonconscious African American stereotypes: Impact on first impression and diagnostic ratings by therapists. *Journal of Consulting and Clinical Psychology* 67(3):387–93.

Agency for Healthcare Research and Quality. (2001). Addressing racial and ethnic disparities in healthcare. Fact sheet accessed from internet site www.ahrq.gov/research/disparit.htm on December 18, 2001.

Allison JJ, Kiefe CI, Centor RM, Box JB, Farmer RM. (1996). Racial differences in the medical treatment of elderly Medicare patients with acute myocardial infarction. *Journal of General Internal Medicine* 11:736–43.

Ayanian JZ, Udvarhelyi IS, Gatsonis CA, Pasho, CL, Epstein AM. (1993). Racial differences in the use of revascularization procedures after coronary angiography. *Journal of the American Medical Association* 269:2642–6.

Ayanian JZ, Weissman JS, Chasan-Taber S, Epstein AM. (1999). Quality of care by race and gender for congestive heart failure and pneumonia. *Medical Care* 37:1260–9.

Bach PB, Cramer LD, Warren JL, Begg CB. (1999). Racial differences in the treatment of early-stage lung cancer. *New England Journal of Medicine* 341:1198–205.

Balsa A, McGuire TG. (2001). Prejudice, uncertainty and stereotypes as sources of health care disparities. Boston University, unpublished manuscript.

Barker-Cummings C, McClellan W, Soucie, JM, Krisher J. (1995). Ethnic differences in the use of peritoneal dialysis as initial treatment for end-stage renal disease. *Journal of the American Medical Association* 274(23):1858–1862.

Bennett CL, Horner RD, Weinstein RA, Dickinson GM, Dehovitz JA, Cohn SE, Kessler HA, Jacobson J, Goetz MB, Simberkoff M, Pitrak D, George WL, Gilman SC, Shapiro MF. (1995). Racial differences in care among hospitalized patients with pneumocystis carinii pneumonia in Chicago, New York, Los Angeles, Miami, and Raleigh-Durham. *Archives of Internal Medicine* 155(15):1586–92.

Bernabei R, Gambassi G, Lapane K, et al. (1998). Management of pain in elderly patients with cancer. *Journal of the American Medical Association* 279:1877–82.

Bloche MG. (2001). Race and discretion in American medicine. *Yale Journal of Health Policy, Law, and Ethics* 1:95–131.

Bobo LD. (2001). Racial attitudes and relations at the close of the twentieth century. In Smelser NJ, Wilson WI, and Mitchell F (Eds.), *America Becoming: Racial Trends and Their Consequences*. Washington, DC: National Academy Press.

Brogan D, Tuttle EP. (1988). Transplantation and the Medicare end-stage renal disease program [Letter]. *New England Journal of Medicine* 319:55.

Brownstein IN, Cheal N, Ackermann SF, Bassford TL, Campos-Outcalt D. (1992). Breast and cervical cancer screening in minority populations: A model for using lay health educators. *Journal of Cancer Education* 7(4):321–326.

Canto JG, Allison JJ, Kiefe CI, Fincher C, Farmer R, Sekar P, Person S, Weissman NW. (2000). Relation of race and sex to the use of reperfusion therapy in Medicare beneficiaries with acute myocardial infarction. *New England Journal of Medicine* 342:1094–1100.

Carrasquillo O, Orav EJ, Brennan TA, Burstin HR. (1999). Impact of language barriers on patient satisfaction in an emergency department. *Journal of General Internal Medicine* 14(2):82–7.

Chin MH, Zhang JX, Merrell K. (1998). Diabetes in the African-American Medicare population: Morbidity, quality of care, and resource utilization. *Diabetes Care* 21(7):1090–1095.

Cooper-Patrick L, Gallo JJ, Gonzales JJ, Vu HT, Powe NR, Nelson C, Ford DE. (1999). Race, gender, and partnership in the patient-physician relationship. *Journal of the American Medical Association* 282(6):583–9.

Cunningham WE, Mosen DM, Morales LS. (2000). Ethnic and racial differences in long-term survival from hospitalization for HIV infection. *Journal of Health Care for the Poor and Underserved* 11(2):163–178.

David RA, Rhee M. (1998). The impact of language as a barrier to effective health care in an underserved urban Hispanic community. *Mount Sinai Journal of Medicine* 65(5-6):393–397.

Derose KP, Baker DW. (2000). Limited English proficiency and Latinos' use of physician services. *Medical Care Research and Review* 57(1):76–91.

Dovidio JF, Brigham JC, Johnson BT, Gaertner SL. (1996). Stereotyping, prejudice, and discrimination: Another look. In Macrae N, Stangor C, and Hewstone M (Eds.), *Stereotypes and Stereotyping* 276–319. New York: Guilford.

Dovidio JF, Gaertner SL. (1998). On the nature of contemporary prejudice: The causes, consequences, and challenges of aversive racism. In Eberhardt J and Fiske ST (Eds.), *Confronting Racism: The Problem and the Response* 3–32. Thousand Oaks, CA: Sage.

Earp JL, Flax VL. (1999). What lay health advisors do: An evaluation of advisors' activities. *Cancer Practice* 7(1):16–21.

Epstein AM, Ayanian JZ, Keogh JH, Noonan SJ, Armistead N, Cleary PO, Weissman JS, David-Kasdan JA, Carlson D, Fuller J, March D, Conti R. (2000). Racial disparities in access to renal transplantation. *New England Journal of Medicine* 343(21):1537–1544.

Exner DV, Dries DL, Domanski MJ, Cohn IN. (2001). Lesser response to angiotensin-converting-enzyme inhibitor therapy in black as compared with white patients with left ventricular dysfunction. *New England Journal of Medicine* 344:1351–1357.

Gaylin DS, Held PJ, Port FK, et al. (1993). The impact of comorbid and sociodemographic factors on access to renal transplantation. *Journal of the American Medical Association* 269:603–608.

Geiger J. (this volume). Racial and ethnic disparities in diagnosis and treatment: A review of the evidence and a consideration of causes.

Giles WH, Anda RF, Casper ML, Escobedo LG, Taylor HA. (1995). Race and sex differences in rates of invasive cardiac procedures in U.S. hospitals. *Archives of Internal Medicine* 155:318–24.

Gomes C, McGuire TG. (2001). Identifying the sources of racial and ethnic disparities in health care use. Unpublished manuscript.

Gornick ME, Egers PW, Reilly TW, Mentnech RM, Fitterman LK, Kucken LE, Vladeck BC. (1996). Effects of race and income on mortality and use of services among Medicare beneficiaries. *New England Journal of Medicine* 335(11):791–799.

Hannan EL, Van Ryn M, Burke J, et al. (1999). Access to coronary artery bypass surgery by race/ethnicity and gender among patients who are appropriate for surgery. *Medical Care* 37:68–77.

Hashimoto OM. (2001). The proposed Patients' Bill of Rights: The case of the missing equal protection clause. *Yale Journal of Health Policy, Law, and Ethics* 1:77–93.

Herholz H, Goff DC, Ramsey DI, Chan FA, Ortiz C, Labarthe DR, Nichaman MZ. (1996). Women and Mexican Americans receive fewer cardiovascular drugs following myocardial infarction than men and non-Hispanic whites: The Corpus Christi Heart Project, 1988–1990. *Journal of Clinical Epidemiology* 49(3):279–87.

Hill MN, Miller NH. (1996). Compliance enhancement. A call for multidisciplinary team approaches. *Circulation* 93(1):4–6.

House JS, Williams D. (2000). Understanding and reducing socioeconomic and racial/ethnic disparities in health. In Smedley BD and Syme SL (Eds.), *Promoting Health: Intervention Strategies from Social and Behavioral Research*. Washington, DC: National Academy Press.

Imperato PJ, Nenner RP, Will TO. (1996). Radical prostatectomy: Lower rates among African American men. *Journal of the National Medical Association* 88(9):589–94.

Institute of Medicine. (2001). *Crossing the Quality Chasm*. Washington, DC: The National Academy Press.

Jackson EJ, Parks CP. (1997). Recruitment and training issues from selected lay health advisor programs among African Americans: A 20-year perspective. *Health Education & Behavior* 24(4):418–43l.

Johnson, PA, Lee TH, Cook EF, Rouan GW, Goldman L. (1993). Effect of race on the presentation and management of patients with acute chest pain. *Annals of Internal Medicine* 118:593–60l.

Jussim, L. (1991). Social perception and social reality: A reflection-construction model. *Psychological Review* 98:54–73.

Kahn KL, Pearson ML, Harrison ER, Desmond KA, Rogers WH, Rubenstein LV, Brook RH, Keeler EB. (1994). Health care for black and poor hospitalized Medicare patients. *Journal of the American Medical Association* 271(15):1169–1174.

Kaplan GA, Everson SA, Lynch JW. (2000). The contribution of social and behavioral research to an understanding of the distribution of disease: A multilevel approach. In Smedley BD and Syme SL (Eds.), *Promoting Health: Intervention Strategies from Social and Behavioral Research.* Washington, DC: National Academy Press.

Kasiske B, London W, Ellison MD. (1998). Race and socioeconomic factors influencing early placement on the kidney transplant waiting list. *Journal of the American Society of Nephrology* 9(11):2142–2147.

Kjellstrand CM. (1988). Age, sex, and race inequality in renal transplantation. *Archives of Internal Medicine* 148(6):1305–9.

Komaromy M, Grumbach K, Drake M, Vranizan K, Lurie N, Keane D, Bindman AB. (1996). The role of black and Hispanic physicians in providing health care for underserved populations. *New England Journal of Medicine* 334:1305–1310.

Korsch BM. (1984). What do patients and parents want to know? What do they need to know? *Pediatrics* 74(5 Pt 2):917–919.

Kressin NR, Petersen LA. (2001). Racial differences in the use of invasive cardiovascular procedures: Review of the literature and prescription for future research. *Annals of Internal Medicine* 135(5):352–366.

Laouri M, Kravitz RL, French WJ, Yang I, Milliken JC, Hilborne L, Wachsner R, Brook RH. (1997). Underuse of coronary revascularization procedures: Application of a clinical method. *Journal of the American College of Cardiology* 29:891–897.

LaVeist TA, Nickerson KJ, Bowie JV. (2000). Attitudes about racism, medical mistrust, and satisfaction with care among African American and white cardiac patients. *Medical Care Research and Review* 57(Supplement 1):146–6l.

Leigh WA, Lillie-Blanton M, Martinez RM, Collins KS. (1999). Managed care in three states: Experiences of low-income African-Americans and Hispanics. *Inquiry* 36(3):318–31.

Lillie-Blanton M, Brodie M, Rowland D, Altman D, McIntosh, M. (2000). Race, ethnicity, and the health care system: Public perceptions and experiences. *Medical Care Research and Review* 57(1):218–235.

Lillie-Blanton M, Martinez RM, Salganicoff A. (2001). Site of medical care: Do racial and ethnic differences persist? *Yale Journal of Health Policy, Law, and Ethics* 1(1):1–17.

Lowe RA, Chhaya S, Nasci K, Gavin LJ, Shaw K, Zwanger ML, Zeccardi JA, Dalsey WC, Abbuhl SB, Feldman H, Berlin JA. (2001). Effect of ethnicity on denial of authorization for emergency department care by managed care gatekeepers. *Academic Emergency Medicine* 8(3):259–66.

Mackie DM, Hamilton DL, Susskind L Rosselli F. (1996). Social psychological foundations of stereotype formation. In Macrae N, Stangor C, and Hewstone M (Eds.), *Stereotypes and stereotyping* (pp. 41–78). New York: Guilford Press.

Manson A. (1988). Language concordance as a determinant of patient compliance and emergency room use in patients with asthma. *Medical Care* 26(12):1119–1128.

Mayberry RM, Mili F, Ofili E. (2000). Racial and ethnic differences in access to medical care. *Medical Care Research and Review* 57(1):108–45.

McMahon LF, Wolfe RA, Huang S, Tedeschi P, Manning W, Edlund MJ. (1999). Racial and gender variation in use of diagnostic colonic procedures in the Michigan Medicare population. *Medical Care* 37(7):712–7.

Mitchell JB, McCormack LA. (1997). Time trends in late-stage diagnosis of cervical cancer: Differences by race/ethnicity and income. *Medical Care* 35(12):1220–4.

Moore RD, Stanton D, Gopalan R, Chaisson RE. (1994). Racial differences in the use of drug therapy for HIV disease in an urban community. *New England Journal of Medicine* 330(11):763–8.

Morin R. (2001). Misperceptions cloud whites' view of blacks. *The Washington Post,* July 11, 2001.

Morrison RS, Wallenstein S, Natale DK, Senzel RS, Huang L. (2000). "We don't carry that" Failure of pharmacies in predominantly nonwhite neighborhoods to stock opioid analgesics. *New England Journal of Medicine* 342(14): 1023–1026.

Mukamel DB, Murthy AS, Weimer DL. (2000). Racial differences in access to high-quality cardiac surgeons. *American Journal of Public Health* 90:1774–1777.

Petersen LA, Wright SM, Peterson ED, Daley J. (2002). Impact of race on cardiac care and outcomes in veterans with acute myocardial infarction. *Medical Care* 40(1Suppl):I-86–96.

Peterson ED, Shaw LK, DeLong ER, Pryor DB, Califf RM, Mark DB. (1997). Racial variation in the use of coronary-vascularization procedures: Are the differences real? Do they matter? *New England Journal of Medicine* 336: 480–6.

Phillips KA, Mayer ML, Aday LA. (2000). Barriers to care among racial/ethnic groups under managed care. *Health Affairs* 19:65–75.

Rice T. (this volume). The impact of cost-containment efforts on racial and ethnic disparities in health care: A conceptualization.

Robert Wood Johnson Foundation. (2001). New survey shows language barriers causing many Spanish-speaking Latinos to skip care. Fact sheet presented at press briefing, December 12, 2001. Washington, DC.

Rodney M, Clasen C, Goldman G, Markert R, Deane D. (1998). Three evaluation methods of a community health advocate program. *Journal of Community Health* 23(5):371–381.

Schneider EC, Leape LL, Weissman JS, Piana RN, Gatsonis C, Epstein AM. (2001). Racial differences in cardiac revascularization rates: Does "overuse" explain higher rates among white patients? *Annals of Internal Medicine* 135(5):328–37.

Schulman KA, Berlin JA, Harless W, et al. (1999). The effect of race and sex on physicians' recommendations for cardiac catheterization. *New England Journal of Medicine* 340:618–626.

Sedlis SP, Fisher VJ, Tice D, Esposito R, Madmon L, Steinberg EH. (1997). Racial differences in performance of invasive cardiac procedures in a Department of Veterans Affairs Medical Center. *Journal of Clinical Epidemiology* 50(8):899–901.

Shapiro MF, Morton SC, McCaffrey DF, Senterfitt JW, Fleishman JA, Perlman IF, Athey LA, Keesey JW, Goldman DP, Berry SH, Bozette SA. (1999). Variations in the care of HIVinfected adults in the United States: Results from the HIV Vost and Services Utilization Study. *Journal of the American Medical Association* 281:2305–75.

Smith DB. (1999). *Health Care Divided: Race and Healing a Nation.* Ann Arbor: The University of Michigan Press.

Tai-Seale M, Freund D, LoSasso A. (2001). Racial disparities in service use among Medicaid beneficiaries after mandatory enrollment in managed care: A difference-in-differences approach. *Inquiry* 38(1):49–59.

U.S. Commission on Civil Rights. (2001). *Funding Federal Civil Rights Enforcement: 2000 and Beyond.* Washington, DC: U.S. Commission on Civil Rights.

van Ryn M. (2002). Research on the provider contribution to race/ethnicity disparities in medical care. *Medical Care* 40(1): I-140–I-151.

van Ryn M, Burke J. (2000). The effect of patient race and socio-economic status on physician's perceptions of patients. *Social Science and Medicine* 50:813–828.

Weisse CS, Sorum PC, Sanders KN, Syat BL. (2001). Do gender and race affect decisions about pain management? *Journal of General Internal Medicine* 16(4)211–217.

Weitzman S, Cooper L, Chambless L, Rosamond W, Clegg L, Marcucci G, Romm F, White A. (1997). Gender, racial, and geographic differences in the performance of cardiac diagnostic and therapeutic procedures for hospitalized acute myocardial infarction in four states. *The American Journal of Cardiology* 79:722–6.

Wenneker MB, Epstein AM. (1989) Racial inequalities in the use of procedures for patients with ischemic heart disease in Massachusetts. *Journal of the American Medical Association* 261:253–7.

Williams DR. (1999). Race, socioeconomic status, and health: The added effects of racism and discrimination. *Annals of the New York Academy of Sciences* 896:173–88.

Williams DR. Rucker TD (2000). Understanding and addressing racial disparities in health care. *Health Care Financing Review* 21:75–90.

Williams JF, Zimmerman JW, Wagner DP, Hawkins M, Knaus W A. (1995). African-American and white patients admitted to the intensive care unit: Is there a difference in therapy and outcome? *Critical Care Medicine* 23(4):626–636.

Witmer A, Seifer SD, Finocchio L, Leslie J, O'Neil EH. (1995). Community health workers: Integral members of the health care work force. *American Journal of Public Health* 85(8):1055–1058.

Woloshin S, Bickell NA, Schwartz LM, Gany F, Welch HG. (1995). Language barriers in medicine in the United States. *Journal of the American Medical Association* 273(9):724–728.

Wood AJJ. (2001). Racial differences in the response to drugs-pointers to genetic differences. *New England Journal of Medicine* 344:1393–1395.

Yergan J, Food AB, LoGerfo JP, Diher P. Relationship between patient race and the intensity of hospital services. *Medical Care* 25:592–603.

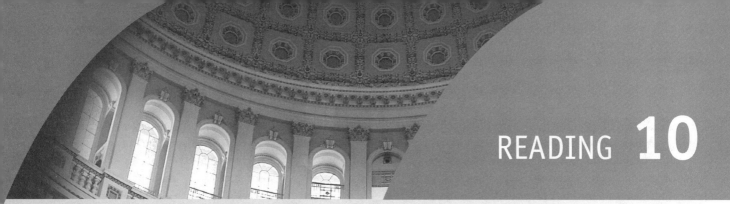

Case Law: *Canterbury v. Spence* (Patient-Oriented Standard of Informed Consent)

Jerry W. CANTERBURY, Appellant, v. William Thornton SPENCE and the Washington Hospital Center, a body corporate, Appellees

UNITED STATES COURT OF APPEALS FOR THE DISTRICT OF COLUMBIA CIRCUIT

December 18, 1969, Argued.

May 19, 1972, Decided.

OPINION: SPOTTSWOOD W. ROBINSON, III, Circuit Judge: This appeal is from a judgment entered in the District Court on verdicts directed for the two appellees at the conclusion of plaintiff-appellant Canterbury's case in chief. His action sought damages for personal injuries allegedly sustained as a result of an operation negligently performed by appellee Spence, a negligent failure by Dr. Spence to disclose a risk of serious disability inherent in the operation, and negligent post-operative care by appellee Washington Hospital Center. On close examination of the record, we find evidence which required submission of these issues to the jury. We accordingly reverse the judgment as to each appellee and remand the case to the District Court for a new trial.

I

The record we review tells a depressing tale. A youth troubled only by back pain submitted to an operation without being informed of a risk of paralysis incidental thereto. A day after the operation he fell from his hospital bed after having been left without assistance while voiding. A few hours after the fall, the lower half of his body was paralyzed, and he had to be operated on again. Despite extensive medical care, he has never been what he was before.

Instead of the back pain, even years later, he hobbled about on crutches, a victim of paralysis of the bowels and urinary incontinence. In a very real sense this lawsuit is an understandable search for reasons. At the time of the events which gave rise to this litigation, appellant was nineteen years of age, a clerk-typist employed by the Federal Bureau of Investigation. In December, 1958, he began to experience severe pain between his shoulder blades.[1] He consulted two general practitioners, but the medications they prescribed failed to eliminate the pain. Thereafter, appellant secured an appointment with Dr. Spence, who is a neurosurgeon.

Dr. Spence examined appellant in his office at some length but found nothing amiss. On Dr. Spence's advice appellant was x-rayed, but the films did not identify any abnormality. Dr. Spence then recommended that appellant undergo a myelogram—a procedure in which dye is injected into the spinal column and traced to find evidence of disease or other disorder—at the Washington Hospital Center. Appellant entered the hospital on February 4, 1959.[2] The myelogram revealed a "filling defect" in the region of the fourth thoracic vertebra. Since a myelogram often does no more than pinpoint the location of an aberration, surgery may be necessary to discover the cause. Dr. Spence told appellant that he would have

---

1. Two months earlier, appellant was hospitalized for diagnostic tests following complaints of weight loss and lassitude. He was discharged with a final diagnosis of neurosis and thereafter given supportive therapy by his then attending physician.

2. The dates stated herein are taken from the hospital records. At trial, appellant and his mother contended that the records were inaccurate, but the one-day difference over which they argued is without significance.

to undergo a laminectomy—the excision of the posterior arch of the vertebra—to correct what he suspected was a ruptured disc. Appellant did not raise any objection to the proposed operation nor did he probe into its exact nature.

Appellant explained to Dr. Spence that his mother was a widow of slender financial means living in Cyclone, West Virginia, and that she could be reached through a neighbor's telephone. Appellant called his mother the day after the myelogram was performed and, failing to contact her, left Dr. Spence's telephone number with the neighbor. When Mrs. Canterbury returned the call, Dr. Spence told her that the surgery was occasioned by a suspected ruptured disc. Mrs. Canterbury then asked if the recommended operation was serious and Dr. Spence replied "Not anymore than any other operation." He added that he knew Mrs. Canterbury was not well off and that her presence in Washington would not be necessary. The testimony is contradictory as to whether during the course of the conversation Mrs. Canterbury expressed her consent to the operation. Appellant himself apparently did not converse again with Dr. Spence prior to the operation.

Dr. Spence performed the laminectomy on February 11[3] at the Washington Hospital Center. Mrs. Canterbury traveled to Washington, arriving on that date but after the operation was over, and signed a consent form at the hospital. The laminectomy revealed several anomalies: a spinal cord that was swollen and unable to pulsate, an accumulation of large tortuous and dilated veins, and a complete absence of epidural fat which normally surrounds the spine. A thin hypodermic needle was inserted into the spinal cord to aspirate any cysts which might have been present, but no fluid emerged. In suturing the wound, Dr. Spence attempted to relieve the pressure on the spinal cord by enlarging the dura—the outer protective wall of the spinal cord—at the area of swelling.

For approximately the first day after the operation appellant recuperated normally, but then suffered a fall and an almost immediate setback. Since there is some conflict as to precisely when or why appellant fell,[4] we reconstruct the events from the evidence most favorable to him.[5] Dr. Spence left orders that appellant was to remain in bed during the process of voiding. These orders were changed to direct that voiding be done out of bed, and the jury could find that the change was made by hospital personnel. Just prior to the fall, appellant summoned a nurse and was given a receptacle for use in voiding, but was then left unattended. Appellant testified that during the course of the endeavor he slipped off the side of the bed, and that there was no one to assist him, or side rail to prevent the fall.

Several hours later, appellant began to complain that he could not move his legs and that he was having trouble breathing; paralysis seems to have been virtually total from the waist down. Dr. Spence was notified on the night of February 12, and he rushed to the hospital. Mrs. Canterbury signed another consent form and appellant was again taken into the operating room. The surgical wound was reopened and Dr. Spence created a gusset to allow the spinal cord greater room in which to pulsate. Appellant's control over his muscles improved somewhat after the second operation but he was unable to void properly. As a result of this condition, he came under the care of a urologist while still in the hospital. In April, following a cystoscopic examination, appellant was operated on for removal of bladder stones, and in May was released from the hospital. He reentered the hospital the following August for a 10-day period, apparently because of his urologic problems. For several years after his discharge he was under the care of several specialists, and at all times was under the care of a urologist. At the time of the trial in April, 1968, appellant required crutches to walk, still suffered from urinal incontinence and paralysis of the bowels, and wore a penile clamp.

In November, 1959 on Dr. Spence's recommendation, appellant was transferred by the F.B.I. to Miami where he could get more swimming and exercise. Appellant worked three years for the F.B.I. in Miami, Los Angeles and Houston, resigning finally in June, 1962. From then until the time of the trial, he held a number of jobs, but had constant trouble finding work because he needed to remain seated and close to a bathroom. The damages appellant claims include extensive pain and suffering, medical expenses, and loss of earnings.

II

Appellant filed suit in the District Court on March 7, 1963, four years after the laminectomy and approximately two years after he attained his majority. The complaint stated several causes of action against each defendant. Against Dr. Spence it alleged, among other things, negligence in the performance of the laminectomy and failure to inform him beforehand of the risk involved. Against the hospital the complaint charged negligent post-operative care in permitting appellant to remain unattended after the laminectomy, in failing to provide a nurse or orderly to assist him at the time of his fall, and in failing to maintain a side rail on his

---

3. The operation was postponed five days because appellant was suffering from an abdominal infection.

4. The one fact clearly emerging from the otherwise murky portrayal by the record, however, is that appellant did fall while attempting to void and while completely unattended.

5. See *Aylor v. Intercounty Constr. Corp.*, 127 U.S.App.D.C. 151, 153, 381 F.2d 930, 932 (1967), and cases cited in footnote 2 thereof.

bed. The answers denied the allegations of negligence and defended on the ground that the suit was barred by the statute of limitations.

Pretrial discovery—including depositions by appellant, his mother, and Dr. Spence—continuances and other delays consumed five years. At trial, disposition of the threshold question whether the statute of limitations had run was held in abeyance until the relevant facts developed.

Appellant introduced no evidence to show medical and hospital practices, if any, customarily pursued in regard to the critical aspects of the case, and only Dr. Spence, called as an adverse witness, testified on the issue of causality. Dr. Spence described the surgical procedures he utilized in the two operations and expressed his opinion that appellant's disabilities stemmed from his pre-operative condition as symptomatized by the swollen, non-pulsating spinal cord. He stated, however, that neither he nor any of the other physicians with whom he consulted was certain as to what that condition was, and he admitted that trauma can be a cause of paralysis. Dr. Spence further testified that even without trauma paralysis can be anticipated "somewhere in the nature of one percent" of the laminectomies performed, a risk he termed "a very slight possibility." He felt that communication of that risk to the patient is not good medical practice because it might deter patients from undergoing needed surgery and might produce adverse psychological reactions which could preclude the success of the operation.

At the close of appellant's case in chief, each defendant moved for a directed verdict and the trial judge granted both motions. The basis of the ruling, he explained, was that appellant had failed to produce any medical evidence indicating negligence on Dr. Spence's part in diagnosing appellant's malady or in performing the laminectomy; that there was no proof that Dr. Spence's treatment was responsible for appellant's disabilities; and that notwithstanding some evidence to show negligent post-operative care, an absence of medical testimony to show causality precluded submission of the case against the hospital to the jury. The judge did not allude specifically to the alleged breach of duty by Dr. Spence to divulge the possible consequences of the laminectomy.

We reverse. The testimony of appellant and his mother that Dr. Spence did not reveal the risk of paralysis from the laminectomy made out a prima facie case of violation of the physician's duty to disclose which Dr. Spence's explanation did not negate as a matter of law. There was also testimony from which the jury could have found that the laminectomy was negligently performed by Dr. Spence, and that appellant's fall was the consequence of negligence on the part of the hospital. The record, moreover, contains evidence of sufficient quantity and quality to tender jury issues as to whether and to what extent any such negligence was causally related to appellant's post-laminectomy condition. These considerations entitled appellant to a new trial.

Elucidation of our reasoning necessitates elaboration on a number of points. In Parts III and IV we explore the origins and rationale of the physician's duty to reasonably inform an ailing patient as to the treatment alternatives available and the risks incidental to them. In Part V, we investigate the scope of the disclosure requirement and in Part VI the physician's privileges not to disclose. In Part VII we examine the role of causality, and in Part VIII the need for expert testimony in non-disclosure litigation. In Part IX we deal with appellees' statute of limitations defense and in Part X we apply the principles discussed to the case at bar.

III

Suits charging failure by a physician[6] adequately to disclose the risks and alternatives of proposed treatment are not innovations in American law. They date back a good half-century,[7] and in the last decade they have multiplied rapidly.[8] There is, nonetheless, disagreement among the courts and the commentators[9] on many major questions, and there is no precedent of our own directly in point.[10] For the tools enabling

---

6. Since there was neither allegation nor proof that the appellee hospital failed in any duty to disclose, we have no occasion to inquire as to whether or under what circumstances such a duty might arise.

7. See, e.g., *Theodore v. Ellis*, 141 La. 709, 75 So. 655, 660 (1917); *Wojciechowski v. Coryell*, 217 S.W. 638, 644 (Mo.App.1920); *Hunter v. Burroughs*, 123 Va. 113, 96 S.E. 360, 366-368 (1918).

8. See the collections in Annot., 79 A.L.R.2d 1028 (1961); Comment, Informed Consent in Medical Malpractice, 55 Calif. L.Rev. 1396, 1397 n. 5 (1967).

9. For references to a considerable body of commentary, see Waltz & Scheuneman, Informed Consent to Therapy, 64 Nw.U.L.Rev. 628 n. 1 (1970).

10. In *Stivers v. George Washington Univ.*, 116 U.S.App.D.C. 29, 320 F.2d 751 (1963), a charge was asserted against a physician and a hospital that a patient's written consent to a bilateral arteriogram was based on inadequate information, but our decision did not touch the legal aspects of that claim. The jury to which the case was tried found for the physician, and the trial judge awarded judgment for the hospital notwithstanding a jury verdict against it. The patient confined the appeal to this court to the judgment entered for the hospital, and in no way implicated the verdict for the physician. We concluded that the verdict constitutes a jury finding that [the physician] was not guilty of withholding relevant information from [the patient] or in the alternative that he violated no duty owed her in telling her what he did tell her or in withholding what he did not tell her...." 116 U.S.App.D.C. at 31, 320 F.2d at 753. The fact that no review of the verdict as to the physician was sought thus became critical. The hospital could not be held derivatively liable on the theory of a master–servant relationship with the physician since the physician himself had been exonerated. And since there was no evidence upon which the verdict against the hospital could properly have been predicated independently, we affirmed the trial judge's action in setting it aside. 116 U.S.App.D.C. at 31-32, 320 F.2d at 753-754. In these circumstances, our opinion in Stivers cannot be taken as either approving or disapproving the handling of the risk-nondisclosure issue between the patient and the physician in the trial court.

resolution of the issues on this appeal, we are forced to begin at first principles.[11]

The root premise is the concept, fundamental in American jurisprudence, that "every human being of adult years and sound mind has a right to determine what shall be done with his own body. . . ."[12] True consent to what happens to one's self is the informed exercise of a choice, and that entails an opportunity to evaluate knowledgeably the options available and the risks attendant upon each.[13] The average patient has little or no understanding of the medical arts, and ordinarily has only his physician to whom he can look for enlightenment with which to reach an intelligent decision.[14] From these almost axiomatic considerations springs the need, and in turn the requirement, of a reasonable divulgence by physician to patient to make such a decision possible.[15]

A physician is under a duty to treat his patient skillfully[16] but proficiency in diagnosis and therapy is not the full measure of his responsibility. The cases demonstrate that the physician is under an obligation to communicate specific information to the patient when the exigencies of reasonable care call for it.[17] Due care may require a physician perceiving symptoms of bodily abnormality to alert the patient to the condition.[18] It may call upon the physician confronting an ailment which does not respond to his ministrations to inform the patient thereof.[19] It may command the physician to instruct the patient as to any limitations to be presently observed for his own welfare,[20] and as to any precautionary therapy he should seek in the future.[21] It may oblige the physician to advise the patient of the need for or desirability of any alternative treatment promising greater benefit than that being pursued.[22] Just as plainly, due care normally demands that the physician warn the patient of any risks to his well-being which contemplated therapy may involve.[23]

The context in which the duty of risk-disclosure arises is invariably the occasion for decision as to whether a particular

---

11. We undertake only a general outline of legal doctrine on the subject and, of course, a discussion and application of the principles which in our view should govern this appeal. The rest we leave for future litigation.

12. *Schloendorff v. Society of New York Hospital*, 211 N.Y. 125, 105 N.E. 92, 93 (1914). See also *Natanson v. Kline*, 186 Kan. 393, 350 P.2d 1093, 1104 (1960), clarified, 187 Kan. 186, 354 P.2d 670 (1960); W. Prosser, Torts § 18 at 102 (3d ed. 1964); Restatement of Torts § 49 (1934).

13. See *Dunham v. Wright*, 423 F.2d 940, 943-946 (3d Cir. 1970) (applying Pennsylvania law); *Campbell v. Oliva*, 424 F.2d 1244, 1250-1251 (6th Cir. 1970) (applying Tennessee law); *Bowers v. Talmage*, 159 So.2d 888 (Fla.App.1963); *Woods v. Brumlop*, 71 N.M. 221, 377 P.2d 520, 524-525 (1962); *Mason v. Ellsworth*, 3 Wash.App. 298, 474 P.2d 909, 915, 918-919 (1970).

14. Patients ordinarily are persons unlearned in the medical sciences. Some few, of course, are schooled in branches of the medical profession or in related fields. But even within the latter group variations in degree of medical knowledge specifically referable to particular therapy may be broad, as for example, between a specialist and a general practitioner, or between a physician and a nurse. It may well be, then, that it is only in the unusual case that a court could safely assume that the patient's insights were on a parity with those of the treating physician.

15. The doctrine that a consent effective as authority to form therapy can arise only from the patient's understanding of alternatives to and risks of the therapy is commonly denominated "informed consent." See, e.g., *Waltz & Scheuneman*, Informed Consent to Therapy, 64 Nw.U.L.Rev. 628, 629 (1970). The same appellation is frequently assigned to the doctrine requiring physicians, as a matter of duty to patients, to communicate information as to such alternatives and risks. See, e.g., Comment, Informed Consent in Medical Malpractice, 55 Calif.L.Rev. 1396 (1967). While we recognize the general utility of shorthand phrases in literary expositions, we caution that uncritical use of the "informed consent" label can be misleading. See, e.g., Plante, An Analysis of "Informed Consent," 36 Ford.L.Rev. 639, 671-72 (1968). In duty-to-disclose cases, the focus of attention is more properly upon the nature and content of the physician's divulgence than the patient's understanding or consent. Adequate disclosure and informed consent are, of course, two sides of the same coin—the former a sine qua non of the latter. But the vital inquiry on duty to disclose relates to the physician's performance of an obligation, while one of the difficulties with analysis in terms of "informed consent" is its tendency to imply that what is decisive is the degree of the patient's comprehension. As we later emphasize, the physician discharges the duty when he makes a reasonable effort to convey sufficient information although the patient, without fault of the physician, may not fully grasp it. See text infra at notes 82-89. Even though the fact-finder may have occasion to draw an inference on the state of the patient's enlightenment, the fact-finding process on performance of the duty ultimately reaches back to what the physician actually said or failed to say. And while the factual conclusion on adequacy of the revelation will vary as between patients—as, for example, between a lay patient and a physician–patient—the fluctuations are attributable to the kind of divulgence which may be reasonable under the circumstances.

16. *Brown v. Keaveny*, 117 U.S.App.D.C. 117, 118, 326 F.2d 660, 661 (1963); *Quick v. Thurston*, 110 U.S.App.D.C. 169, 171, 290 F.2d 360, 362, 88 A.L.R.2d 299 (en banc 1961); *Rodgers v. Lawson*, 83 U.S.App.D.C. 281, 282, 170 F.2d 157, 158 (1948).

17. See discussion in McCoid, *The Care Required of Medical Practitioners*, 12 Vand.L.Rev. 549, 586-97 (1959).

18. See *Union Carbide & Carbon Corp. v. Stapleton*, 237 F.2d 229, 232 (6th Cir. 1956); *Maertins v. Kaiser Foundation Hosp.*, 162 Cal.App.2d 661, 328 P.2d 494, 497 (1958); *Doty v. Canterbury v. Spence* Page 11 of 11 *Lutheran Hosp. Ass'n*, 110 Neb. 467, 194 N.W. 444, 445, 447 (1923); *Tvedt v. Haugen*, 70 N.D. 338, 294 N.W. 183, 187 (1940). See also *Dietze v. King*, 184 F. Supp. 944, 948, 949 (E.D.Va.1960); *Dowling v. Mutual Life Ins. Co.*, 168 So.2d 107, 116 (La.App.1964), writ refused, 247 La. 248, 170 So.2d 508 (1965).

19. See *Rahn v. United States*, 222 F. Supp. 775, 780-781 (S.D.Ga.1963) (applying Georgia law); *Baldor v. Rogers*, 81 So.2d 658, 662, 55 A.L.R.2d 453 (Fla.1955); *Manion v. Tweedy*, 257 Minn. 59, 100 N.W.2d 124, 128, 129 (1959); *Tvedt v. Haugen*, supra note 18, 294 N.W. at 187; *Ison v. McFall*, 55 Tenn.App. 326, 400 S.W.2d 243, 258 (1964); *Kelly v. Carroll*, 36 Wash.2d 482, 219 P.2d 79, 88, 19 A.L.R.2d 1174, cert. denied, 340 U.S. 892, 71 S. Ct. 208, 95 L. Ed. 646 (1950).

20. *Newman v. Anderson*, 195 Wis. 200, 217 N.W. 306 (1928). See also *Whitfield v. Daniel Constr. Co.*, 226 S.C. 37, 83 S.E.2d 460, 463 (1954).

21. *Beck v. German Klinik*, 78 Iowa 696, 43 N.W. 617, 618 (1889); *Pike v. Honsinger*, 155 N.Y. 201, 49 N.E. 760, 762 (1898); *Doan v. Griffith*, 402 S.W.2d 855, 856 (Ky.1966).

22. The typical situation is where a general practitioner discovers that the patient's malady calls for specialized treatment, whereupon the duty generally arises to advise the patient to consult a specialist. See the cases collected in Annot., 35 A.L.R.3d 349 (1971). See also *Baldor v. Rogers*, supra note 19, 81 So.2d at 662; *Garafola v. Maimonides Hosp.*, 22 A.D.2d 85, 253 N.Y.S.2d 856, 858, 28 A.L.R.3d 1357 (1964); aff'd, 19 N.Y.2d 765, 279 N.Y.S.2d 523, 226 N.E.2d 311, 28 A.L.R.3d 1362 (1967); McCoid, *The Care Required of Medical Practitioners*, 12 Vand.L.Rev. 549, 597-98 (1959).

23. See, e.g., *Wall v. Brim*, 138 F.2d 478, 480-481 (5th Cir. 1943), consent issue tried on remand and verdict for plaintiff aff'd., 145 F.2d 492 (5th Cir. 1944), cert. denied, 324 U.S. 857, 65 S. Ct. 858, 89 L. Ed. 1415 (1945); *Belcher v. Carter*, 13 Ohio App.2d 113, 234 N.E.2d 311, 312 (1967); *Hunter v. Burroughs*, supra note 7, 96 S.E. at 366; Plante, An Analysis of "Informed Consent," 36 Ford.L.Rev. 639, 653 (1968).

treatment procedure is to be undertaken. To the physician, whose training enables a self-satisfying evaluation, the answer may seem clear, but it is the prerogative of the patient, not the physician, to determine for himself the direction in which his interests seem to lie.[24] To enable the patient to chart his course understandably, some familiarity with the therapeutic alternatives and their hazards becomes essential.[25]

A reasonable revelation in these respects is not only a necessity but, as we see it, is as much a matter of the physician's duty. It is a duty to warn of the dangers lurking in the proposed treatment, and that is surely a facet of due care.[26] It is, too, a duty to impart information which the patient has every right to expect.[27] The patient's reliance upon the physician is a trust of the kind which traditionally has exacted obligations beyond those associated with armslength transactions.[28] His dependence upon the physician for information affecting his well-being, in terms of contemplated treatment, is well-nigh abject. As earlier noted, long before the instant litigation arose, courts had recognized that the physician had the responsibility of satisfying the vital informational needs of the patient.[29] More recently, we ourselves have found "in the fiducial qualities of [the physician–patient] relationship the physician's duty to reveal to the patient that which in his best interests it is important that he should know."[30] We now find, as a part of the

physician's overall obligation to the patient, a similar duty of reasonable disclosure of the choices with respect to proposed therapy and the dangers inherently and potentially involved.[31]

This disclosure requirement, on analysis, reflects much more of a change in doctrinal emphasis than a substantive addition to malpractice law. It is well established that the physician must seek and secure his patient's consent before commencing an operation or other course of treatment.[32] It is also clear that the consent, to be efficacious, must be free from imposition upon the patient.[33] It is the settled rule that therapy not authorized by the patient may amount to a tort—a common law battery—by the physician.[34] And it is evident that it is normally impossible to obtain a consent worthy of the name unless the physician first elucidates the options and the perils for the patient's edification.[35] Thus the physician has long borne a duty, on pain of liability for unauthorized treatment, to make adequate disclosure to the patient.[36] The evolution of the obligation to communicate for the patient's benefit as well as the physician's protection has hardly involved an extraordinary restructuring of the law.

IV

Duty to disclose has gained recognition in a large number of American jurisdictions,[37] but more largely on a different rationale. The majority of courts dealing with the problem have

24. See text supra at notes 12-13.

25. See cases cited supra notes 14-15.

26. See text supra at notes 17-23.

27. Some doubt has been expressed as to ability of physicians to suitably communicate their evaluations of risks and the advantages of optional treatment, and as to the lay patient's ability to understand what the physician tells him. Karchmer, Informed Consent: A Plaintiff's Medical Malpractice "Wonder Drug," 31 Mo.L.Rev. 29, 41 (1966). We do not share these apprehensions. The discussion need not be a disquisition, and surely the physician is not compelled to give his patient a short medical education; the disclosure rule summons the physician only to a reasonable explanation. See Part V, infra. That means generally informing the patient in nontechnical terms as to what is at stake: the therapy alternatives open to him, the goals expectably to be achieved, and the risks that may ensue from particular treatment and no treatment. See *Stinnett v. Price*, 446 S.W.2d 893, 894, 895 (Tex.Civ.App.1969). So informing the patient hardly taxes the physician, and it must be the exceptional patient who cannot comprehend such an explanation at least in a rough way.

28. That element comes to the fore in litigation involving contractual and property dealings between physician and patient. See, e.g., *Campbell v. Oliva*, supra note 13, 424 F.2d at 1250; In re Bourquin's Estate, 161 Cal.App.2d 289, 326 P.2d 604, 610 (1958); *Butler v. O'Brien*, 8 Ill.2d 203, 133 N.E.2d 274, 277 (1956); *Woodbury v. Woodbury*, 141 Mass. 329, 5 N.E. 275, 278, 279 (1886); *Clinton v. Miller*, 77 Okl. 173, 186 P. 932, 933 (1919); *Hodge v. Shea*, 252 S.C. 601, 168 S.E.2d 82, 84, 87 (1969).

29. See, e.g., *Sheets v. Burman*, 322 F.2d 277, 279-280 (5th Cir. 1963); *Hudson v. Moore*, 239 Ala. 130, 194 So. 147, 149 (1940); *Guy v. Schuldt*, 236 Ind. 101, 138 N.E.2d 891, 895 (1956); *Perrin v. Rodriguez*, 153 So. 555, 556-557 (La.App.1934); *Schmucking v. Mayo*, 183 Minn. 37, 235 N.W. 633 (1931); *Thompson v. Barnard*, 142 S.W.2d 238, 241 (Tex.Civ.App.1940), aff'd, 138 Tex. 277, 158 S.W.2d 486 (1942).

30. *Emmett v. Eastern Dispensary & Cas. Hosp.*, 130 U.S.App.D.C. 50, 54, 396 F.2d 931, 935 (1967), See also, Swan, The California Law of Malpractice of Physicians, Surgeons, and Dentists, 33 Calif.L.Rev. 248, 251 (1945).

31. See cases cited supra notes 16-28; *Berkey v. Anderson*, 1 Cal.App.3d 790, 82 Cal.Rptr. 67, 78 (1970); Smith, Antecedent Grounds of Liability in the Practice of Surgery, 14 Rocky Mt.L.Rev. 233, 249-50 (1942); Swan, The California Law of Malpractice of Physicians, Surgeons, and Dentists, 33 Calif.L.Rev. 248, 251 (1945); Note, 40 Minn.L.Rev. 876, 879-80 (1956).

32. See cases collected in Annot., 56 A.L.R.2d 695 (1967). Where the patient is incapable of consenting, the physician may have to obtain consent from someone else. See, e.g., *Bonner v. Moran*, 75 U.S.App.D.C. 156, 157-158, 126 F.2d 121, 122-123, 139 A.L.R. 1366 (1941).

33. See Restatement (Second) of Torts §§ 55-58 (1965).

34. See, e.g., *Bonner v. Moran*, supra note 32, 75 U.S.App.D.C. at 157, 126 F.2d at 122, and cases collected in Annot., 56 A.L.R.2d 695, 697-99 (1957). See also Part IX, infra.

35. See cases cited supra note 13. See also McCoid, The Care Required of Medical Practitioners, 12 Vand.L.Rev. 549, 587-91 (1959).

36. We discard the thought that the patient should ask for information before the physician is required to disclose. Caveat emptor is not the norm for the consumer of medical services. Duty to disclose is more than a call to speak merely on the patient's request, or merely to answer the patient's questions; it is a duty to volunteer, if necessary, the information the patient needs for intelligent decision. The patient may be ignorant, confused, overawed by the physician or frightened by the hospital, or even ashamed to inquire. See generally Note, Restructuring Informed Consent: Legal Therapy for the Doctor-Patient Relationship, 79 Yale L.J. 1533, 1545-51 (1970). Perhaps relatively few patients could in any event identify the relevant questions in the absence of prior explanation by the physician. Physicians and hospitals have patients of widely divergent socio-economic backgrounds, and a rule which presumes a degree of sophistication which many members of society lack is likely to breed gross inequities. See Note, Informed Consent as a Theory of Medical Liability, 1970 Wis.L.Rev. 879, 891-97.

37. The number is reported at 22 by 1967. Comment, Informed Consent in Medical Malpractice, 55 Calif.L.Rev. 1396, 1397, and cases cited in n. 5 (1967).

made the duty depend on whether it was the custom of physicians practicing in the community to make the particular disclosure to the patient.[38] If so, the physician may be held liable for an unreasonable and injurious failure to divulge, but there can be no recovery unless the omission forsakes a practice prevalent in the profession.[39] We agree that the physician's noncompliance with a professional custom to reveal, like any other departure from prevailing medical practice,[40] may give rise to liability to the patient. We do not agree that the patient's cause of action is dependent upon the existence and nonperformance of a relevant professional tradition.

There are, in our view, formidable obstacles to acceptance of the notion that the physician's obligation to disclose is either germinated or limited by medical practice. To begin with, the reality of any discernible custom reflecting a professional consensus on communication of option and risk information to patients is open to serious doubt.[41] We sense the danger that what in fact is no custom at all may be taken as an affirmative custom to maintain silence, and that physician-witnesses to the so-called custom may state merely their personal opinions as to what they or others would do under given conditions.[42] We cannot gloss over the inconsistency between reliance on a general practice respecting divulgence and, on the other hand, realization that the myriad of variables among patients[43] makes each case so different that its omission can rationally be justified only by the effect of its individual circumstances.[44] Nor can we ignore the fact that to bind the disclosure obligation to medical usage is to arrogate the decision on revelation to the physician alone.[45] Respect for the patient's right of self-determination on particular therapy[46] demands a standard set by law for physicians rather than one which physicians may or may not impose upon themselves.[47]

More fundamentally, the majority rule overlooks the graduation of reasonable-care demands in Anglo-American jurisprudence and the position of professional custom in the hierarchy. The caliber of the performance exacted by the reasonable-care standard varies between the professional and non-professional worlds, and so also the role of professional custom. "With but few exceptions," we recently declared, "society demands that everyone under a duty to use care observe minimally a general standard."[48] "Familiarly expressed judicially," we added, "the yardstick is that degree of care which a reasonably prudent person would have exercised under the same or similar circumstances."[49] "Beyond this," however, we emphasized, "the law requires those engaging in activities requiring unique knowledge and ability to give a performance commensurate with the undertaking."[50] Thus physicians treating the sick must perform at higher levels than non-physicians in order to meet the reasonable care standard in its special application to physicians[51]—"that degree of care and skill ordinarily exercised by the profession in [the physician's] own or similar localities."[52] And practices adopted by the profession have indispensable value as evidence tending to establish just what that degree of care and skill is.[53]

We have admonished, however, that "the special medical standards[54] are but adaptions of the general standard to a group who are required to act as reasonable men possessing their medical talents presumably would."[55] There is, by the same token, no basis for operation of the special medical standard where the physician's activity does not bring his medical knowledge and skills peculiarly into play.[56] And

---

38. See, e.g., *DiFilippo v. Preston*, 3 Storey 539, 53 Del. 539, 173 A.2d 333, 339 (1961); *Haggerty v. McCarthy*, 344 Mass. 136, 181 N.E.2d 562, 565, 566 (1962); *Roberts v. Young*, 369 Mich. 133, 119 N.W.2d 627, 630 (1963); *Aiken v. Clary*, 396 S.W.2d 668, 675, 676 (Mo.1965). As these cases indicate, majority rule courts hold that expert testimony is necessary to establish the custom.

39. See cases cited supra note 38.

40. See, e.g., W. Prosser, Torts § 33 at 171 (3d ed. 1964).

41. See, e.g., Comment, Informed Consent in Medical Malpractice, 55 Calif.L.Rev. 1396, 1404-05 (1967); Comment, Valid Consent to Medical Treatment: Need the Patient Know?, 4 Duquesne L.Rev. 450, 458-59 (1966); Note, 75 Harv.L.Rev. 1445, 1447 (1962).

42. Comment, Informed Consent in Medical Malpractice, 55 Calif.L.Rev. 1396, 1404 (1967); Note, 75 Harv.L.Rev. 1445, 1447 (1962).

43. For example, the variables which may or may not give rise to the physician's privilege to withhold risk information for therapeutic reasons. See text Part VI, infra.

44. Note, 75 Harv.L.Rev. 1445, 1447 (1962).

45. E.g., W. Prosser, Torts § 32 at 168 (3d ed. 1964); Comment, Informed Consent in Medical Malpractice, 55 Calif.L.Rev. 1396, 1409 (1967).

46. See text supra at notes 12-13.

47. See *Berkey v. Anderson*, supra note 31, 82 Cal.Rptr. at 78; Comment, Informed Consent in Medical Malpractice, 55 Calif.L.Rev. 1396, 1409-10 (1967). Medical custom bared in the cases indicates the frequency with which the profession has not engaged in self-imposition. See, e.g., cases cited supra note 23.

48. *Washington Hosp. Center v. Butler*, 127 U.S.App.D.C. 379, 383, 384 F.2d 331, 335 (1967).

49. Id.

50. Id.

51. Id.

52. *Rodgers v. Lawson*, supra note 16, 83 U.S.App.D.C. at 282, 170 F.2d at 158. See also *Brown v. Keaveny*, supra note 16, 117 U.S.App.D.C. at 118, 326 F.2d at 661; *Quick v. Thurston*, supra note 16, 110 U.S.App.D.C. at 171, 290 F.2d at 362.

53. E.g., *Washington Hosp. Center v. Butler*, supra note 48, 127 U.S.App.D.C. at 383, 384 F.2d at 335. See also cases cited infra note 119.

54. Id. at 383 ns. 10-12, 384 F.2d at 335 ns. 10-12. [**30]

55. Id. at 384 n. 15, 384 F.2d at 336 n. 15.

56. E.g., *Lucy Webb Hayes Nat. Training School v. Perotti*, 136 U.S.App.D.C. 122, 127-129, 419 F.2d 704, 710-711 (1969); *Monk v. Doctors Hosp.*, 131 U.S.App.D.C. 174, 177, 403 F.2d 580, 583 (1968); *Washington Hosp. Center v. Butler*, supra note 48.

where the challenge to the physician's conduct is not to be gauged by the special standard, it follows that medical custom cannot furnish the test of its propriety, whatever its relevance under the proper test may be.[57] The decision to unveil the patient's condition and the chances as to remediation, as we shall see, is ofttimes a non-medical judgment[58] and, if so, is a decision outside the ambit of the special standard. Where that is the situation, professional custom hardly furnishes the legal criterion for measuring the physician's responsibility to reasonably inform his patient of the options and the hazards as to treatment.

The majority rule, moreover, is at war with our prior holdings that a showing of medical practice, however probative, does not fix the standard governing recovery for medical malpractice.[59] Prevailing medical practice, we have maintained, has evidentiary value in determinations as to what the specific criteria measuring challenged professional conduct are and whether they have been met,[60] but does not itself define the standard.[61] That has been our position in treatment cases, where the physician's performance is ordinarily to be adjudicated by the special medical standard of due care.[62] We see no logic in a different rule for nondisclosure cases, where the governing standard is much more largely divorced from professional considerations.[63]

And surely in nondisclosure cases the fact-finder is not invariably functioning in an area of such technical complexity that it must be bound to medical custom as an inexorable application of the community standard of reasonable care.[64]

Thus we distinguished, for purposes of duty to disclose, the special and general-standard aspects of the physician–patient relationship. When medical judgment enters the picture and for that reason the special standard controls, prevailing medical practice must be given its just due. In all other instances, however, the general standard exacting ordinary care applies, and that standard is set by law. In summary, the physi-

cian's duty to disclose is governed by the same legal principles applicable to others in comparable situations, with modifications only to the extent that medical judgment enters the picture.[65] We hold that the standard measuring performance of that duty by physicians, as by others, is conduct which is reasonable under the circumstances.[66]

V

Once the circumstances give rise to a duty on the physician's part to inform his patient, the next inquiry is [**33] the scope of the disclosure the physician is legally obliged to make. The courts have frequently confronted this problem but no uniform standard defining the adequacy of the divulgence emerges from the decisions. Some have said "full" disclosure,[67] a norm we are unwilling to adopt literally. It seems obviously prohibitive and unrealistic to expect physicians to discuss with their patients every risk of proposed treatment—no matter how small or remote[68]—and generally unnecessary from the patient's viewpoint as well. Indeed, the cases speaking in terms of "full" disclosure appear to envision something less than total disclosure,[69] leaving unanswered the question of just how much.

The larger number of courts, as might be expected, have applied tests framed with reference to prevailing fashion within the medical profession.[70] Some have measured the disclosure by "good medical practice,"[71] others by what a reasonable practitioner would have bared under the circumstances,[72] and still others by what medical custom in the community would demand.[73] We have explored this rather considerable body of

---

57. *Washington Hosp. Center v. Butler*, supra note 48, 127 U.S.App.D.C. at 387-388, 384 F.2d at 336-337. See also cases cited infra note 59.

58. See Part V, infra.

59. *Washington Hosp. Center v. Butler*, supra note 48, 127 U.S.App.D.C. at 387-388, 384 F.2d at 336-337; *Garfield Memorial Hosp. v. Marshall*, 92 U.S.App.D.C. 234, 240, 204 F.2d 721, 726-727, 37 A.L.R.2d 1270 (1953); *Byrom v. Eastern Dispensary & Cas. Hosp.*, 78 U.S.App.D.C. 42, 43, 136 F.2d 278, 279 (1943).

60. E.g., *Washington Hosp. Center v. Butler*, supra note 48, 127 U.S.App.D.C. at 383, 384 F.2d at 335. See also cases cited infra note 119.

61. See cases cited supra note 59.

62. See cases cited supra note 59.

63. See Part V, infra.

64. Comment, Informed Consent in Medical Malpractice, 55 Calif.L.Rev. 1396, 1405 (1967).

65. See Part VI, infra.

66. See Note, 75 Harv.L.Rev. 1445, 1447 (1962). See also authorities cited supra notes 17-23.

67. E.g., *Salgo v. Leland Stanford Jr. Univ. Bd. of Trustees*, 154 Cal.App.2d 560, 317 P.2d 170, 181 (1957); *Woods v. Brumlop*, supra note 13, 377 P.2d at 524-525.

68. See *Stottlemire v. Cawood*, 213 F. Supp. 897, 898 (D.D.C.), new trial denied, 215 F. Supp. 266 (1963); *Yeates v. Harms*, 193 Kan. 320, 393 P.2d 982, 991 (1964), on rehearing, 194 Kan. 675, 401 P.2d 659 (1965); *Bell v. Umstattd*, 401 S.W.2d 306, 313 (Tex.Civ.App.1966); Waltz & Scheuneman, Informed Consent to Therapy, 64 Nw.U.L.Rev. 628, 635-38 (1970).

69. See, Comment, Informed Consent in Medical Malpractice, 55 Calif.L.Rev. 1396, 1402-03 (1967).

70. E.g., *Shetter v. Rochelle*, 2 Ariz.App. 358, 409 P.2d 74, 86 (1965), modified, 2 Ariz.App. 607, 411 P.2d 45 (1966); *Ditlow v. Kaplan*, 181 So.2d 226, 228 (Fla.App.1965); *Williams v. Menehan*, 191 Kan. 6, 379 P.2d 292, 294 (1963); *Kaplan v. Haines*, 96 N.J.Super. 242, 232 A.2d 840, 845 (1967) aff'd, 51 N.J. 404, 241 A.2d 235 (1968); *Govin v. Hunter*, 374 P.2d 421, 424 (Wyo.1962). This is not surprising since, as indicated, the majority of American jurisdictions find the source, as well as the scope, of duty to disclose in medical custom. See text supra at note 38.

71. *Shetter v. Rochelle*, supra note 70, 409 P.2d at 86.

72. E.g., *Ditlow v. Kaplan*, supra note 70, 181 So.2d at 228; *Kaplan v. Haines*, supra note 70, 232 A.2d at 845.

73. E.g., *Williams v. Menehan*, supra note 70, 379 P.2d at 294; *Govin v. Hunter*, supra note 70, 374 P.2d at 424.

law but are unprepared to follow it. The duty to disclose, we have reasoned, arises from phenomena apart from medical custom and practice.[74] The latter, we think, should no more establish the scope of the duty than its existence. Any definition of scope in terms purely of a professional standard is at odds with the patient's prerogative to decide on projected therapy himself.[75] That prerogative, we have said, is at the very foundation of the duty to disclose,[76] and both the patient's right to know and the physician's correlative obligation to tell him are diluted to the extent that its compass is dictated by the medical profession.[77]

In our view, the patient's right of self-decision shapes the boundaries of the duty to reveal. That right can be effectively exercised only if the patient possesses enough information to enable an intelligent choice. The scope of the physician's communications to the patient, then, must be measured by the patient's need,[78] and that need is the information material to the decision. Thus the test for determining whether a particular peril must be divulged is its materiality to the patient's decision: all risks potentially affecting the decision must be unmasked.[79] And to safeguard the patient's interest in achieving his own determination on treatment, the law must itself set the standard for adequate disclosure.[80]

Optimally for the patient, exposure of a risk would be mandatory whenever the patient would deem it significant to his decision, either singly or in combination with other risks. Such a requirement, however, would summon the physician to second-guess the patient, whose ideas on materiality could hardly be known to the physician. That would make an undue demand upon medical practitioners, whose conduct, like that of others, is to be measured in terms of reasonableness. Consonantly with orthodox negligence doctrine, the physician's liability for nondisclosure is to be determined on the basis of foresight, not hindsight; no less than any other aspect of negligence, the issue on nondisclosure must be approached from the viewpoint of the reasonableness of the physician's divulgence in terms of what he knows or should know to be the patient's informational needs. If, but only if, the fact-finder can say that the physician's communication was unreasonably

inadequate is an imposition of liability legally or morally justified.[81]

Of necessity, the content of the disclosure rests in the first instance with the physician. Ordinarily it is only he who is in position to identify particular dangers; always he must make a judgment, in terms of materiality, as to whether and to what extent revelation to the patient is called for. He cannot know with complete exactitude what the patient would consider important to his decision, but on the basis of his medical training and experience he can sense how the average, reasonable patient expectably would react.[82] Indeed, with knowledge of, or ability to learn, his patient's background and current condition, he is in a position superior to that of most others—attorneys, for example—who are called upon to make judgments on pain of liability in damages for unreasonable miscalculation.[83]

From these considerations we derive the breadth of the disclosure of risks legally to be required. The scope of the standard is not subjective as to either the physician or the patient; it remains objective with due regard for the patient's informational needs and with suitable leeway for the physician's situation. In broad outline, we agree that "[a] risk is thus material when a reasonable person, in what the physician knows or should know to be the patient's position, would be likely to attach significance to the risk or cluster of risks in deciding whether or not to forego the proposed therapy."[84]

The topics importantly demanding a communication of information are the inherent and potential hazards of the proposed treatment, the alternatives to that treatment, if any, and the results likely if the patient remains untreated. The factors contributing significance to the dangerousness of a medical technique are, of course, the incidence of injury and the degree of the harm threatened.[85] A very small chance of death or serious disablement may well be significant; a potential disability which dramatically outweighs the potential benefit of the

---

74. See Part III, supra.

75. See text supra at notes 12–13.

76. See Part III, supra.

77. For similar reasons, we reject the suggestion that disclosure should be discretionary with the physician. See Note, 109 U.Pa.L.Rev. 768, 772–73 (1961).

78. See text supra at notes 12–15.

79. See Waltz & Scheuneman, Informed Consent to Therapy, 64 N.W.U.L.Rev. 628, 639–41 (1970).

80. See Comment, Informed Consent in Medical Malpractice, 55 *Canterbury v. Spence* Page 23 of 23 Calif.L.Rev. 1396, 1407–10 (1967).

---

81. See Waltz & Scheuneman, Informed Consent to Therapy, 64 N.W.U.L.Rev. 628, 639–40 (1970).

82. Id.

83. Id.

84. Id. at 640. The category of risks which the physician should communicate is, of course, no broader than the complement he could communicate. See *Block v. McVay*, 80 S.D. 469, 126 N.W.2d 808, 812 (1964). The duty to divulge may extend to any risk he actually knows, but he obviously cannot divulge any of which he may be unaware. Nondisclosure of an unknown risk does not, strictly speaking, present a problem in terms of the duty to disclose although it very well might pose problems in terms of the physician's duties to have known of it and to have acted accordingly. See Waltz & Scheuneman, Informed Consent to Therapy, 64 N.W.U.L.Rev. 628, 630–35 (1970). We have no occasion to explore problems of the latter type on this appeal.

85. See Comment, Informed Consent in Medical Malpractice, 55 Calif.L.Rev. 1396, 1407 n. 68 (1967).

therapy or the detriments of the existing malady may summon discussion with the patient.[86]

There is no bright line separating the significant from the insignificant; the answer in any case must abide a rule of reason. Some dangers—infection, for example—are inherent in any operation; there is no obligation to communicate those of which persons of average sophistication are aware.[87] Even more clearly, the physician bears no responsibility for discussion of hazards the patient has already discovered,[88] or those having no apparent materiality to patients' decision on therapy.[89] The disclosure doctrine, like others marking lines between permissible and impermissible behavior in medical practice, is in essence a requirement of conduct prudent under the circumstances. Whenever nondisclosure of particular risk information is open to debate by reasonable-minded men, the issue is for the finder of the facts.[90]

VI

Two exceptions to the general rule of disclosure have been noted by the courts. Each is in the nature of a physician's privilege not to disclose, and the reasoning underlying them is appealing. Each, indeed, is but a recognition that, as important as is the patient's right to know, it is greatly outweighed by the magnitudinous circumstances giving rise to the privilege. The first comes into play when the patient is unconscious or otherwise incapable of consenting, and harm from a failure to treat is imminent and outweighs any harm threatened by the proposed treatment. When a genuine emergency of that sort arises, it is settled that the impracticality of conferring with the patient dispenses with need for it.[91] Even in situations of that character, the physician should, as current law requires, attempt to secure a relative's consent if possible,[92] but if time is too short to accommodate discussion, obviously the physician should proceed with the treatment.[93]

The second exception obtains when risk-disclosure poses such a threat of detriment to the patient as to become unfeasible or contraindicated from a medical point of view. It is recognized that patients occasionally become so ill or emotionally distraught on disclosure as to foreclose a rational decision, or complicate or hinder the treatment, or perhaps even pose psychological damage to the patient.[94] Where that is so, the cases have generally held that the physician is armed with a privilege to keep the information from the patient,[95] and we think it clear that portents of that type may justify the physician in action he deems medically warranted. The critical inquiry is whether the physician responded to a sound medical judgment that communication of the risk information would present a threat to the patient's well-being.

The physician's privilege to withhold information for therapeutic reasons must be carefully circumscribed, however, for otherwise it might devour the disclosure rule itself. The privilege does not accept the paternalistic notion that the physician may remain silent simply because divulgence might prompt the patient to forego therapy the physician feels the patient really needs.[96] That attitude presumes instability or perversity for even the normal patient, and runs counter to the foundation

---

86. See *Bowers v. Talmage*, supra note 13 (3% chance of death, paralysis or other injury, disclosure required); *Scott v. Wilson*, 396 S.W.2d 532 (Tex.Civ.App.1965), aff'd, 412 S.W.2d 299 (Tex.1967) (1% chance of loss of hearing, disclosure required). Compare, where the physician was held not liable. *Stottlemire v. Cawood*, supra note 68, (1/800,000 chance of aplastic anemia); *Yeates v. Harms*, supra note 68 (1.5% chance of loss of eye); *Starnes v. Taylor*, 272 N.C. 386, 158 S.E.2d 339, 344 (1968) (1/250 to 1/500 chance of perforation of esophagus).

87. *Roberts v. Young*, supra note 38, 119 N.W.2d at 629-630; *Starnes v. Taylor*, supra note 86, 158 S.E.2d at 344; Comment, Informed Consent in Medical Malpractice, 55 Calif.L.Rev. 1396, 1407 n. 69 (1967); Note, 75 Harv.L.Rev. 1445, 1448 (1962).

88. *Yeates v. Harms*, supra note 68, 393 P.2d at 991; *Fleishman v. Richardson-Merrell, Inc.*, 94 N.J.Super. 90, 226 A.2d 843, 845-846 (1967). See also *Natanson v. Kline*, supra note 12, 350 P.2d at 1106.

89. See text supra at note 84. And compare to the contrary, Oppenheim, Informed Consent to Medical Treatment, 11 Clev.-Mar. L.Rev. 249, 264-65 (1962); Comment, Valid Consent to Medical Treatment: Need the Patient Know, 4 Duquesne L.Rev. 450, 457-58 (1966), a position we deem unrealistic. On the other hand, we do not subscribe to the view which holds that only risks which would cause the patient to forego the treatment must be divulged, see Johnson, Medical Malpractice—Doctrines of Res Ipsa Loquitur and Informed Consent, 37 U.Colo.L.Rev. 182, 185-91 (1965); Comment, Informed Consent in Medical Malpractice, 55 Calif.L.Rev. 1396, 1407 n. 68 (1967); Note, 75 Harv.L.Rev. 1445, 1446-47 (1962), for such a principle ignores the possibility that while a single risk might not have that effect, two or more might do so. Accord, Waltz & Scheuneman, Informed Consent to Therapy, 64 Nw.U.L.Rev. 628, 635-41 (1970).

90. E.g., *Bowers v. Talmage*, supra note 13, 159 So.2d at 889; *Aiken v. Clary*, supra note 38, 396 S.W.2d at 676; *Hastings v. Hughes*, 59 Tenn.App. 98, 438 S.W.2d 349, 352 (1968).

91. E.g., *Dunham v. Wright*, supra note 13, 423 F.2d at 941-942 (applying Pennsylvania law); *Koury v. Follo*, 272 N.C. 366, 158 S.E.2d 548, 555 (1968); *Woods v. Brumlop*, supra note 13, 377 P.2d at 525; *Gravis v. Physicians & Surgeons Hosp.*, 415 S.W.2d 674, 677, 678 (Tex.Civ.App.1967).

92. Where the complaint in suit is unauthorized treatment of a patient legally or factually incapable of giving consent, the established rule is that, absent an emergency, the physician must obtain the necessary authority from a relative. See, e.g., *Bonner v. Moran*, supra note 32, 75 U.S.App.D.C. at 157-158, 126 F.2d at 122-123 (15-year old child). See also *Koury v. Follo*, supra note 91 (patient a baby).

93. Compare, e.g., Application of President & Directors of Georgetown College, 118 U.S.App.D.C. 80, 331 F.2d 1000, rehearing en banc denied, 118 U.S.App.D.C. 90, 331 F.2d 1010, cert. denied, *Jones v. President and Directors of Georgetown College, Inc.*, 377 U.S. 978, 84 S. Ct. 1883, 12 L. Ed. 2d 746 (1964).

94. See, e.g., *Salgo v. Leland Stanford Jr. Univ. Bd. Of Trustees*, supra note 67, 317 P.2d at 181 (1957); Waltz & Scheuneman, Informed Consent to Therapy, 64 Nw.U.L.Rev. 628, 641-43 (1970).

95. E.g., *Roberts v. Wood*, 206 F. Supp. 579, 583 (S.D.Ala.1962); *Nishi v. Hartwell*, 52 Haw. 188, 473 P.2d 116, 119, 52 Haw. 296 (1970); *Woods v. Brumlop*, supra note 13, 377 P.2d at 525; *Ball v. Mallinkrodt Chem. Works*, 53 Tenn.App. 218, 381 S.W.2d 563, 567-568 (1964).

96. E.g., *Scott v. Wilson*, supra note 86, 396 S.W.2d at 534-535; Comment, Informed Consent in Medical Malpractice, 55 Calif.L.Rev. 1396, 1409-10 (1967); Note, 75 Harv.L.Rev. 1445, 1448 (1962).

principle that the patient should and ordinarily can make the choice for himself.[97] Nor does the privilege contemplate operation save where the patient's reaction to risk information, as reasonably foreseen by the physician, is menacing.[98] And even in a situation of that kind, disclosure to a close relative with a view to securing consent to the proposed treatment may be the only alternative open to the physician.[99]

VII

No more than breach of any other legal duty does nonfulfillment of the physician's obligation to disclose alone establish liability to the patient. An unrevealed risk that should have been made known must materialize, for otherwise the omission, however unpardonable, is legally without consequence. Occurrence of the risk must be harmful to the patient, for negligence unrelated to injury is nonactionable.[100] And, as in malpractice actions generally,[101] there must be a causal relationship between the physician's failure to adequately divulge and damage to the patient.[102]

A causal connection exists when, but only when, disclosure of significant risks incidental to treatment would have resulted in a decision against it.[103] The patient obviously has no complaint if he would have submitted to the therapy notwithstanding awareness that the risk was one of its perils. On the other hand, the very purpose of the disclosure rule is to protect the patient against consequences which, if known, he would have avoided by foregoing the treatment.[104] The more difficult question is whether the factual issue on causality calls for an objective or a subjective determination.

It has been assumed that the issue is to be resolved according to whether the fact-finder believes the patient's testimony that he would not have agreed to the treatment if he had known of the danger which later ripened into injury.[105] We think a technique which ties the factual conclusion on causation simply to the assessment of the patient's credibility is unsatisfactory. To be sure, the objective of risk-disclosure is preservation of the patient's interest in intelligent self-choice on proposed treatment, a matter the patient is free to decide for any reason that appeals to him.[106] When, prior to commencement of therapy, the patient is sufficiently informed on risks and he exercises his choice, it may truly be said that he did exactly what he wanted to do. But when causality is explored at a postinjury trial with a professedly uninformed patient, the question whether he actually would have turned the treatment down if he had known the risks is purely hypothetical: "Viewed from the point at which he had to decide, would the patient have decided differently had he known something he did not know?"[107] And the answer which the patient supplies hardly represents more than a guess, perhaps tinged by the circumstance that the uncommunicated hazard has in fact materialized.[108]

In our view, this method of dealing with the issue on causation comes in second-best. It places the physician in jeopardy of the patient's hindsight and bitterness. It places the fact-finder in the position of deciding whether a speculative answer to a hypothetical question is to be credited. It calls for a subjective determination solely on testimony of a patient-witness shadowed by the occurrence of the undisclosed risk.[109]

Better it is, we believe, to resolve the causality issue on an objective basis: in terms of what a prudent person in the patient's position would have decided if suitably informed of all perils bearing significance.[110] If adequate disclosure could reasonably be expected to have caused that person to decline the treatment because of the revelation of the kind of risk or danger that resulted in harm, causation is shown, but otherwise not.[111] The patient's testimony is relevant on that score of course but it would not threaten to dominate the findings. And since that testimony would probably be appraised congruently with the fact-finder's belief in its reasonableness, the case for a wholly objective standard for passing on causation is

---

97. See text supra at notes 12-13.

98. Note, 75 Harv.L.Rev. 1445, 1448 (1962).

99. See *Fiorentino v. Wenger*, 26 A.D.2d 693, 272 N.Y.S.2d 557, 559 (1966), appeal dismissed, 18 N.Y.2d 908, 276 N.Y.S.2d 639, 223 N.E.2d 46 (1966), reversed on other grounds, 19 N.Y.2d 407, 280 N.Y.S.2d 373, 227 N.E.2d 296 (1967). See also note 92, supra.

100. *Becker v. Colonial Parking, Inc.*, 133 U.S.App.D.C. 213, 219-220, 409 F.2d 1130, 1136-1137 (1969); *Richardson v. Gregory*, 108 U.S.App.D.C. 263, 266-267, 281 F.2d 626, 629-630 (1960); *Arthur v. Standard Eng'r. Co.*, 89 U.S.App.D.C. 399, 401, 193 F.2d 903, 905, 32 A.L.R.2d 408 (1951), cert. denied, 343 U.S. 964, 72 S. Ct. 1057, 96 L. Ed. 1361 (1952); *Industrial Savs. Bank v. People's Funeral Serv. Corp.*, 54 App.D.C. 259, 260, 296 F. 1006, 1007 (1924).

101. See *Morse v. Moretti*, 131 U.S.App.D.C. 158, 403 F.2d 564 (1968); *Kosberg v. Washington Hosp. Center, Inc.*, 129 U.S.App.D.C. 322, 324, 394 F.2d 947, 949 (1968); *Levy v. Vaughan*, 42 U.S. App. D.C. 146, 153, 157 (1914).

102. *Shetter v. Rochelle*, supra note 70, 409 P.2d at 82-85; Waltz & Scheuneman, Informed Consent to Therapy, 64 Nw.U.L.Rev. 628, 646 (1970).

103. *Shetter v. Rochelle*, supra note 70, 409 P.2d at 83-84. See also *Natanson v. Kline*, supra note 12, 350 P.2d at 1106-1107; *Hunter v. Burroughs*, supra note 7, 96 S.E. at 369.

104. See text supra at notes 23-35, 74-79.

105. Plante, An Analysis of "Informed Consent," 36 Fordham L.Rev. 639, 666-67 (1968); Waltz & Scheuneman, Informed Consent to Therapy, 64 Nw.U.L.Rev. 628, 646-48 (1970); Comment, Informed Consent in Medical Malpractice, 55 Calif.L.Rev. 1396, 1411-14 (1967).

106. See text supra at notes 12-13.

107. Waltz & Scheuneman, Informed Consent to Therapy, 64 Nw.U.L.Rev. 628, 647 (1970).

108. Id. at 647.

109. Id. at 646.

110. Id. at 648.

111. See cases cited supra note 103.

strengthened. Such a standard would in any event ease the fact-finding process and better assure the truth as its product.

VIII

In the context of trial of a suit claiming inadequate disclosure of risk information by a physician, the patient has the burden of going forward with evidence tending to establish prima facie the essential elements of the cause of action, and ultimately the burden of proof—the risk of nonpersuasion[112]—on those elements.[113] These are normal impositions upon moving litigants, and no reason why they should not attach in nondisclosure cases is apparent. The burden of going forward with evidence pertaining to a privilege not to disclose,[114] however, rests properly upon the physician. This is not only because the patient has made out a prima facie case before an issue on privilege is reached, but also because any evidence bearing on the privilege is usually in the hands of the physician alone. Requiring him to open the proof on privilege is consistent with judicial policy laying such a burden on the party who seeks shelter from an exception to a general rule and who is more likely to have possession of the facts.[115]

As in much malpractice litigation,[116] recovery in nondisclosure lawsuits has hinged upon the patient's ability to prove through expert testimony that the physician's performance departed from medical custom. This is not surprising since, as we have pointed out, the majority of American jurisdictions have limited the patient's right to know to whatever boon can be found in medical practice.[117] We have already discussed our disagreement with the majority rationale.[118] We now delineate our view on the need for expert testimony in nondisclosure cases. There are obviously important roles for medical testimony in such cases, and some roles which only medical evidence can fill. Experts are ordinarily indispensable to identify and elucidate for the fact-finder the risks of therapy and the consequences of leaving existing maladies untreated. They are normally needed on issues as to the cause of any injury or disability suffered by the patient and, where privileges are asserted, as to the existence of any emergency claimed and the

nature and seriousness of any impact upon the patient from risk-disclosure. Save for relative infrequent instances where questions of this type are resolvable wholly within the realm of ordinary human knowledge and experience, the need for the expert is clear.[119]

The guiding consideration our decisions distill, however, is that medical facts are for medical experts[120] and other facts are for any witnesses—expert or not—having sufficient knowledge and capacity to testify to them.[121] It is evident that many of the issues typically involved in nondisclosure cases do not reside peculiarly within the medical domain. Lay witness testimony can competently establish a physician's failure to disclose particular risk information, the patient's lack of knowledge of the risk, and the adverse consequences following the treatment.[122] Experts are unnecessary to a showing of the materiality of a risk to a patient's decision on treatment, or to the reasonably, expectable effect of risk disclosure on the decision.[123] These conspicuous examples of permissible uses of nonexpert testimony illustrate the relative freedom of broad

---

112. See 9 J. Wigmore, Evidence § 2485 (3d ed. 1940).

113. See, e.g., *Morse v. Moretti*, supra note 101, 131 U.S.App.D.C. at 158, 403 F.2d at 564; *Kosberg v. Washington Hosp. Center, Inc.*, supra note 101, 129 U.S.App.D.C. at 324, 394 F.2d at 949; *Smith v. Reitman*, 128 U.S.App.D.C. 352, 353, 389 F.2d 303, 304 (1967).

114. See Part VI, supra.

115. See 9 J. Wigmore, Evidence § 2486, 2488, 2489 (3d ed. 1940). See also *Raza v. Sullivan*, 139 U.S.App.D.C. 184, 186-188, 432 F.2d 617, 619-621 (1970), cert. denied, 400 U.S. 992, 91 S. Ct. 458, 27 L. Ed. 2d 440 (1971).

116. See cases cited infra note 119.

117. See text supra at notes 37-39.

118. See Part IV, supra.

119. *Lucy Webb Hayes Nat. Training School v. Perotti*, supra note 56, 136 U.S.App.D.C. at 126-127, 419 F.2d at 708-709 (hospital's failure to install safety glass in psychiatric ward); *Alden v. Providence Hosp.*, 127 U.S.App.D.C. 214, 217, 382 F.2d 163, 166 (1967) (caliber of medical diagnosis); *Brown v. Keaveny*, supra note 16, 117 U.S.App.D.C. at 118, 326 F.2d at 661 (caliber of medical treatment); *Quick v. Thurston*, supra note 16, 110 U.S.App.D.C. at 171-173, 290 F.2d at 362-364 (sufficiency of medical attendance and caliber of medical treatment); *Rodgers v. Lawson*, supra note 16, 83 U.S.App.D.C. at 285-286, 170 F.2d at 161-162 (sufficiency of medical attendance, and caliber of medical diagnosis and treatment); *Byrom v. Eastern Dispensary & Cas. Hosp.*, supra note 59, 78 U.S.App.D.C. at 43, 136 F.2d at 279 (caliber of medical treatment), *Christie v. Callahan*, 75 U.S.App.D.C. 133, 136, 124 F.2d 825, 828 (1941) (caliber of medical treatment); *Carson v. Jackson*, 52 App.D.C. 51, 55, 281 F. 411, 415 (1922) (caliber of medical treatment).

120. See cases cited supra note 119.

121. *Lucy Webb Hayes Nat. Training School v. Perotti*, supra note 56, 136 U.S.App.D.C. at 127-129, 419 F.2d at 709-711 (permitting patient to wander from closed to open section of psychiatric ward); *Monk v. Doctors Hosp.*, supra note 56, 131 U.S.App.D.C. at 177, 403 F.2d at 583 (operation of electro-surgical machine); *Washington Hosp. Center v. Butler*, supra note 48 (fall by unattended x-ray patient); *Young v. Fishback*, 104 U.S.App.D.C. 372, 373, 262 F.2d 469, 470 (1958) (bit of gauze left at operative site); *Garfield Memorial Hosp. v. Marshall*, supra note 59, 92 U.S.App.D.C. at 240, 204 F.2d at 726 (newborn baby's head striking operating table); *Goodwin v. Hertzberg*, 91 U.S.App.D.C. 385, 386, 201 F.2d 204, 205 (1952) (perforation of urethra); *Byrom v. Eastern Dispensary & Cas. Hosp.*, supra note 59, 78 U.S.App.D.C. at 43, 136 F.2d at 279 (failure to further diagnose and treat after unsuccessful therapy); *Grubb v. Groover*, 62 App.D.C. 305, 306, 67 F.2d 511, 512 (1933), cert. denied, 291 U.S. 660, 54 S. Ct. 377, 78 L. Ed. 1052 (1934) (burn while unattended during x-ray treatment). See also *Furr v. Herzmark*, 92 U.S.App.D.C. 350, 353-354, 206 F.2d 468, 470-471 (1953); *Christie v. Callahan*, supra note 119, 75 U.S.App.D.C. at 136, 124 F.2d at 828; *Sweeney v. Erving*, 35 App.D.C. 57, 62, 43 L.R.A., N.S. 734 (1910), aff'd, 228 U.S. 233, 33 S. Ct. 416, 57 L. Ed. 815 (1913).

122. See Waltz & Scheuneman, Informed Consent to Therapy, 64 Nw.U.L.Rev. 628, 645, 647 (1970); Comment, Informed Consent in Medical Malpractice, 55 Calif.L.Rev. 1396, 1410-11 (1967).

123. See Waltz & Scheuneman, Informed Consent to Therapy, 64 Nw.U.L.Rev. 628, 639-40 (1970); Comment, Informed Consent in Medical Malpractice, 55 Calif.L.Rev. 1396, 1411 (1967).

areas of the legal problem of risk nondisclosure from the demands for expert testimony that shackle plaintiffs' other types of medical malpractice litigation.[124]

IX

We now confront the question whether appellant's suit was barred, wholly or partly, by the statute of limitations. The statutory periods relevant to this inquiry are one year for battery actions[125] and three years for those charging negligence.[126] For one a minor when his cause of action accrues, they do not begin to run until he has attained his majority.[127] Appellant was nineteen years old when the laminectomy and related events occurred, and he filed his complaint roughly two years after he reached twenty-one. Consequently, any claim in suit subject to the one-year limitation came too late.

Appellant's causes of action for the allegedly faulty laminectomy by Dr. Spence and allegedly careless post-operative care by the hospital present no problem. Quite obviously, each was grounded in negligence and so was governed by the three-year provision.[128] The duty-to-disclose claim appellant asserted against Dr. Spence, however, draws another consideration into the picture. We have previously observed that an unauthorized operation constitutes a battery, and that an uninformed consent to an operation does not confer the necessary authority.[129] If, therefore, appellant had at stake no more than a recovery of damages on account of a laminectomy intentionally done without intelligent permission, the statute would have interposed a bar.

It is evident, however, that appellant had much more at stake.[130] His interest in bodily integrity commanded protection, not only against an intentional invasion by an unauthorized operation[131] but also against a negligent invasion by his physician's dereliction of duty to adequately disclose.[132] Appellant has asserted and litigated a violation of that duty throughout the case.[133] That claim, like the others, was governed by the three-year period of limitation applicable to negligence actions[134] and was unaffected by the fact that its alternative was barred by the one-year period pertaining to batteries.[135]

X

This brings us to the remaining question, common to all three causes of action: whether appellant's evidence was of such caliber as to require a submission to the jury. On the first, the evidence was clearly sufficient to raise an issue as to whether Dr. Spence's obligation to disclose information on risks was reasonably met or was excused by the surrounding circumstances. Appellant testified that Dr. Spence revealed to him nothing suggesting a hazard associated with the laminectomy. His mother testified that, in response to her specific inquiry, Dr. Spence informed her that the laminectomy was no more serious than any other operation. When, at trial, it developed from Dr. Spence's testimony that paralysis can be expected in one percent of laminectomies, it became the jury's responsibility to decide whether that peril was of sufficient magnitude to bring the disclosure duty into play.[136] There was no emergency to frustrate an opportunity to disclose,[137] and Dr. Spence's expressed opinion that disclosure would have been unwise did not foreclose a contrary conclusion by the jury. There was no evidence that appellant's emotional makeup was such that concealment of the risk of paralysis was medically

---

124. One of the chief obstacles facing plaintiffs in malpractice cases has been the difficulty, and all too frequently the apparent impossibility, of securing testimony from the medical profession. See, e.g., *Washington Hosp. Center v. Butler*, supra note 48, 127 U.S.App.D.C. at 386 n. 27, 384 F.2d at 338 n. 27; *Brown v. Keaveny*, supra note 16, 117 U.S.App.D.C. at 118, 326 F.2d at 661 (dissenting opinion); *Huffman v. Lindquist*, 37 Cal.2d 465, 234 P.2d 34, 46 (1951) (dissenting opinion); Comment, Informed Consent in Medical Malpractice, 55 Calif.L.Rev. 1396, 1405-06 (1967); Note, 75 Harv.L.Rev. 1445, 1447 (1962).

125. D.C.Code § 12-301(4) (1967).

126. D.C.Code § 12-301(8), specifying a three-year limitation for all actions not otherwise provided for. Suits seeking damages for negligent personal injury or property damage are in this category. *Finegan v. Lumbermens Mut. Cas. Co.*, 117 U.S.App.D.C. 276, 329 F.2d 231 (1963); *Keleket X-Ray Corp. v. United States*, 107 U.S.App.D.C. 138, 275 F.2d 167 (1960); *Hanna v. Fletcher*, 97 U.S.App.D.C. 310, 313, 231 F.2d 469, 472, 58 A.L.R.2d 847, cert. denied, *Gichner Iron Works, Inc. v. Hanna*, 351 U.S. 989, 76 S. Ct. 1051, 100 L. Ed. 1501 (1956).

127. D.C.Code § 12-302(a)(1) (1967). See also *Carson v. Jackson*, supra note 119, 52 App.D.C. at 53, 281 F. at 413.

128. See cases cited supra note 126.

129. See text supra at notes 32-36.

130. For discussions of the differences between battery and negligence actions, see, McCoid, A Reappraisal of Liability for Unauthorized Medical Treatment, 41 Minn.L.Rev. 381, 423-25 (1957); Comment, Informed Consent in Medical Malpractice, 55 Calif.L.Rev. 1396, 1399-1400 n. 18 (1967); Note 75 Harv.L.Rev. 1445, 1446 (1962).

131. See *Natanson v. Kline*, supra note 12, 350 P.2d at 1100; Restatement (Second) of Torts §§ 13, 15 (1965).

132. The obligation to disclose, as we have said, is but a part of the physician's general duty to exercise reasonable care for the benefit of his patient. See Part III, supra.

133. Thus we may distinguish *Morfessis v. Baum*, 108 U.S.App.D.C. 303, 305, 281 F.2d 938, 940 (1960), where an action labeled one for abuse of process was, on analysis, found to be really one for malicious prosecution. [**60]

134. See *Maercklein v. Smith*, 129 Colo. 72, 266 P.2d 1095, 1097-1098 (en banc 1954); *Hershey v. Peake*, 115 Kan. 562, 223 P. 1113 (1924); *Mayor v. Dowsett*, 240 Or. 196, 400 P.2d 234, 250-251 (en banc 1965); McCoid, A Reappraisal of Liability for Unauthorized Medical Treatment, 41 Minn.L.Rev. 381, 424-25, 434 (1957); McCoid, The Care Required of Medical Practitioners, 12 Vand.L.Rev. 586-87 (1959); Plante, An Analysis of "Informed Consent," 36 Fordham L.Rev. 639, 669-71 (1968); Comment, Informed Consent in Medical Malpractice, 55 Calif.L.Rev. 1396, 1399-4100 n. 18 (1967); Note, 75 Harv.L.Rev. 1445, 1446 (1962). *Canterbury v. Spence* Page 38 of 38.

135. See *Mellon v. Seymoure*, 56 App.D.C. 301, 303, 12 F.2d 836, 837 (1926); *Pedesky v. Bleiberg*, 251 Cal.App.2d 119, 59 Cal.Rptr. 294 (1967).

136. See text supra at notes 81-90.

137. See text supra at notes 91-92.

sound.[138] Even if disclosure to appellant himself might have bred ill consequences, no reason appears for the omission to communicate the information to his mother, particularly in view of his minority.[139] The jury, not Dr. Spence, was the final arbiter of whether nondisclosure was reasonable under the circumstances.[140]

Proceeding to the next cause of action, we find evidence generating issues as to whether Dr. Spence performed the laminectomy negligently and, if so, whether that negligence contributed causally to appellant's subsequent disabilities. A report Dr. Spence prepared after the second operation indicated that at the time he felt that too-tight sutures at the laminectomy site might have caused the paralysis. While at trial Dr. Spence voiced the opinion that the sutures were not responsible, there were circumstances lending support to his original view. Prior to the laminectomy, appellant had [*795] none of the disabilities of which he now complains.

The disabilities appeared almost immediately after the laminectomy. The gusset Dr. Spence made on the second operation left greater room for the spinal cord to pulsate, and this alleviated appellant's condition somewhat. That Dr. Spence's in-trial opinion was hardly the last word is manifest from the fact that the team of specialists consulting on appellant was unable to settle on the origin of the paralysis. We are advertent to Dr. Spence's attribution of appellant's disabilities to his condition preexisting the laminectomy, but that was a matter for the jury. And even if the jury had found that theory acceptable, there would have remained the question whether Dr. Spence aggravated the preexisting condition. A tort-feasor takes his victim as he finds him, and negligence intensifying an old condition creates liability just as surely as negligence precipitating a new one.[141] It was for the jury to say, on the whole

evidence, just what contributions appellant's preexisting condition and Dr. Spence's medical treatment respectively made to the disabilities.

In sum, judged by legal standards, the proof militated against a directed verdict in Dr. Spence's favor. True it is that the evidence did not furnish ready answers on the dispositive factual issues, but the important consideration is that appellant showed enough to call for resolution of those issues by the jury. As in *Sentilles v. Inter-Carribbean Shipping Corporation*,[142] a case resembling this one, the Supreme Court stated, The jury's power to draw the inference that the aggravation of petitioner's tubercular condition, evident so shortly after the accident, was in fact caused by that accident, was not impaired by the failure of any medical witness to testify that it was in fact the cause. Neither can it be impaired by the lack of medical unanimity as to the respective likelihood of the potential causes of the aggravation, or by the fact that other potential causes of aggravation existed and were not conclusively negated by the proofs. The matter does not turn on the use of a particular form of words by the physicians in giving their testimony.

The members of the jury, not the medical witnesses, were sworn to make a legal determination of the question of causation. They were entitled to take all the circumstances, including the medical testimony into consideration.[143]

We conclude, lastly, that the case against the hospital should also have gone to the jury. The circumstances surrounding appellant's fall—the change in Dr. Spence's order that appellant be kept in bed,[144] the failure to maintain a side rail on appellant's bed, and the absence of any attendant while appellant was attempting to relieve himself—could certainly suggest to jurors a dereliction of the hospital's duty to exercise reasonable care for the safety and well-being of the patient.[145] On the issue of causality, the evidence was uncontradicted that appellant progressed after the operation until the fall but, a few hours thereafter, his condition had deteriorated, and there were complaints of paralysis and respiratory difficulty. That falls tend to cause or aggravate injuries is, of course, common knowledge, which in our view the jury was at liberty to utilize.[146] To this may be added Dr. Spence's testimony that

138. See Part VI, supra. With appellant's prima facie case of violation of duty to disclose, the burden of introducing evidence showing a privilege was on Dr. Spence. See text supra at notes 114-115. Dr. Spence's opinion—that disclosure is medically unwise—was expressed as to patients generally, and not with reference to traits possessed by appellant. His explanation was: I think that I always explain to patients the operations are serious, and I feel that any operation is serious. I think that I would not tell patients that they might be paralyzed because of the small percentage, one per cent, that exists. There would be a tremendous percentage of people that would not have surgery and would not therefore be benefited by it, the tremendous percentage that get along very well, 99 per cent.

139. See Part VI, supra. Since appellant's evidence was that neither he nor his mother was informed by Dr. Spence of the risk of paralysis from the laminectomy, we need not decide whether a parent's consent to an operation on a nineteen-year-old is ordinarily required. Compare *Bonner v. Moran*, supra note 32, 75 U.S.App.D.C. at 157-158, 126 F.2d at 122-123.

140. See Part V, supra.

141. *Bourne v. Washburn*, 142 U.S.App.D.C. 332, 336, 441 F.2d 1022, 1026 (1971); *Clark v. Associated Retail Credit Men*, 70 App.D.C. 183, 187, 105 F.2d 62, 66 (1939); *Baltimore & O.R.R. v. Morgan*, 35 App.D.C. 195, 200-201 (1910); *Washington A. & M. V. Ry. v. Lukens*, 32 App.D.C. 442, 453-454 (1909).

142. 361 U.S. 107, 80 S. Ct. 173, 4 L. Ed. 2d 142 (1959).

143. Id. at 109-110, 80 S. Ct. at (footnote omitted).

144. Even if Dr. Spence himself made the change, the result would not vary as to the hospital. It was or should have been known by hospital personnel that appellant had just undergone a serious operation. A jury might fairly conclude that at the time of the fall he was in no condition to be left to fend for himself. Compare *Washington Hosp. Center v. Butler*, supra note 48, 127 U.S.App.D.C. at 385, 384 F.2d at 337.

145. Compare id. See also cases cited supra note 121.

146. See id. at 383-385, 384 F.2d at 335-337.

paralysis can be brought on by trauma or shock. All told, the jury had available a store of information enabling an intelligent resolution of the issues respecting the hospital.[147]

We realize that, when appellant rested his case in chief, the evidence scarcely served to put the blame for appellant's disabilities squarely on one appellee or the other. But this does not mean that either could escape liability at the hand of the jury simply because appellant was unable to do more. As ever so recently we ruled, "a showing of negligence by each of two (or more) defendants with uncertainty as to which caused the harm does not defeat recovery but passes the burden to the tortfeasor for each to prove, if he can, that he did not cause the harm."[148] In the case before us, appellant's evidentiary presentation on negligence survived the claims of legal insufficiency, and appellees should have been put to their proof.[149]

Reversed and remanded for a new trial.

---

148. *Bowman v. Redding & Co.*, 145 U.S.App.D.C. 294, 305, 449 F.2d 956, 967 (1971).

149. Appellant's remaining points on appeal require no elaboration. He contends that his counsel, not the trial judge, should have conducted the voir dire examination of prospective jurors, but that matter lay within the discretion of the judge, Fed.R.Civ.P. 47(a). He argues that Mrs. Canterbury, a rebuttal witness, should not have been excluded from the courtroom during other stages of the trial. That also was within the trial judge's discretion and, in any event, no prejudice from the exclusion appears. He complains of the trial judge's refusal to admit into evidence bylaws of the hospital pertaining to written consent for surgery, and the judge's refusal to permit two physicians to testify as to medical custom and practice on the same general subject. What we have already said makes it unnecessary for us to deal further with those complaints.

---

147. See id.

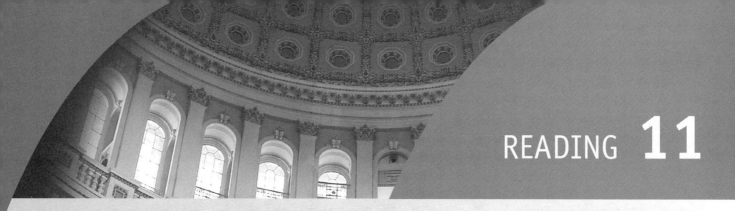

Case Law: *Jones v. Chicago* (Managed Care Liability for Institutional Negligence)

SHEILA JONES, Indiv. and as Mother and Next Friend of Shawndale Jones, a Minor, Appellant, v. CHICAGO HMO LTD. OF ILLINOIS, Appellee.

Opinion filed May 18, 2000.

JUSTICE BILANDIC delivered the opinion of the court:

This appeal asks whether a health maintenance organization (HMO) may be held liable for institutional negligence. We answer in the affirmative.

The plaintiff, Sheila Jones (Jones), individually and as the mother of the minor, Shawndale Jones, brought this medical malpractice action against the defendants, Chicago HMO Ltd. of Illinois (Chicago HMO), Dr. Robert A. Jordan and another party. The Joneses were members of Chicago HMO, an HMO. Dr. Jordan was a contract physician of Chicago HMO and the primary care physician of Shawndale.

The circuit court of Cook County awarded summary judgment in favor of Chicago HMO on all three counts of Jones' second amended complaint. Count I charges Chicago HMO with institutional negligence. Count II charges Chicago HMO with vicarious liability for Dr. Jordan's alleged negligence under the doctrine of apparent authority. Count III charges Chicago HMO with breach of contract. The circuit court also entered a finding pursuant to Supreme Court Rule 304(a) (155 Ill. 2d R. 304(a)). On appeal, the appellate court affirmed the grant of summary judgment as to counts I and III, but reversed the grant of summary judgment as to count II, remanding that claim for further proceedings. 301 Ill. App. 3d 103. We allowed Jones' petition for leave to appeal (177 Ill. 2d R. 315). Because Chicago HMO does not challenge the appellate court's reversal of count II, only counts I and III are at issue in this appeal.

Two organizations filed amicus curiae briefs with the permission of this court. See 155 Ill. 2d R. 345. The Illinois Association of Health Maintenance Organizations filed a brief in support of Chicago HMO. The Illinois Trial Lawyers Association filed a brief in support of Jones. For the reasons explained below, we affirm the summary judgment as to count III, breach of contract, but we reverse the summary judgment as to count I, institutional negligence, and remand that claim for further proceedings.

FACTS

In reviewing an award of summary judgment, we must view the facts in the light most favorable to the nonmoving party. *Petrovich v. Share Health Plan of Illinois, Inc.*, 188 Ill. 2d 17, 30-31 (1999). The following facts thus emerge.

On January 18, 1991, Jones' three-month-old daughter Shawndale was ill. Jones called Dr. Jordan's office, as she had been instructed to do by Chicago HMO. Jones related Shawndale's symptoms, specifically that she was sick, was constipated, was crying a lot and felt very warm. An assistant advised Jones to give Shawndale some castor oil. When Jones insisted on speaking with Dr. Jordan, the assistant stated that Dr. Jordan was not available but would return her call. Dr. Jordan returned Jones' call late that evening. After Jones described the same symptoms to Dr. Jordan, he also advised Jones to give castor oil to Shawndale.

On January 19, 1991, Jones took Shawndale to a hospital emergency room because her condition had not improved. Chicago HMO authorized Shawndale's admission. Shawndale was diagnosed with bacterial meningitis, secondary to bilateral otitis media, an ear infection. As a result of the meningitis, Shawndale is permanently disabled.

The medical expert for the plaintiff, Dr. Richard Pawl, stated in his affidavit and deposition testimony that Dr. Jordan had deviated from the standard of care. In Dr. Pawl's opinion, upon being advised of a three-month-old infant who is warm, irritable and constipated, the standard of care requires a physician to schedule an immediate appointment to see the infant or, alternatively, to instruct the parent to obtain immediate medical care for the infant through another physician. Dr. Pawl gave no opinion regarding whether Chicago HMO was negligent.

Although Jones filed this action against Chicago HMO, Dr. Jordan and another party, this appeal concerns only counts I and III of Jones' second amended complaint, which are directed against Chicago HMO. Count I charges Chicago HMO with institutional negligence for, *inter alia*, (1) negligently assigning Dr. Jordan as Shawndale's primary care physician while he was serving an overloaded patient population, and (2) negligently adopting procedures that required Jones to call first for an appointment before visiting the doctor's office or obtaining emergency care. Count III charges Chicago HMO with breach of contract and is based solely on Chicago HMO's contract with the Department of Public Aid. Chicago HMO moved for summary judgment on both counts. Jones and Chicago HMO submitted various depositions, affidavits and exhibits in support of their positions.

Chicago HMO is a for-profit corporation. During all pertinent times, Chicago HMO was organized as an independent practice association model HMO under the Illinois Health Maintenance Organization Act (Ill. Rev. Stat. 1991, ch. 111½, par. 1401 *et seq.*).

In her deposition testimony, Jones described how she first enrolled in Chicago HMO while living in Park Forest. A Chicago HMO representative visited her home. According to Jones, he "was telling me what it was all about, that HMO is better than a regular medical card and everything so I am just listening to him and signing my name and stuff on the papers. *** I asked him what kind of benefits you get out of it and stuff, and he was telling me that it is better than a regular card."

The "HMO ENROLLMENT UNDERSTANDING" form signed by Jones in 1987 stated: "I understand that all my medical care will be provided through the Health Plan once my application becomes effective." Jones remembered that, at the time she signed this form, the Chicago HMO representative told her "you have got to call your doctor and stuff before you see your doctor; and before you go to the hospital, you have got to call."

Jones testified that when she later moved to Chicago Heights another Chicago HMO representative visited her home. This meeting was not arranged in advance. It occurred because the representative was "in the building knocking from door to door." Jones informed the representative that she was already a member.

When Jones moved to Chicago Heights, she did not select Dr. Jordan as Shawndale's primary care physician. Rather, Chicago HMO assigned Dr. Jordan to her. Jones explained:

"They gave me *** Dr. Jordan. They didn't ask me if I wanted a doctor. They gave me him.

      * * *

*** They told me that he was a good doctor *** for the kids because I didn't know what doctor to take my kids to because I was staying in Chicago Heights so they gave me him so I started taking my kids there to him."

Dr. Mitchell J. Trubitt, Chicago HMO's medical director, testified at his deposition that Dr. Jordan was under contract with Chicago HMO for two sites, Homewood and Chicago Heights. The service agreement for the Homewood site was first entered into on May 5, 1987. The service agreement for the Chicago Heights site was first entered into on February 1, 1990. Dr. Jordan was serving both patient populations in January of 1991 when Shawndale became ill.

Dr. Trubitt stated that, before Chicago HMO and Dr. Jordan executed the Chicago Heights service agreement, another physician serviced that area. Chicago HMO terminated that physician for failing to provide covered immunizations. At the time that Chicago HMO terminated that physician, Dr. Jordan agreed "to go into the [Chicago Heights] area and serve the patients." Chicago HMO then assigned to Dr. Jordan all of the patients of that physician. Dr. Trubitt explained:

"Q. So then with the elimination of [the other physician], Dr. Jordan then—were the members notified that Dr. Jordan would be their [primary care physician] from that point on?
A. Yes.
Q. They weren't given a choice?
A. At that point in the area there was no choice.
Q. So they weren't given a choice?
A. They were directed to Dr. Jordan."

Dr. Trubitt also explained that Dr. Jordan was Chicago HMO's only physician who was willing to serve the public aid membership in Chicago Heights. Dr. Trubitt characterized this lack of physicians as "a problem" for Chicago HMO.

Dr. Jordan testified at his deposition that, in January of 1991, he was a solo practitioner. He divided his time equally between his offices in Homewood and Chicago Heights. Dr. Jordan was under contract with Chicago HMO for both sites. In addition, Dr. Jordan was under contract with 20 other HMOs, and he maintained his own private practice of non-HMO patients. Dr. Jordan estimated that he was designated the primary care physician of 3,000 Chicago HMO members and 1,500 members of other HMOs. In contrast to Dr. Jordan's estimate, Chicago HMO's own "Provider Capitation Summary Reports" listed Dr. Jordan as being the primary care provider of 4,527 Chicago HMO patients as of December 1, 1990.

Jones' legal counsel and Dr. Trubitt engaged in the following colloquy concerning patient load:

"Q. In entering into an agreement with a provider, is any consideration given to the number of patients to be designated as the primary provider for?

A Yes, there is consideration given to that element in terms of volume of patients that he is capable of handling.

Q. And who determines the volume of patients he is capable of handling? The Chicago HMO or the provider or—

A. There is some guidelines that HCFA provides.

Q. Who provides?

A. HCFA. The Health [Care Finance Administration], the governmental health and welfare.

Q. Do you happen to know what those limits are with respect to pediatricians?

A. I am going to say I believe they are 3,500 patients to a primary care physician. The number can be expanded depending on the number of physicians in the office and the number of hours of operation.

Q. So you can't tell me whether or not if Dr. Jordan had 6,000 or 6,500 that would be an unusually large number?

A. If he himself had it.

Q. It would be unusually large?

A. It would.

Q. And that would be of some concern to the Chicago HMO, right?

A. Well, yes, if he had those."

In January of 1991, Dr. Jordan employed four part-time physicians, in addition to himself. This included an obstetrician/gynecologist, an internist, a family practitioner and a pediatrician. Dr. Jordan, however, did not explain in what capacities these physicians served. The record contains no further information regarding these physicians.

The record also contains evidence concerning Chicago HMO procedures for obtaining health care. Chicago HMO's "Member Handbook" told members in need of medical care to "*Call your Chicago HMO doctor first* when you experience an emergency or begin to feel sick." (Emphasis in original.) Also, Chicago HMO gave its contract physicians a "Provider

Manual." The manual contains certain provisions with which the providers are expected to comply. The manual contains a section entitled, "The Appointment System/Afterhours Care," which states that all HMO sites are statutorily required to maintain an appointment system for their patients.

Dr. Trubitt testified that Chicago HMO encouraged its providers to maintain an appointment system and also "to retain open spaces on their schedules so that patients who came in as walk-ins could be seen." Retaining space on the schedule for walk-ins was recommended because it offers quicker access to care, keeping patients out of the emergency room with its increased costs, and because, historically, the Medicaid patient population often did not make or keep appointments.

Dr. Jordan related that his office worked on an appointment system and had its own written procedures and forms for handling patient calls and appointments. When a patient called and Dr. Jordan was not in the office, written forms were used by his staff or his answering service to relay the information to him. If Dr. Jordan was in the office, the procedure was as follows:

"Q. *** [I]f it was a routine appointment for the purpose of having a routine shot or checkup, [the office staff] could make the appointment themselves?

A. Yes.

Q. But if the caller calls and says there is some problem, then they would take the temperature and find out the complaints and refer that call to you; is that correct?

A. That's correct.

Q. And you were the one who would make the determination as to whether or not to schedule an appointment, is that correct?

A. Medical decision, yes.

Q. Medical decision. And I assume there were times when people would call and after you reviewed the information and talked to them that you decided that they didn't need the appointment; is that correct?

A. Of course.

Q. In other words, you would perform some type of triage over the telephone; is that correct?

A. Yes."

Three agreements appear in the record. First, Chicago HMO and the Department of Public Aid entered into a 1990 "AGREEMENT FOR FURNISHING HEALTH SERVICES." This agreement was "for the delivery of medical services to Medicaid recipients on a prepaid capitation basis." Jones and her children, Medicaid recipients, fall within the agreement's definition of beneficiaries.

The preamble to the agreement stated that Chicago HMO "is organized primarily for the purpose of providing health care services." It continued: "[Chicago HMO] warrants that it is able to provide the medical care and services required under this Agreement in accordance with prevailing community standards, and is able to provide these services promptly, efficiently, and economically."

Article V of the agreement described various duties of Chicago HMO, as follows. Chicago HMO "shall provide or arrange to have provided all covered services to all Beneficiaries under this Agreement." Chicago HMO "shall provide all Beneficiaries with medical care consistent with prevailing community standards." In addition, a section entitled "Choice of Physicians" provided in relevant part:

"[Chicago HMO] shall afford to each Beneficiary a health professional who will supervise and coordinate his care, and, to the extent feasible within appropriate limits established by [Chicago HMO] and approved by the Department, shall afford the Beneficiary a choice of a physician.

There shall be at least one full-time equivalent, board eligible physician to every 1,200 enrollees, including one full-time equivalent, board certified primary care physician for each 2,000 enrollees. *** There shall be *** one pediatrician for each 2,000 enrollees under age 17."

Another article V duty stated that, although Chicago HMO may furnish the services required by the agreement by means of subcontractors, Chicago HMO "shall remain responsible for the performance of the subcontractors."

Regarding appointments, this agreement stated that Chicago HMO "shall encourage members to be seen by appointment, except in emergencies." The agreement also stated that "[m]embers with more serious or urgent problems not deemed emergencies shall be triaged and provided same day service, if necessary," and that "emergency treatment shall be available on an immediate basis, seven days a week, 24-hours a day." Finally, the agreement directed that Chicago HMO "shall have an established policy that scheduled patients shall not routinely wait for more than one hour to be seen by a provider and no more than six appointments shall be made for each primary care physician per hour."

The record also contains a second agreement, a 1990 "MEDICAL GROUP SERVICE AGREEMENT" between Chicago HMO and Dr. Jordan, that lists a Chicago Heights office address for Dr. Jordan. This agreement described numerous duties of Dr. Jordan. Pertinent here, Dr. Jordan would provide to Chicago HMO subscribers specified medical services "of good quality and in accordance with accepted medical and hospital standards of the community." Pursuant to a "PUBLIC AID AMENDMENT TO THE MEDICAL GROUP SERVICE AGREEMENT," Dr. Jordan agreed to "abide by any conditions imposed by [Chicago HMO] as part of [Chicago HMO's] agreement with [the Department]."

The third agreement appearing of record is a second "MEDICAL GROUP SERVICE AGREEMENT" between Chicago HMO and Dr. Jordan. This agreement was entered into in 1987 and lists a Homewood office address for Dr. Jordan.

Both agreements between Chicago HMO and Dr. Jordan provided for a capitation method of compensation. Under capitation, Chicago HMO paid Dr. Jordan a fixed amount of money for each member who selected Dr. Jordan as the member's primary care provider. In exchange, Dr. Jordan agreed to render health care to his enrolled Chicago HMO members in accordance with the Chicago HMO health plan. Dr. Jordan was paid the same monthly capitation fee per member regardless of the services he rendered. For example, for each female patient under two years old, Chicago HMO paid Dr. Jordan $34.19 per month regardless of whether he treated that patient. In addition, Chicago HMO utilized an incentive fund for Dr. Jordan. Certain costs such as inpatient hospital costs were paid from this fund. Chicago HMO would then pay Dr. Jordan 60% of any remaining, unused balance of the fund at the end of each year.

As earlier noted, the appellate court affirmed the circuit court's grant of summary judgment in favor of Chicago HMO as to count I, institutional negligence, and as to count III, breach of contract. 301 Ill. App. 3d 103. We are asked to decide whether Chicago HMO was properly awarded summary judgment on these two counts.

ANALYSIS

We conduct *de novo* review of an award of summary judgment. *Olson v. Etheridge*, 177 Ill. 2d 396, 404 (1997). Summary judgment is proper where the pleadings, depositions, admissions, affidavits and exhibits on file, when viewed in the light most favorable to the nonmoving party, show that there is no genuine issue as to any material fact and that the moving party is entitled to judgment as a matter of law. *Busch v. Graphic Color Corp.*, 169 Ill. 2d 325, 333 (1996). Summary judgment is a drastic remedy and should be allowed only when the right of the moving party is clear and free from doubt. *Colvin v. Hobart Brothers*, 156 Ill. 2d 166, 169-70 (1993).

This court first addressed a question of whether an HMO could be held liable for medical malpractice in *Petrovich v. Share Health Plan of Illinois, Inc.*, 188 Ill. 2d 17, 29 (1999). *Petrovich*, however, involved different legal theories of liability than those presented here. *Petrovich* held that an HMO may be held vicariously liable for the medical malpractice of its independent-contractor physicians under both the doctrines of apparent authority and implied authority. *Petrovich*, 188 Ill. 2d 17. In contrast, this appeal focuses on whether an

HMO may be held liable under the theory of institutional negligence.

I. Institutional Negligence

Institutional negligence is also known as direct corporate negligence. Since the landmark decision of *Darling v. Charleston Community Memorial Hospital*, 33 Ill. 2d 326 (1965), Illinois has recognized that *hospitals* may be held liable for institutional negligence. *Darling* acknowledged an independent duty of hospitals to assume responsibility for the care of their patients. Ordinarily, this duty is administrative or managerial in character. *Advincula v. United Blood Services*, 176 Ill. 2d 1, 28 (1996) (and authorities cited therein). To fulfill this duty, a hospital must act as would a "reasonably careful hospital" under the circumstances. *Advincula*, 176 Ill. 2d at 29. Liability is predicated on the hospital's own negligence, not the negligence of the physician.

Underlying the tort of institutional negligence is a recognition of the comprehensive nature of hospital operations today. The hospital's expanded role in providing health care services to patients brings with it increased corporate responsibilities. As *Darling* explained: "Present-day hospitals, as their manner of operation plainly demonstrates, do far more than furnish facilities for treatment. They regularly employ on a salary basis a large staff of physicians, nurses and interns, as well as administrative and manual workers, and they charge patients for medical care and treatment, collecting for such services, if necessary, by legal action." *Darling*, 33 Ill. 2d at 332. Expounding on the point, this court later stated: "[A] modern hospital *** is an amalgam of many individuals not all of whom are licensed medical practitioners. Moreover, it is clear that at times a hospital functions far beyond the narrow sphere of medical practice." *Greenberg v. Michael Reese Hospital*, 83 Ill. 2d 282, 293 (1980). Thus, in recognizing hospital institutional negligence as a cause of action, *Darling* merely applied principles of common law negligence to hospitals in a manner that comports with the true scope of their operations. See *Darling*, 33 Ill. 2d at 331 (noting that the duty in negligence cases is always the same, to conform to the legal standard of reasonable conduct in light of the apparent risk).

In accordance with the preceding rationale, we now hold that the doctrine of institutional negligence may be applied to HMOs. This court in *Petrovich* acknowledged the potential for applying this theory to HMOs. See *Petrovich*, 188 Ill. 2d at 30 (and authorities cited therein). A court in another jurisdiction has likewise extended the theory of hospital institutional negligence to HMOs. *Shannon v. McNulty*, 718 A.2d 828 (Pa. Super. Ct. 1998). It did so out of a recognition that HMOs, like hospitals, consist of an amalgam of many individuals who play various roles in order to provide comprehensive health care services to their members. *Shannon*, 718 A.2d at 835-36. Moreover, because HMOs undertake an expansive role in arranging for and providing health care services to their members, they have corresponding corporate responsibilities as well. *Shannon*, 718 A.2d at 835-36; see *Petrovich*, 188 Ill. 2d at 28, 33-40 (recognizing that HMOs act as health care providers and attempt to contain the costs of health care); 215 ILCS 125/1-2(9) (West 1998) (defining an HMO as "any organization formed *** to provide or arrange for one or more health care plans under a system which causes any part of the risk of health care delivery to be borne by the organization or its providers"); *Official Lists Current Amicus Briefs of Labor Department on Medical Malpractice*, 68 U.S.L.W. 2249-50 (November 2, 1999) (noting that, according to the United States Department of Labor, HMOs wear "three different hats," one of which is "medical provider"). Our nationwide research has revealed no decision expressing a contrary view, and Chicago HMO makes no argument against extending the doctrine of institutional negligence to HMOs. Hence, we conclude that the law imposes a duty upon HMOs to conform to the legal standard of reasonable conduct in light of the apparent risk. See *Darling*, 33 Ill. 2d at 331. To fulfill this duty, an HMO must act as would a "reasonably careful" HMO under the circumstances. See *Advincula*, 176 Ill. 2d at 29.

Having determined that institutional negligence is a valid claim against HMOs, we turn to the parties' arguments in this case. Jones contends that Chicago HMO is not entitled to summary judgment on her claim of institutional negligence. She asserts that genuine issues of material fact exist as to whether Chicago HMO (1) negligently assigned more enrollees to Dr. Jordan than he was capable of serving, and (2) negligently adopted procedures requiring Jones to call first for an appointment before visiting the doctor's office.

Chicago HMO argues that Jones' claim of institutional negligence cannot proceed because she failed to provide sufficient evidence delineating the standard of care required of an HMO in these circumstances. In particular, Chicago HMO contends that Jones should have presented expert testimony on the standard of care required of an HMO.

Jones responds that she has provided sufficient evidence showing the standard of care required of an HMO in these circumstances. She argues further that her claim does not require expert testimony on this point. In support, Jones relies on *Darling*, where a claim of institutional negligence was allowed against a hospital without expert testimony because other evidence established the hospital's standard of care. *Darling*, 33 Ill. 2d 326.

Given that the parties' dispute centers on standard of care evidence and the need for expert testimony, we briefly review the roles of the standard of care and expert testimony in negligence cases. We then discuss *Darling* and its progeny.

The elements of a negligence cause of action are a duty owed by the defendant to the plaintiff, a breach of that duty, and an injury proximately caused by the breach. *Cunis v. Brennan*, 56 Ill. 2d 372, 374 (1974). The standard of care, also known as the standard of conduct, falls within the duty element. Dean Prosser has explained:

"It is better to reserve 'duty' for the problem of the relation between individuals which imposes upon one a legal obligation for the benefit of the other, and to deal with particular conduct in terms of a legal standard of what is required to meet the obligation. In other words, 'duty' is a question of whether the defendant is under any obligation for the benefit of the particular plaintiff; and in negligence cases, the duty is always the same, to conform to the legal standard of reasonable conduct in light of the apparent risk. *What the defendant must do, or must not do, is a question of the standard of conduct required to satisfy the duty*. The distinction is one of convenience only, and it must be remembered that the two are correlative, and one cannot exist without the other.

A duty, in negligence cases, may be defined as an obligation, to which the law will give recognition and effect, to conform to a particular standard of conduct toward another." (Emphasis added.) W. Prosser, Torts, at 324 (4th ed. 1971).

In an ordinary negligence case, the standard of care required of a defendant is to act as would an "'ordinarily careful person'" or a "'reasonably prudent' person." *Advincula v. United Blood Services*, 176 Ill. 2d 1, 22 (1996), quoting *Cunis*, 56 Ill. 2d at 376. No expert testimony is required in a case of ordinary negligence. See *Advincula*, 176 Ill. 2d at 24.

In contrast, in a professional negligence case, the standard of care required of a defendant is to act as would an "ordinarily careful professional." *Advincula*, 176 Ill. 2d at 23. Pursuant to this standard of care, professionals are expected to use the same degree of knowledge, skill and ability as an ordinarily careful professional would exercise under similar circumstances. *Advincula*, 176 Ill. 2d at 23-24. Expert testimony is usually required in a case of professional negligence. *Advincula*, 176 Ill. 2d at 24, 38. Expert testimony is necessary to establish both (1) the standard of care expected of the professional and (2) the professional's deviation from the standard. See *Purtill v. Hess*, 111 Ill. 2d 229, 242 (1986). The rationale for requiring expert testimony is that a lay juror is not skilled in the profession and thus is not equipped to determine what constitutes reasonable care in professional conduct without the help of expert testimony. *Advincula*, 176 Ill. 2d at 24; see *Purtill*, 111 Ill.

2d at 246. In Illinois, a professional standard of care has been applied in cases involving a variety of both medical and non-medical professions, such as law and dentistry. *Advincula*, 176 Ill. 2d at 23-24 (and cases cited therein).

The foregoing principles of law establish that the crucial difference between ordinary negligence and professional malpractice actions is the necessity of expert testimony to establish the standard of care and that its breach was the cause of the plaintiff's injury. Although not applicable to this case, there are exceptions to the requirement of expert testimony in professional negligence cases. For example, in instances where the professional's conduct is so grossly negligent or the treatment so common that a lay juror could readily appraise it, no expert testimony or other such relevant evidence is required. *Advincula*, 176 Ill. 2d at 24 (and cases cited therein); *Walski v. Tiesenga*, 72 Ill. 2d 249, 257 (1978) (noting that examples of this exception in medical malpractice cases include instruments left in a patient's body after surgery and X-ray burns); see also *Ohligschlager v. Proctor Community Hospital*, 55 Ill. 2d 411 (1973) (holding that a drug manufacturer's instructions provided the proper standard of care with which to measure the conduct of a physician).

As Jones correctly notes, the institutional negligence of hospitals can also be determined without expert testimony in some cases. The standard of care evidence required to bring an action for institutional negligence against a hospital is best understood by a review of the relevant case law.

In *Darling v. Charleston Community Memorial Hospital*, 33 Ill. 2d 326 (1965), the plaintiff had his leg placed in a cast at the defendant hospital. While remaining at the hospital, he suffered a serious case of gangrene. He ultimately lost his leg below the knee. The plaintiff brought an action directly against the hospital for failing to have trained nurses monitor his condition and for failing to review his treatment. In support of his argument that the hospital breached the standard of care required of hospitals in this regard, the plaintiff presented evidence that the hospital breached its own bylaws, as well as the state's licensing regulations and the "Standards for Hospital Accreditation." *Darling*, 33 Ill. 2d at 330-32. A jury returned a verdict for the plaintiff, and this court affirmed. *Darling*, 33 Ill. 2d at 328.

As earlier noted, this court in *Darling* recognized an independent duty of hospitals to assume responsibility for the care of their patients. Relevant here, *Darling* also held that the hospital bylaws, licensing regulations, and standards for hospital accreditation were sufficient evidence with which to establish the hospital's standard of care. *Darling* likened this evidence to evidence of custom, which may also be used to determine a hospital's standard of care. The jury was therefore entitled to conclude from the plaintiff's evidence that the hospital had breached its duty to the plaintiff. *Darling*, 33 Ill. 2d at 330-33.

In *Greenberg v. Michael Reese Hospital*, 83 Ill. 2d 282 (1980), a group of plaintiffs sued the hospital for injuries that they sustained as a result of being X-rayed without a protective shield. As standard of care evidence, the plaintiffs presented an expert witness who was a health physicist specializing in the effects of radiation. The hospital challenged the qualifications of plaintiffs' expert, claiming that, since he was not a physician practicing in any school of medicine, he could not testify concerning conduct that involves a medical judgment. This court held that the affidavit of the plaintiffs' nonphysician expert was sufficient to withstand the hospital's motion for summary judgment. *Greenberg*, 83 Ill. 2d at 293-94. Although the expert was not a medical practitioner, he was highly qualified and familiar with radiation therapy in hospitals. This court deemed "it appropriate to the diversity inherent in hospital administration that a broad range of evidence be available to establish the applicable standard of care." *Greenberg*, 83 Ill. 2d at 293.

More recently, this court in *Advincula v. United Blood Services*, 176 Ill. 2d 1, 29 (1996), stated that the standard of care required of a hospital in a case of institutional negligence may be shown by a wide variety of evidence, including, but not limited to, expert testimony, hospital bylaws, statutes, accreditation standards, custom and community practice. *Advincula* explained that this variety of evidence is appropriate given the inherent diversity in hospital administrative and managerial actions, only a portion of which involves the exercise of medical judgment. *Advincula*, 176 Ill. 2d at 32-34. *Advincula* further explained, however, that the tort of institutional negligence "does not encompass, whatsoever, a hospital's responsibility for the conduct of its *** medical professionals." *Advincula*, 176 Ill. 2d at 31. Rather, in cases against hospitals based on vicarious liability for the conduct of medical professionals, the standard of care remains the standard applied to all professionals, *i.e.*, to use the same degree of knowledge, skill and ability as an ordinarily careful professional would exercise under similar circumstances. *Advincula*, 176 Ill. 2d at 30, 31.

Darling and its progeny have firmly established that, in an action for institutional negligence against a hospital, the standard of care applicable to a hospital may be proved via a number of evidentiary sources, and expert testimony is not always required. *Advincula*, 176 Ill. 2d at 29-34; *Greenberg*, 83 Ill. 2d at 293-94; *Darling*, 33 Ill. 2d at 330-33. We likewise conclude that, in an action for institutional negligence against an HMO, the standard of care applicable to an HMO may be proved through a number of evidentiary sources, and expert testimony is not

necessarily required. Accordingly, expert testimony concerning the standard of care required of an HMO is not a prerequisite to Jones' claim. Nonetheless, Jones, as the plaintiff here, still bears the burden of establishing the standard of care required of an HMO through other, proper evidentiary sources. We must therefore evaluate the evidence presented on this point to determine whether Jones' claim withstands Chicago HMO's motion for summary judgment. In deciding whether Jones' standard of care evidence is sufficient, we look to whether that evidence can equip a lay juror to determine what constitutes the standard of care required of a "reasonably careful HMO" under the circumstances of this case.

A. Patient Load

We first consider Jones' assertion that Chicago HMO negligently assigned more patients to Dr. Jordan than he was capable of serving. Parenthetically, we note that this assertion involves an administrative or managerial action by Chicago HMO, not the professional conduct of its physicians. Therefore, this claim properly falls within the purview of HMO institutional negligence. Jones argues that the standard of care evidence in the record is sufficient to support her claim. She points to Dr. Trubitt's testimony, as well as the contract between Chicago HMO and the Department of Public Aid.

Dr. Trubitt was the medical director for Chicago HMO. He testified that, when Chicago HMO entered into agreements with primary care physicians, it considered the number of patients that the physician is capable of handling. The HMO would look to federal "guidelines" in making this determination. Based on those guidelines, Dr. Trubitt expressed 3,500 as the maximum number of patients that should be assigned to any one primary care physician. He stated that, if Dr. Jordan himself had 6,000 or more patients, then that would be an unusually large number and of concern to Chicago HMO.

We agree with Jones that Dr. Trubitt's testimony is proper and sufficient evidence of the standard of care on this issue. According to Dr. Trubitt, an HMO should not assign more than 3,500 patients to any single primary care physician. Chicago HMO even concedes in its brief that the maximum patient load to which Dr. Trubitt testified "represent[s] a 'standard of care' whose violation could affect the quality of patient care." This particular standard of care evidence, setting forth a limit of 3,500 patients per primary care physician, is adequate to equip a lay juror to determine what constitutes the standard of care required of a "reasonably careful HMO" under the circumstances of this case. Whether Dr. Trubitt relied on an unidentified federal regulation or some other source in arriving at a maximum patient load of 3,500 is of no consequence. It is enough that Chicago HMO, through its medical director, admitted that it used the 3,500 limit as a guide in assigning patient loads. See *Darling*, 33 Ill. 2d at 330-33 (holding that the hospital's own bylaws may be used to establish the hospital's standard of care).

Chicago HMO, however, submits that there is no evidence in the record that Dr. Jordan's patient load exceeded 3,500. We disagree. Chicago HMO's "Provider Capitation Summary Reports" listed Dr. Jordan as being the primary care provider of 4,527 Chicago HMO members as of December 1, 1990. Thus, Chicago HMO's own records show Dr. Jordan's patient load as exceeding the 3,500 limit by more than 1,000 patients. In addition, Dr. Jordan estimated that he himself was designated the primary care physician for an additional 1,500 members of other HMOs. He also maintained his own private practice of non-HMO patients. This evidence supports Jones' theory that Dr. Jordan had more than 6,000 HMO patients.

Chicago HMO, in support of its position, points to Dr. Jordan's testimony that he employed four part-time physicians in his office. We disagree with Chicago HMO concerning the significance of this testimony. Although Dr. Jordan testified that he employed four part-time physicians, he never explained in what capacities these physicians served. In fact, the record contains no further information regarding these physicians. Notably, the agreements between Chicago HMO and Dr. Jordan do not refer to any physicians other than Dr. Jordan himself. The evidence in the record, therefore, supports Jones' theory that Chicago HMO negligently assigned more than 3,500 patients to Dr. Jordan himself. At best, the testimony regarding the four part-time physicians creates a genuine issue of material fact as to how many patients Dr. Jordan actually served himself. Consequently, this limited information in the record about part-time physicians does not entitle Chicago HMO to summary judgment. As earlier noted, it is well established that summary judgment is a drastic remedy and should be awarded only where the right of the moving party is clear and free from doubt.

Chicago HMO also submits that Jones' claim of patient overload must fail because there is no evidence of a causal connection between the number of patients that Dr. Jordan was serving and his failure to schedule an appointment to see Shawndale. We disagree. We can easily infer from this record that Dr. Jordan's failure to see Shawndale resulted from an inability to serve an overloaded patient population. A lay juror can discern that a physician who has thousands more patients than he should will not have time to service them all in an appropriate manner.

We note, moreover, that additional evidence in the record supports Jones' claim. The record indicates that Chicago HMO was actively soliciting new members door-to-door around the same time that it lacked the physicians willing to serve those members. Jones described how she first enrolled in Chicago HMO while living in Park Forest. A Chicago HMO representative visited her home and persuaded her to become a member, telling her that Chicago HMO "is better than a regular medical card." When Jones later moved to Chicago Heights, another Chicago HMO representative visited her home. Jones explained that this meeting was not arranged in advance. Rather, the representative was "in the building knocking from door to door." Jones also testified that, when she moved to Chicago Heights, Chicago HMO assigned Dr. Jordan to her and did not give her a choice of primary care physicians.

The latter aspect of Jones' testimony was supported by Dr. Trubitt. He explained that, before Chicago HMO and Dr. Jordan executed the Chicago Heights service agreement, another physician serviced that area. When Chicago HMO terminated that other physician, Dr. Jordan agreed "to go into the [Chicago Heights] area and serve the patients." Chicago HMO then assigned to Dr. Jordan all of the patients of that physician. Chicago HMO directed its members to Dr. Jordan; they had no other choice of a physician because "[a]t that point in the area there was no choice." According to Dr. Trubitt, Dr. Jordan was Chicago HMO's only physician who was willing to serve the public aid membership in Chicago Heights. Dr. Trubitt stated that this lack of physicians was "a problem" for Chicago HMO.

The record further reflects that Chicago HMO directed its Chicago Heights members to Dr. Jordan, even though it knew that Dr. Jordan worked at that location only half the time. Chicago HMO entered into two service agreements with Dr. Jordan, the first for a Homewood site in 1987, and the second for the Chicago Heights site in 1990. Dr. Trubitt indicated that Chicago HMO and Dr. Jordan executed the Chicago Heights service agreement at the time that Chicago HMO terminated the other physician. Dr. Jordan confirmed that, in January of 1991, he was dividing his time equally between his two offices. All of the foregoing evidence supports Jones' theory that Chicago HMO acted negligently in assigning more enrollees to Dr. Jordan than he was capable of handling.

Jones also relies on the contract between Chicago HMO and the Department of Public Aid as standard of care evidence. That contract stated that Chicago HMO shall have one full-time equivalent primary care physician for every 2,000 enrollees. We need not address in this appeal whether this contractual provision may serve as standard of care evidence. Our role here is to determine whether Chicago HMO is entitled to summary judgment on the patient overload aspect of the institutional negligence claim. Even if this contractual provision is removed from consideration, Chicago HMO is not entitled to summary judgment. Accordingly, we express no opinion on whether this provision may properly serve as standard of care evidence.

One final matter with respect to patient load remains to be considered. Chicago HMO contends that imposing a duty on HMOs to ascertain how many patients their doctors are serving would be unreasonably burdensome. Chicago HMO asserts that only physicians, and not HMOs, should have the duty to determine if the physician has too many patients.

To determine whether a duty exists in a certain instance, a court considers the following factors: (1) the reasonable foreseeability of injury, (2) the likelihood of injury, (3) the magnitude of the burden of guarding against the injury, and (4) the consequences of placing that burden upon the defendant. *Deibert v. Bauer Brothers Construction Co.*, 141 Ill. 2d 430, 437-38 (1990); *Kirk v. Michael Reese Hospital & Medical Center*, 117 Ill. 2d 507, 526 (1987). Lastly, the existence of a duty turns in large part on public policy considerations. *Ward v. K mart Corp.*, 136 Ill. 2d 132, 151 (1990); see *Mieher v. Brown*, 54 Ill. 2d 539, 545 (1973). Whether a duty exists is a question of law to be determined by the court. *Cunis*, 56 Ill. 2d at 374.

Here, given the circumstances of this case, we hold that Chicago HMO had a duty to its enrollees to refrain from assigning an excessive number of patients to Dr. Jordan. HMOs contract with primary care physicians in order to provide and arrange for medical care for their enrollees. It is thus reasonably foreseeable that assigning an excessive number of patients to a primary care physician could result in injury, as that care may not be provided. For the same reason, the likelihood of injury is great. Nor would imposing this duty on HMOs be overly burdensome. Here, for example, Chicago HMO needed only to review its "Provider Capitation Summary Reports" to obtain the number of patients that it had assigned to Dr. Jordan. This information is likely to be available to all HMOs, as they must know the number of patients that a physician is serving in order to compute the physician's monthly capitation payments. The HMO may also simply ask the physician how many patients the physician is serving. Finally, the remaining factors favor placing this burden on HMOs as well. Public policy would not be well served by allowing HMOs to assign an excessive number of patients to a primary care physician and then "wash their hands" of the matter. The central consequence of placing this burden on HMOs is HMO accountability for their own actions. This court in *Petrovich* recognized that HMO accountability is needed to counterbalance the HMO goal of cost containment and, where applicable, the inherent drive of an HMO to achieve profits. *Petrovich*, 188 Ill. 2d at 29.

In conclusion, Chicago HMO is not entitled to summary judgment on Jones' claim of institutional negligence for assigning too many patients to Dr. Jordan.

B. Appointment Procedures

We next consider Jones' assertion that Chicago HMO negligently adopted procedures requiring Jones to call first for an appointment before visiting the doctor's office or obtaining emergency care. Jones fails to develop this argument in her brief. In particular, she points to no evidence in the record as providing the standard of care required of an HMO in developing appointment procedures. This claim cannot proceed without standard of care evidence. Chicago HMO is therefore entitled to summary judgment with respect to this portion of Jones' claim of institutional negligence.

II. Breach of Contract

Jones argues that Chicago HMO is not entitled to summary judgment on her breach of contract claim. This claim, set forth in count III of Jones' complaint, is based solely on the contract between Chicago HMO and the Department of Public Aid. Jones is not a signatory to this contract, but rather a beneficiary. Jones, however, expressly disclaims any reliance on a third-party beneficiary theory of liability. Instead, Jones insists that she may maintain an action for damages against Chicago HMO as if she were a party to the agreement.

The appellate court held that summary judgment was properly awarded to Chicago HMO on this claim because Jones is not a party to the contract at issue. The appellate court also noted that Jones' theory of liability in this regard was "murky at best." 301 Ill. App. 3d at 115.

We hold that Chicago HMO is entitled to summary judgment on count III. The record discloses that Jones is not a party to the contract that she seeks to enforce. Rather, the contracting parties are Chicago HMO and the Department. Nonetheless, Jones insists that she may maintain a cause of action on that contract, while also disclaiming any reliance on a third-party beneficiary theory of liability. Jones' position is not correct as a matter of law. See *Olson v. Etheridge*, 177 Ill. 2d 396, 404 (1997) (explaining third-party beneficiary theory); 17A Am. Jur. 2d *Contracts* §§ 435, 437 (2d ed. 1991) (noting that a nonparty to a contract must sue under a third-party beneficiary theory). We also agree with the appellate court that the theory presented by Jones on this point is not clear.

III. Breach of Warranty

Jones lastly argues that she should be permitted to pursue a breach of warranty claim against Chicago HMO. She asserts that count III can be construed as raising this claim. Chicago

HMO counters that Jones has waived any breach of warranty claim by failing to raise it in the courts below. We agree with Chicago HMO. Issues raised for the first time on appeal are waived. *Employers Insurance v. Ehlco Liquidating Trust*, 186 Ill. 2d 127, 161 (1999). Our review of the record reveals that Jones did not raise this claim in either the circuit court or the appellate court. Nor did Jones raise this issue in her petition for leave to appeal. We thus conclude that Jones has waived any claim of breach of warranty.

CONCLUSION

An HMO may be held liable for institutional negligence. Chicago HMO is not entitled to summary judgment on Jones' claim charging Chicago HMO with institutional negligence for assigning more enrollees to Dr. Jordan than he was capable of serving. We therefore reverse the award of summary judgment to Chicago HMO on count I of Jones' second amended complaint and remand that claim to the circuit court for further proceedings. As to count III, we affirm the award of summary judgment to Chicago HMO.

The judgments of the appellate and circuit courts are affirmed in part and reversed in part and the cause is remanded to the circuit court.

Judgments affirmed in part and reversed in part
[Concurring and dissenting opinions omitted.]

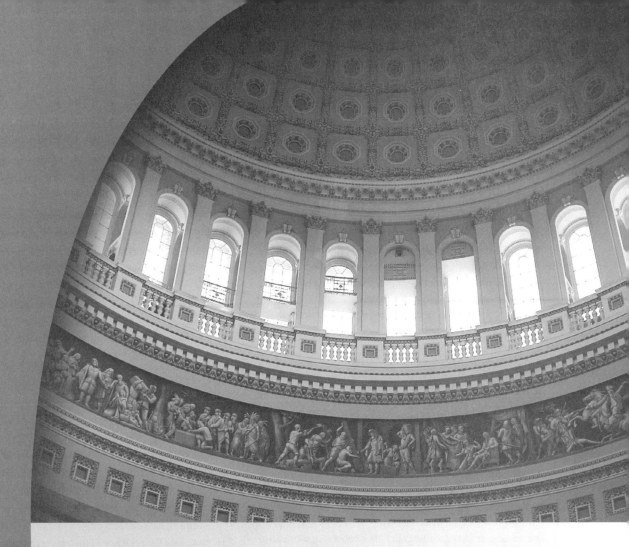

PART III

Policy, Law, Medicine, and Ethics

The readings in Part 3 collectively intersect at the crossroads of policy, law, medicine, and ethics and represent a broad subset of health policy and law that received relatively little attention in the textbook. The readings open with two articles—one by Carol Levine titled "Analyzing Pandora's Box: The History of Bioethics" and one titled "Public Health Ethics: Mapping the Terrain" by James Childress and colleagues. These articles provide context for the readings that follow and delineate the differences between medical ethics and public health ethics.

The readings then turn to two enormous health policy and law issues that implicate both medical and public health ethics: the right to a legal abortion and the right of individuals to determine the timing and other circumstances surrounding their death. The right to an abortion and the right to die are two incredibly polarizing issues, and raise fascinating and complex questions about the roles of ethics and medical technology in the shaping of health policy and law.

In *Roe v. Wade*—one of the United States Supreme Court's most widely known and commonly misunderstood opinions—the Court determined that the U.S. Constitution includes the right to obtain an abortion, with certain restrictions. In *Planned Parenthood v. Casey*, the Court invalidated *Roe*'s "trimester framework" and altered the legal analysis applicable to state abortion laws but left intact *Roe*'s defining feature, namely, the determination that the right to obtain an abortion is a constitutional protection. The next reading—the statutory text of the federal Partial Birth Abortion Ban Act—sets the stage for the Supreme Court's opinion in *Gonzales v. Carhart*, which considers the constitutionality of the Act.

The remainder of the readings in Part 3 concern the constitutional right to withdraw life-sustaining treatment (*Cruzan v. Director, Missouri Department of Health*) and the right to physician-assisted suicide (*Washington v. Glucksberg* and *Vacco v. Quill*, in which the Supreme Court ruled against two theories meant to confer a federal right to physician-assisted suicide). The readings conclude with a mini-case study of Oregon's effort to implement a right to physician-assisted suicide through its Death With Dignity Act. The statute and implementing regulations are reproduced, as are an Oregon report on usage of the right and the Supreme Court's opinion (*Gonzalez v. Oregon*) on whether the state law withstands constitutional scrutiny.

IN THIS SECTION

Carol Levine, "Analyzing Pandora's Box: The History of Bioethics" from *The Ethics of Bioethics*

James Childress et al., "Public Health Ethics: Mapping the Terrain"

Case law: *Roe v. Wade* (constitutional right to abortion)

Case law: *Planned Parenthood v. Casey* (validity of Pennsylvania abortion statute)

The Partial Birth Abortion Ban Act

Case law: *Gonzales v. Carhart* (constitutionality of the Partial Birth Abortion Ban Act)

Case law: *Cruzan v. Director, Missouri Department of Health* (constitutional right to withdraw life-sustaining treatment)

Case law: *Washington v. Glucksberg* (physician-assisted suicide)

Case law: *Vacco v. Quill* (physician-assisted suicide)

The Oregon Death With Dignity Act statute, regulations, and state's report on its use

Case law: *Gonzalez v. Oregon* (physician-assisted suicide)

Analyzing Pandora's Box: The History of Bioethics, from *The Ethics of Bioethics*

Carol Levine

Source: Analyzing Pandora's Box: The History of Bioethics, Carol Levine, M.A., from *The Ethics of Bioethics: Mapping the Moral Landscape*, The Johns Hopkins University Press, Baltimore, MD (2007).

The definitive history of bioethics has yet to be written. That is not surprising since bioethics in its modern American incarnation is only about fifty years old. But the future historian will have a mountain of source material, for nearly everyone involved in the field has written about some clinical dilemma, legal ruling, policy option, philosophical analysis, or personal experience. All the many public commissions and advisory boards that have examined specific issues have produced a flood of documents.

The future historian will also have the benefit of several publications by some of the major participants themselves—notably books by David Rothman (1992), Al Jonsen (1998), H. Tristram Engelhardt Jr. (1996), and members of the Kennedy Institute of Ethics (Walter and Klein, 2003) and articles by Stephen Toulmin (1988), Daniel Callahan (1999, 2005). Renée C. Fox and Judith P. Swazey (2005), David Thomasma (2002), and Daniel Kevles (2000), among others. The various editions of the *Encyclopedia of Bioethics* (1978, 1995, 2003) are a rich resource. Some accounts criticize bioethics in terms of its founding principles and current practice (Stevens 2000; Evans 2002; Short 2003; and Smith 2002), seeing capitulation to the demands of transplantation or other technology (Stevens), hubris (Evans and Smith). or plain misreading of the basic philosophical texts (Short).

There are also a few attempts to revise the conventional wisdom about some of the early debates. For example, it is often stated that the Report of the Harvard Ad Hoc Committee to Examine the Definition of Brain Death developed the concept of "brain death" in 1968 to facilitate procuring organs for transplantation. In reviewing the original documents, especially the papers of Henry Beecher, one of the most prominent committee members, and interviews with surviving members, Gary Belkin concluded that "a more careful history of the Report pushes interest in transplantation to the side, and sees it as a subset of the primary problem of coma and hopelessness" (Belkin 2003, 357). It is likely that future historians may also revise other articles of faith within bioethics about early decisions and reports.

Increasingly, writing about bioethics analyzes not just the issues that concern the field, but the field itself. What started as a largely academic, fairly modest endeavor has moved rapidly onto the center stage of media, political, and public attention. While some of the ideas were radical for their time, and bioethics at its beginnings had many elements of a social movement, institutionalization set in rather quickly.

As a participant over the past thirty years in some of the major ethical debates, I do not claim to be totally objective. Nevertheless, I hope to provide in this chapter as unbiased a view as possible, relying on my own experience and those elements of the historical record that are easily available. The founding fathers (and they were indeed mostly fathers or Fathers) would undoubtedly be amazed that their efforts had created so much controversy. The widespread interest in matters bioethical today confirms the premise that bioethics addresses critical issues affecting the way we live and die; however, some of the internal focus also threatens to distract attention from the issues themselves. Will this revolution, like so many others, end by eating its own children?

WHERE DID BIOETHICS COME FROM?

This question can be answered in two ways: the origin of the term and the origin of the field. The term *bioethics* itself was born twice—in Wisconsin and in Washington, D.C. Influenced by the work of land ethicist and conservationist Aldo Leopold (1949), Van Rensselaer Potter, a cancer specialist at the University of Wisconsin, published an article in 1970 called "Bioethics, the Science of Survival." In it he proposed "bioethics" as a global movement integrating concern for the environment and ethics (Potter 1970). He extended these views in his book *Bioethics: A Bridge to the Future* (1971), which proposed bioethics as a link between science and humanities. Later, as Potter saw mainstream bioethics focusing more on technology and genetics, he modified his original term and called his position "global bioethics" (Potter 1998). Without using the term, Hans Jonas, a German philosopher-in-exile who taught at the New School for Social Research for many years, focused on many of the same issues in his philosophical writing, especially the "imperative of responsibility" to sustain the planet for future generations (Jonas 1984).

As Peter Whitehouse, Potter's student and disciple, put it, "The original formulation of bioethics by Van Rensselaer Potter included a profound commitment to the future that the world desperately needs bioethicists to rediscover" (Whitehouse 2003, W26). Potter's concerns were relatively dormant within bioethics for many years but have surfaced recently in the controversy over genetic manipulation of food and other environmental issues and a more global focus in the field.

Also in 1970 Sargent Shriver, husband of Eunice Kennedy Shriver, came up with the term *bioethics* in discussions with André Hellegers, a Dutch physician and Jesuit priest, and others about the creation of an institute at Georgetown University that would apply moral philosophy to medical dilemmas (Reich 1994, 1995). These discussions resulted in the creation in 1971 of the Joseph and Rose Kennedy Center for the Study of Human Reproduction and Bioethics, now known as the Kennedy Institute of Ethics. While Potter's use of *bioethics* was the first to be published, it was the Kennedy Institute's use of the term, focusing on medicine and an institutional base for scholarly discussion, which came to dominate the field.

What were the origins of bioethics as a field of inquiry? An anthropologist might observe that its followers tell different creation stories. In one version, bioethics in Western thought starts with the Hippocratic corpus. Another goes back to the British physician Thomas Percival's 1803 book *Medical Ethics*, which argued for professional codes of ethics and which influenced the first American codes of medical ethics a half century later. Early codes of ethics were largely but not exclusively focused on the guild aspects of medicine and mutual obligations among practitioners.

When it comes to America in the mid-twentieth century, the creation stories are often summarized in a word— "Nuremberg," "Tuskegee," "Willowbrook," and more. All of these stand for part of but not the whole story. In its foundational beliefs in individual autonomy, bioethics had a distinctly American cast. In warning against American "bioethics imperialism," however, Moreno (2004) cites the experience of Weimar Germany in the early 1930s when a few physicians created a journal called *Ethics* to discuss various theories of eugenics, then the dominant social philosophy of medicine. Moreno calls the devolution of this journal into a Nazi tract for racial purification a warning that an intellectual movement can slide into disaster.

Hanauske-Abel (1996) interprets the situation differently. Rather than the German medical community being a "victim of circumstances," he contends that it set its own course. Medical organizations voluntarily placed the resources and loyalties of their profession at the service of the state. Within a short period in 1933 doctors in some respects even outpaced the Nazi regime in enthusiastically carrying out eugenic sterilizations. (Several other countries, including the United States, permitted forced sterilization, with the imprimatur of the U.S. Supreme Court's 1927 decision in *Buck v. Bell*, into the 1960s [Kevles 2000].)

Moreover, in 1931 a federal law in Germany was passed that clearly specified the obligations of physicians and the rights of patients in medical research (Sass 1983). Even stricter in some ways than the Nuremberg Code that followed the trial of German doctors in 1947, these rules were not repealed under the Nazis. Nevertheless, in the Nazi period German physicians carried out some of the most heinous and cruel abuses ever conducted under medical aegis. If their digression illustrates one overriding theme, it is that medical ethics is inextricably entwined with the social and political forces of its time and place.

In our time and our place, bioethics emerged in the late 1950s and 1960s, a turbulent era in which authorities of all kinds—parental, academic, political, medical, military—were challenged. In this version of the creation story, one need name only the key events of the period to realize the impact on all sectors of society: Vatican II, with its appeal to modernize the Catholic Church; the Vietnam War and its dissenters; college campuses turned into battlefields; the birth control pill that revolutionized women's control over reproduction; various rights movements, starting with civil rights for black Americans, then women's rights, gay and lesbian rights, abortion rights, disability rights, animal rights, and more. Some of these social movements directly affected the emergence of bioethics; others contributed to the general tenor of the times.

This was also a period in which scientific advances were creating startling and often unsettling new possibilities in controlling and facilitating reproduction, modifying behavior, and understanding genetics. People who would have died in earlier eras could be sustained on life-prolonging machinery, not just feeding tubes but also dialysis machines and ventilators. Extremely premature infants could be kept alive, albeit with significant health problems. Decisions had to be made about allocating kidney dialysis machines, then a scarce resource. Organ transplantation became feasible, if there were enough organs to transplant. So many of these inventions have become so commonplace and so accepted, and in some cases inappropriately used, that it is worth remembering that they did not always exist. The agonizing decisions that make up so much of modern bioethics discussion are the outcomes of modern technology introduced with great hopes but little forethought. In this brave new world most physicians assumed, as they had for centuries, that they were the only appropriate decision makers. Against this background it seemed inevitable that patients would begin to challenge physicians' authority.

Partnership in decision making is now often presented as the ideal, especially given the often overwhelming amount and easy access to medical information of variable quality. But when bioethics emerged, physicians had almost total control of information and decision-making power. The women's movement of the 1960s and 1970s was a front-line attack on this patriarchal and authoritarian model. In the "good old days" of the 1950s doctors frequently performed "one-step" mastectomies—breast biopsies followed immediately by radical surgery without the patient's knowledge or consent (Lerner 2001). Why trouble the little woman, they said, when I can just tell her husband what I am going to do? In the early 1980s women's groups succeeded in getting state legislation requiring informed consent and disclosure of alternatives for breast cancer treatments. The right to be heard and to be treated as full moral and political agents was not just a rallying cry; it was at the core of the women's movement.

In recalling his early days in promoting a patient-centered ethic as opposed to a physician-dominated ethic, Veatch says: "The arrogance of the medical professional claiming that he or she (mostly 'he') had the authority to decide, even against a patient's wishes, what was best for the patient was morally in-

defensible. Physicians were deciding not only that continued tortuous life support was in a dying person's best interest but that the physician's 'order' justified continued infliction of that torture. That ethic seemed so wrong, so contrary to any moral decency, that it was only natural to challenge it in the name of patients' rights" (Veatch 2002, 345).

Those who determined to provide some reflection on all these issues—the founders of bioethics—came largely from a religious or philosophical background or were philosophically inclined physicians or scientists. Among the physicians were Eric Cassell, Fritz Redlich, Robert Morison, and Robert F. Murray Jr. Scientists included Theodosius Dobzhansky, Rene Dubos, and Ernst Mayr. Among the most prominent nonscientists were Richard McCormick, a Jesuit priest; Warren Reich, a Catholic philosopher; K. Danner Clouser, the first philosopher to teach ethics in a medical school (Pennsylvania State University); and Sam Gorovitz, a philosopher at Case Western Reserve University. Prominent Protestant theologians involved in bioethics included William F. May of Southern Methodist University. James Gustafson of the University of Chicago. Ralph Potter of the Harvard Divinity School, Stanley Hauerwas, now at Duke University Divinity School, and Paul Ramsey of Princeton University, whose book *The Patient as Person* (1970) was a major statement of the primary goal of medicine. Joseph Fletcher, an Episcopalian priest turned atheist, taught at Harvard Divinity School and then at the University of Virginia; his 1954 book *Morals and Medicine,* and his 1966 work *Situation Ethics,* offered an approach in which rules were meant to be reviewed, not necessarily followed and in which decisions should be made on the basis of a Christian love.

In 1969 in Hastings-on-Hudson, New York, Daniel Callahan, a philosopher and former editor of the liberal Catholic journal *Commonweal,* and Willard Gaylin, a psychiatrist, formed the Institute of Society, Ethics, and the Life Sciences, later changed to the Hastings Center. Institutes, centers, and departments of medical ethics and medical humanities sprang up around the country soon after. The Kennedy Institute was a collection of scholars working and teaching more or less independently. The Hastings Center had a different model: it convened research groups from among its fellows (elected from scholars and others around the country) and led by a staff member. The Hastings Center chose the independent "think tank" model but only after considering and rejecting university affiliation (Callahan 1999). As a staff member and participant in Hastings Center meetings from 1975 to 1987, I can attest to their abstract nature and rarefied tenor during the early years, the absence of media interest, and the limited dissemination of the results, either through publication in the *Hastings Center Report* or another scholarly journal or book. The meetings were often stimulating and spirited but in the way that seminars can be stimulating and academic debates can be spirited. There wasn't a twenty-second sound bite to be heard. Nor can I recall more than a handful of conversations that escaped the bounds of civility.

The university-based model had certain advantages for the early bioethics ventures. Affiliation brought credibility, an administrative and financial home (although supporting funds had to be raised), academic appointments for scholars, and often access to medical schools and clinical services. On the other hand, university affiliations placed bioethics squarely in the academic world with all its "ivory tower" connotations, and subjected bioethics to the vagaries of university politics and policies. Medical centers connected with universities usually have their own administrations and priorities; integrating bioethics into a world controlled by physicians required the ability to get along in this environment, not always a comfortable position for a nonmedical outsider. Universities welcomed bioethics because they saw an opportunity to be in the forefront of a new wave of public interest and government funding.

Scholars had varying reasons to take this new career path but were influenced by a combination of the compelling and stimulating nature of the questions being discussed and dissatisfaction with the prevailing currents in disciplines such as philosophy. As Thomasma recalled, "ethics was not where the action was in philosophy . . . and applied philosophy was the lowest possible kind of philosophy in the hierarchy of the department" (Thomasma 2002, 339). In the title of a classic article, Stephen Toulmin, a British philosopher of science, put it bluntly: medicine saved ethics (1982).

Once scholars began to find new homes in universities, they began to do what scholars in any field do: they banded together, sought funding, found new outlets for their writing, convened conferences, and promoted their interests among students and administrators. New journals appeared linking medicine and ethics, such as the *Journal of Medicine and Philosophy, Theoretical Medicine and Bioethics,* and *Perspectives in Biology and Medicine.*

The Society for Health and Human Values (SHHV) was established by a collaboration of the Protestant and Methodist United Ministries in Education in 1970. The Society was funded by the National Endowment for the Humanities and the Russell Sage Foundation. Edmund Pellegrino, a physician, became the chairman of the Institute on Human Values in Medicine, which was focused on education in medical schools. After much deliberation about the advantages and disadvantages of having separate societies with similar missions, in January 1998 the SHHV merged with the American Society for Bioethics and the Society for Bioethics Consultation (SBC)

to form the American Society for Bioethics and Humanities (ASBH). The ASBH now has over fifteen hundred individual and institutional members. Future historians of bioethics organizations will find eleven linear feet of shelf space devoted to the archives of the SHHV at the University of Texas Medical Branch in Galveston.

If one were to list all the names of all the people who were involved in bioethics in these early years, the list would include at most seventy-five to one hundred people, nearly all with academic appointments in philosophy, theology, or medicine. When Al Jonsen convened a conference on "The Birth of Bioethics" in 1992, he limited the invitations to "pioneers"— those who had been named in the first edition of the *Bibliography of Bioethics* (1975) and continued to work in the field—a total of sixty people (Jonsen 1993). Only a few women (Karen Lebacqz of the Pacific Institute of Religion, Patricia King of Georgetown Law Center, Sissela Bok of Harvard, Ruth Macklin of Case Western Reserve University and then the Hastings Center, and Loretta Kopelman of East Carolina University) and a few lawyers (King, Harold Edgar of Columbia University, and Alexander Morgan Capron) were involved. Renee Fox of the University of Pennsylvania and Judith Swazey of Boston University represented the social sciences. Robert Murray, a medical geneticist at Howard University, and King were the only prominent African Americans, and other minority groups were not represented at all.

In their early years bioethics programs depended on the generosity of individuals (the Kennedys) or foundations (Rockefeller Foundation, Russell Sage Foundation, Ford Foundation, and others). Government support came from the National Library of Medicine and the National Endowment for the Humanities. There was little or no corporate support.

Several events brought bioethics out of the seminar room into the glare of politicians, the public, and the media. The first was a series of congressional hearings convened by Senator Walter Mondale, a fellow of the Hastings Center, in 1975 around issues of experimentation that resulted in the establishment of the National Commission for the Protection of Human Subjects of Biomedical and Behavioral Research and ultimately the system of institutional review boards (IRBs) that has oversight over federally funded research. Research scandals were the impetus for the National Commission—Beecher's 1966 article on unethical experimentation in the United States, the 1972 revelations about the forty-year history of the Tuskegee syphilis study, and concerns about fetal experimentation and prisoners as research subjects. The National Commission was the first of six (so far) national commissions under different names and sponsorships; it proved, according to Albert Dzur and Daniel Levin, that "bioethics and advisory commissions were made for each other" (2004, 334).

The second event to bring attention to bioethics was the case of Karen Ann Quinlan, a young New Jersey woman who in 1975 suffered irreversible brain damage and whose parents sought to have her ventilator removed. The 1976 decision in the legal case led to the creation of ethics committees in hospitals around the country to advise on end-of-life dilemmas and other controversies. Along with bioethics representation on IRBs to review research protocols, bioethicists were enlisted as members of these hospital or institutional ethics committees. Bioethics began to look less and less like the solitary pursuit of truth and justice and more like employment as the designated ethics hitter on a variety of clinical and policy teams.

Other events also played a role. As early as 1962 the public became aware of resource allocation issues when Shana Alexander, a journalist, published an article in *Life* magazine, then a leading source of America's news and public opinion, called "They Decide Who Lives, Who Dies." (The thirtieth anniversary of this publication was the occasion for Jonsen's "Birth of Bioethics" conference.) The subject was the deliberations of a Seattle hospital committee, which included non-physicians, charged with deciding which of the several candidates for the new and scarce kidney dialysis machines would get them. The use of "social worth" criteria by the "God Committee" became a flashpoint for controversy. When a person with end-stage kidney disease was dialyzed in the halls of Congress, legislators bowed to public opinion and created the federal End-Stage Renal Disease (ESRD) program under Medicare. They justified this exception for a single disease as an interim step before national health insurance was passed. When the ESRD program was begun in 1973, it served 10,000 people on dialysis; there are now more than 320,000 patients, and the number and the cost keep growing.

In 1984 the "Baby Doe" rules were promulgated to address the care and treatment of infants born with birth defects. This issue, raised by the specific case of an Indiana baby whose parents opted against surgery, on the advice of physicians, brought to the fore questions of parental rights, decision making on behalf of an incompetent person, and the role of concepts such as "best interests of the child." The first rules, based on section 504 of the Rehabilitation Act of 1973, were replaced in 1985 by rules based on amendments to the Child Abuse and Protection and Treatment Act. In order to receive federal funding, states must have in place procedures for reporting and addressing cases of withholding "medically indicated" treatment. Even now, these rules are controversial (Kopelman 2005).

The National Commission for the Protection of Human Subjects of Biomedical and Behavioral Research and the var-

ious commissions that followed brought what had been an academic or a clinically focused enterprise squarely into the public policy arena. The Quinlan case brought the kind of agonizing decision that had been largely unexamined and private into the open and into the media. The Seattle dialysis committee raised awareness of allocation issues. And the Baby Doe rules started a public discussion of the appropriate care of infants born with serious birth defects who would have died in earlier periods.

These shifts created the at times uneasy and ill-defined role of bioethics in public policy and clinical decision making. For all that bioethicists proclaim that they do not "make decisions" but only "lay out the options and the moral reasoning behind them," and only "advise" on public policy, there continue to be critics who assign ulterior motives or believe that bioethicists have no special expertise in determining what is ethical and what is not.

THE EARLIEST BIOETHICS ISSUES

In the early years, as bioethics was defining itself; it also got to choose its agenda, in contrast to the situation today, when to a large degree the bioethics agenda follows the news or policy makers' or corporate interests. Although some individuals have written extensively on important social and political questions in medicine, such as health care for the uninsured or disparities in health care based on race or ethnicity or the inadequacy of the acute care model of health care for an aging population, or firearm-related violence (Turner 2005), these problems have not been at the core of bioethics. On the other hand, other topics—stem cell research comes to mind—are almost obsessively pursued.

As already noted, one of the first issues to be raised on the new bioethics agenda was research ethics. This came about less as an echo of Nuremberg than as publicity about domestic scandals. Nevertheless, the Nazi experience was clearly a stimulus for Jay Katz, a psychiatrist who had lost family members in the Holocaust. In an apt description of the path of many at the time and even later, Katz says that he "wandered into bioethics" in the 1960s at Yale University's Law School. Recalling his first public lecture on human experimentation in 1965, he says that the senior physicians—his colleagues—in the audience were not pleased: "[They] told me afterwards, in polite but no uncertain *terms,* that the subject of human experimentation was not something to talk about and surely not in the way I had done it" (Katz 1994, 89). The cardinal sin that Katz had committed—less than two decades after the Nuremberg trials of Nazi doctors—was to suggest that there were complexities in the relationships between physician–investigators and patient–subjects and that disclosure of risks and obtaining of consent ought to be part of the research process.

The areas chosen by the Hastings Center as its focus were death and dying, genetics, reproductive biology and population issues, and behavior control (Callahan 1999, 60). All these issues (with the possible exception of population control) are still with us, albeit in different forms. Research on fetuses—one of the original stimuli for the creation of the National Commission—is governed by federal regulations; stem cell research has taken its place as one of the most divisive issues. In vitro fertilization, still thought of as science fiction in the 1960s, is now so commonplace that a whole industry has built up around strollers and other supplies for twin and triplet babies. Yet in 1978 the birth of Louise Brown, the first IVF baby, was a media sensation. Despite the U.S. Supreme Court decision in *Roe v. Wade* in 1973, legal abortion remains bitterly debated. Other permutations of reproductive technology—multiple births and births to older women, for example—are newer examples of the older debates about what is "natural" and to what extent medicine can or should control human reproduction.

When Willard Gaylin, co-founder of the Hastings Center, published a serious article with the tabloid title of "The Frankenstein Myth Becomes a Reality: We Have the Awful Knowledge to Make Exact Copies of Human Beings," cloning was still another science fiction theme (Gaylin 1972). While no one has yet cloned a human being, success in cloning animals (real, not fraudulent) has brought the possibility to the bioethics agenda, this time for real.

Some of the early debates on behavior control—psychosurgery, for example—have been resolved and that infamous procedure ceased to be performed. But others continue. The use of drugs to make children less hyperactive or to enhance athletic or academic performance are current issues with historical resonance. Of all the scientific advances, genetics is undoubtedly the one with the most dramatic implications. Early debates around genetics focused on screening—the possibility of stigmatizing or misleading populations such as African Americans by encouraging sickle cell screening, for example—employed techniques that, compared with knowledge about the human genome, seem primitive. Yet the basic question remains: What are the appropriate uses of genetic knowledge, especially given its uncertainties and implications for other aspects of a person's life? While early debates focused on detecting genes that cause disease, today's debates focus more on genetics to enhance human possibilities.

One of the Hastings Center's earliest research groups was devoted to "Death and Dying." That phrase, along with "terminal" illness, is now outmoded and bioethicists and others talk about end-of-life care. One of the earliest essays published in the *Hastings Center Report* (June 1971) was William F. May's "On Not Facing Death Alone: The Trauma of Dying Need Not Mean the Eclipse of the Human." Decades later, we are still trying to put that ideal into practice. Undoubtedly hospice and now palliative care have made a difference for some people, yet for many others death is still accompanied by unwanted and ineffective interventions, unrelieved pain and suffering, and a loss of personal dignity and autonomy. Advocates have moved from urging people to sign living wills to recommending advance directives and especially health care proxies, but no one has figured out a way to make people who do not want to think about death take that step and to ensure that those wishes are followed or, as the President's Council on Bioethics argues (2005), set aside on the grounds of the "authenticity of the person that is, not the person that was" (122). These legal documents are probably neither as flawed as critics would have it nor as fail-safe as proponents would like to believe.

International population control was on the agenda of the early bioethics movement, at least at the Hastings Center. Undoubtedly some of that interest came from the Rockefeller Foundation's own efforts to introduce family planning in developing countries, but the fear of explosive population growth was high all around, fueled in part by Paul Ehrlich's influential 1968 book *The Population Bomb*. The Hastings research group focused on ethical issues in governmental programs that encouraged sterilization in countries like India.

Apart from this issue, international dilemmas and public health concerns generally were not high on the early U.S. bioethics agenda. Today there is a much less parochial vision (Keenan 2005) and many contacts with colleagues in other countries. Some issues resonate more deeply with European colleagues, such as broad philosophical concepts such as the goals of medicine (Callahan 1999) or the ethics of genetically enhanced food. Asian and African societies still, for the most part, have desperate gaps in resources and coexisting Western and traditional medical systems. Many American bioethicists today urge the field to turn its attention to issues of fairness—what the rich and developed countries owe to the world's poorest people and to understanding cultural differences. By and large, however, bioethics in this country remains focused on domestic concerns, and often those that raise "interesting" but uncommon dilemmas. Even in the international context Western bioethics is still dominant. The IRB system has been established, with modifications, in all countries doing clinical research that will eventually be submitted to the Food and Drug Administration for approval.

In the 1970s and early 1980s infectious diseases were largely considered to have been controlled (except in far-off places like Africa). Medicine's successes had lulled its practitioners into complacency, and infectious diseases had never been high on the bioethics agenda. The advent of HIV/AIDS brought new and unsettling issues concerning the relationship between public health and personal liberties and the obligations of professionals to put themselves at risk by treating patients, as well as confronting their own beliefs about drug use and homosexuality. Now that effective pharmaceutical therapies are available in the United States, most but not all the bioethicists who continue to be interested in HIV/AIDS focus on the equitable allocation of antiretroviral drugs in Africa and Asia or on clinical trials in developing countries. Meanwhile, the epidemic continues at home, especially among young minority women and men. The ethical issues underlying prevention programs based on abstinence only, the pernicious role of stigma, or the power imbalance between men and women in "negotiating" safe sex are seldom discussed outside the public health world and rarely in ethics terms.

In addition to HIV/AIDS, the newest issues in bioethics concern terrorism and its threats to public health and individual liberties. The possible use of biological weapons and governmental efforts to combat terrorism have raised new questions for bioethics. Concern about medical participation in torture and interrogation of terror suspects in the Iraq war is an important related issue, one that goes to the heart of medical professional ethics. Although there is considerable continuity between the early days of bioethics and the present, the examples of HIV/AIDS and bioterrorism are reminders that the issues bioethics confronts can be new and urgent as well as old and familiar.

WHO SPEAKS FOR BIOETHICS AND IN WHAT LANGUAGE?

Even as bioethics was created as a new discipline in academia and medicine, some tensions were apparent at the outset. There was no department of bioethics to which interested people could apply for jobs or study. No one was a bioethicist; one's primary allegiance was to philosophy, medicine, nursing, theology, or law. As a consultant for the Institute on Human Values in Medicine, David Thomasma "was struck by how many philosophers were reluctant to 'leave' their own departments and disciplines and take up residency in a medical school or health sciences center" (Thomasma 2002, 335). Undoubtedly even fewer physicians were willing to leave the medical setting for a philosophy department. Veatch was probably the first person to choose the new field over his early academic training in pharmacology and his doctorate in ethics from the Harvard Divinity School to become the first staff person at the Institute of Society, Ethics, and the life Sciences, with the title of "Associate for Medical Ethics" (Veatch 2002, 347).

From the beginning there have been tensions between clinicians and nonclinicians. Clinicians sometimes felt that their intimate knowledge of medicine, the hospital setting, and patients (as opposed to persons) privileged their views. This was particularly apparent in the development of clinical ethics, which discussed individual cases at the bedside or close to it. Nonclinicians, for their part, saw themselves as "outsiders" and believed that their perspective was more objective and brought structure to the discussion of moral dilemmas rather than letting them play out in idiosyncratic ways. Some nonclinicians took so zealously to their "white coats" that they began to sound more like doctors than doctors, some of whom learned to like the language of ethics or at least the language of autonomy and beneficence.

As Callahan points out (1999, 64), "the relationship [of bioethics] with the social sciences has always been somewhat troubled." Some of this may stem, he suggests, from the perception among social scientists that they were being replaced by ethicists on medical faculties, and that bioethicists do not take seriously enough the rigorous methods and broad perspectives of social science. And it is true, he says, that some bioethicists believe that social science knowledge is not decisive for moral judgments (the "is" is not an "ought" argument). For their part, some social scientists have been fairly caustic about bioethics. Charles Bosk, one of the most astute social science observers of medical practice and a frequent writer on ethical issues, titled one of his articles "Professional Ethicist Available: Logical, Secular, Friendly" (1999). If anything, the tension between bioethics and social sciences has not only abated. it seems to have reversed. Bioethicists today are likely to be enamored of data, and social scientists often are eager to apply their skills to bioethics issues.

Another type of dissension arose between philosophers and theologians or specialists in religious studies. Philosophers. working from a secular tradition based on texts from Locke to Rawls, sought to find grounds to justify or prohibit actions based on reason and moral arguments. The result was an appeal to principles, most influentially codified by Beauchamp and Childress (2001), as "beneficence, respect for persons, and justice." "Principlism" has been criticized since the 1980s, and autonomy, the corollary of respect for persons, is now beaten down at every turn, although there does not seem to be a movement to restore absolute authority over medical decision making to physicians. The principles approach, however, remains an important part of the bioethics canon.

For the most part theologians, whatever their denomination, looked to religious authority and traditional values for answers to modern dilemmas. This discussion did not remain a binary division for long; soon other types of value systems were suggested to fill the gaps—virtue ethics, feminist ethics, nursing ethics, narrative ethics, casuistry, for example. The earlier division between philosophers and theologians has a new incarnation in the division between bioethics as seen from a religious and politically conservative perspective (as in the President's Council on Bioethics, originally led by Leon Kass) and the academic tradition, which has been more secular and politically liberal in its interpretations.

These variations reflect, according to Belkin and Brandt (2001, 6), "a seemingly timeless tension between rules and circumstance, between an attempt at moral deliberation that derives ethics from larger theory, rules, or basic principles, or one that builds moral conclusions or consensus through responding to the particular circumstances or moral intuitions that appear in the context of a given case." Belkin and Brandt suggest a "historical ethics," one that attends to "the histories and historical assumptions that make a particular view compelling" (6–7). A historical ethics can bring more voices to the question, focus more on the process of moral deliberation rather than just the "right" answer, and can shift from abstract terms and concepts to the way in which experiences and practices are established in culture. Belkin and Brandt say: "The power of bioethical formulations is in their resonance with experience, in their consistency with how attitudes toward suffering, expectations about medicine, customs of establishing desert and entitlement, get formed, cohere, and change" (8). In giving "one cheer for bioethics," Churchill and Schenck (2005, 390) point to the importance of attending to the "moral experience of patients and practitioners" who may be "morally wise" although not "ethically learned."

In the public commission realm, Dzur and Levin (2004) see a tension between the competing visions of these groups as either "agenda-setting" or providing expertise. Agenda-setters, they say, "want to spark, guide, and learn from public debate," while experts "want answers and solutions that they can communicate to the public" (334). Critics such as Cheryl Noble (1982) argue against the idea that bioethicists have some sort of moral expertise. "Moral problems," she says, "are everybody's business" (7). Reflecting on his experience as assistant director of the President's Commission on the Protection of Human Subjects of Biomedical and Behavioral Research, Alan Weisbard concluded that staff philosophers' methods and standards were "better suited to the halls of academe than the halls of Congress" (Weisbard 1987, 783), Dzur and Levin believe that "bioethicists serving on a commission or on the staff do not have to think the same way as the average American. Instead, their pressing task is to clarify the terms of the debate" (349). "Although inevitable, the distance between the formal, small group, expert discourse of commissions and informal, widespread, public discourse must be traversed energetically and creatively" (353).

The relationship between medical humanities and bioethics is another area in which different approaches exist. Perhaps some of the tension results from differing perceptions of the definition of "medical humanities" and its place in the curriculum. For those trained in literary theory and criticism, fiction and poetry about doctors and patients comprise the core of medical humanities. Those trained in philosophy, history, and anthropology, on the other hand, see their disciplines as medical humanities as well. These fields are perhaps more easily included under the "bioethics" rubric, which tends to see literature as enrichment rather than enlightenment.

Although there is much overlap, Howard Brody, a physician, says that "the tension between bioethical and literary goals seems unavoidable . . . in the question of ambiguity" (Brody 1991, 99). Ethics seeks to strip away layers of ambiguity to find a core that can be understood in terms of agreed-upon concepts and principles. Literature, on the other hand, revels in ambiguity. "Ethics, it seems, wants us to see face to face, while literature bids us peer through a glass, darkly." Nevertheless, Brody asserts that ethics and literature can be better meshed by getting beyond an overreliance on a single approach like principles and incorporating virtues and cases. Like Belkin and Brandt, Brody says that "ethical problems do not simply have a logic—they have a history; they have narrative meaning; and they occur within a social and cultural context" (109).

Yet another tension exists between what might be called, without intending any disparagement, "elitists" and "popularizers." In the early years bioethics was clearly a forum led by and for scholars and theorists whose primary audience was their colleagues. There were a few exceptions; Callahan, for example, had been an editor and he developed the *Hastings Center Report* as an interdisciplinary publication for interested citizens. The *Report*, however, was sometimes not the first choice for writers who preferred to be published in their own disciplinary journals. "Ordinary" people, for example, individuals who had experienced the dilemmas under discussion, were not typically invited to the bioethics table. Their perspective was deemed too idiosyncratic, too biased. If it did nothing else for bioethics, the advent of HIV/AIDS made it essential to bring affected individuals to bioethics discussions. No discussion of public health or prevention measures in the mid-1980s could be effective without understanding and attending to the views of advocates from the gay community. We now have "consumers" on almost every policy group.

With the growth of media interest, including TV, radio, and op-ed columns, many bioethicists believed that it was well within their mission to use these opportunities to explain the particular dilemma to the general public. This was easier to do in the early days when almost everyone could be a generalist of sorts; today, given the way some bioethicists have specialized and the way that the media do not distinguish one specialist from another, it is harder to accomplish. It is one thing for a TV producer on deadline to recognize that a story about a new cancer drug probably requires an oncologist to comment; it is quite another for that producer to know that the bioethicist-on-call has spent years mastering the facts and issues in genetics and has only a passing knowledge of the ethics of drug research.

Some bioethicists became quite adept at translating complex arguments into short and catchy statements; others disdain such efforts as trivializing and over-simplifying serious matters. While mass media undoubtedly bring these issues home in powerful ways, they also tend to focus on extreme views and treat all points of view as equally valid. The result is that the public gets a skewed view of a particular issue and bioethics as well. The nuanced view that bioethicists may bring to an issue, with a thoughtful discussion of various alternatives, is lost in the confrontational format. Without any other source of information, it is easy to see why people may consider a bioethicist just another opinionated talking head.

The media also create a pressure to come up with a quick response for the six o'clock news before all the facts of a particular case are known and before the thoughtful analysis that is supposed to characterize bioethics can take place. This was not so in the early years, when for the most part issues could be discussed for weeks or months before any public pronouncement was made. There is a certain headiness for academics when they are pursued by the media, but it is often followed by dismay at the result. The media's lack of appreciation of the way bioethicists analyze a dilemma and their search for the snappy comeback is balanced by bioethicists' general lack of understanding of how the media work and how to fine-tune an argument to fit the format.

A final source of tension, perhaps the one most at issue today, is the relationship between funding source and independent views. Even in the early years, proposals were often tailored to the interests of the funder, whether that was the government or a private foundation. However, the initial interest in the topic usually came from the institution or scholar seeking funding. not the other way around. And there were few instances of a funder seeking to direct the results. (They could, however, withhold their support for future projects.) Whether individuals selectively censored their own thinking to satisfy what they understood as funders' goals is another question. I did not see that happen, but it is certainly a possibility.

With the growth of corporate support and the use of bioethicists as consultants by pharmaceutical companies, managed care companies, and other large for-profit enterprises, the situation has changed. In these instances bioethicists are asked to give their advice or opinion on a specific matter, or series of issues of interest to the sponsor. That places them in a difficult position but not one that is automatically a conflict of interest. Nevertheless, bioethicists, says Elliott (2005, 382), risk becoming a "branch of the advice industry" or "window dressers" (Takala 2005). This issue will be covered in more detail in other chapters and is particularly important as career paths are increasingly oriented toward the corporate sector.

THE PERSISTENCE OF CHANGE

In the relatively short history of American bioethics, there is both continuity and change. Continuity pervades most of the basic issues that bioethics addresses: care at the end of life, genetics, reproduction, and research ethics. Some new issues have been added, such as HIV/AIDS (and the potential for other new infectious diseases), and bioterrorism. There are, to conclude, some issues that have always been present but have risen to new levels of urgency. Economics is the prime example. Very few of the early discussions specifically focused on money, although it was always in the background. Now it is often the first, and sometimes the only, issue raised in, for example, discussions of new technologies and allocation of health care resources. The "elephant in the living room" of course is the existence in the most expensive health care system in the world of 45 million people without health insurance.

The growth of international bioethics, and even media attention, are important ways to expand the reach of bioethics and at the same time incorporate a range of views. By extending its reach and its audience, however, bioethics has become more politicized, and it runs the risk of becoming just another shrill voice in the cacophony of public discourse, rather than a clear and objective voice of reason. This is no reason to withdraw from political debates but a caution about keeping one's role clear, expressing one's views in ordinary (but surely precise) language, and keeping the focus on the issue, not the personalities.

What lies ahead? On one hand, there will undoubtedly be more diversity in the people who choose bioethics as a professional field and more diversity of disciplines and views among bioethicists (Fox and Swazey 2005). This trend enriches the field. On the other hand, there may be even less basic agreement on what constitutes the field and how it should carry out its goals. As Stephen Toulmin pointed out, "The problems of medical ethics are like the contents of Pandora's box. Now they are out, it will be years before they are rounded up, labeled, and properly corralled" (1988, 15). It is worth remembering that the last spirit released from Pandora's Box was Hope, sent to heal the wounds inflicted by all the evil spirits of disease and sorrow imprisoned in the box. While the early bioethicists have begun the task of healing, it is up to current and future practitioners to continue it.

ACKNOWLEDGMENTS

I would like to thank Kathleen Powderly for advice on the structure and content of this chapter. I would also like to apologize to all those who contributed to the growth of bioethics but whose names are not mentioned. As a matter of justice, they should have been acknowledged; but expediency won out.

REFERENCES

Baker, R. 2005. Getting agreement: How bioethics got started. *Hastings Center Report* May–June:50–51.

Beauchamp, T. L., and Childress, J. F. 2001. *Principles of Biomedical Ethics.* 5th ed. (Originally published in 1979.) New York: Simon and Schuster.

Beecher, H. K. 1966. Ethics and clinical research. *New England Journal of Medicine* 274 (June 16):1354–60.

Belkin, G. S. 2003. Brain death and the historical understanding of bioethics. *Journal of the History of Medicine* 58(3):325–61.

Belkin, G, S., and Brandt, A. M. 2001. Bioethics: Using its historical and social context. *International Anesthesiology Clinics* 39(3):1–11.

Bosk, C. L. 1999. Professional bioethicist available: Logical, secular, friendly. *Daedalus* 128(4):47–68.

Brody, H. 1991. Literature and bioethics: Different approaches? *Literature and Medicine* 10:98–110.

Callahan, D. 1999. The Hastings Center and the early years of bioethics. *Kennedy Institute of Ethics Journal* 9(1): 53–71.

———. 2005. Bioethics and the culture wars. *Cambridge Quarterly of Healthcare Ethics* 14:424–31.

Churchill, L. R., and Schenck, D. 2005. One cheer for bioethics: Engaging the moral experiences of patients and practitioners beyond the big decisions. *Cambridge Quarterly of Healthcare Ethics* 14:389–403.

Dzur, A. W., and Levin, D. 2004. The "nation's conscience": Assessing bioethics commissions as public forums. *Kennedy Institute of Ethics Journal* 14(4):333–60.

Elliott, C. 2005. The soul of a new machine: Bioethicists in the bureaucracy. *Cambridge Quarterly of Healthcare Ethics* 14:379–84.

Engelhardt. H. T, Jr. 1996. The *Foundations of Bioethics.* 2nd ed. (Originally published in 1986.) New York: Oxford University Press.

Evans. J. H. 2002. *Playing God? Human Genetic Engineering and the Rationalization of Public Bioethical Debate.* Chicago: University of Chicago Press.

Fox, R. C., and Swazey, J. P. 2005. Examining American bioethics: Its problems and prospects. *Cambridge Quarterly of Healthcare Ethics* 14:361–73.

Gaylin, W. 1972. The Frankenstein myth becomes a reality: We have the awful knowledge to make exact copies of human beings. *New York Times Magazine.* March 5:12–13 ff.

Hanauske-Abel, H. M. 1996. Not a slippery slope or sudden subversion: German medicine and National Socialism in 1933. *British Medical Journal* 313(7070):1453–63.

Jonas, H. 1984. The *Imperative of Responsibility: In Search of an Ethics for the Technological Age.* Chicago: University of Chicago Press. (Originally published in German in 1979.)

Jonsen, A. R., ed. 1993. The birth of bioethics. Special Supplement, *Hastings Center Report* 23(6):S1–S15.

———. 1998. *The Birth of Bioethics.* New York: Oxford University Press.

———. 2000. *A Short History of Medical Ethics.* New York: Oxford University Press.

Katz, J. 1994. Reflections on unethical experiments and the beginnings of bioethics in the United States. *Kennedy Institute of Ethics Journal* 4(2):85–92.

Keenan, J. F. 2005. Developments in bioethics from the perspective of HIV/AIDS. *Cambridge Quarterly of Healthcare Ethics* 14:416–23.

Kevles, D. 2000. The historical contingency of bioethics. The *Princeton Journal of Bioethics* 3(1):51–58.

Kopelman, L. 2005. Are the 21-year-old Baby Doe rules misunderstood or mistaken? *Pediatrics* 115:797–802.

Leopold, A. R. 1949. *A Sand County Almanac.* Reissued 1986. New York: Random House.

Lerner, B. H. 2001. *The Breast Cancer Wars: Hope, Fear, and the Pursuit of a Cure in Twentieth-Century America.* New York: Oxford University Press.

Martensen, R. 2001. The history of bioethics: An essay review. *Journal of the History of Medicine* 56(2):168–75.

May, W. F. 1971. On not facing death alone: The trauma of dying need not mean the eclipse of the human. *Hastings Center Report* 1:6–7.

Moreno. J. 2004. Bioethics imperialism. *ASBH Exchange.* Fall: 2.

Noble, C. 1982. Ethics and experts. *Hastings Center Report* 12(3):7–9.

Potter, V. R. 1970. Bioethics: The science of survival. *Perspectives in Biology and Medicine* 14:127–53.

———. 1971. *Bioethics: A Bridge to the Future.* Englewood Cliffs, NJ: Prentice Hall.

———. 1998. *Global Bioethics: Building on the Leopold Legacy.* East Lansing: Michigan State University Press.

Potter, V. R., and Whitehouse, P. J. 1998. Deep and global bioethics for a livable third millennium. *The Scientist* 12.1 (January 5). www.the-scientist.com/yr1998/jan/opin_980105.html.

President's Council on Bioethics. 2005. *Taking Care: Ethical Caregiving in Our Aging Society.* Washington. DC. Available at www.bioethics.gov.

Ramsey, P. 1970. *The Patient as Person.* New Haven: Yale University Press.

Reich, W. T. 1994. The word "bioethics": Its birth and the legacies who shaped it. *Kennedy Institute of Ethics Journal* 4(4):319–55.

———. 1995. The word "bioethics": The struggle over its earliest meaning. *Kennedy Institute of Ethics Journal* 5(1): 19–34.

Rothman. D. 1992. *Strangers at the Bedside: A History of How Law and Bioethics Transformed Medical Decision Making.* New York: Basic Books.

Sass, H. M. 1983. *Reichsrundschreiben* 1931: Pre-Nuremberg German regulations concerning new therapy and human experimentation. *Journal of Medicine and Philosophy* 8:99–111.

Short, B. W. 2003. History "lite" in modern American bioethics. *Issues in Law and Medicine* 19(1):45–76.

Smith. W. J. 2002. *Culture of Death: The Assault on Medical Ethics in America.* San Francisco: Encounter Books.

Stevens, M. L. T. 2000. *Bioethics in America: Origins and Cultural Politics.* Baltimore: Johns Hopkins University Press.

Takala, T. 2005. Demagogues, firefighters, and window dressers; Who are we and what should we be? *Cambridge Quarterly of Healthcare Ethics* 14:385–88.

Thomasma, D. C. 2002. Early bioethics. *Cambridge Quarterly of Healthcare Ethics* 11:335–43.

Toulmin, S. 1982. How medicine saved the life of ethics. *Perspectives in Biology and Medicine* 25(4):736–50.

———. 1988. Medical ethics in its American context: An historical survey. *Annals of the New York Academy of Sciences* 530:7–15.

Turner, L. 2005. Bioethics, social class, and the sociological imagination. *Cambridge Quarterly of Healthcare Ethics* 14:374–78.

Veatch, R. M. 2002. The birth of bioethics: Autobiographical reflections of a patient person. *Cambridge Quarterly of Healthcare Ethics* 11:344–52.

Walter, J. K., and Klein, E. P., eds. 2003. *The Story of Bioethics: From Seminal Works to Contemporary Exploration.* Washington, DC: Georgetown University Press.

Weisbard, A. J. 1987. The role of philosophers in the public policy process: A view from the President's Commission. *Ethics* 97(4):776–85.

Whitehouse. P. 2003. The rebirth of bioethics: Extending the original formulations of Van Rensselaer Potter. *American Journal of Bioethics* 3(4): W26–W31.

Public Health Ethics: Mapping the Terrain

James F. Childress, Ruth R. Faden, Ruth D. Gaare, Lawrence O. Gostin, Jeffrey Kahn,
Richard J. Bonnie, Nancy E. Kass, Anna C. Mastroianni, Jonathan D. Moreno, and Phillip Nieburg

Source: Courtesy of the Jornal of Law, Medicine, and Ethics.
Public Health Ethics: Mapping the Terrain. James F. Childress,
Ruth R. Faden, Ruth D. Gaare, Lawrence O. Gostin, Jeffrey
Kahn, Richard J. Bonnie, Nancy E. Kass, Anna C. Mastroianni,
Jonathan D. Moreno, and Phillip Nieburg. *Journal of Law,*
Medicine & Ethics, 30 (2002):170–178.

Public health ethics, like the field of public health it addresses, traditionally has focused more on practice and particular cases than on theory, with the result that some concepts, methods, and boundaries remain largely undefined. This paper attempts to provide a rough conceptual map of the terrain of public health ethics. We begin by briefly defining public health and identifying general features of the field that are particularly relevant for a discussion of public health ethics.

Public health is primarily concerned with the health of the entire population, rather than the health of individuals. Its features include an emphasis on the promotion of health and the prevention of disease and disability; the collection and use of epidemiological data, population surveillance, and other forms of empirical quantitative assessment; a recognition of the multidimensional nature of the determinants of health; and a focus on the complex interactions of many factors—biological, behavioral, social, and environmental—in developing effective interventions.

How can we distinguish public health from medicine? While medicine focuses on the treatment and cure of individual patients, public health aims to understand and ameliorate the causes of disease and disability in a population. In addition, whereas the physician–patient relationship is at the center of medicine, public health involves interactions and relationships among many professionals and members of the community as well as agencies of government in the development, implementation, and assessment of interventions. From this starting point, we can suggest that public health systems consist of all the people and actions, including laws, policies, practices, and activities, that have the primary purpose of protecting and improving the health of the public.[1] While we need not assume that public health systems are tightly structured or centrally directed, we recognize that they include a wide range of governmental, private and non-profit organizations, as well as professionals from many disciplines, all of which (alone and together) have a stake in and an effect on a community's health. Government has a unique role in public health because of its responsibility, grounded in its police powers, to protect the public's health and welfare, because it alone can undertake certain interventions, such as regulation, taxation, and the expenditure of public funds, and because many, perhaps most, public health programs are public goods that cannot be optimally provided if left to individuals or small groups.

The Institute of Medicine's landmark 1988 definition of public health provides additional insight: "Public health is what we, as a society, do collectively to assure the conditions in which people can be healthy."[2] The words "what we, as a society, do collectively" suggest the need for cooperative behavior and relationships built on overlapping values and trust. The words "to assure the conditions in which people can be healthy" suggest a far-reaching agenda for public health that focuses attention not only on the medical needs of individuals, but on fundamental social conditions that affect population levels of morbidity and mortality. From an ethical standpoint, public health activities are generally understood to be teleological (end-oriented) and consequentialist—the health of the public is the primary end that is sought and the primary outcome for measuring success.[3] Defining and measuring "health" is not easy, as we will emphasize below, but, in addition, "public" is a complex concept with at least three dimensions that are important for our discussion of ethics.

First, public can be used to mean the "numerical public," i.e., the target population. In view of public health's goal of producing net health benefits for the population, this meaning of public is very important. In measurement and analysis, the "numerical public" reflects the utilitarian view that each individual counts as one and only one. In this context, ethical analysis focuses on issues in measurement, many of which raise considerations of justice. For example, how should we define a population, how should we compare gains in life expectancy with gains in health-related quality of life, and whose values should be used in making those judgments?

Second, public is what we collectively do through government and public agency—we can call this "political public." Government provides much of the funding for a vast array of public health functions, and public health professionals in governmental roles are the focal point of much collective activity. In the United States, as Lawrence Gostin notes, government "is compelled by its role as the elected representative of the community to act affirmatively to promote the health of the people," even though it "cannot unduly invade individuals' rights in the name of the communal good."[4] The government is a central player in public health because of the collective responsibility it must assume and implement. The state's use of its police powers for public health raises important ethical questions, particularly about the justification and limits of governmental coercion and about its duty to treat all citizens equally in exercising these powers. In a liberal, pluralistic democracy, the justification of coercive policies, as well as other policies, must rest on moral reasons that the public in whose name the policies are carried out could reasonably be expected to accept.[5]

Third, public, defined as what we do collectively in a broad sense, includes all forms of social and community action affecting public health—we can call this "communal public." Ethical analysis on this level extends beyond the political public. People collectively, outside of government and with private funds, often have greater freedom to undertake public health interventions since they do not have to justify their actions to the political public. However, their actions are still subject to various moral requirements, including, for instance, respect for individual autonomy, liberty, privacy and confidentiality, and transparency in disclosure of conflicts of interest.

GENERAL MORAL CONSIDERATIONS

In providing a map of the terrain of public health ethics, we do not suggest that there is a consensus about the methods and content of public health ethics.[6] Controversies persist about theory and method in other areas of applied or practical ethics, and it should not be surprising that variety also prevails in public health ethics.[7] The terrain of public health ethics includes a loose set of general moral considerations—clusters of moral concepts and norms that are variously called values, principles, or rules—that are arguably relevant to public health. Public health ethics, in part, involves ongoing efforts to specify and to assign weights to these general moral considerations in the context of particular policies, practices, and actions, in order to provide concrete moral guidance.

Recognizing general moral considerations in public health ethics does not entail a commitment to any particular theory or method. What we describe and propose is compatible with several approaches. To take one major example, casuistical reasoning (examining the relevant similarities and differences between cases) is not only compatible with, but indispensable to our conception of public health ethics. Not only do—or should—public health agents examine new situations they confront in light of general moral considerations, but they should also focus on a new situation's relevant similarities to and differences from paradigm or precedent cases—cases that have gained a relatively settled moral consensus. Whether a relatively settled moral consensus is articulated first in a general moral consideration or in precedent cases does not constitute a fundamental issue—both are relevant. Furthermore, some of the precedents may concern how general moral considerations are interpreted, specified, and balanced in some public health activity, especially where conflicts emerge.

Conceptions of morality usually recognize a formal requirement of universalizability in addition to a substantive requirement of attention to human welfare. Whatever language is used, this formal feature requires that we treat similar cases in a similar way. This requirement undergirds casuistical reasoning in morality as well as in law. In public health ethics, for example, any recommendations for an HIV screening policy must take into account both past precedents in screening for other infectious diseases and the precedents the new policy will create for, say, screening for genetic conditions. Much of the moral argument will hinge on which similarities and differences between cases are morally relevant, and that argument will often, though not always, appeal to general moral considerations.[8] We can establish the relevance of a set of these considerations in part by looking at the kinds of moral appeals that public health agents make in deliberating about and justifying their actions as well as at debates about moral issues in public health. The relevant general moral considerations include:

- Producing benefits;
- avoiding, preventing, and removing harms;
- producing the maximal balance of benefits over harms and other costs (often called utility);
- distributing benefits and burdens fairly (distributive justice) and ensuring public participation, including the participation of affected parties (procedural justice);
- respecting autonomous choices and actions, including liberty of action;
- protecting privacy and confidentiality;
- keeping promises and commitments;
- disclosing information as well as speaking honestly and truthfully (often grouped under transparency); and
- building and maintaining trust.

Several of these general moral considerations—especially benefiting others, preventing and removing harms, and utility—provide a *prima facie* warrant for many activities in pursuit of the goal of public health. It is sufficient for our purposes to note that public health activities have their grounding in general moral considerations, and that public health identifies one major broad benefit that societies and governments ought to pursue. The relation of public health to the whole set of general moral considerations is complex. Some general moral considerations support this pursuit; institutionalizing several others may be a condition for or means to public health (we address this point later when we discuss human rights and public health); and yet, in particular cases, some of the same general moral considerations may limit or constrain what may be done in pursuit of public health. Hence, conflicts may occur among these general moral considerations.

The content of these various general moral considerations can be divided and arranged in several ways—for instance, some theories may locate one or more of these concepts under others. But, whatever theory one embraces, the whole set of general moral considerations roughly captures the moral content of public health ethics. It then becomes necessary to address several practical questions. First, how can we make these general moral considerations more specific and concrete in order to guide action? Second, how can we resolve conflicts among them? Some of the conflicts will concern how much weight and significance to assign to the ends and effects of protecting and promoting public health relative to the other considerations that limit and constrain ways to pursue such outcomes. While each general moral consideration may limit and constrain public health activities in some circumstances;

for our purposes, justice or fairness, respect for autonomy and liberty, and privacy and confidentiality are particularly noteworthy in this regard.

Specifying and Weighting General Moral Considerations

We do not present a universal public health ethic. Although arguably these general moral considerations find support in various societies and cultures, an analysis of the role of cultural context in public health ethics is beyond the scope of this paper. Instead, we focus here on public health ethics in the particular setting of the United States, with its traditions, practices, and legal and constitutional requirements, all of which set directions for and circumscribe public health ethics. (Below we will indicate how this conception of public health ethics relates to human rights.)

General moral considerations have two major dimensions. One is their meaning and range or scope; the other is their weight or strength. The first determines the extent of conflict among them—if their range or scope is interpreted in certain ways, conflicts may be increased or reduced. The second dimension determines when different considerations yield to others in cases of conflict.

Specifying the meaning and range or scope of general moral considerations—the first dimension—provides increasingly concrete guidance in public health ethics. A common example is specifying respect for autonomy by rules of voluntary, informed consent. However, it would be a mistake to suppose that respect for autonomy requires consent in all contexts of public health or to assume that consent alone sufficiently specifies the duty to respect autonomy in public health settings. Indeed, specifying the meaning and scope of general moral considerations entails difficult moral work. Nowhere is this more evident in public health ethics than with regard to considerations of justice. Explicating the demands of justice in allocating public health resources and in setting priorities for public health policies, or in determining whom they should target, remains among the most daunting challenges in public health ethics.

The various general moral considerations are not absolute. Each may conflict with another and each may have to yield in some circumstances. At most, then, these general moral considerations identify features of actions, practices, and policies that make them *prima facie* or presumptively right or wrong, i.e., right or wrong, all other things being equal. But since any particular action, practice, or policy for the public's health may also have features that infringe one or more of these general moral considerations, it will be necessary to determine which of them has priority. Some argue for a lexical or serial ordering, in which one general moral consideration, while not generally absolute, has priority over another. For instance, one theory might hold that protecting or promoting public health always has priority over privacy, while another might hold that individual liberty always has priority over protecting or promoting public health. Neither of these priority rules is plausible, and any priority rule that is plausible will probably involve tight or narrow specifications of the relevant general moral considerations to reduce conflicts. From our standpoint, it is better to recognize the need to balance general moral considerations in particular circumstances when conflicts arise. We cannot determine their weights in advance, only in particular contexts that may affect their weights—for instance, promises may not have the same moral weights in different contexts.

Resolving Conflicts Among General Moral Considerations

We do not believe it is possible to develop an algorithm to resolve all conflicts among general moral considerations. Such conflicts can arise in multiple ways. For example, it is common in public health practice and policy for conflicts to emerge between privacy and justice (for instance, the state collects and records private information in disease registries about individuals in order to allocate and provide access to resources for appropriate prevention and treatment services), or between different conceptions of justice (for instance, a government with a finite public health budget must decide whether to dedicate resources to vaccination or to treatment of conditions when they arise). In this paper, however, we focus on one particular permutation of conflicts among general moral considerations that has received the most attention in commentary and in law. This is the conflict between the general moral considerations that are generally taken to instantiate the goal of public health—producing benefits, preventing harms, and maximizing utility—and those that express other moral commitments. For conflicts that assume this structure, we propose five "justificatory conditions": effectiveness, proportionality, necessity, least infringement, and public justification. These conditions are intended to help determine whether promoting public health warrants overriding such values as individual liberty or justice in particular cases.

Effectiveness

It is essential to show that infringing one or more general moral considerations will probably protect public health. For instance, a policy that infringes one or more general moral considerations in the name of public health but has little chance of realizing its goal is ethically unjustified.

Proportionality

It is essential to show that the probable public health benefits outweigh the infringed general moral considerations—this condition is sometimes called proportionality. For instance, the policy may breach autonomy or privacy and have undesirable consequences. All of the positive features and benefits must be balanced against the negative features and effects.

Necessity

Not all effective and proportionate policies are necessary to realize the public health goal that is sought. The fact that a policy will infringe a general moral consideration provides a strong moral reason to seek an alternative strategy that is less morally troubling. This is the logic of a *prima facie* or presumptive general moral consideration. For instance, all other things being equal, a policy that provides incentives for persons with tuberculosis to complete their treatment until cured will have priority over a policy that forcibly detains such persons in order to ensure the completion of treatment. Proponents of the forcible strategy have the burden of moral proof. This means that the proponents must have a good faith belief, for which they can give supportable reasons, that a coercive approach is necessary. In many contexts, this condition does not require that proponents provide empirical evidence by actually trying the alternative measures and demonstrating their failure.[9]

Least Infringement

Even when a proposed policy satisfies the first three justificatory conditions—that is, it is effective, proportionate, and essential in realizing the goal of public health—public health agents should seek to minimize the infringement of general moral considerations. For instance, when a policy infringes autonomy, public health agents should seek the least restrictive alternative; when it infringes privacy, they should seek the least intrusive alternative; and when it infringes confidentiality, they should disclose only the amount and kind of information needed, and only to those necessary, to realize the goal.[10] The justificatory condition of least infringement could plausibly be interpreted as a corollary of necessity—for instance, a proposed coercive measure must be necessary in degree as well as in kind.

Public Justification

When public health agents believe that one of their actions, practices, or policies infringes one or more general moral considerations, they also have a responsibility, in our judgment, to explain and justify that infringement, whenever possible, to the relevant parties, including those affected by the infringement. In the context of what we called "political public," public health agents should offer public justification for policies in terms that fit the overall social contract in a liberal, pluralistic democracy. This transparency stems in part from the requirement to treat citizens as equals and with respect by offering moral reasons, which in principle they could find acceptable, for policies that infringe general moral considerations. Transparency is also essential to creating and maintaining public trust; and it is crucial to establishing accountability. (Below we elaborate a process-oriented approach to public accountability that goes beyond public justification to include, as an expression of justice and fairness, input from the relevant affected parties in the formulation of policy.)

Screening Program Example

An extended example may illustrate how these moral justificatory conditions function in public health ethics. Let us suppose that public health agents are considering whether to implement a screening program for HIV infection, tuberculosis, another infectious or contagious disease, or a genetic condition (see Table 13-1 for some morally relevant features of screening programs).

The relevant justificatory conditions will require public health agents to consider whether any proposed program will be likely to realize the public health goal that is sought (effectiveness), whether its probable benefits will outweigh the infringed general moral considerations (proportionality), whether the policy is essential to realize the end (necessity), whether it involves the least infringement possible consistent with realizing the goal that is sought (least infringement), and whether it can be publicly justified. These conditions will give priority to selective programs over universal ones if the selective programs will realize the goal (as we note below, questions may arise about universality within selected categories, such as pregnant women), and to voluntary programs over mandatory ones if the voluntary programs will realize the goal.[11]

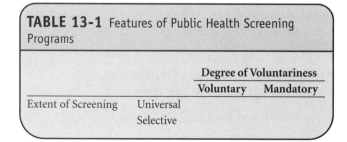

TABLE 13-1 Features of Public Health Screening Programs

		Degree of Voluntariness	
		Voluntary	Mandatory
Extent of Screening	Universal		
	Selective		

Different screening programs may fail close scrutiny in light of one or more of these conditions. For instance, neither mandatory nor voluntary universal screening for HIV infection can meet these conditions in the society as a whole. Some voluntary and some mandatory selective screening programs for HIV infection can be justified, while others cannot. Mandatory screening of donated blood, organs, sperm, and ova is easily justified, and screening of individuals may also be justified in some settings where they can expose others to bodily fluids and potential victims cannot protect themselves. The question of whether and under what conditions screening of pregnant women for HIV infection should be instituted has been particularly controversial. Even before the advent of effective treatment for HIV infection and the identification of zidovudine (AZT) as effective in reducing the rate of perinatal transmission, there were calls for mandatory screening of pregnant women, especially in "high risk" communities. These calls were defeated by sound arguments that such policies entailed unjustifiable violations of autonomy, privacy, and justice.[12] In effect, the recommended policies failed to satisfy any of the justificatory conditions we have proposed here.

However, once it was established that zidovudine could interrupt maternal-fetal transmission of HIV, the weight of the argument shifted in the direction of instituting screening programs of some type. The focus of the debate became the tensions between the public health interests in utility and efficiency, which argued for mandatory, selective screening in high-risk communities, and considerations of liberty, privacy, and justice, which argued for voluntary, universal screening.[13]

In many situations, the most defensible public health policy for screening and testing *expresses* community rather than *imposes* it. Imposing community involves mandating or compelling testing through coercive measures. By contrast, expressing community involves taking steps to express solidarity with individuals, to protect their interests, and to gain their trust. Expressing community may include, for example, providing communal support, disclosing adequate information, protecting privacy and confidentiality, and encouraging certain choices. This approach seeks to make testing a reasonable, and perhaps moral, choice for individuals, especially by engendering public trust, rather than making it compulsory. Several diseases that might be subjected to screening for public health reasons involve stigma, and breaches of privacy and confidentiality may put individuals' employment and insurance at risk. Expressing community is often an appropriate strategy for public health, and, *ceteris paribus,* it has priority over imposing community through coercive policies.

PROCESSES OF PUBLIC ACCOUNTABILITY

Our discussion of the fifth justificatory condition—public justification—focused on providing public reasons for policies that infringe general moral considerations; this condition is particularly applicable in the political context. While public accountability includes public justification, it is broader—it is prospective as well as retrospective. It involves soliciting input from the relevant publics (the numerical, political, and communal publics) in the process of formulating public health policies, practices, and actions, as well as justifying to the relevant publics what is being undertaken. This is especially, but not only, important when one of the other *prima facie* general moral considerations is infringed, as with coercive protective measures to prevent epidemics. At a minimum, public accountability involves transparency in openly seeking information from those affected and in honestly disclosing relevant information to the public; it is indispensable for engendering and sustaining public trust, as well as for expressing justice.[14]

Public accountability regarding health promotion or priority-setting for public health funding additionally might involve a more developed fair process. Noting that in a pluralistic society we are likely to find disagreement about which principles should govern issues such as priority-setting in health care, Norman Daniels calls for a fair process that includes the following elements: transparency and publicity about the reasons for a decision; appeals to rationales and evidence that fair-minded patties would agree are relevant; and procedures for appealing and revising decisions in light of challenges by various stakeholders. He explains why this process can facilitate social learning: "Since we may not be able to construct principles that yield fair decisions ahead of time, we need a process that allows us to develop those reasons over time as we face real cases."[15]

Public accountability also involves acknowledging the more complex relationship between public health and the public, one that addresses fundamental issues such as those involving characterization of risk and scientific uncertainty. Because public health depends for its success on the satisfaction of deeply personal health goals of individuals and groups in the population, concepts such as "health" and "risk" cannot be understood or acted upon on the basis of *a priori*, formal definitions or scientific analysis. Public accountability recognizes that the fundamental conceptualization of these terms is a critical part of the basic formulation of public health goals and problems to be addressed. This means that the public, along with scientific experts, plays an important role in the *analysis* of public health issues, as well as in the development and assessment of appropriate *strategies* for addressing them.

Risk characterization provides a helpful example. A National Research Council report, *Understanding Risk: Informing Decisions in a Democratic Society*, concluded that risk characterization is not properly understood if defined only as a summary of scientific information; rather, it is the outcome of a complex analytic-deliberative process—"a decision-driven activity, directed toward informing choices and solving problems."[16] The report explains that scientific analysis, which uses rigorous, replicable methods, brings new information into the process, and that deliberation helps to frame analysis by posing new questions and new ways of formulating problems, with the result that risk characterization is the output of a recursive process, not a linear one, and is a decision-driven activity.

Assessment of the health risks of dioxin illustrates this process. While scientific analysis provides information about the dose-response relationship between dioxin exposure and possible human health effects, public health focuses on the placement of waste incinerators and community issues in which dioxin is only one of many hazardous chemicals involved and cancer only one of many outcomes of concern. The critical point is that good risk characterization results from a process that "not only gets the science right," but also "gets the right science."[17]

Public health accountability addresses the responsibility of public health agents to work with the public and scientific experts to identify, define, and understand at a fundamental level the threats to public health, and the risks and benefits of ways to address them. The appropriate level of public involvement in the analytic-deliberative process depends on the particular public health problem.

Public accountability requires an openness to public deliberation and imposes an obligation on decision-makers to provide honest information and justifications for their decisions. No ethical principle can eliminate the fact that individual interests must sometimes yield to collective needs. Public accountability, however, ensures that such trade-offs will be made openly, with an explicit acknowledgment that individuals' fundamental well-being and values are at stake and that reasons, grounded in ethics, will be provided to those affected by the decisions.[18] It provides a basis for public trust, even when policies infringe or appear to infringe some general moral considerations.

PUBLIC HEALTH INTERVENTIONS VS. PATERNALISTIC INTERVENTIONS

An important empirical, conceptual, and normative issue in public health ethics is the relationship between protecting and promoting the health of individuals and protecting and promoting public health. Although public health is directed to the health of populations, the indices of population health, of course, include an aggregation of the health of individuals. But suppose the primary reason for some restrictions on the liberties of individuals is to prevent harm to those whose actions are substantially voluntary and do not affect others adversely. The ethical question then is, when can paternalistic interventions (defined as interventions designed to protect or benefit individuals themselves against their express wishes) be ethically justified if they infringe general moral considerations such as respect for autonomy, including liberty of action?

Consider the chart in Table 13-2: An individual's actions may be substantially voluntary (competent, adequately informed, and free of controlling influences) or non-voluntary (incompetent, inadequately informed, or subject to controlling influences). In addition, those actions may be self-regarding (the adverse effects of the actions fall primarily on the individual himself or herself) or other-regarding (the adverse effects of the actions fall primarily on others).

Paternalism in a morally interesting and problematic sense arises in the first quadrant (marked by the number "1" in Table 13-2)—where the individual's actions are both voluntary and self-regarding. According to John Stuart Mill, whose *On Liberty* has inspired this chart, other-regarding conduct not only affects others adversely, but also affects them directly and without "their free, voluntary, and undeceived consent and participation."[19] If others, in the maturity of their faculties, consent to an agent's imposition of risk, then the agent's actions are not other-regarding in Mill's sense.

Whether an agent's other-regarding conduct is voluntary or non-voluntary, the society may justifiably intervene in various ways, including the use of coercion, to reduce or prevent the imposition of serious risk on others. Societal intervention in non-voluntary self-regarding conduct is considered weak (or soft) paternalism, if it is paternalistic at all, and it is easily justified. By contrast, societal interference in voluntary self-regarding conduct would be strong (or hard) paternalism.

Coercive intervention in the name of strong paternalism would be insulting and disrespectful to individuals because it would override their voluntary actions for their own benefit, even though their actions do not harm others. Such interventions are thus very difficult to justify in a liberal, pluralistic democracy.

Because of this difficulty, proponents of public health sometimes contend that the first quadrant is really a small class of cases because individuals' risky actions are, in most cases, other-regarding or non-voluntary, or both. Thus, they insist, even if we assume that strong or hard paternalism cannot be ethically justified, the real question is whether most public health interventions in personal life plans and risk budgets are paternalistic at all, at least in the morally problematic sense.

To a great extent, the question is where we draw the boundaries of the self and its actions; that is, whether various influences on agents so determine their actions that they are not voluntary, and whether the adverse effects of those actions extend beyond the agents themselves. Such boundary drawing involves empirical, conceptual, and normative questions that demand attention in public health ethics. On the one hand, it is not sufficient to show that social-cultural factors influence an individual's actions; it is necessary to show that those influences render that individual's actions substantially non-voluntary and warrant societal interventions to protect him or her. Controversies about the strong influence of food marketing on diet and weight (and, as a result, on the risk of disease and death) illustrate the debates about this condition.

On the other hand, it is not sufficient to show that an individual's actions have some adverse effects on others; it is necessary to show that those adverse effects on others are significant enough to warrant overriding the individual's liberty. Controversies about whether the state should require motorcyclists to wear helmets illustrate the debates about this condition. These controversies also show how the inclusion of the financial costs to society and the emotional costs to, say, observers and rescue squads can appear to make virtually any intervention non-paternalistic. But even if these adverse financial and emotional effects on others are morally relevant as a matter of social utility, it would still be necessary to show that they are significant enough to justify the intervention.

Either kind of attempt to reduce the sphere of autonomous, self-regarding actions, in order to warrant interventions in the name of public health, or, more broadly, social utility, can sometimes be justified, but either attempt must be subjected to careful scrutiny. Sometimes both may represent rationalization and bad faith as public health agents seek to evade the stringent demands of the general moral consideration of respect for autonomy. Requiring consistency across an

TABLE 13-2 Two Models of Stigma

		Adverse Effects of Individuals' Actions	
		Self-Regarding	Other-Regarding
Voluntariness of Individuals' Actions	Voluntary	1	2
	Non-voluntary	3	4

array of cases may provide a safeguard against rationalization and bad faith, particularly when motives for intervention may be mixed.

Much of this debate reflects different views about whether and when strong paternalistic interventions can be ethically justified. In view of the justificatory conditions identified earlier, relevant factors will include the nature of the intervention, the degree to which it infringes an individual's fundamental values, the magnitude of the risk to the individual apart from the intervention (either in terms of harm or lost benefit), and so forth. For example, even though the authors of this paper would disagree about some cases, we agree that strong paternalistic interventions that do not threaten individuals' core values and that will probably protect them against serious risks are more easily justifiable than strong paternalistic interventions that threaten individuals' core values and that will reduce only minor risks. Of course, evaluating actual and proposed policies that infringe general moral considerations becomes very complicated when both paternalistic and public health reasons exist for, and are intertwined in, those policies.

SOCIAL JUSTICE, HUMAN RIGHTS, AND HEALTH

We have noted potential and actual conflicts between promoting the good of public health and other general moral considerations. But it is important not to exaggerate these conflicts. Indeed, the societal institutionalization of other general moral considerations in legal rights and social-cultural practices generally contributes to public health. Social injustices expressed in poverty, racism, and sexism have long been implicated in conditions of poor health. In recent years, some evidence suggests that societies that embody more egalitarian conceptions of socioeconomic justice have higher levels of health than ones that do not.[20] Public health activity has traditionally encompassed much more than medicine and health care. Indeed, historically much of the focus of public health has been on the poor and on the impact of squalor and sanitation on health. The focus today on the social determinants of health is in keeping with this tradition. The data about social determinants are impressive even though not wholly uncontroversial. At any rate, they are strong enough to warrant close attention to the ways conditions of social justice contribute to the public's health.

Apart from social justice, some in public health argue that embodying several other general moral considerations, especially as articulated in human rights, is consistent with and may even contribute to public health. For example, Jonathan Mann contended that public health officials now have two fundamental responsibilities—protecting and promoting public health and protecting and promoting human rights. Sometimes public health programs burden human rights, but human rights violations "have adverse effects on physical, mental, and social well-being" and "promoting and protecting human rights is inextricably linked with promoting and protecting health."[21] Mann noted, and we concur, that, ultimately, "ethics and human rights derive from a set of quite similar, if not identical, core values," several of which we believe are captured in our loose set of general moral considerations.[22] Often, as we have suggested, the most effective ways to protect public health respect general moral considerations rather than violate them, employ voluntary measures rather than coercive ones, protect privacy and confidentiality, and, more generally, express rather than impose community. Recognizing that promoting health and respecting other general moral considerations or human rights may be mutually supportive can enable us to create policies that avoid or at least reduce conflicts.

While more often than not public health and human rights—or general moral considerations not expressed in human rights—do not conflict and may even be synergistic, conflicts do sometimes arise and require resolution.[23] Sometimes, in particular cases, a society cannot simultaneously realize its commitments to public health and to certain other general moral considerations, such as liberty, privacy, and confidentiality. We have tried to provide elements of a framework for thinking through and resolving such conflicts. This process needs to be transparent in order to engender and sustain public trust.

ACKNOWLEDGMENTS

This work was supported by a grant from The Greenwall Foundation. Other project participants were John D. Arras and Paul A. Lombardo, both of the University of Virginia, and Donna T. Chen of the National Institute of Mental Health and Department of Bioethics, National Institutes of Health.

REFERENCES

1. Our definition builds on the definition of health systems offered by the World Health Organization: Health systems include "all the activities whose primary purpose is to promote, restore, or maintain health." See *World Health Report 2000 Health Systems: Improving Performance* (Geneva: World Health Organization, 2000): at 5.

2. Committee for the Study of the Future of Public Health, Division of Health Care Services, Institute of Medicine, *The Future of Public Health* (Washington, D.C.: National Academy Press, 1988): at 1.

3. We recognize that there are different views about the ultimate moral justification for the social institution of public health. For example, some communitarians appear to support public health as an instrumental goal to achieve community. Others may take the view that the state has a duty to ensure the public's health as a matter of social justice. Although these different interpretations and others are very important for some purposes, they do not seriously affect the conception of public health ethics that we are developing, as long as public health agents identify and inform others of their various goals.

4. L.O. Gostin, *Public Health Law: Power, Duty, Restraint* (Berkeley: University of California Press; New York: The Milbank Memorial Fund, 2000): at 20.

5. T. Nagel, "Moral Epistemology," in R.E. Bulger, E.M. Bobby, and H.V. Fineberg, eds., Committee on the Social and Ethical Impacts of Developments in Biomedicine, Division of Health Sciences Policy, Institute of Medicine, *Society's Choices: Social and Ethical Decision Making in Biomedicine* (Washington, D.C.: National Academy Press, 1995): 201–14.

6. For some other approaches, see P. Nieburg, R. Gaare-Bernheim, and R. Bonnie, "Ethics and the Practice of Public Health," in R.A. Goodman et al., eds., *Law in Public Health Practice* (New York: Oxford University Press, in press), and N.E. Kass, "An Ethics Framework for Public Health," *American Journal of Public Health*, 91 (2001): 1776–82.

7. We do not explore here the overlaps among public health ethics, medical ethics, research ethics, and public policy ethics, although some areas of overlap and difference will be evident throughout the discussion. Further work is needed to address some public health activities that fall within overlapping areas for instance, surveillance, outbreak investigations, and community-based interventions may sometimes raise issues in the ethics of research involving human subjects.

8. Recognizing universalizability by attending to past precedents and possible future precedents does not preclude a variety of experiments, for instance, to determine the best ways to protect the public's health. Thus, it is not inappropriate for different states, in our federalist system, to try different approaches, as long as each of them is morally acceptable.

9. This justificatory condition is probably the most controversial. Some of the authors of this paper believe that the language of "necessity" is too strong. Whatever language is used, the point is to avoid a purely utilitarian strategy that accepts only the first two conditions of effectiveness and proportionality and to ensure that the non-utilitarian general moral considerations set some *prima facie* limits and constraints and establish moral priorities, *ceteris paribus*.

10. For another version of these justificatory conditions, see T.L Beauchamp and J.F. Childress, *Principles of Biomedical Ethics*, 5th ed. (New York: Oxford University Press, 2001): at 19–21. We observe that some of these justificatory conditions are quite similar to the justificatory conditions that must be met in U.S. constitutional law when there is strict scrutiny because,

for instance, a fundamental liberty is at stake. In such cases, the government must demonstrate that it has a "compelling interest," that its methods are strictly necessary to achieve its objectives, and that it has adopted the "least restrictive alternative." See Gostin, *supra* note 4, at 80–81.

11. Of course, this chart is oversimplified, particularly in identifying only voluntary and mandatory options. For a fuller discussion, see R. Faden, M. Powers, and N. Kass, "Warrants for Screening Programs: Public Health, Legal and Ethical Frameworks," in R. Faden, G. Geller, and M. Powers, eds., *AIDS, Women and the Next Generation* (New York: Oxford University Press, 1991): 3–26.

12. Working Group on HIV Testing of Pregnant Women and Newborns, "HIV Infection, Pregnant Women, and Newborns," *Journal of the American Medical Association*, 264, no. 18 (1990): 2416–20.

13. See Faden, Geller, and Powers, *supra* note 11; Gostin, *supra* note 4, at 199–201.

14. In rare cases, it may be ethically justifiable to limit the disclosure of some information for a period of time (for example, when there are serious concerns about national security; about the interpretation, certainty, or reliability of public health data; or about the potential negative effects of disclosing the information, such as with suicide clusters).

15. N. Daniels, "Accountability for Reasonableness," *British Medical Journal*, 321 (2000): 1300–01, at 1301.

16. P.C. Stern and H.V. Fineberg, eds., Committee on Risk Characterization, Commission on Behavioral and Social Sciences and Education, National Research Council, *Understanding Risk: Informing Decisions in a Democratic Society* (Washington, D.C.: National Academy Press, 1996): at 155.

17. *Id.* at 16–17, 156.

18. See, for example, N. Daniels and J. Sabin, "Limits to Health Care: Fair Procedures, Democratic Deliberation, and the Legitimacy Problem for Insurers," *Philosophy and Public Affairs*, 26 (Fall 1997): 303–50, at 350.

19. J.S. Mill, *On Liberty*, ed. G. Himmelfarb (Harmondsworth, England: Penguin Books, 1976): at 71. For this chart, see J.F. Childress, *Who Should Decide? Paternalism in Health Care* (New York: Oxford University Press, 1982): at 193.

20. See, for example, the discussion in I. Kawachi, B.P. Kennedy, and R.G. Wilkinson, eds., *Income Inequality and Health*, vol. 1 of *The Society and Population Health Reader* (New York: The New Press, 2000).

21. J.M. Mann. "Medicine and Public Health, Ethics and Human Rights," *The Hastings Center Report*, 27 (May-June 1997): 6–13, at 11–12. Contrast Gostin, *supra* note 4, at 21. For a fuller analysis and assessment of Mann's work, see L. O. Gostin, "Public Health, Ethics, and Human Rights: A Tribute to the Late Jonathan Mann," S.P. Marks, "Jonathan Mann's Legacy to the 21st Century: The Human Rights Imperative for Public Health," and L.O. Gostin, "A Vision of Health and Human Rights for the 21st Century: A Continuing Discussion with Stephen P. Marks," *Journal of Law, Medicine, and Ethics*, 29, no. 2 (2001): 121–40.

22. Mann, *supra* note 21, at 10. Mann thought that the language of ethics could guide individual behavior, while the language of human rights could best guide societal-level analysis and response. See Mann, *supra* note 21, at 8; Marks, *supra* note 21, at 131–38. We disagree with this separation and instead note the overlap of ethics and human rights, but we endorse the essence of Mann's position on human rights.

23. See Gostin, *supra* note 4, at 21.

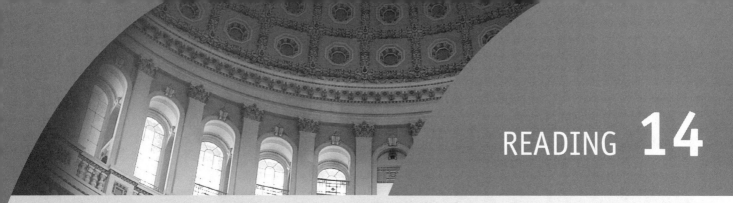

Case Law:
Roe v. Wade (Constitutional Right to Abortion)

Roe et al. v. Wade, **District Attorney of Dallas County**

Case #410 U.S. 113

Appeal From The United States District Court For The Northern District Of Texas

NO. 70-18. Argued December 13, 1971—Reargued October 11, 1972—Decided January 22, 1973

BLACKMUN, J., delivered the opinion of the Court, in which BURGER, C. J., and DOUGLAS, BRENNAN, STEWART, MARSHALL, and POWELL, JJ., joined. BURGER, C. J., post, p. 207, DOUGLAS, J., post, p. 209, and STEWART, J., post, p. 167, filed concurring opinions. WHITE, J., filed a dissenting opinion, in which REHNQUIST, J., joined, post, p. 221. REHNQUIST, J., filed a dissenting opinion, post, p. 171.

MR. JUSTICE BLACKMUN delivered the opinion of the court.

This Texas federal appeal and its Georgia companion, *Doe v. Bolton,* post, p. 179, present constitutional challenges to state criminal abortion legislation. The Texas statutes under attack here are typical of those that have been in effect in many states for approximately a century. The Georgia statutes, in contrast, have a modern cast and are a legislative product that, to an extent at least, obviously reflects the influences of recent attitudinal change, of advancing medical knowledge and techniques, and of new thinking about an old issue.

We forthwith acknowledge our awareness of the sensitive and emotional nature of the abortion controversy, of the vigorous opposing views, even among physicians, and of the deep and seemingly absolute convictions that the subject inspires. One's philosophy, one's experiences, one's exposure to the raw edges of human existence, one's religious training, one's attitudes toward life and family and their values, and the moral standards one establishes and seeks to observe, are all likely to influence and to color one's thinking and conclusions about abortion.

In addition, population growth, pollution, poverty, and racial overtones tend to complicate and not to simplify the problem.

Our task, of course, is to resolve the issue by constitutional measurement, free of emotion and of predilection. We seek earnestly to do this, and, because we do, we have inquired into, and in this opinion place some emphasis upon, medical and medical–legal history and what that history reveals about man's attitudes toward the abortion procedure over the centuries. We bear in mind, too, Mr. Justice Holmes' admonition in his now-vindicated dissent in *Lochner v. New York,* 198 U.S. 45, 76 (1905): "(The Constitution) is made for people of fundamentally differing views, and the accident of our finding certain opinions natural and familiar or novel and even shocking ought not to conclude our judgment upon the question whether statutes embodying them conflict with the constitution of the United States."

I

The Texas statutes that concern us here are Arts. 1191-1194 and 1196 of the State's Penal Code. /1/ These make it a crime to "procure an abortion," as therein defined, or to attempt one, except with respect to "an abortion procured or attempted by medical advice for the purpose of saving the life of the mother." Similar statutes are in existence in a majority of the States. /2/

Texas first enacted a criminal abortion statute in 1854. Texas laws 1854, c. 49, sec. 1, set forth in 3 H. Gammel, Laws of Texas 1502 (1898). This was soon modified into language that has remained substantially unchanged to the present time. See Texas Penal Code of 1857, C. 7, Arts. 531-536; G. Paschel, Laws of Texas, Arts. 2192-2197 (1866); Texas Rev. Stat., c. 8, Arts. 536-541 (1879); Texas Rev. Crim. Stat., Arts. 1071-1076 (1911). The final article in each of these compilations provided the same exception, as does the present Article 1196, for an abortion by "medical advice for the purpose of saving the life of the mother." /3/

II

Jane Roe, /4/ a single woman who was residing in Dallas County, Texas, instituted this federal action in March 1970 against the District Attorney of the county. She sought a declaratory judgment that the Texas criminal abortion statutes were unconstitutional on their face, and an injunction restraining the defendant from forcing the statutes.

Roe alleged that she was unmarried and pregnant; that she wished to terminate her pregnancy by an abortion "performed by a competent, licensed physician, under safe, clinical conditions"; that she was unable to get a "legal" abortion in Texas because her life did not appear to be threatened by the continuation of her pregnancy; and that she could not afford to travel to another jurisdiction in order to secure a legal abortion under safe conditions. She claimed that the Texas statutes were unconstitutionally vague and that they abridged her right of personal privacy, protected by the First, Fourth, Fifth, Ninth, and Fourteenth amendments. By an amendment to her complaint Roe purported to sue "on behalf of herself and all other women" similarly situated.

James Hubert Hallford, a licensed physician, sought and was granted leave to intervene in Roe's action. In his complaint he alleged that he had been arrested previously for violations of the Texas abortion statutes and that two such prosecutions were pending against him. He described conditions of patients who came to him seeking abortions, and he claimed that for many cases he, as a physician, was unable to determine whether they fell within or outside the exception recognized by Article 1196. He alleged that, as a consequence, the statutes were vague and uncertain, in violation of the Fourteenth Amendment, and that they violated his own and his patients' rights to privacy in the doctor–patient relationship and his own right to practice medicine, rights he claimed were guaranteed by the First, Fourth, Fifth, Ninth, and Fourteenth amendments.

John and Mary Doe, /5/ a married couple, filed a companion complaint to that of Roe. They also named the District Attorney as defendant, claimed like constitutional deprivations, and sought declaratory and injunctive relief. The Does alleged that they were a childless couple; that Mrs. Doe was suffering from a "neural-chemical" disorder; that her physician had "advised her to avoid pregnancy until such time as her condition has materially improved" (although a pregnancy at the present time would not present "a serious risk" to her life); that, pursuant to medical advice, she had discontinued use of birth control pills; and that if she should become pregnant, she would want to terminate the pregnancy by an abortion performed by a competent, licensed physician under safe, clinical conditions. By an amendment to their complaint, the Does purported to sue "on behalf of themselves and all couples similarly situated."

The two actions were consolidated and heard together by a duly convened three-judge district court. The suits thus presented the situations of the pregnant single woman, the childless couple, with the wife not pregnant, and the licensed practicing physician, all joining in the attack on the Texas criminal abortion statutes. Upon the filing of affidavits, motions were made for dismissal and for summary judgment. The court held that Roe and members of her class, and Dr. Hallford, had standing to sue and presented justiciable controversies, but that the Does had failed to allege facts sufficient to state a present controversy and did not have standing. It concluded that, with respect to the requests for a declaratory judgment, abstention was not warranted. On the merits, the District Court held that the "fundamental right of single women and married persons to choose whether to have children is protected by the Ninth Amendment, through the Fourteenth Amendment," and that the Texas criminal abortion statutes were void on their face because they were both unconstitutionally vague and constituted an overbroad infringement of the plaintiffs' Ninth Amendment rights. The court then held that abstention was warranted with respect to the requests for an injunction. It therefore dismissed the Does' complaint, declared the abortion statutes void, and dismissed the application for injunctive relief. 314 F. Supp. 1217, 1225 (ND Tex. 1970).

The plaintiffs Roe and Doe and the intervenor Hallford, pursuant to 28 U.S.C. 1253, have appealed to this Court from that part of the District Court's judgment denying the injunction. The defendant district attorney had purported to cross-appeal, pursuant to the same statute, from the court's grant of declaratory relief to Roe and Hallford. Both sides also have taken protective appeals to the United States Court of Appeals for the Fifth Circuit. That court ordered the appeals held in abeyance pending decision here. We postponed decision on jurisdiction to the hearing on the merits. 402 U.S. 941 (1971).

III

It might have been preferable if the defendant, pursuant to our Rule 20, had presented to us a petition for certiorari before judgment in the Court of Appeals with respect to the granting of the plaintiffs' prayer for declaratory relief. Our decisions in *Mitchell v. Donovan*, 398 U.S. 427 (1970), and *Gunn v. University Committee*, 399 U.S. 383 (1970), are to the effect that 1253 does not authorize an appeal to this Court from the grant or denial of declaratory relief alone. We conclude, nevertheless, that those decisions do not foreclose our review of both the injunctive and the declaratory aspects of a case of this kind when it is properly here, as this one is, on appeal under 1253 from specific denial of injunctive relief, and the arguments as to both aspects are necessarily identical. See *Carter v. Jury Comm'n*, 396 U.S. 320 (1970); *Florida Lime Growers v. Jacobsen*, 362 U.S. 73, 80-81 (1960). It would be destructive of time and energy for all concerned were we to rule otherwise. Cf. *Doe v. Bolton*, post, p. 179.

IV

We are next confronted with issues of justiciability, standing, and abstention. Have Roe and the Does established that "personal stake in the outcome of the controversy," *Baker v. Carr*, 369 U.S. 186, 204 (1962), that insures that "the dispute sought to be adjudicated will be presented in an adversary context and in a form historically viewed as capable of judicial resolution," *Flast v. Cohen*, 392 U.S. 83, 101 (1968), and *Sierra Club v. Morton*, 405 U.S. 727, 732 (1972)? And what effect did the pendency of criminal abortion charges against Dr. Hallford in state court have upon the propriety of the federal court's granting relief to him as a plaintiff-intervenor?

A. Jane Roe. Despite the use of the pseudonym, no suggestion is made that Roe is a fictitious person. For purposes of her case, we accept as true, and as established, her existence; her pregnant state, as of the inception of her suit in March 1970 and as late as May 21 of that year when she filed an alias affidavit with the District Court; and her inability to obtain a legal abortion in Texas.

Viewing Roe's case as of the time of its filing and thereafter until as late May, there can be little dispute that it then presented a case or controversy and that, wholly apart from the class aspects, she, as a pregnant single woman thwarted by the Texas criminal abortion laws, had standing to challenge those statutes. *Abele v. Markle*, 452 F.2D 1121, 1125 (CA2 1971); *Crossen v. Breckenridge*, 446 F.2d 833, 838-839 (CA6 1971); *Poe v. Menghini*, 339 F. Supp. 986, 990-991 (Kan. 1972). See *Truax v. Raich*, 239 U.S. 33 (1915). Indeed, we do not read the appellee's brief as really asserting anything to the contrary. The

"logical nexus between the status asserted ant the claim sought to be adjudicated," *Flast v. Cohen*, 392 U.S.,At 102, and the necessary degree of contentiousness, *Golden v. Zwickler*, 394 U.S. 103 (1969), are both present.

The appellee notes, however, that the record does not disclose that Roe was pregnant at the time of the District Court hearing on May 22, 1970, /6/ or on the following June 17 when the court's opinion and judgment were filed. And he suggests that Roe's case must now be moot because she and all other members of her class are no longer subject to any 1970 pregnancy.

The usual rule in federal cases is that an actual controversy must exist at stages of appellate or certiorari review, and not simply at the date the action is initiated. *United States v. Munsingwear, Inc.*, 340 U.S. 36 (1950); *Golden v. Zwickler, supra*; *SEC v. Medical Committee for Human Rights*, 404 U.S. 403 (1972).

But when, as here, pregnancy is a significant fact in the litigation, the normal 266-day human gestation period is so short that the pregnancy will come to term before the usual appellate process is complete. If that termination makes a case moot, pregnancy litigation seldom will survive much beyond the trial stage, and appellate review will be effectively denied. Our law should not be that rigid. Pregnancy often comes more than once to the same woman, and in the general population, if man is to survive, it will always be with us. Pregnancy provides a classic justification for a conclusion of nonmootness. It truly could be "capable of repetition, yet evading review." *Southern Pacific Terminal Co. v. ICC*, 219 U.S. 498, 515 (1911). See *Moore v. Ogilvie*, 394 U.S. 814, 816 (1969); *Carroll v. Princess Anne*, 393 U.S. 175, 178-179 (1968); *United States v. W. T. Grant Co.*, 345 U.S. 629, 632-633 (1953).

We, therefore, agree with the District Court that Jane Roe had standing to undertake this litigation, that she presented a justiciable controversy, and that the termination of her 1970 pregnancy has not rendered her case moot.

B. Dr. Hallford. The doctor's position is different. he entered Roe's litigation as a plaintiff-intervenor, alleging in his complaint that he: "in the past has been arrested for violating the Texas abortion laws and at the present time stands charged by indictment with violating said laws in the criminal district court of Dallas county, Texas to-wit: (1) *The State of Texas vs. James H. Hallford*, No. C-69-5307-IH, and (2) *The State of Texas vs. James H. Hallford*, No. C-69-2524-H. In both cases the defendant is charged with abortion . . . ." In his application for leave to intervene, the doctor made like representations as to the abortion charges pending in the state court. These representations were also repeated in the affidavit he executed and filed in support of his motion for summary judgment.

Dr. Hallford is, therefore, in the position of seeking, in a federal court, declaratory and injunctive relief with respect to the same statutes under which he stands charged in criminal prosecutions simultaneously pending in state court. Although he stated that he has been arrested in the past for violating the State's abortion laws, he makes no allegation of any substantial and immediate threat to any federally protected right that cannot be asserted in his defense against the state prosecution. Neither is there any allegation of harassment or bad-faith prosecution. In order to escape the rule articulated in the cases cited in the next paragraph of this opinion that, absent harassment and bad faith, a defendant in a pending state criminal case cannot affirmatively challenge in federal court the statutes under which the State is prosecuting him, Dr. Hallford seeks to distinguish his status as a present state defendant from his status as a "potential future defendant" and to assert only the latter for standing purposes here.

We see no merit in that distinction. Our decision in *Samuels v. Mackell*, 401 U.S. 66 (1971), compels the conclusion that the District Court erred when it granted declaratory relief to Dr. Hallford instead of refraining from so doing. The court, of course, was correct in refusing to grant injunctive relief to the doctor. The reasons supportive of that action, however, are those expressed in *Samuels v. Mackell*, supra, and in *Younger v. Harris*, 401 U.S. 37 (1971); *Boyle v. Landry*, 401 U.S. 77 (1971); *Perez v. Ledesma*, 401 U.S. 82 (1971); and *Byrne v. Karalexis*, 401 U.S. 216 (1971). See also *Dombrowski v. Pfister*, 380 U.S. 479 (1965). We note, in passing, that Younger and its companion cases were decided after the three-judge District Court decision in this case.

Dr. Hallford's complaint in intervention, therefore, is to be dismissed. /7/ He is remitted to his defenses in the state criminal proceedings against him. We reverse the judgment of the District Court insofar as it granted Dr. Hallford relief and failed to dismiss his complaint in intervention.

C. The Does. In view of our ruling as to Roe's standing in her case, the issue of the Does' standing in their case has little significance. The claims they assert are essentially the same as those of Roe, and they attack the same statutes. Nevertheless, we briefly note the Does' posture.

Their pleadings present them as a childless married couple, the woman not being pregnant, who have no desire to have children at this time because of their having received medical advice that Mrs. Doe should avoid pregnancy, and for "other highly personal reasons." But they "fear . . . they may face the prospect of becoming parents," and if pregnancy ensues, they "would want to terminate" it by an abortion. They assert an inability to obtain an abortion legally in Texas and, consequently, the prospect of obtaining an illegal abortion there or of going outside Texas to some place where the procedure could be obtained legally and competently.

We thus have as plaintiffs a married couple who have, as their asserted immediate and present injury, only an alleged "detrimental effect upon (their) marital happiness" because they are forced to "the choice of refraining from normal sexual relations or of endangering Mary Doe's health through a possible pregnancy." Their claim is that sometime in the future Mrs. Doe might become pregnant because of possible failure of contraceptive measures, and at that time in the future she might want an abortion that might then be illegal under the Texas statutes.

This very phrasing of the Does' position reveals its speculative character. Their alleged injury rests on possible future unpreparedness for parenthood, and possible future impairment of health. Any one or more of these several possibilities may not take place and all may not combine. In the Does' estimation, these possibilities might have some real or imagined impact upon their marital happiness. But we are not prepared to say that the bare allegation of so indirect an injury is sufficient to present an actual case or controversy. *Younger v. Harris*, 401 U.S., at 41-42; *Golden v. Zwickler*, 394 U.S., at 109-110; *Abele v. Markle*, 452 F.2d, at 1124-1125; *Crossen v. Breckenridge*, 446 F.2d, at 839. The Does' claim falls far short of those resolved otherwise in the cases that the Does urge upon us, namely, *Investment Co. Institute v. Camp*, 401 U.S. 617 (1971); *Data Processing Service v. Camp*, 397 U.S. 150 (1970); and *Epperson v. Arkansas*, 393 U.S. 97 (1968). See Also *Truax v. Raich*, 239 U.S. 33 (1915).

The Does therefore are not appropriate plaintiffs in this litigation. Their complaint was properly dismissed by the District Court, and we affirm that dismissal.

V

The principal thrust of appellant's attack on the Texas statutes is that they improperly invade a right, said to be possessed by the pregnant woman, to choose to terminate her pregnancy. Appellant would discover this right in the concept of personal "liberty" embodied in the Fourteenth Amendment's due process clause; or in personal, marital, familial, and sexual privacy said to be protected by the Bill of Rights or its penumbras, see *Griswold v. Connecticut*, 381 U.S. 479 (1965); *Eisenstaedt v. Baird*, 405 U.S. 438 (1972); id., at 460 (WHITE, J., concurring in result); or among those rights reserved to the people by the Ninth Amendment, *Griswold v. Connecticut*, 381 U.S., at 486 (Goldberg, J., concurring). Before addressing this claim, we feel it desirable briefly to survey, in several aspects, the history of abortion, for such insight as that history may afford us, and then to examine the state purposes and interests behind the criminal abortion laws.

VI

It perhaps is not generally appreciated that the restrictive criminal abortion laws in effect in a majority of States today are of relatively recent vintage. Those laws, generally proscribing abortion or its attempt at any time during pregnancy except when necessary to preserve the pregnant woman's life, are not of ancient or even of common-law origin. Instead, they derive from statutory changes effected, for the most part, in the latter half of the 19th century.

1. Ancient attitudes. These are not capable of precise determination. We are told that at the time of the Persian Empire abortifacients were known and that criminal abortions were severely punished. /8/ We are also told, however, that abortion was practiced in Greek times as well as in the Roman Era, /9/ and that "it was resorted to without scruple." /10/ The Ephesian, Soranos, often described as the greatest of the ancient gynecologists, appears to have been generally opposed to Rome's prevailing free-abortion practices. He found it necessary to think first of the life of the mother, and he resorted to abortion when, upon this standard, he felt the procedure advisable. /11/ Greek and Roman law afforded little protection to the unborn. If abortion was prosecuted in some places, it seems to have been based on a concept of a violation of the father's right to his offspring. Ancient religion did not bar abortion. /12/

2. The Hippocratic Oath. What then of the famous Oath that has stood so long as the ethical guide of the medical profession and that bears the name of the great Greek (460 (?)-377 (?) B.C.), who had been described as the Father of Medicine, the "wisest and the greatest practitioner of his art," and the "most important and most complete medical personality of antiquity," who dominated the medical schools of his time, and who typified the sum of the medical knowledge of the past? /13/ The Oath varies somewhat according to the particular translation, but in any translation the content is clear: "I will give no deadly medicine to anyone if asked, nor suggest any such counsel; and in like manner I will not give to a woman a pessary to produce abortion," /14/ or "I will neither give a deadly drug to anybody if asked for it, nor will I make a suggestion to this effect. Similarly, I will not give to a woman an abortive remedy." /15/

Although the Oath is not mentioned in any of the principal briefs in this case or in *Doe v. Bolton*, post, p. 179, it represents the apex of the development of strict ethical concepts in medicine, and its influence endures to this day. Why did not the authority of Hippocrates dissuade abortion practice in his time and that of Rome? The late Dr. Edelstein provides us with a theory: /16/ The Oath was not uncontested even in Hippocrates' day; only the Pythagorean school of philosophers frowned upon the related act of suicide. Most Greek thinkers, on the other hand, commended abortion, at least prior to viability. See Plato, *Republic*, V, 461; Aristotle, *Politics*, VII, 1335b 25. For the Pythagoreans, however, it was a matter of dogma. For them the embryo was animate from the moment of conception, and abortion meant destruction of a living being. The abortion clause of the Oath, therefore, "echoes Pythagorean doctrines," and "in no other stratum of Greek opinion were such views held or proposed in the same spirit of uncompromising austerity." /17/

Dr. Edelstein then concludes that the Oath originated in a group representing only a small segment of Greek opinion and that it certainly was not accepted by all ancient physicians. He points out that medical writings down to Galen (A.D. 130-200) "give evidence of the violation of almost every one of its injunctions." /18/ But with the end of antiquity a decided change took place. Resistance against suicide and against abortion became common. The Oath came to be popular. The emerging teachings of Christianity were in agreement with the Pythagorean ethic. The Oath "became the nucleus of all medical ethics" and "was applauded as the embodiment of truth." Thus, suggests Dr. Edelstein, it is "a Pythagorean manifesto and not the expression of an absolute standard of medical conduct." /19/

This, it seems to us, is a satisfactory and acceptable explanation of the Hippocratic Oath's apparent rigidity. It enables us to understand, in historical context, a long-accepted and reversed statement of medical ethics.

3. The common law. It is undisputed that at common law, abortion performed before "quickening"—the first recognizable movement of the fetus in utero, appearing usually from the 16th to the 18th week of pregnancy /20/ —was not an indictable offense. /21/ The absence of a common-law crime for pre-quickening abortion appears to have developed from a confluence of earlier philosophical, theological, and civil and canon law concepts of when life begins. These disciplines variously approached the question in terms of the point at which the embryo or fetus became "formed" or recognizably human, or in terms of when a "person" came into being, that is, infused with a "soul" or "animated." A loose consensus evolved in early English law that these events occurred at some point between conception and live birth. /22 This was "mediate animation." Although Christian theology and the canon law came to fix the point of animation at 40 days for a male and 80 days for a female, a view that persisted until the 19th century, there was otherwise little agreement about the precise time of formation or animation. There was agreement, however, that prior to this point the fetus was to be regarded as part of the mother,

and its destruction, therefore, was not homicide. Due to continued uncertainty about the precise time when animation occurred, to the lack of any empirical basis for the 40-80-day view, and perhaps to Aquinas' definition of movement as one of the two first principles of life, Bracton focused upon quickening as the critical point. The significance of quickening was echoed by later common-law scholars and found its way into the received common law in this country.

Whether abortion of a quick fetus was a felony at common law, or even a lesser crime, is still disputed. Bracton, writing early in the 13th century, thought it homicide. /23/ But the later and predominant view, following the great common-law scholars, has been that it was, at most, a lesser offense. In a frequently cited passage, Coke took the position that abortion of a woman "quick with child" is "a great misprision, and no murder." /24/ Blackstone followed, saying that while abortion after quickening had once been considered manslaughter (though not murder), "modern law" took a less severe view. /25/ A recent review of the common-law precedents argues, however, that those precedents contradict Coke and that even post-quickening abortion was never established as a common-law crime. /26/ This is of some importance because while most American courts ruled, in holding or dictum, that abortion of an unquickened fetus was not criminal under their received common law, /27/ others followed Coke in stating that abortion of a quick fetus was a "misprision," a term they translated to mean "misdemeanor." /28/ That their reliance on Coke on this aspect of the law was uncritical and, apparently in all the reported cases, dictum (due probably to the paucity of common-law prosecutions for post-quickening abortion), makes it now appear doubtful that abortion was ever firmly established as a common-law crime even with respect to the destruction of a quick fetus.

4. The English statutory law. England's first criminal abortion statute, Lord Ellenborough's Act, 43 Geo. 3, c. 58, came in 1803. It made abortion of a quick fetus, 1, a capital crime, but in 2 it provided lesser penalties for the felony of abortion before quickening, and thus preserved the "quickening" distinction. This contrast was continued in the general revision of 1828, 9 Geo. 4, c. 31, 13. It disappeared, however, together with the death penalty, in 1837, 7 Will. 4 & 1 Vict., c. 85, 6, and did not reappear in the Offenses Against the Person Act of 1861, 24 & 25 Vict., c. 100, 59, that formed the core of English antiabortion law until the liberalizing reforms of 1967. In 1929, the Infant Life (Preservation) Act, 19 & 20 Geo. 5, c. 34, came into being. Its emphasis was upon the destruction of "the life of a child capable of being born alive." It made a willful act performed with the necessary intent a felony. It contained a proviso that one was not to be found guilty of the offense "un-

less it is proved that the act which caused the death of the child was not done in good faith for the purpose only of preserving the life of the mother."

A seemingly notable development in the English law was the case of *Rex v. Bourne*, 1939. 1 K.B. 687. This case apparently answered in the affirmative the question whether an abortion necessary to preserve the life of the pregnant woman was excepted from the criminal penalties of the 1861 act. In his instructions to the jury, Judge Macnaghten referred to the 1929 Act, and observed that that Act related to "the case where a child is killed by a willful act at the time when it is being delivered in the ordinary course of nature." ID., at 691. He concluded that the 1861 Act's use of the word "unlawfully," imported the same meaning expressed by the specific proviso in the 1929 Act, even though there was no mention of preserving the mother's life in the 1861 Act. He then construed the phrase "preserving the life of the mother" broadly, that is, "in a reasonable sense," to include a serious and permanent threat to the mother's health, and instructed the jury to acquit Dr. Bourne if it found he had acted in a good-faith belief that the abortion was necessary for this purpose. Id., at 693-694. The jury did acquit.

Recently, Parliament enacted a new abortion law. This is the Abortion Act of 1967, 15 & 16 Eliz. 2, c. 87. The act permits a licensed physician to perform an abortion where two other licensed physicians agree (a) "that the continuance of the pregnancy would involve risk to the life of the pregnant woman, or of injury to the physical or mental health of the pregnant woman or any existing children of her family, greater than if the pregnancy were terminated" or (b) "that there is a substantial risk that if the child were born it would suffer from such physical or mental abnormalities as to be seriously handicapped." The Act also provides that, in making this determination, "account may be taken of the pregnant woman's actual or reasonably foreseeable environment." It also permits a physician, without the concurrence of others, to terminate a pregnancy where he is of the good-faith opinion that the abortion "is immediately necessary to save the life or to prevent grave permanent injury to the physical or mental health of the pregnant woman."

5. The American law. In this country, the law in effect in all but a few States until mid-19th century was the pre-existing English common law. Connecticut, the first state to enact abortion legislation, adopted in 1821 that part of Lord Ellenborough's Act that related to a woman "quick with child." /29/ The death penalty was not imposed. Abortion before quickening was made a crime in that State only in 1860. /30/ In 1828, New York enacted legislation /31/ that, in two respects, was to serve as a model for

early anti-abortion statutes. First, while barring destruction of an unquickened fetus as well as a quick fetus, it made the former only a misdemeanor, but the latter second-degree manslaughter. Second, it incorporated a concept of therapeutic abortion by providing that an abortion was excused if it "shall have been necessary to preserve the life of such mother, or shall have been advised by two physicians to be necessary for such purpose." By 1840, when Texas had received the common law, /32/ only eight American States had statutes dealing with abortion. /33/ It was not until after the war between the states that legislation began generally to replace the common law. Most of these initial statutes dealt severely with abortion after quickening but were lenient with it before quickening. Most punished attempts equally with completed abortions. While many statutes included the exception for an abortion thought by one or more physicians to be necessary to save the mother's life, that provision soon disappeared and the typical law required that the procedure actually be necessary for that purpose.

Gradually, in the middle and late 19th century the quickening distinction disappeared from the statutory law of most States and the degree of the offense and the penalties were increased. By the end of the 1950's, a large majority of the jurisdictions banned abortion, however and whenever performed, unless done to save or preserve the life of the mother. /34/ The exceptions, Alabama and the District of Columbia, permitted abortion to preserve the mother's health. /35/ Three States permitted abortions that were not "unlawfully" performed or that were not "without lawful justification," leaving interpretation of those standards to the courts. /36/ In the past several years, however, a trend toward liberalization of abortion statutes has resulted in adoption, by about one-third of the States, of less stringent laws, most of them patterned after the Ali Model Penal Code, 230.3, /37/ set forth as appendix b to the opinion in *Doe v. Bolton*, post, p. 205.

It is thus apparent that at common law, at the time of the adoption of our Constitution, and throughout the major portion of the 19th century, abortion was viewed with less disfavor than under most American statutes currently in effect. Phrasing it another way, a woman enjoyed a substantially broader right to terminate a pregnancy than she does in most States today. At least with respect to the early stage of pregnancy, and very possibly without such a limitation, the opportunity to make this choice was present in this country well into the 19th century. Even later, the law continued for some time to treat less punitively an abortion procured in early pregnancy.

6. The position of The American Medical Association. The anti-abortion mood prevalent in this country in the late 19th century was shared by the medical profession. Indeed, the at-

titude of the profession may have played a significant role in the enactment of stringent criminal abortion legislation during the period.

An AMA Committee on criminal abortion was appointed in May 1857. It presented its report, 12 Trans. of the Am. Med. Assn. 73-78 (1859), to the Twelfth Annual Meeting. That report observed that the Committee had been appointed to investigate criminal abortion "with a view to its general suppression." It deplored abortion and its frequency and it listed three causes of "this general demoralization":

"the first of these causes is a wide-spread popular ignorance of the true character of the crime—a belief, even among mothers themselves, that the foetus is not alive till after the period of quickening.
"The second of the agents alluded to is the fact that the profession themselves are frequently supposed careless of foetal life."
"the third reason of the frightful extent of this crime is found in the grave defects of our laws, both common and statute, as regards the independent and actual existence of the child before birth, as a living being. These errors, which are sufficient in most instances to prevent conviction, are based, and only based, upon mistaken and exploded medical dogmas. With strange inconsistency, the law fully acknowledges the foetus in utero and its inherent rights, for civil purposes; while personally and as criminally affected, it fails to recognize it, and to its life as yet denies all protection." Id., at 75-76.

The Committee then offered, and the Association adopted, resolutions protesting "against such unwarrantable destruction of human life," calling upon state legislatures to revise their abortion laws, and requesting the cooperation of state medical societies "in pressing the subject." Id., at 28, 78.

In 1871, a long and vivid report was submitted by the Committee on Criminal Abortion. It ended with the observation, "We had to deal with human life. In a matter of less importance we could entertain no compromise. An honest judge on the bench would call things by their proper names. We could do no less." 22 Trans. of the Am. Med. Assn. 258 (1871). It proffered resolutions, adopted by the association, id., at 38-39, recommending, among other things, that it "be unlawful and unprofessional for any physician to induce abortion or premature labor, without the concurrent opinion of at least one respectable consulting physician, and then always with a view to the safety of the child—if that be possible," and calling "the attention of the clergy of all denominations to the perverted views of morality entertained by a large class of females—aye, and men also, on this important question."

Except for periodic condemnation of the criminal abortionist, no further formal AMA action took place until 1967. In that year, the Committee on Human Reproduction urged the adoption of a stated policy of opposition to induced abortion, except when there is "documented medical evidence" of a threat to the health or life of the mother, or that the child "may be born with incapacitating physical deformity or mental deficiency," or that a pregnancy "resulting from legally established statutory or forcible rape or incest may constitute a threat to the mental or physical health of the patient," two other physicians "chosen because of their recognized professional competence have examined the patient and have concurred in writing," and the procedure "is performed in a hospital accredited by the Joint Commission on Accreditation of Hospitals." The providing of medical information by physicians to state legislatures in their consideration of legislation regarding therapeutic abortion was "to be considered consistent with the principles of ethics of the American Medical Association." This recommendation was adopted by the House of Delegates. Proceedings of the AMA House of Delegates 40-51 (June 1967).

In 1970, after the introduction of a variety of proposed resolutions, and of a report from its board of trustees, a reference committee noted "polarization of the medical profession on this controversial issue"; division among those who had testified; a difference of opinion among AMA councils and committees; "the remarkable shift in testimony" in six months, felt to be influenced "by the rapid changes in state laws and by the judicial decisions which tend to make abortion more freely available;" and a feeling "that this trend will continue." On June 25, 1970, the House of Delegates adopted preambles and most of the resolutions proposed by the reference committee. The preambles emphasized "the best interests of the patient," "sound clinical judgment," and "informed patient consent," in contrast to "mere acquiescence to the patient's demand." The resolutions asserted that abortion is a medical procedure that should be performed by a licensed physician in an accredited hospital only after consultation with two other physicians and in conformity with state law, and that no party to the procedure should be required to violate personally held moral principles. /38/ Proceedings of the AMA house of delegates 220 (June 1970). The AMA Judicial Council rendered a complementary opinion. /39/

7. The position of the American Public Health Association. In October 1970, the executive board of the APHA adopted Standards for Abortion Services. These were five in number.

"a. Rapid and simple abortion referral must be readily available through state and local public health departments, medical societies, or other nonprofit organizations.

"b. An important function of counseling should be to simplify and expedite the provision of abortion services; it should not delay the obtaining of these services.

"c. Psychiatric consultation should not be mandatory. As in the case of other specialized medical services, psychiatric consultation should be sought for definite indications and not on a routine basis.

"d. A wide range of individuals from appropriately trained, sympathetic volunteers to highly skilled physicians may qualify as abortion counselors.

"e. Contraception and/or sterilization should be discussed with each abortion patient." Recommended Standards For Abortion Services, 61 *Am. J. Pub. Health* 396 (1971).

Among factors pertinent to life and health risks associated with abortion were three that "are recognized as important":10

"a. The skill of the physician,

"b. The environment in which the abortion is performed, and above all

"c. The duration of pregnancy, as determined by uterine size and confirmed by menstrual history." Id., at 397.

It was said that "a well-equipped hospital" offers more protection "to cope with unforeseen difficulties than an office or clinic without such resources . . . the factor of gestational age is of overriding importance." Thus, it was recommended that abortions in the second trimester and early abortions in the presence of existing medical complications be performed in hospitals as inpatient procedures. For pregnancies in the first trimester, abortion in the hospital with or without overnight stay "is probably the safest practice." An abortion in an extramural facility, however, is an acceptable alternative "provided arrangements exist in advance to admit patients promptly if unforeseen complications develop." Standards for an abortion facility were listed. It was said that at present abortions should be performed by physicians or osteopaths who are licensed to practice and who have "adequate training." Id., at 398.

8. The position of the American Bar Association. At its meeting in February 1972 the ABA House of Delegates approved, with 17 opposing votes, the Uniform Abortion Act that had been drafted and approved the preceding August by the Conference of Commissioners on Uniform State Laws. 58 A.B.A.J. 380 (1972). We set forth the Act in full in the margin. /40/ The Conference has appended an enlightening Prefatory Note. /41/

VII

Three reasons have been advanced to explain historically the enactment of criminal abortion laws in the 19th century and to justify their continued existence.

It has been argued occasionally that these laws were the product of a Victorian social concern to discourage illicit sexual conduct. Texas, however, does not advance this justification in the present case, and it appears that no court or commentator has taken the argument seriously. /42/ The appellants and amici contend, moreover, that this is not a proper state purpose at all and suggest that, if it were, the Texas statutes are overbroad in protecting it since the law fails to distinguish between married and unwed mothers.

A second reason is concerned with abortion as a medical procedure. When most criminal abortion laws were first enacted, the procedure was a hazardous one for the woman. /43/ This was particularly true prior to the development of antisepsis. Antiseptic techniques, of course, were based on discoveries by Lister, Pasteur, and others first announced in 1867, but were not generally accepted and employed until about the turn of the century. Abortion mortality was high. Even after 1900, and perhaps until as late as the development of antibiotics in the 1940's, standard modern techniques such as dilation and curettage were not nearly so safe as they are today. Thus, it has been argued that a State's real concern in enacting a criminal abortion law was to protect the pregnant woman, that is, to restrain her from submitting to a procedure that placed her life in serious jeopardy.

Modern medical techniques have altered this situation. Appellants and various amici refer to medical data indicating that abortion in early pregnancy, that is, prior to the end of the first trimester, although not without its risk, is now relatively safe. Mortality rates for women undergoing early abortions, where the procedure is legal, appear to be as low as or lower than the rates for normal childbirth. /44/ Consequently, any interest of the State in protecting the woman from an inherently hazardous procedure except when it would be equally dangerous for her to forgo it, has largely disappeared. Of course, important state interests in the areas of health and medical standards do remain. The State has a legitimate interest in seeing to it that abortion, like any other medical procedure, is performed under circumstances that insure maximum safety for the patient. This interest obviously extends at least to the performing physician and his staff, to the facilities involved, to the availability of after-care, and to adequate provision for any complication or emergency that might arise. The prevalence of high mortality rates at illegal "abortion mills" strengthens, rather than weaken, the State's interest in regulating the conditions under which abortions are performed. Moreover, the risk to the woman increases as her pregnancy continues. Thus, the State retains a definite interest in protecting the woman's own health and safety when an abortion is proposed at a late stage of pregnancy.

The third reason is the State's interest—some phrase it in terms of duty—in protecting prenatal life. Some of the argument for this justification rests on the theory that a new human life is present from the moment of conception. /45/ The State's interest and general obligation to protect life then extends, it is argued, to prenatal life. Only when the life of the pregnant mother herself is at stake, balanced against the life she carries within her, should the interest of the embryo or fetus not prevail. Logically, of course, a legitimate state interest in this area need not stand or fall on acceptance of the belief that life begins at conception or at some other point prior to live birth. In assessing the State's interest, recognition may be given to the less rigid claim that as long as at least potential life is involved, the state may assert interests beyond the protection of the pregnant woman alone.

Parties challenging state abortion laws have sharply disputed in some courts the contention that a purpose of these laws, when enacted, was to protect prenatal life. /46/ Pointing to the absence of legislative history to support the contention, they claim that most state laws were designed solely to protect the woman. Because medical advances have lessened this concern, at least with respect to abortion in early pregnancy, they argue that with respect to such abortions the laws can no longer be justified by any state interest. There is some scholarly support for this view of original purpose. /47/ The few state courts called upon to interpret their laws in the late 19th and early 20th centuries did focus on the State's interest in protecting the woman's health rather than in preserving the embryo and fetus. /48/ Proponents of this view point out that in many States, including Texas, /49/ by statute or judicial interpretation, the pregnant woman herself could not be prosecuted for self-abortion or for cooperating in an abortion performed upon her by another. /50/ They claim that adoption of the "quickening through received common law and state statutes tacitly recognizes the greater health hazards inherent in late abortion and impliedly repudiates the theory that life begins at conception.

It is with these interests, and the weight to be attached to them, that this case is concerned.

VIII

The Constitution does not explicitly mention any right of privacy. In a line of decisions, however, going back perhaps as far as *Union Pacific R. Co. v. Botsford*, 141 U.S. 250, 251 (1891), the Court has recognized that a right of personal privacy, or a guarantee of certain areas or zones of privacy, does exist under the Constitution. In varying contexts, the Court or individual Justices have, indeed, found at least the roots of that right in the First Amendment, *Stanley v. Georgia*, 394 U.S. 557, 564 (1969);

in the Fourth And Fifth Amendments, *Terry v. Ohio*, 392 U.S. 1, 8-9 (1968), *Katz v. United States*, 389 U.S. 347, 350 (1967), *Boyd v. United States*, 116 U.S. 616 (1886), see *Olmstead v. United States*, 277 U.S. 438, 478 (1928) (Brandeis, J., Dissenting); in the penumbras of the Bill of Rights, *Griswold v. Connecticut*, 381 U.S., at 484-485; in the Ninth Amendment, id., at 486 (Goldberg, J., concurring); or in the concept of liberty guaranteed by the first section of the Fourteenth Amendment, see *Meyer v. Nebraska*, 262 U.S. 390, 399 (1923). These decisions make it clear that only personal rights that can be deemed "fundamental" or "implicit in the concept of ordered liberty," *Palko v. Connecticut*, 302 U.S. 319, 325 (1937), are included in this guarantee of personal privacy. They also make it clear that the right has some extension to activities relating to marriage, *Loving v. Virginia*, 388 U.S. 1, 12 (1967); procreation, *Skinner v. Oklahoma*, 316 U.S. 535, 541-542 (1942); contraception, *Eisenstadt v. Baird*, 405 U.S., at 453-454; id., at 460, 463-465 (WHITE J., Concurring In Result); family relationships, *Prince v. Massachusetts*, 321 U.S. 158, 166 (1944); and child rearing and education, *Pierce v. Society of Sisters*, 268 U.S. 510, 535 (1925), *Meyer v. Nebraska, Supra.*

This right of privacy, whether it be founded in the Fourteenth Amendment's concept of personal liberty and restrictions upon state action, as we feel it is, or, as the District Court determined, in the Ninth Amendment's reservation of rights to the people, is broad enough to encompass a woman's decision whether or not to terminate her pregnancy. The detriment that the State would impose upon the pregnant woman by denying this choice altogether is apparent. Specific and direct harm medically diagnosable even in early pregnancy may be involved. Maternity, or additional offspring, may force upon the woman a distressful life and future. Psychological harm may be imminent. Mental and physical health may be taxed by child care. There is also the distress, for all concerned, associated with the unwanted child, and there is the problem of bringing a child into a family already unable, psychologically and otherwise, to care for it. In other cases, as in this one, the additional difficulties and continuing stigma of unwed motherhood may be involved. All these are factors the woman and her responsible physician necessarily will consider in consultation.

On the basis of elements such as these, appellant and some amici argue that the woman's right is absolute and that she is entitled to terminate her pregnancy at whatever time, in whatever way, and for whatever reason she alone chooses. With this we do not agree. Appellant's arguments that Texas either has no valid interest at all in regulating the abortion decision, or no interest strong enough to support any limitation upon the woman's sole determination, are unpersuasive. The Court's decisions recognizing a right of privacy also acknowledge that some state regulation in areas protected by that right is appropriate. As noted above, a State may properly assert important interests in safeguarding health, in maintaining medical standards, and in protecting potential life. At some point in pregnancy, these respective interests become sufficiently compelling to sustain regulation of the factors that govern the abortion decision. The privacy right involved, therefore, cannot be said to be absolute. In fact, it is not clear to us that the claim asserted by some amici that one has an unlimited right to do with one's body as one pleases bears a close relationship to the right of privacy previously articulated in the Court's decisions. The Court has refused to recognize an unlimited right of this kind in the past. *Jacobson v. Massachusetts*, 197 U.S. 11 (1905) (vaccination); *Buck v. Bell*, 274 U.S. 200 (1927) (Sterilization).

We, therefore, conclude that the right of personal privacy includes the abortion decision, but that this right is not unqualified and must be considered against important state interests in regulation.

We note that those federal and state courts that have recently considered abortion law challenges have reached the same conclusion. A majority, in addition to the District Court in the present case, have held state laws unconstitutional, at least in part, because of vagueness or because of overbreadth and abridgment of rights. *Abele v. Markle*, 342 F. Supp. 800 (Conn. 1972), appeal docketed, No. 72-56; *Abele v. Markle*, 351 F. Supp. 224 (Conn. 1972), appeal docketed, No. 72-730; *Doe v. Bolton*, 319 F. Supp. 1048 (ND Ga. 1970), appeal decided today, post, p. 179; *Doe v. Scott*, 321 F. Supp. 1385 (ND Ill. 1971), appeal docketed, No. 70-105; *Poe v. Menghini*, 339 F. Supp. 986 (Kan. 1972); *Ywca v. Kugler*, 342 F. Supp. 1048 (NJ 1972); *Babbitz v. Mccann*, 310 F. Supp. 293 (ED Wis. 1970), appeal dismissed, 400 U.S. 1 (1970); *People v. Belous*, 71 Cal.2d 954, 458 P.2d 194 (1969), cert. denied, 397 U.S. 915 (1970); *State v. Barquet*, 262 So.2d 431 (Fla. 1972).

Others have sustained state statutes. *Crossen v. Attorney General*, 344 F. Supp. 587 (ED Ky. 1972), appeal docketed, No. 72-256; *Rosen v. Louisiana State Board of Medical Examiners*, 318 F. Supp. 1217 (ED La. 1970), appeal docketed, No. 70-42; *Corkey v. Edwards*, 322 F. Supp. 1248 (WDNC 1971), appeal docketed, No. 71-92; *Steinberg v. Brown*, 321 F. Supp. 741 (ND Ohio 1970); *Doe v. Rampton* (Utah 1971), appeal docketed, No. 71-5666; *Cheaney v. State*, ___ Ind. ___, 285 N.E.2d 265 (1972); *Spears v. State*, 257 So.2d 876 (Miss. 1972); *State v. Munson*, 86 S.D. 663, 201 N.W.2d 123 (1972), appeal docketed, No. 72-631.

Although the results are divided, most of these courts have agreed that the right of privacy, however based, is broad enough to cover the abortion decision; that the right, nonetheless, is not absolute and is subject to some limitations; and that at some point the state interests as to protection of health, medical standards, and prenatal life, become dominant. We agree with this approach.

Where certain "fundamental rights" are involved, the Court has held that regulation limiting these rights may be justified only by a "compelling state interest," *Kramer v. Union Free School District*, 395 U.S. 621, 627 (1969); *Shapiro v. Thompson*, 394 U.S. 618, 634 (1969), *Sherbert v. Verner*, 374 U.S. 398, 406 (1963), and that legislative enactments must be narrowly drawn to express only the legitimate state interests at stake. *Griswold v. Connecticut*, 381 U.S., at 485; *Aptheker v. Secretary of State*, 378 U.S. 500, 508 (1964); *Cantwell v. Connecticut*, 310 U.S. 296, 307-308 (1940); see *Eisenstadt v. Baird*, 405 U.S., at 460, 463-464 (WHITE, J., concurring in result).

In the recent abortion cases, cited above, courts have recognized these principles. Those striking down state laws have generally scrutinized the State's interests in protecting health and potential life, and have concluded that neither interest justified broad limitations on the reasons for which a physician and his pregnant patient might decide that she should have an abortion in the early stages of pregnancy. Courts sustaining state laws have held that the State's determinations to protect health or prenatal life are dominant and constitutionally justifiable.

IX

The District Court held that the appellee failed to meet his burden of demonstrating that the Texas statute's infringement upon Roe's rights was necessary to support a compelling state interest, and that, although the appellee presented "several compelling justifications for state presence in the area of abortions," the statutes outstripped these justifications and swept "far beyond any areas of compelling state interest." 314 F. Supp., at 1222-1223. Appellant and appellee both contest that holding. Appellant, as has been indicated, claims an absolute right that bars any state imposition of criminal penalties in the area. Appellee argues that the State's determination to recognize and protect prenatal life from and after conception constitutes a compelling state interest. As noted above, we do not agree fully with either formulation.

A. The appellee and certain amici argue that the fetus is a "person" within the language and meaning of the Fourteenth Amendment. In support of this, they outline at length and in detail the well-known facts of fetal development. If this suggestion of personhood is established, the appellant's case, of course, collapses, for the fetus' right to life would then be guaranteed specifically by the Amendment. The appellant conceded as much on reargument. /51/ On the other hand, the appellee conceded on reargument /52/ that no case could be cited that

holds that a fetus is a person within the meaning of the Fourteenth Amendment.

The Constitution does not define "person" in so many words. Section 1 of the Fourteenth Amendment contains three references to person. The first, in defining "citizens," speaks of "persons born or naturalized in the United States." The word also appears both in the Due Process Clause and in the Equal Protection Clause. "Person" is used in other places in the Constitution: in the listing of qualifications for Representatives and Senators, Art. I, sec. 2, cl. 2, and 3, cl. 3; in the Apportionment Clause, Art. I, 2, cl. 3; /53/ in the Migration and Importation provision, Art. I, 9, cl. 1; in the Emolument Clause, Art. I, 9, cl. 8; in the Electors Provisions, Art. II, 1 cl. 2, and the superseded cl. 3; in the provision outlining qualifications for the office of President, Art. II, 1, cl. 5; in the Extradition provision, Art. IV, 2, cl. 2, and the superseded Fugitive Slave Clause 3; and in the Fifth, Twelfth, and Twenty-Second Amendments, as well as in 2 and 3 of the Fourteenth Amendment. But in nearly all these instances, the use of the word is such that it has application only postnatally. None indicates, with any assurance, that it has any possible pre-natal application. /54/

All this, together with our observation, supra, that throughout the major portion of the 19th century prevailing legal abortion practices were far freer than they are today, persuades us that the word "person," as used in the Fourteenth Amendment, does not include the unborn. /55/ This is in accord with the results reached in those few cases where the issue has been squarely presented. *Mcgarvey v. Magee Womens Hospital*, 340 F. Supp. 751 (WD Pa. 1972); *Byrn v. New York City Health & Hospitals Corp.*, 31 N.Y.2d 194, 286 N.E.2d 887 (1972), appeal docketed, No. 72-434; *Abele v. Markle*, 351 F. Supp. 224 (Conn. 1972), appeal docketed, No. 72-730. Cf. *Cheaney v. State*,— Ind., at— , 285 N.E.2d At 270; *Montana v. Rogers*, 278 F.2d 68, 72 (CA7 1960), aff'd sub nom. *Montana v. Kennedy*, 366 U.S. 308 (1961); *Keeler v. Superior Court*, 2 Cal. 3d 619, 470 P.2d 617 (1970); *State v. Dickinson*, 28 Ohio St.2d 65, 275 N.E. 2d 599 (1971). Indeed, our decision in *United States v. Vuitch*, 402 U.S. 62 (1971), inferentially is to the same effect, for we there would not have indulged in statutory interpretation favorable to abortion in specified circumstances if the necessary consequence was the termination of life entitled to fourteenth amendment protection.

This conclusion, however, does not of itself fully answer the contentions raised by Texas, and we pass on to other considerations.

B. The pregnant woman cannot be isolated in her privacy. She carries an embryo and, later, a fetus, if one accepts the medical definitions of the developing young in the human uterus. See *Dorland's Illustrated Medical Dictionary* 478-479, 547 (24th ed.

1965). The situation therefore is inherently different from marital intimacy, or bedroom possession of obscene material, or marriage, or procreation, or education, with which Eisenstaedt and Griswold, Stanley, Loving, Skinner, and Pierce and Meyer were respectively concerned. As we have intimated above, it is reasonable and appropriate for a State to decide that at some point in time another interest, that of health of the mother or that of potential human life, becomes significantly involved. The woman's privacy is no longer sole and any right of privacy she possesses must be measured accordingly.

Texas urges that, apart from the Fourteenth Amendment, life begins at conception and is present throughout pregnancy, and that, therefore, the State has a compelling interest in protecting that life from and after conception. We need not resolve the difficult question of when life begins. When those trained in the respective disciplines of medicine, philosophy, and theology are unable to arrive at any consensus, the judiciary, at this point in the development of man's knowledge, is not in a position to speculate as to the answer.

It should be sufficient to note briefly the wide divergence of thinking on this most sensitive and difficult question. There has always been strong support for the view that life does not begin until live birth. This was the belief of the stoics. /56/ It appears to be the predominant, though not the unanimous, attitude of the Jewish faith. /57/ It may be taken to represent also the position of a large segment of the Protestant community, insofar as that can be ascertained; organized groups that have taken a formal position on the abortion issue have generally regarded abortion as a matter for the conscience of the individual and her family. /58/ As we have noted, the common law found greater significance in quickening. Physicians and their scientific colleagues have regarded that event with less interest and have tended to focus either upon conception, upon live birth, or upon the interim point at which the fetus becomes "viable," that is, potentially able to live outside the mother's womb, albeit with artificial aid. /59/ Viability is usually placed at about seven months (28 weeks) but may occur earlier, even at 24 weeks. /60/ The Aristotelian theory of "mediate animation," that held sway throughout the Middle Ages and the Renaissance in Europe, continued to be official Roman Catholic dogma until the 19th century, despite opposition to this "ensoulment" theory from those in the Church who would recognize the existence of life from the moment of conception. /61/ The latter is now, of course, the official belief of the Catholic Church. As one brief amicus discloses, this is a view strongly held by many non-Catholics as well, and by many physicians. Substantial problems for precise definition of this view are posed, however, by new embryological data that purport to indicate that conception is a "process" over time, rather than an

event, and by new medical techniques such as menstrual extraction, the "morning-after" pill, implantation of embryos, artificial insemination, and even artificial wombs. /62/

In areas other than criminal abortion, the law has been reluctant to endorse any theory that life, as we recognize it, begins before live birth or to accord legal rights to the unborn except in narrowly defined situations and except when the rights are contingent upon live birth. For example, the traditional rule of tort law denied recovery for prenatal injuries even though the child was born alive. /63/ That rule has been changed in almost every jurisdiction. In most States, recovery is said to be permitted only if the fetus was viable, or at least quick, when the injuries were sustained, though few courts have squarely so held. /64/ In a recent development, generally opposed by the commentators, some States permit the parents of a stillborn child to maintain an action for wrongful death because of prenatal injures. /65/ Such an action, however, would appear to be one to vindicate the parents' interest and is thus consistent with the view that the fetus, at most, represents only the potentiality of life. Similarly, unborn children have been recognized as acquiring rights or interests by way of inheritance or other devolution of property, and have been represented by guardians ad litem. /66/ Perfection of the interests involved, again, has generally been contingent upon live birth. In short, the unborn have never been recognized in the law as persons in the whole sense.

X

In view of all this, we do not agree that, by adopting one theory of life, Texas may override the rights of the pregnant woman that are at stake. We repeat, however, that the State does have an important and legitimate interest in preserving and protecting the health of the pregnant woman, whether she be a resident of the State or a nonresident who seeks medical consultation and treatment there, and that it has still another important and legitimate interest in protecting the potentiality of human life. These interests are separate and distinct. Each grows in substantiality as the woman approaches term and, at a point during pregnancy, each becomes "compelling."

With respect to the State's important and legitimate interest in the health of the mother, the "compelling" point, in the light of present medical knowledge, is at approximately the end of the first trimester. This is so because of the now-established medical fact, referred to above at 149, that until the end of the first trimester mortality in abortion may be less than mortality in normal childbirth. It follows that, from and after this point, a State may regulate the abortion procedure to the extent that the regulation reasonably relates to the preservation and protection of maternal health. Examples of permissible state regulation in this area are requirements as to the qualifications of the person who is to perform the abortion; as to the licensure of that person; as to the facility in which the procedure is to be performed, that is, whether it must be a hospital or may be a clinic or some other place of less-than-hospital status; as to the licensing of the facility; and the like.

This means, on the other hand, that, for the period of pregnancy prior to this "compelling" point, the attending physician, in consultation with his patient, is free to determine, without regulation by the State, that, in his medical judgment, the patient's pregnancy should be terminated. If that decision is reached, the judgment may be effectuated by an abortion free of interference by the State.

With respect to the State's important and legitimate interest in potential life, the "compelling" point is at viability. This is so because the fetus then presumably has the capability of meaningful life outside the mother's womb. State regulation protective of fetal life after viability thus has both logical and biological justifications. If the State is interested in protecting fetal life after viability, it may go so far as to proscribe abortion during that period, except when it is necessary to preserve the life or health of the mother.

Measured against these standards, Art. 1196 of the Texas penal code, in restricting legal abortions to those "procured or attempted by medical advice for the purpose of saving the life of the mother," sweeps too broadly. The statute makes no distinction between abortions performed early in pregnancy and those performed later, and it limits to a single reason, "saving" the mother's life, the legal justification for the procedure. The statute, therefore, cannot survive the constitutional attack made upon it here.

This conclusion makes it unnecessary for us to consider the additional challenge to the Texas statute asserted on grounds of vagueness. See *United States v. Vuitch*, 402 U.S., at 67-72.

XI

To summarize and to repeat:

1. A state criminal abortion statute of the current Texas type, that excepts from criminality only a lifesaving procedure on behalf of the mother, without regard to pregnancy stage and without recognition of the other interests involved, is violative of the Due Process Clause of the Fourteenth Amendment.

(a) For the stage prior to approximately the end of the first trimester, the abortion decision and its effectuation must be left to the medical judgment of the pregnant woman's attending physician.

(b) For the stage subsequent to approximately the end of the first trimester, the State, in promoting its interest in the health of the mother, may, if it chooses, regulate the abortion procedure in ways that are reasonably related to maternal health.

(c) For the stage subsequent to viability, the State in promoting its interest in the potentiality of human life may, if it chooses, regulate, and even proscribe, abortion except where it is necessary, in appropriate medical judgment, for the preservation of the life or health of the mother.

2. The State may define the term "physician," as it has been employed in the preceding paragraphs of this Part XI of this opinion, to mean only a physician currently licensed by the state, and may proscribe any abortion by a person who is not a physician as so defined.

In *Doe v. Bolton*, post, p. 179, procedural requirements contained in one of the modern abortion statutes are considered. That opinion and this one, of course, are to be read together. /67/

This holding, we feel, is consistent with the relative weights of the respective interests involved, with the lessons and examples of medical and legal history, with the lenity of the common law, and with the demands of the profound problems of the present day. The decision leaves the State free to place increasing restrictions on abortion as the period of pregnancy lengthens, so long as those restrictions are tailored to the recognized state interests. The decision vindicates the right of the physician to administer medical treatment according to his professional judgment up to the points where important state interests provide compelling justifications for intervention. Up to those points, the abortion decision in all its aspects is inherently, and primarily, a medical decision, and basic responsibility for it must rest with the physician. If an individual practitioner abuses the privilege of exercising proper medical judgment, the usual remedies, judicial and intra-professional, are available.

XII

Our conclusion that Art. 1196 is unconstitutional means, of course, that the Texas abortion statutes, as a unit, must fall. The exception of Art. 1196 cannot be struck down separately, for then the State could be left with a statute proscribing all abortion procedures no matter how medically urgent the case.

Although the District Court granted appellant Roe declaratory relief, it stopped short of issuing an injunction against enforcement of the Texas statutes. The court has recognized that different considerations enter into a federal court's decision as to declaratory relief, on the one hand, and injunctive relief, on the other. *Zwickler v. Koota*, 389 U.S. 241, 252-255 (1967); *Dombrowski v. Pfister*, 380 U.S. 479 (1965). We are not dealing with a statute that, on its face, appears to abridge free expression, an area of particular concern under Dombrowski and refined in *Younger v. Harris*, 401 U.S., At 50.

We find it unnecessary to decide whether the District Court erred in withholding injunctive relief, for we assume the Texas prosecutorial authorities will give full credence to this decision that the present criminal abortion statutes of that State are unconstitutional.

The judgment of the District Court as to intervenor Hallford is reversed, and Dr. Hallford's complaint in intervention is dismissed. In all other respects, the judgment of the district court is affirmed. Costs are allowed to the appellee.

It is so ordered.

[Concurring and dissenting opinions omitted.]

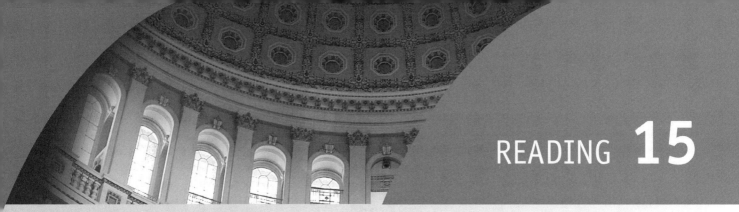

Case Law: *Planned Parenthood v. Casey* (Validity of Pennsylvania Abortion Statute)

PLANNED PARENTHOOD OF SOUTHEASTERN PENNSYLVANIA, et al., PETITIONERS 91-744 v. ROBERT P. CASEY, et al., etc. PETITIONERS 91-902

SUPREME COURT OF THE UNITED STATES

Nos. 91-744 and 91-902

ON WRITS OF CERTIORARI TO THE UNITED STATES COURT OF APPEALS FOR THE THIRD CIRCUIT

[June 29, 1992]

O'CONNOR, KENNEDY, and SOUTER, JJ., announced the judgment of the Court and delivered the opinion of the Court with respect to Parts I, II, III, V-A, V-C, and VI, in which BLACKMUN and STEVENS, JJ., joined, an opinion with respect to Part V-E, in which STEVENS, J., joined, and an opinion with respect to Parts IV, V-B, and V-D. STEVENS, J., filed an opinion concurring in part and dissenting in part, *post,* p. 911. BLACKMUN, J., filed an opinion concurring in part, concurring in the judgment in part, and dissenting in part, *post,* p. 922. REHNQUIST, C. J., filed an opinion concurring in the judgment in part and dissenting in part, in which WHITE, SCALIA, and THOMAS, JJ., joined, *post,* p. 944. SCALIA, J., filed an opinion concurring in the judgment in part and dissenting in part, in which REHNQUIST, C. J., and WHITE and THOMAS, JJ., joined, *post,* p. 979.

Liberty finds no refuge in a jurisprudence of doubt. Yet 19 years after our holding that the Constitution protects a woman's right to terminate her pregnancy in its early stages, *Roe* v. *Wade,* 410 U.S. 113 (1973), that definition of Liberty is still questioned. Joining the respondents as *amicus curiae,* the United States, as it has done in five other cases in the last decade, again asks us to overrule *Roe.* See Brief for Respondents 104-117; Brief for United States as *Amicus Curiae* 8.

At issue in these cases are five provisions of the Pennsylvania Abortion Control Act of 1982 as amended in 1988 and 1989. 18 Pa. Cons. Stat. §§ 3203-3220 (1990). Relevant portions of the Act are set forth in the appendix. *Infra,* at 60. The Act requires that a woman seeking an abortion give her informed consent prior to the abortion procedure, and specifies that she be provided with certain information at least 24 hours before the abortion is performed. § 3205. For a minor to obtain an abortion, the Act requires the informed consent of one of her parents, but provides for a judicial bypass option if the minor does not wish to or cannot obtain a parent's consent. § 3206. Another provision of the Act requires that, unless certain exceptions apply, a married woman seeking an abortion must sign a statement indicating that she has notified her husband of her intended abortion. § 3209. The Act exempts compliance with these three requirements in the event of a "medical emergency," which is defined in § 3203 of the Act. See §§ 3203, 3205(a), 3206(a), 3209(c). In addition to the above provisions regulating the performance of abortions, the Act imposes certain reporting requirements on facilities that provide abortion services. §§ 3207(b), 3214(a), 3214(f).

Before any of these provisions took effect, the petitioners, who are five abortion clinics and one physician representing himself as well as a class of physicians who provide abortion services, brought this suit seeking declaratory and injunctive relief. Each provision was challenged as unconstitutional on its face. The District Court entered a preliminary injunction against the enforcement of the regulations, and, after a 3 day bench trial, held all the provisions at issue here unconstitutional, entering a permanent injunction against Pennsylvania's enforcement of them. 744 F.Supp. 1323 (ED Pa. 1990). The Court of Appeals for the Third Circuit affirmed in part and reversed in part, upholding all of the regulations except for the husband notification requirement. 947 F. 2d 682 (1991). We granted certiorari. 502 U.S. ____ (1992).

The Court of Appeals found it necessary to follow an elaborate course of reasoning even to identify the first premise to use to determine whether the statute enacted by Pennsylvania meets constitutional standards. See 947 F. 2d, at 687-698. And at oral argument in this Court, the attorney for the parties challenging the statute took the position that none of the enactments can be upheld without overruling *Roe* v. *Wade*. Tr. of Oral Arg. 5-6. We disagree with that analysis; but we acknowledge that our decisions after *Roe* cast doubt upon the meaning and reach of its holding. Further, the Chief Justice admits that he would overrule the central holding of *Roe* and adopt the rational relationship test as the sole criterion of constitutionality. See *post*, at ____. State and federal courts as well as legislatures throughout the Union must have guidance as they seek to address this subject in conformance with the Constitution. Given these premises, we find it imperative to review once more the principles that define the rights of the woman and the legitimate authority of the State respecting the termination of pregnancies by abortion procedures.

After considering the fundamental constitutional questions resolved by *Roe*, principles of institutional integrity, and the rule of *stare decisis*, we are led to conclude this: the essential holding of *Roe* v. *Wade* should be retained and once again reaffirmed.

It must be stated at the outset and with clarity that *Roe's* essential holding, the holding we reaffirm, has three parts. First is a recognition of the right of the woman to choose to have an abortion before viability and to obtain it without undue interference from the State. Before viability, the State's interests are not strong enough to support a prohibition of abortion or the imposition of a substantial obstacle to the woman's effective right to elect the procedure. Second is a confirmation of the State's power to restrict abortions after fetal viability, if the law contains exceptions for pregnancies which endanger a woman's life or health. And third is the principle that the State has legitimate interests from the outset of the pregnancy in protecting the health of the woman and the life of the fetus that may become a child. These principles do not contradict one another; and we adhere to each.

Constitutional protection of the woman's decision to terminate her pregnancy derives from the Due Process Clause of the Fourteenth Amendment. It declares that no State shall "de-prive any person of life, liberty, or property, without due process of law." The controlling word in the case before us is "liberty." Although a literal reading of the Clause might suggest that it governs only the procedures by which a State may deprive persons of liberty, for at least 105 years, at least since *Mugler* v. *Kansas*, 123 U.S. 623, 660-661 (1887), the Clause has been understood to contain a substantive component as well, one "barring certain government actions regardless of the fairness of the procedures used to implement them." *Daniels* v. *Williams*, 474 U.S. 327, 331 (1986). As Justice Brandeis (joined by Justice Holmes) observed, "[d]espite arguments to the contrary which had seemed to me persuasive, it is settled that the due process clause of the Fourteenth Amendment applies to matters of substantive law as well as to matters of procedure. Thus all fundamental rights comprised within the term liberty are protected by the Federal Constitution from invasion by the States." *Whitney* v. *California*, 274 U.S. 357, 373 (1927) (Brandeis, J., concurring). "[T]he guaranties of due process, though having their roots in Magna Carta's '*per legem terrae*' and considered as procedural safeguards 'against executive usurpation and tyranny,' have in this country 'become bulwarks also against arbitrary legislation.'" *Poe* v. *Ullman*, 367 U.S. 497, 541 (1961) (Harlan, J., dissenting from dismissal on jurisdictional grounds) (quoting *Hurtado* v. *California*, 110 U.S. 516, 532 (1884)).

The most familiar of the substantive liberties protected by the Fourteenth Amendment are those recognized by the Bill of Rights. We have held that the Due Process Clause of the Fourteenth Amendment incorporates most of the Bill of Rights against the States. See, *e. g.*, *Duncan* v. *Louisiana*, 391 U.S. 145, 147-148 (1968). It is tempting, as a means of curbing the discretion of federal judges, to suppose that liberty encompasses no more than those rights already guaranteed to the individual against federal interference by the express provisions of the first eight amendments to the Constitution. See *Adamson* v. *California*, 332 U.S. 46, 68-92 (1947) (Black, J., dissenting). But of course this Court has never accepted that view.

It is also tempting, for the same reason, to suppose that the Due Process Clause protects only those practices, defined at the most specific level, that were protected against government interference by other rules of law when the Fourteenth Amendment was ratified. See *Michael H.* v. *Gerald D.*, 491 U.S. 110, 127-128, n. 6 (1989) (opinion of Scalia, J.). But such a view would be inconsistent with our law. It is a promise of the Constitution that there is a realm of personal liberty which the government may not enter. We have vindicated this principle before. Marriage is mentioned nowhere in the Bill of Rights and interracial marriage was illegal in most States in the 19th century, but the Court was no doubt correct in finding it to be an aspect of liberty protected against state interference by the substantive component of the Due Process Clause in *Loving* v. *Virginia*, 388 U.S. 1, 12 (1967) (relying, in an opinion for eight Justices, on the Due Process Clause). Similar examples may be found in *Turner* v. *Safley*, 482 U.S. 78, 94-99 (1987); in *Carey* v. *Population Services International*, 431 U.S. 678, 684-686 (1977); in *Griswold* v. *Connecticut*, 381 U.S. 479, 481-482 (1965), as well as in the separate opinions of a majority of the Members of the Court in that case, *id.*, at 486-488 (Goldberg J., joined by Warren, C. J., and Brennan, J., concurring) (expressly relying on due process), *id.*, at 500-502 (Harlan, J., concurring in judgment) (same), *id.*, at 502-507 (White, J., concurring in judgment) (same); in *Pierce* v. *Society of Sisters*, 268 U.S. 510, 534-535 (1925); and in *Meyer* v. *Nebraska*, 262 U.S. 390, 399-403 (1923).

Neither the Bill of Rights nor the specific practices of States at the time of the adoption of the Fourteenth Amendment marks the outer limits of the substantive sphere of liberty which the Fourteenth Amendment protects. See U. S. Const., Amend. 9. As the second Justice Harlan recognized:

> "[T]he full scope of the liberty guaranteed by the Due Process Clause cannot be found in or limited by the precise terms of the specific guarantees elsewhere provided in the Constitution. This 'liberty' is not a series of isolated points pricked out in terms of the taking of property; the freedom of speech, press, and religion; the right to keep and bear arms; the freedom from unreasonable searches and seizures; and so on. It is a rational continuum which, broadly speaking, includes a freedom from all substantial arbitrary impositions and purposeless restraints, . . . and which also recognizes, what a reasonable and sensitive judgment must, that certain interests require particularly careful scrutiny of the state needs asserted to justify their abridgment." *Poe* v. *Ullman, supra*, at 543 (Harlan, J., dissenting from dismissal on jurisdictional grounds).

Justice Harlan wrote these words in addressing an issue the full Court did not reach in *Poe* v. *Ullman*, but the Court adopted his position four Terms later in *Griswold* v. *Connecticut, supra*. In *Griswold*, we held that the Constitution does not permit a State to forbid a married couple to use contraceptives. That same freedom was later guaranteed, under the Equal Protection Clause, for unmarried couples. See *Eisenstadt* v. *Baird*, 405 U.S. 438 (1972). Constitutional protection was extended to the sale and distribution of contraceptives in *Carey* v. *Population Services International, supra*. It is settled now, as

it was when the Court heard arguments in *Roe* v. *Wade*, that the Constitution places limits on a State's right to interfere with a person's most basic decisions about family and parenthood, see *Carey* v. *Population Services International, supra; Moore* v. *East Cleveland*, 431 U.S. 494 (1977); *Eisenstadt* v. *Baird, supra; Loving* v. *Virginia, supra; Griswold* v. *Connecticut, supra; Skinner* v. *Oklahoma ex rel. Williamson*, 316 U.S. 535 (1942); *Pierce* v. *Society of Sisters, supra; Meyer* v. *Nebraska, supra*, as well as bodily integrity. See, *e. g., Washington* v. *Harper*, 494 U.S. 210, 221-222 (1990); *Winston* v. *Lee*, 470 U.S. 753 (1985); *Rochin* v. *California*, 342 U.S. 165 (1952).

The inescapable fact is that adjudication of substantive due process claims may call upon the Court in interpreting the Constitution to exercise that same capacity which by tradition courts always have exercised: reasoned judgment. Its boundaries are not susceptible of expression as a simple rule. That does not mean we are free to invalidate state policy choices with which we disagree; yet neither does it permit us to shrink from the duties of our office. As Justice Harlan observed:

> "Due process has not been reduced to any formula; its content cannot be determined by reference to any code. The best that can be said is that through the course of this Court's decisions it has represented the balance which our Nation, built upon postulates of respect for the liberty of the individual, has struck between that liberty and the demands of organized society. If the supplying of content to this Constitutional concept has of necessity been a rational process, it certainly has not been one where judges have felt free to roam where unguided speculation might take them. The balance of which I speak is the balance struck by this country, having regard to what history teaches are the traditions from which it developed as well as the traditions from which it broke. That tradition is a living thing. A decision of this Court which radically departs from it could not long survive, while a decision which builds on what has survived is likely to be sound. No formula could serve as a substitute, in this area, for judgment and restraint." *Poe* v. *Ullman*, 367 U. S., at 542 (Harlan, J., dissenting from dismissal on jurisdictional grounds).

See also *Rochin* v. *California, supra*, at 171-172 (Frankfurter, J., writing for the Court) ("To believe that this judicial exercise of judgment could be avoided by freezing 'due process of law' at some fixed stage of time or thought is to suggest that the most important aspect of constitutional adjudication is a function for inanimate machines and not for judges").

Men and women of good conscience can disagree, and we suppose some always shall disagree, about the profound moral and spiritual implications of terminating a pregnancy, even in its earliest stage. Some of us as individuals find abortion offensive to our most basic principles of morality, but that cannot control our decision. Our obligation is to define the liberty of all, not to mandate our own moral code. The underlying constitutional issue is whether the State can resolve these philosophic questions in such a definitive way that a woman lacks all choice in the matter, except perhaps in those rare circumstances in which the pregnancy is itself a danger to her own life or health, or is the result of rape or incest.

It is conventional constitutional doctrine that where reasonable people disagree the government can adopt one position or the other. See, *e. g.*, *Ferguson* v. *Skrupa*, 372 U.S. 726 (1963); *Williamson* v. *Lee Optical of Oklahoma, Inc.*, 348 U.S. 483 (1955). That theorem, however, assumes a state of affairs in which the choice does not intrude upon a protected liberty. Thus, while some people might disagree about whether or not the flag should be saluted, or disagree about the proposition that it may not be defiled, we have ruled that a State may not compel or enforce one view or the other. See *West Virginia State Bd. of Education* v. *Barnette*, 319 U.S. 624 (1943); *Texas* v. *Johnson*, 491 U.S. 397 (1989).

Our law affords constitutional protection to personal decisions relating to marriage, procreation, contraception, family relationships, child rearing, and education. *Carey* v. *Population Services International*, 431 U. S., at 685. Our cases recognize "the right of the *individual*, married or single, to be free from unwarranted governmental intrusion into matters so fundamentally affecting a person as the decision whether to bear or beget a child." *Eisenstadt* v. *Baird, supra*, at 453 (emphasis in original). Our precedents "have respected the private realm of family life which the state cannot enter." *Prince* v. *Massachusetts*, 321 U.S. 158, 166 (1944). These matters, involving the most intimate and personal choices a person may make in a lifetime, choices central to personal dignity and autonomy, are central to the liberty protected by the Fourteenth Amendment. At the heart of liberty is the right to define one's own concept of existence, of meaning, of the universe, and of the mystery of human life. Beliefs about these matters could not define the attributes of personhood were they formed under compulsion of the State.

These considerations begin our analysis of the woman's interest in terminating her pregnancy but cannot end it, for this reason: though the abortion decision may originate within the zone of conscience and belief, it is more than a philosophic exercise. Abortion is a unique act. It is an act fraught with consequences for others: for the woman who must live with the implications of her decision; for the persons who perform and assist in the procedure; for the spouse, family, and society which must confront the knowledge that these procedures exist, procedures some deem nothing short of an act of violence against innocent human life; and, depending on one's beliefs, for the life or potential life that is aborted. Though abortion is conduct, it does not follow that the State is entitled to proscribe it in all instances. That is because the liberty of the woman is at stake in a sense unique to the human condition and so unique to the law. The mother who carries a child to full term is subject to anxieties, to physical constraints, to pain that only she must bear. That these sacrifices have from the beginning of the human race been endured by woman with a pride that ennobles her in the eyes of others and gives to the infant a bond of love cannot alone be grounds for the State to insist she make the sacrifice. Her suffering is too intimate and personal for the State to insist, without more, upon its own vision of the woman's role, however dominant that vision has been in the course of our history and our culture. The destiny of the woman must be shaped to a large extent on her own conception of her spiritual imperatives and her place in society.

It should be recognized, moreover, that in some critical respects the abortion decision is of the same character as the decision to use contraception, to which *Griswold* v. *Connecticut*, *Eisenstadt* v. *Baird*, and *Carey* v. *Population Services International*, afford constitutional protection. We have no doubt as to the correctness of those decisions. They support the reasoning in *Roe* relating to the woman's liberty because they involve personal decisions concerning not only the meaning of procreation but also human responsibility and respect for it. As with abortion, reasonable people will have differences of opinion about these matters. One view is based on such reverence for the wonder of creation that any pregnancy ought to be welcomed and carried to full term no matter how difficult it will be to provide for the child and ensure its well being. Another is that the inability to provide for the nurture and care of the infant is a cruelty to the child and an anguish to the parent. These are intimate views with infinite variations, and their deep, personal character underlay our decisions in *Griswold*, *Eisenstadt*, and *Carey*. The same concerns are present when the woman confronts the reality that, perhaps despite her attempts to avoid it, she has become pregnant.

It was this dimension of personal liberty that *Roe* sought to protect, and its holding invoked the reasoning and the tradition of the precedents we have discussed, granting protection to substantive liberties of the person. *Roe* was, of course, an extension of those cases and, as the decision itself indicated, the separate States could act in some degree to further their own legitimate interests in protecting pre-natal life. The extent to which the legislatures of the States might act to outweigh the interests of the woman in choosing to terminate her pregnancy was a subject of debate both in *Roe* itself and in decisions following it.

While we appreciate the weight of the arguments made on behalf of the State in the case before us, arguments which in their ultimate formulation conclude that *Roe* should be overruled, the reservations any of us may have in reaffirming the central holding of *Roe* are outweighed by the explication of individual liberty we have given combined with the force of *stare decisis*. We turn now to that doctrine.

The obligation to follow precedent begins with necessity, and a contrary necessity marks its outer limit. With Cardozo, we recognize that no judicial system could do society's work if it eyed each issue afresh in every case that raised it. See B. Cardozo, The Nature of the Judicial Process 149 (1921). Indeed, the very concept of the rule of law underlying our own Constitution requires such continuity over time that a respect for precedent is, by definition, indispensable. See Powell, Stare Decisis and Judicial Restraint, 1991 Journal of Supreme Court History 13, 16. At the other extreme, a different necessity would make itself felt if a prior judicial ruling should come to be seen so clearly as error that its enforcement was for that very reason doomed.

Even when the decision to overrule a prior case is not, as in the rare, latter instance, virtually foreordained, it is common wisdom that the rule of *stare decisis* is not an "inexorable command," and certainly it is not such in every constitutional case, see *Burnet* v. *Coronado Oil Gas Co.*, 285 U.S. 393, 405-411 (1932) (Brandeis, J., dissenting). See also *Payne* v. *Tennessee*, 501 U. S. ____, ____ (1991) (slip op., at ___) (Souter, J., joined by Kennedy, J., concurring); *Arizona* v. *Rumsey*, 467 U.S. 203, 212 (1984). Rather, when this Court reexamines a prior holding, its judgment is customarily informed by a series of prudential and pragmatic considerations designed to test the consistency of overruling a prior decision with the ideal of the rule of law, and to gauge the respective costs of reaffirming and overruling a prior case. Thus, for example, we may ask whether the rule has proved to be intolerable simply in defying practical workability, *Swift & Co.* v. *Wickham*, 382 U.S. 111, 116 (1965); whether the rule is subject to a kind of reliance that would lend a special hardship to the consequences of overruling and add inequity to the cost of repudiation, *e. g., United States* v. *Title Ins. & Trust Co.*, 265 U.S. 472, 486 (1924); whether related principles of law have so far developed as to have left the old rule no more than a remnant of abandoned doctrine, see *Patterson* v. *McLean Credit Union*, 491 U.S. 164, 173-174 (1989);

or whether facts have so changed or come to be seen so differently, as to have robbed the old rule of significant application or justification, *e. g., Burnet, supra*, at 412 (Brandeis, J., dissenting).

So in this case we may inquire whether *Roe's* central rule has been found unworkable; whether the rule's limitation on state power could be removed without serious inequity to those who have relied upon it or significant damage to the stability of the society governed by the rule in question; whether the law's growth in the intervening years has left *Roe's* central rule a doctrinal anachronism discounted by society; and whether *Roe's* premises of fact have so far changed in the ensuing two decades as to render its central holding somehow irrelevant or unjustifiable in dealing with the issue it addressed.

Although *Roe* has engendered opposition, it has in no sense proven "unworkable," see *Garcia* v. *San Antonio Metropolitan Transit Authority*, 469 U.S. 528, 546 (1985), representing as it does a simple limitation beyond which a state law is unenforceable. While *Roe* has, of course, required judicial assessment of state laws affecting the exercise of the choice guaranteed against government infringement, and although the need for such review will remain as a consequence of today's decision, the required determinations fall within judicial competence.

The inquiry into reliance counts the cost of a rule's repudiation as it would fall on those who have relied reasonably on the rule's continued application. Since the classic case for weighing reliance heavily in favor of following the earlier rule occurs in the commercial context, see *Payne* v. *Tennessee, supra*, at ____ (slip op., at ___), where advance planning of great precision is most obviously a necessity, it is no cause for surprise that some would find no reliance worthy of consideration in support of *Roe*.

While neither respondents nor their *amici* in so many words deny that the abortion right invites some reliance prior to its actual exercise, one can readily imagine an argument stressing the dissimilarity of this case to one involving property or contract. Abortion is customarily chosen as an unplanned response to the consequence of unplanned activity or to the failure of conventional birth control, and except on the assumption that no intercourse would have occurred but for *Roe's* holding, such behavior may appear to justify no reliance claim. Even if reliance could be claimed on that unrealistic assumption, the argument might run, any reliance interest would be *de minimis*. This argument would be premised on the hypothesis that reproductive planning could take virtually immediate account of any sudden restoration of state authority to ban abortions.

To eliminate the issue of reliance that easily, however, one would need to limit cognizable reliance to specific instances of sexual activity. But to do this would be simply to refuse to face the fact that for two decades of economic and social developments, people have organized intimate relationships and made choices that define their views of themselves and their places in society, in reliance on the availability of abortion in the event that contraception should fail. The ability of women to participate equally in the economic and social life of the Nation has been facilitated by their ability to control their reproductive lives. See, *e.g.*, R. Petchesky, Abortion and Woman's Choice 109, 133, n. 7 (rev. ed. 1990). The Constitution serves human values, and while the effect of reliance on *Roe* cannot be exactly measured, neither can the certain cost of overruling *Roe* for people who have ordered their thinking and living around that case be dismissed.

No evolution of legal principle has left *Roe*'s doctrinal footings weaker than they were in 1973. No development of constitutional law since the case was decided has implicitly or explicitly left *Roe* behind as a mere survivor of obsolete constitutional thinking.

It will be recognized, of course, that *Roe* stands at an intersection of two lines of decisions, but in whichever doctrinal category one reads the case, the result for present purposes will be the same. The *Roe* Court itself placed its holding in the succession of cases most prominently exemplified by *Griswold* v. *Connecticut*, 381 U.S. 479 (1965), see *Roe*, 410 U. S., at 152-153. When it is so seen, *Roe* is clearly in no jeopardy, since subsequent constitutional developments have neither disturbed, nor do they threaten to diminish, the scope of recognized protection accorded to the liberty relating to intimate relationships, the family, and decisions about whether or not to beget or bear a child. See, *e.g.*, *Carey* v. *Population Services International*, 431 U.S. 678 (1977); *Moore* v. *East Cleveland*, 431 U.S. 678 (1977).

Roe, however, may be seen not only as an exemplar of *Griswold* liberty but as a rule (whether or not mistaken) of personal autonomy and bodily integrity, with doctrinal affinity to cases recognizing limits on governmental power to mandate medical treatment or to bar its rejection. If so, our cases since *Roe* accord with *Roe*'s view that a State's interest in the protection of life falls short of justifying any plenary override of individual liberty claims. *Cruzan* v. *Director, Missouri Dept. of Health*, 497 U.S. 261,278 (1990); Cf., *e.g.*, *Riggins* v. *Nevada*, 504 U.S. ____, ____ (1992) (slip. op., at 7); *Washington* v. *Harper*, 494 U.S. 210 (1990); see also, *e.g.*, *Rochin* v. *California*, 342 U.S. 165 (1952); *Jacobson* v. *Massachusetts*, 197 U.S. 11, 24-30 (1905).

Finally, one could classify *Roe* as *sui generis*. If the case is so viewed, then there clearly has been no erosion of its central determination. The original holding resting on the concur-

rence of seven Members of the Court in 1973 was expressly affirmed by a majority of six in 1983, see *Akron* v. *Akron Center for Reproductive Health, Inc.*, 462 U.S. 416 (1983) *(Akron I)*, and by a majority of five in 1986, see *Thornburgh* v. *American College of Obstetricians and Gynecologists*, 476 U.S. 747 (1986), expressing adherence to the constitutional ruling despite legislative efforts in some States to test its limits. More recently, in *Webster* v. *Reproductive Health Services*, 492 U.S. 490 (1989), although two of the present authors questioned the trimester framework in a way consistent with our judgment today, see *id.*, at 518 (Rehnquist C. J., joined by White, and Kennedy, JJ.); *id.*, at 529 (O'Connor, J., concurring in part and concurring in judgment), a majority of the Court either decided to reaffirm or declined to address the constitutional validity of the central holding of *Roe*. See *Webster*, 492 U. S., at 521 (Rehnquist, C. J., joined by White and Kennedy, JJ.); *id.*, at 525-526 (O'Connor, J., concurring in part and concurring in judgment); *id.*, at 537, 553 (Blackmun, J., joined by Brennan and Marshall, JJ., concurring in part and dissenting in part); *id.*, at 561-563 (Stevens, J., concurring in part and dissenting in part).

Nor will courts building upon *Roe* be likely to hand down erroneous decisions as a consequence. Even on the assumption that the central holding of *Roe* was in error, that error would go only to the strength of the state interest in fetal protection, not to the recognition afforded by the Constitution to the woman's liberty. The latter aspect of the decision fits comfortably within the framework of the Court's prior decisions including *Skinner* v. *Oklahoma ex rel. Williamson*, 316 U.S. 535 (1942), *Griswold, supra*, *Loving* v. *Virginia*, 388 U.S. 1 (1967), and *Eisenstadt* v. *Baird*, 405 U.S. 438 (1972), the holdings of which are "not a series of isolated points," but mark a "rational continuum." *Poe* v. *Ullman*, 367 U. S., at 543 (1961) (Harlan, J., dissenting). As we described in *Carey* v. *Population Services International*, *supra*, the liberty which encompasses those decisions "includes 'the interest in independence in making certain kinds of important decisions.' While the outer limits of this aspect of [protected liberty] have not been marked by the Court, it is clear that among the decisions that an individual may make without unjustified government interference are personal decisions 'relating to marriage, procreation, contraception, family relationships, and child rearing and education.' " *Id.*, at 684-685 (citations omitted).

The soundness of this prong of the *Roe* analysis is apparent from a consideration of the alternative. If indeed the woman's interest in deciding whether to bear and beget a child had not been recognized as in *Roe*, the State might as readily restrict a woman's right to choose to carry a pregnancy to term as to terminate it, to further asserted state interests in population control, or eugenics, for example. Yet *Roe* has been sensibly relied upon to counter any such suggestions. *E.g., Arnold* v. *Board of Education of Escambia County, Ala.,* 880 F. 2d 305, 311 (CA11 1989) (relying upon *Roe* and concluding that government officials violate the Constitution by coercing a minor to have an abortion); *Avery* v. *County of Burke,* 660 F. 2d 111, 115 (CA4 1981) (county agency inducing teenage girl to undergo unwanted sterilization on the basis of misrepresentation that she had sickle cell trait); see also *In re Quinlan,* 70 N.J. 10, 355 A. 2d 647, cert. denied *sub nom. Garger* v. *New Jersey,* 429 U.S. 922 (1976) (relying on *Roe* in finding a right to terminate medical treatment). In any event, because *Roe*'s scope is confined by the fact of its concern with postconception potential life, a concern otherwise likely to be implicated only by some forms of contraception protected independently under *Griswold* and later cases, any error in *Roe* is unlikely to have serious ramifications in future cases.

We have seen how time has overtaken some of *Roe*'s factual assumptions: advances in maternal health care allow for abortions safe to the mother later in pregnancy than was true in 1973, see *Akron I, supra,* at 429, n. 11, and advances in neonatal care have advanced viability to a point somewhat earlier. Compare *Roe,* 410 U. S., at 160, with *Webster, supra,* at 515-516 (opinion of Rehnquist, C.J.); see *Akron I, supra,* at 457, and n. 5 (O'Connor, J., dissenting). But these facts go only to the scheme of time limits on the realization of competing interests, and the divergences from the factual premises of 1973 have no bearing on the validity of *Roe*'s central holding, that viability marks the earliest point at which the State's interest in fetal life is constitutionally adequate to justify a legislative ban on nontherapeutic abortions. The soundness or unsoundness of that constitutional judgment in no sense turns on whether viability occurs at approximately 28 weeks, as was usual at the time of *Roe,* at 23 to 24 weeks, as it sometimes does today, or at some moment even slightly earlier in pregnancy, as it may if fetal respiratory capacity can somehow be enhanced in the future. Whenever it may occur, the attainment of viability may continue to serve as the critical fact, just as it has done since *Roe* was decided; which is to say that no change in *Roe*'s factual underpinning has left its central holding obsolete, and none supports an argument for overruling it.

The sum of the precedential inquiry to this point shows *Roe*'s underpinnings unweakened in any way affecting its central holding. While it has engendered disapproval, it has not been unworkable. An entire generation has come of age free to assume *Roe*'s concept of liberty in defining the capacity of women to act in society, and to make reproductive decisions; no erosion of principle going to liberty or personal autonomy has left *Roe*'s central holding a doctrinal remnant; *Roe* por-

tends no developments at odds with other precedent for the analysis of personal liberty; and no changes of fact have rendered viability more or less appropriate as the point at which the balance of interests tips. Within the bounds of normal *stare decisis* analysis, then, and subject to the considerations on which it customarily turns, the stronger argument is for affirming *Roe*'s central holding, with whatever degree of personal reluctance any of us may have, not for overruling it.

In a less significant case, *stare decisis* analysis could, and would, stop at the point we have reached. But the sustained and widespread debate *Roe* has provoked calls for some comparison between that case and others of comparable dimension that have responded to national controversies and taken on the impress of the controversies addressed. Only two such decisional lines from the past century present themselves for examination, and in each instance the result reached by the Court accorded with the principles we apply today.

The first example is that line of cases identified with *Lochner* v. *New York,* 198 U.S. 45 (1905), which imposed substantive limitations on legislation limiting economic autonomy in favor of health and welfare regulation, adopting, in Justice Holmes' view, the theory of *laissez faire. Id.,* at 75 (Holmes, J., dissenting). The *Lochner* decisions were exemplified by *Adkins* v. *Children's Hospital of D.C.,* 261 U.S. 525 (1923), in which this Court held it to be an infringement of constitutionally protected liberty of contract to require the employers of adult women to satisfy minimum wage standards. Fourteen years later, *West Coast Hotel Co.* v. *Parrish,* 300 U.S. 379 (1937), signaled the demise of *Lochner* by overruling *Adkins.* In the meantime, the Depression had come and, with it, the lesson that seemed unmistakable to most people by 1937, that the interpretation of contractual freedom protected in *Adkins* rested on fundamentally false factual assumptions about the capacity of a relatively unregulated market to satisfy minimal levels of human welfare. See *West Coast Hotel Co., supra,* at 399. As Justice Jackson wrote of the constitutional crisis of 1937 shortly before he came on the bench, "The older world of *laissez faire* was recognized everywhere outside the Court to be dead." R. Jackson, The Struggle for Judicial Supremacy 85 (1941). The facts upon which the earlier case had premised a constitutional resolution of social controversy had proved to be untrue, and history's demonstration of their untruth not only justified but required the new choice of constitutional principle that *West Coast Hotel* announced. Of course, it was true that the Court lost something by its misperception, or its lack of prescience, and the Court packing crisis only magnified the loss; but the clear demonstration that the facts of economic life were different from those previously assumed warranted the repudiation of the old law.

The second comparison that 20th century history invites is with the cases employing the separate but equal rule for applying the Fourteenth Amendment's equal protection guarantee. They began with *Plessy* v. *Ferguson*, 163 U.S. 537 (1896), holding that legislatively mandated racial segregation in public transportation works no denial of equal protection, rejecting the argument that racial separation enforced by the legal machinery of American society treats the black race as inferior. The *Plessy* Court considered "the underlying fallacy of the plaintiff's argument to consist in the assumption that the enforced separation of the two races stamps the colored race with a badge of inferiority. If this be so, it is not by reason of anything found in the act, but solely because the colored race chooses to put that construction upon it." *Id.*, at 551. Whether, as a matter of historical fact, the Justices in the *Plessy* majority believed this or not, see *id.*, at 557, 562 (Harlan, J., dissenting), this understanding of the implication of segregation was the stated justification for the Court's opinion. But this understanding of the facts and the rule it was stated to justify were repudiated in *Brown* v. *Board of Education*, 347 U.S. 483 (1954). As one commentator observed, the question before the Court in *Brown* was "whether discrimination inheres in that segregation which is imposed by law in the twentieth century in certain specific states in the American Union. And that question has meaning and can find an answer only on the ground of history and of common knowledge about the facts of life in the times and places aforesaid." Black, The Lawfulness of the Segregation Decisions, 69 Yale L. J. 421, 427 (1960).

The Court in *Brown* addressed these facts of life by observing that whatever may have been the understanding in *Plessy*'s time of the power of segregation to stigmatize those who were segregated with a "badge of inferiority," it was clear by 1954 that legally sanctioned segregation had just such an effect, to the point that racially separate public educational facilities were deemed inherently unequal. 374 U.S., at 494-495. Society's understanding of the facts upon which a constitutional ruling was sought in 1954 was thus fundamentally different from the basis claimed for the decision in 1896. While we think *Plessy* was wrong the day it was decided, see *Plessy, supra,* at 552-564 (Harlan, J., dissenting), we must also recognize that the *Plessy* Court's explanation for its decision was so clearly at odds with the facts apparent to the Court in 1954 that the decision to reexamine *Plessy* was on this ground alone not only justified but required.

West Coast Hotel and *Brown* each rested on facts, or an understanding of facts, changed from those which furnished the claimed justifications for the earlier constitutional resolutions. Each case was comprehensible as the Court's response to facts that the country could understand, or had come to understand already, but which the Court of an earlier day, as its own declarations disclosed, had not been able to perceive. As the decisions were thus comprehensible they were also defensible, not merely as the victories of one doctrinal school over another by dint of numbers (victories though they were), but as applications of constitutional principle to facts as they had not been seen by the Court before. In constitutional adjudication as elsewhere in life, changed circumstances may impose new obligations, and the thoughtful part of the Nation could accept each decision to overrule a prior case as a response to the Court's constitutional duty.

Because the case before us presents no such occasion it could be seen as no such response. Because neither the factual underpinnings of *Roe*'s central holding nor our understanding of it has changed (and because no other indication of weakened precedent has been shown) the Court could not pretend to be reexamining the prior law with any justification beyond a present doctrinal disposition to come out differently from the Court of 1973. To overrule prior law for no other reason than that would run counter to the view repeated in our cases, that a decision to overrule should rest on some special reason over and above the belief that a prior case was wrongly decided. See, *e.g., Mitchell* v. *W. T. Grant*, 416 U.S. 600, 636 (1974) (Stewart, J., dissenting) ("A basic change in the law upon a ground no firmer than a change in our membership invites the popular misconception that this institution is little different from the two political branches of the Government. No misconception could do more lasting injury to this Court and to the system of law which it is our abiding mission to serve"); *Mapp* v. *Ohio*, 367 U.S. 643, 677 (1961) (Harlan, J., dissenting).

The examination of the conditions justifying the repudiation of *Adkins* by *West Coast Hotel* and *Plessy* by *Brown* is enough to suggest the terrible price that would have been paid if the Court had not overruled as it did. In the present case, however, as our analysis to this point makes clear, the terrible price would be paid for overruling. Our analysis would not be complete, however, without explaining why overruling *Roe*'s central holding would not only reach an unjustifiable result under principles of *stare decisis*, but would seriously weaken the Court's capacity to exercise the judicial power and to function as the Supreme Court of a Nation dedicated to the rule of law. To understand why this would be so it is necessary to understand the source of this Court's authority, the conditions necessary for its preservation, and its relationship to the country's understanding of itself as a constitutional Republic.

The root of American governmental power is revealed most clearly in the instance of the power conferred by the Constitution upon the Judiciary of the United States and specifically upon this Court. As Americans of each succeeding generation are rightly told, the Court cannot buy support for its decisions by spending money and, except to a minor degree, it cannot independently coerce obedience to its decrees. The Court's power lies, rather, in its legitimacy, a product of substance and perception that shows itself in the people's acceptance of the Judiciary as fit to determine what the Nation's law means and to declare what it demands.

The underlying substance of this legitimacy is of course the warrant for the Court's decisions in the Constitution and the lesser sources of legal principle on which the Court draws. That substance is expressed in the Court's opinions, and our contemporary understanding is such that a decision without principled justification would be no judicial act at all. But even when justification is furnished by apposite legal principle, something more is required. Because not every conscientious claim of principled justification will be accepted as such, the justification claimed must be beyond dispute. The Court must take care to speak and act in ways that allow people to accept its decisions on the terms the Court claims for them, as grounded truly in principle, not as compromises with social and political pressures having, as such, no bearing on the principled choices that the Court is obliged to make. Thus, the Court's legitimacy depends on making legally principled decisions under circumstances in which their principled character is sufficiently plausible to be accepted by the Nation.

The need for principled action to be perceived as such is implicated to some degree whenever this, or any other appellate court, overrules a prior case. This is not to say, of course, that this Court cannot give a perfectly satisfactory explanation in most cases. People understand that some of the Constitution's language is hard to fathom and that the Court's Justices are sometimes able to perceive significant facts or to understand principles of law that eluded their predecessors and that justify departures from existing decisions. However upsetting it may be to those most directly affected when one judicially derived rule replaces another, the country can accept some correction of error without necessarily questioning the legitimacy of the Court.

In two circumstances, however, the Court would almost certainly fail to receive the benefit of the doubt in overruling prior cases. There is, first, a point beyond which frequent overruling would overtax the country's belief in the Court's good faith. Despite the variety of reasons that may inform and justify a decision to overrule, we cannot forget that such a decision is usually perceived (and perceived correctly) as, at the least, a statement that a prior decision was wrong. There is a limit to the amount of error that can plausibly be imputed to prior courts. If that limit should be exceeded, disturbance of prior rulings would be taken as evidence that justifiable reex-

amination of principle had given way to drives for particular results in the short term. The legitimacy of the Court would fade with the frequency of its vacillation.

That first circumstance can be described as hypothetical; the second is to the point here and now. Where, in the performance of its judicial duties, the Court decides a case in such a way as to resolve the sort of intensely divisive controversy reflected in *Roe* and those rare, comparable cases, its decision has a dimension that the resolution of the normal case does not carry. It is the dimension present whenever the Court's interpretation of the Constitution calls the contending sides of a national controversy to end their national division by accepting a common mandate rooted in the Constitution.

The Court is not asked to do this very often, having thus addressed the Nation only twice in our lifetime, in the decisions of *Brown* and *Roe*. But when the Court does act in this way, its decision requires an equally rare precedential force to counter the inevitable efforts to overturn it and to thwart its implementation. Some of those efforts may be mere unprincipled emotional reactions; others may proceed from principles worthy of profound respect. But whatever the premises of opposition may be, only the most convincing justification under accepted standards of precedent could suffice to demonstrate that a later decision overruling the first was anything but a surrender to political pressure, and an unjustified repudiation of the principle on which the Court staked its authority in the first instance. So to overrule under fire in the absence of the most compelling reason to reexamine a watershed decision would subvert the Court's legitimacy beyond any serious question. Cf. *Brown* v. *Board of Education*, 349 U.S. 294, 300 (1955) (*Brown II*) ("[I]t should go without saying that the vitality of th[e] constitutional principles [announced in *Brown* v. *Board of Education*, 347 U.S. 483 (1954),] cannot be allowed to yield simply because of disagreement with them").

The country's loss of confidence in the judiciary would be underscored by an equally certain and equally reasonable condemnation for another failing in overruling unnecessarily and under pressure. Some cost will be paid by anyone who approves or implements a constitutional decision where it is unpopular, or who refuses to work to undermine the decision or to force its reversal. The price may be criticism or ostracism, or it may be violence. An extra price will be paid by those who themselves disapprove of the decision's results when viewed outside of constitutional terms, but who nevertheless struggle to accept it, because they respect the rule of law. To all those who will be so tested by following, the Court implicitly undertakes to remain steadfast, lest in the end a price be paid for nothing. The promise of constancy, once given, binds its maker for as long as the power to stand by the decision survives and the understanding of the issue has not changed so fundamentally as to render the commitment obsolete. From the obligation of this promise this Court cannot and should not assume any exemption when duty requires it to decide a case in conformance with the Constitution. A willing breach of it would be nothing less than a breach of faith, and no Court that broke its faith with the people could sensibly expect credit for principle in the decision by which it did that.

It is true that diminished legitimacy may be restored, but only slowly. Unlike the political branches, a Court thus weakened could not seek to regain its position with a new mandate from the voters, and even if the Court could somehow go to the polls, the loss of its principled character could not be retrieved by the casting of so many votes. Like the character of an individual, the legitimacy of the Court must be earned over time. So, indeed, must be the character of a Nation of people who aspire to live according to the rule of law. Their belief in themselves as such a people is not readily separable from their understanding of the Court invested with the authority to decide their constitutional cases and speak before all others for their constitutional ideals. If the Court's legitimacy should be undermined, then, so would the country be in its very ability to see itself through its constitutional ideals. The Court's concern with legitimacy is not for the sake of the Court but for the sake of the Nation to which it is responsible.

The Court's duty in the present case is clear. In 1973, it confronted the already divisive issue of governmental power to limit personal choice to undergo abortion, for which it provided a new resolution based on the due process guaranteed by the Fourteenth Amendment. Whether or not a new social consensus is developing on that issue, its divisiveness is no less today than in 1973, and pressure to overrule the decision, like pressure to retain it, has grown only more intense. A decision to overrule *Roe*'s essential holding under the existing circumstances would address error, if error there was, at the cost of both profound and unnecessary damage to the Court's legitimacy, and to the Nation's commitment to the rule of law. It is therefore imperative to adhere to the essence of *Roe*'s original decision, and we do so today.

From what we have said so far it follows that it is a constitutional liberty of the woman to have some freedom to terminate her pregnancy. We conclude that the basic decision in *Roe* was based on a constitutional analysis which we cannot now repudiate. The woman's liberty is not so unlimited, however, that from the outset the State cannot show its concern for the life of the unborn, and at a later point in fetal development the State's interest in life has sufficient force so that the right of the woman to terminate the pregnancy can be restricted.

That brings us, of course, to the point where much criticism has been directed at *Roe*, a criticism that always inheres when the Court draws a specific rule from what in the Constitution is but a general standard. We conclude, however, that the urgent claims of the woman to retain the ultimate control over her destiny and her body, claims implicit in the meaning of liberty, require us to perform that function. Liberty must not be extinguished for want of a line that is clear. And it falls to us to give some real substance to the woman's liberty to determine whether to carry her pregnancy to full term.

We conclude the line should be drawn at viability, so that before that time the woman has a right to choose to terminate her pregnancy. We adhere to this principle for two reasons. First, as we have said, is the doctrine of *stare decisis*. Any judicial act of line drawing may seem somewhat arbitrary, but *Roe* was a reasoned statement, elaborated with great care. We have twice reaffirmed it in the face of great opposition. See *Thornburgh* v. *American College of Obstetricians & Gynecologists*, 476 U. S., at 759; *Akron I*, 462 U. S., at 419–420. Although we must overrule those parts of *Thornburgh* and *Akron I* which, in our view, are inconsistent with *Roe*'s statement that the State has a legitimate interest in promoting the life or potential life of the unborn, see *infra*, at ___, the central premise of those cases represents an unbroken commitment by this Court to the essential holding of *Roe*. It is that premise which we reaffirm today.

The second reason is that the concept of viability, as we noted in *Roe*, is the time at which there is a realistic possibility of maintaining and nourishing a life outside the womb, so that the independent existence of the second life can in reason and all fairness be the object of state protection that now overrides the rights of the woman. See *Roe* v. *Wade*, 410 U. S., at 163. Consistent with other constitutional norms, legislatures may draw lines which appear arbitrary without the necessity of offering a justification. But courts may not. We must justify the lines we draw. And there is no line other than viability which is more workable. To be sure, as we have said, there may be some medical developments that affect the precise point of viability, see *supra*, at ___, but this is an imprecision within tolerable limits given that the medical community and all those who must apply its discoveries will continue to explore the matter. The viability line also has, as a practical matter, an element of fairness. In some broad sense it might be said that a woman who fails to act before viability has consented to the State's intervention on behalf of the developing child.

The woman's right to terminate her pregnancy before viability is the most central principle of *Roe* v. *Wade*. It is a rule of law and a component of liberty we cannot renounce.

On the other side of the equation is the interest of the State in the protection of potential life. The *Roe* Court recognized the State's "important and legitimate interest in protecting the potentiality of human life." *Roe, supra,* at 162. The weight to be given this state interest, not the strength of the woman's interest, was the difficult question faced in *Roe.* We do not need to say whether each of us, had we been Members of the Court when the valuation of the State interest came before it as an original matter, would have concluded, as the *Roe* Court did, that its weight is insufficient to justify a ban on abortions prior to viability even when it is subject to certain exceptions. The matter is not before us in the first instance, and coming as it does after nearly 20 years of litigation in *Roe's* wake we are satisfied that the immediate question is not the soundness of *Roe's* resolution of the issue, but the precedential force that must be accorded to its holding. And we have concluded that the essential holding of *Roe* should be reaffirmed.

Yet it must be remembered that *Roe* v. *Wade* speaks with clarity in establishing not only the woman's liberty but also the State's "important and legitimate interest in potential life." *Roe, supra,* at 163. That portion of the decision in *Roe* has been given too little acknowledgement and implementation by the Court in its subsequent cases. Those cases decided that any regulation touching upon the abortion decision must survive strict scrutiny, to be sustained only if drawn in narrow terms to further a compelling state interest. See, *e. g., Akron I, supra,* at 427. Not all of the cases decided under that formulation can be reconciled with the holding in *Roe* itself that the State has legitimate interests in the health of the woman and in protecting the potential life within her. In resolving this tension, we choose to rely upon *Roe,* as against the later cases.

Roe established a trimester framework to govern abortion regulations. Under this elaborate but rigid construct, almost no regulation at all is permitted during the first trimester of pregnancy; regulations designed to protect the woman's health, but not to further the State's interest in potential life, are permitted during the second trimester; and during the third trimester, when the fetus is viable, prohibitions are permitted provided the life or health of the mother is not at stake. *Roe* v. *Wade, supra,* at 163-166. Most of our cases since *Roe* have involved the application of rules derived from the trimester framework. See, *e. g., Thornburgh* v. *American College of Obstetricians and Gynecologists, supra; Akron I, supra.*

The trimester framework no doubt was erected to ensure that the woman's right to choose not become so subordinate to the State's interest in promoting fetal life that her choice exists in theory but not in fact. We do not agree, however, that the trimester approach is necessary to accomplish this objective. A framework of this rigidity was unnecessary and in its later interpretation sometimes contradicted the State's permissible exercise of its powers.

Though the woman has a right to choose to terminate or continue her pregnancy before viability, it does not at all follow that the State is prohibited from taking steps to ensure that this choice is thoughtful and informed. Even in the earliest stages of pregnancy, the State may enact rules and regulations designed to encourage her to know that there are philosophic and social arguments of great weight that can be brought to bear in favor of continuing the pregnancy to full term and that there are procedures and institutions to allow adoption of unwanted children as well as a certain degree of state assistance if the mother chooses to raise the child herself. " '[T]he Constitution does not forbid a State or city, pursuant to democratic processes, from expressing a preference for normal childbirth.' " *Webster* v. *Reproductive Health Services,* 492 U.S., at 511 (opinion of the Court) (quoting *Poelker* v. *Doe,* 432 U.S. 519, 521 (1977)). It follows that States are free to enact laws to provide a reasonable framework for a woman to make a decision that has such profound and lasting meaning. This, too, we find consistent with *Roe's* central premises, and indeed the inevitable consequence of our holding that the State has an interest in protecting the life of the unborn.

We reject the trimester framework, which we do not consider to be part of the essential holding of *Roe.* See *Webster* v. *Reproductive Health Services, supra,* at 518 (opinion of Rehnquist, C. J.); *id.,* at 529 (O'Connor, J., concurring in part and concurring in judgment) (describing the trimester framework as "problematic"). Measures aimed at ensuring that a woman's choice contemplates the consequences for the fetus do not necessarily interfere with the right recognized in *Roe,* although those measures have been found to be inconsistent with the rigid trimester framework announced in that case. A logical reading of the central holding in *Roe* itself, and a necessary reconciliation of the liberty of the woman and the interest of the State in promoting prenatal life, require, in our view, that we abandon the trimester framework as a rigid prohibition on all previability regulation aimed at the protection of fetal life. The trimester framework suffers from these basic flaws: in its formulation it misconceives the nature of the pregnant woman's interest; and in practice it undervalues the State's interest in potential life, as recognized in *Roe.* As our jurisprudence relating to all liberties save perhaps abortion has recognized, not every law which makes a right more difficult to exercise is, *ipso facto,* an infringement of that right. An example clarifies the point. We have held that not every ballot access limitation amounts to an infringement of the right to vote. Rather, the States are granted substantial flexibility in establishing the framework within which voters choose the candidates for whom they wish to vote. *Anderson* v. *Celebrezze,* 460 U.S. 780, 788 (1983); *Norman* v. *Reed,* 502 U. S. ___ (1992).

The abortion right is similar. Numerous forms of state regulation might have the incidental effect of increasing the cost or decreasing the availability of medical care, whether for abortion or any other medical procedure. The fact that a law which serves a valid purpose, one not designed to strike at the right itself, has the incidental effect of making it more difficult or more expensive to procure an abortion cannot be enough to invalidate it. Only where state regulation imposes an undue burden on a woman's ability to make this decision does the power of the State reach into the heart of the liberty protected by the Due Process Clause. See *Hodgson* v. *Minnesota*, 497 U.S. 417, 458-459 (1990) (O'Connor, J., concurring in part and concurring in judgment in part); *Ohio* v. *Akron Center for Reproductive Health*, 497 U.S. 502, (1990) (*Akron II*) (opinion of Kennedy, J.) *Webster* v. *Reproductive Health Services, supra,* at 530 (O'Connor, J., concurring in part and concurring in judgment); *Thornburgh* v. *American College of Obstetricians and Gynecologists*, 476 U. S., at 828 (O'Connor, J., dissenting); *Simopoulos* v. *Virginia*, 462 U.S. 506, 520 (1983) (O'Connor, J., concurring in part and concurring in judgment); *Planned Parenthood Assn. of Kansas City* v. *Ashcroft*, 462 U.S. 476, 505 (1983) (O'Connor, J., concurring in judgment in part and dissenting in part); *Akron I*, 462 U. S., at 464 (O'Connor, J., joined by White and Rehnquist, JJ., dissenting); *Bellotti* v. *Baird,* 428 U.S. 132, 147 (1976) (*Bellotti I*).

For the most part, the Court's early abortion cases adhered to this view. In *Maher* v. *Roe*, 432 U.S. 464, 473-474 (1977), the Court explained: "*Roe* did not declare an unqualified 'constitutional right to an abortion,' as the District Court seemed to think. Rather, the right protects the woman from unduly burdensome interference with her freedom to decide whether to terminate her pregnancy." See also *Doe* v. *Bolton,* 410 U.S. 179, 198 (1973) ("[T]he interposition of the hospital abortion committee is unduly restrictive of the patient's rights"); *Bellotti I, supra*, at 147 (State may not "impose undue burdens upon a minor capable of giving an informed consent"); *Harris* v. *McRae*, 448 U.S. 297, 314 (1980) (citing *Maher, supra*). Cf. *Carey* v. *Population Services International,* 431 U. S., at 688 ("[T]he same test must be applied to state regulations that burden an individual's right to decide to prevent conception or terminate pregnancy by substantially limiting access to the means of effectuating that decision as is applied to state statutes that prohibit the decision entirely").

These considerations of the nature of the abortion right illustrate that it is an overstatement to describe it as a right to decide whether to have an abortion "without interference from the State," *Planned Parenthood of Central Mo.* v. *Danforth*, 428 U.S. 52, 61 (1976). All abortion regulations interfere to some

degree with a woman's ability to decide whether to terminate her pregnancy. It is, as a consequence, not surprising that despite the protestations contained in the original *Roe* opinion to the effect that the Court was not recognizing an absolute right, 410 U. S., at 154-155, the Court's experience applying the trimester framework has led to the striking down of some abortion regulations which in no real sense deprived women of the ultimate decision. Those decisions went too far because the right recognized by *Roe* is a right "to be free from unwarranted governmental intrusion into matters so fundamentally affecting a person as the decision whether to bear or beget a child." *Eisenstadt* v. *Baird,* 405 U. S., at 453. Not all governmental intrusion is of necessity unwarranted; and that brings us to the other basic flaw in the trimester framework: even in *Roe*'s terms, in practice it undervalues the State's interest in the potential life within the woman.

Roe v. *Wade* was express in its recognition of the State's "important and legitimate interest[s] in preserving and protecting the health of the pregnant woman [and] in protecting the potentiality of human life." 410 U. S., at 162. The trimester framework, however, does not fulfill *Roe*'s own promise that the State has an interest in protecting fetal life or potential life. *Roe* began the contradiction by using the trimester framework to forbid any regulation of abortion designed to advance that interest before viability. *Id.,* at 163. Before viability, *Roe* and subsequent cases treat all governmental attempts to influence a woman's decision on behalf of the potential life within her as unwarranted. This treatment is, in our judgment, incompatible with the recognition that there is a substantial state interest in potential life throughout pregnancy. Cf. *Webster,* 492 U. S., at 519 (opinion of Rehnquist, C. J.); *Akron I, supra,* at 461 (O'Connor, J., dissenting).

The very notion that the State has a substantial interest in potential life leads to the conclusion that not all regulations must be deemed unwarranted. Not all burdens on the right to decide whether to terminate a pregnancy will be undue. In our view, the undue burden standard is the appropriate means of reconciling the State's interest with the woman's constitutionally protected liberty.

The concept of an undue burden has been utilized by the Court as well as individual members of the Court, including two of us, in ways that could be considered inconsistent. See, e. g., *Hodgson* v. *Minnesota,* 497 U. S., at ___ (O'Connor, J., concurring in part and concurring in judgment); *Akron II*, 497 U. S., at ___ (opinion of Kennedy, J.); *Thornburgh* v. *American College of Obstetricians and Gynecologists*, 476 U. S., at 828-829 (O'Connor, J., dissenting); *Akron I, supra,* at 461-466 (O'Connor, J., dissenting); *Harris* v. *McRae, supra,* at 314;

Maher v. *Roe, supra,* at 473; *Beal* v. *Doe,* 432 U.S. 438, 446 (1977); *Bellotti I, supra,* at 147. Because we set forth a standard of general application to which we intend to adhere, it is important to clarify what is meant by an undue burden.

A finding of an undue burden is a shorthand for the conclusion that a state regulation has the purpose or effect of placing a substantial obstacle in the path of a woman seeking an abortion of a nonviable fetus. A statute with this purpose is invalid because the means chosen by the State to further the interest in potential life must be calculated to inform the woman's free choice, not hinder it. And a statute which, while furthering the interest in potential life or some other valid state interest, has the effect of placing a substantial obstacle in the path of a woman's choice cannot be considered a permissible means of serving its legitimate ends. To the extent that the opinions of the Court or of individual Justices use the undue burden standard in a manner that is inconsistent with this analysis, we set out what in our view should be the controlling standard. Cf. *McCleskey* v. *Zant,* 499 U.S. ___ (1991) (slip op., at 20) (attempting to "define the doctrine of abuse of the writ with more precision" after acknowledging tension among earlier cases). In our considered judgment, an undue burden is an unconstitutional burden. See *Akron II, supra,* at ___ (opinion of Kennedy, J.). Understood another way, we answer the question, left open in previous opinions discussing the undue burden formulation, whether a law designed to further the State's interest in fetal life which imposes an undue burden on the woman's decision before fetal viability could be constitutional. See, *e. g., Akron I, supra,* at 462-463 (O'Connor, J., dissenting). The answer is no.

Some guiding principles should emerge. What is at stake is the woman's right to make the ultimate decision, not a right to be insulated from all others in doing so. Regulations which do no more than create a structural mechanism by which the State, or the parent or guardian of a minor, may express profound respect for the life of the unborn are permitted, if they are not a substantial obstacle to the woman's exercise of the right to choose. See *infra,* at ___ ___ (addressing Pennsylvania's parental consent requirement). Unless it has that effect on her right of choice, a state measure designed to persuade her to choose childbirth over abortion will be upheld if reasonably related to that goal. Regulations designed to foster the health of a woman seeking an abortion are valid if they do not constitute an undue burden.

Even when jurists reason from shared premises, some disagreement is inevitable. Compare *Hodgson,* 497 U. S., at ___ (opinion of Kennedy, J.) with *id.,* at _____ (O'Connor, J., concurring in part and concurring in judgment in part). That is to

be expected in the application of any legal standard which must accommodate life's complexity. We do not expect it to be otherwise with respect to the undue burden standard. We give this summary:

(a) To protect the central right recognized by *Roe* v. *Wade* while at the same time accommodating the State's profound interest in potential life, we will employ the undue burden analysis as explained in this opinion. An undue burden exists, and therefore a provision of law is invalid, if its purpose or effect is to place a substantial obstacle in the path of a woman seeking an abortion before the fetus attains viability.

(b) We reject the rigid trimester framework of *Roe* v. *Wade.* To promote the State's profound interest in potential life, throughout pregnancy the State may take measures to ensure that the woman's choice is informed, and measures designed to advance this interest will not be invalidated as long as their purpose is to persuade the woman to choose childbirth over abortion. These measures must not be an undue burden on the right.

(c) As with any medical procedure, the State may enact regulations to further the health or safety of a woman seeking an abortion. Unnecessary health regulations that have the purpose or effect of presenting a substantial obstacle to a woman seeking an abortion impose an undue burden on the right.

(d) Our adoption of the undue burden analysis does not disturb the central holding of *Roe* v. *Wade,* and we reaffirm that holding. Regardless of whether exceptions are made for particular circumstances, a State may not prohibit any woman from making the ultimate decision to terminate her pregnancy before viability.

(e) We also reaffirm *Roe*'s holding that "subsequent to viability, the State in promoting its interest in the potentiality of human life may, if it chooses, regulate, and even proscribe, abortion except where it is necessary, in appropriate medical judgment, for the preservation of the life or health of the mother." *Roe* v. *Wade,* 410 U. S., at 164-165.

These principles control our assessment of the Pennsylvania statute, and we now turn to the issue of the validity of its challenged provisions.

The Court of Appeals applied what it believed to be the undue burden standard and upheld each of the provisions except for the husband notification requirement. We agree generally with this conclusion, but refine the undue burden analysis in accordance with the principles articulated above. We now consider the separate statutory sections at issue.

Because it is central to the operation of various other requirements, we begin with the statute's definition of medical emergency. Under the statute, a medical emergency is

> "[t]hat condition which, on the basis of the physician's good faith clinical judgment, so complicates the medical condition of a pregnant woman as to necessitate the immediate abortion of her pregnancy to avert her death or for which a delay will create serious risk of substantial and irreversible impairment of a major bodily function." 18 Pa. Cons. Stat. (1990). § 3203.

Petitioners argue that the definition is too narrow, contending that it forecloses the possibility of an immediate abortion despite some significant health risks. If the contention were correct, we would be required to invalidate the restrictive operation of the provision, for the essential holding of *Roe* forbids a State from interfering with a woman's choice to undergo an abortion procedure if continuing her pregnancy would constitute a threat to her health. 410 U. S., at 164. See also *Harris* v. *McRae*, 448 U. S., at 316.

The District Court found that there were three serious conditions which would not be covered by the statute: preeclampsia, inevitable abortion, and premature ruptured membrane. 744 F. Supp., at 1378. Yet, as the Court of Appeals observed, 947 F. 2d, at 700-701, it is undisputed that under some circumstances each of these conditions could lead to an illness with substantial and irreversible consequences. While the definition could be interpreted in an unconstitutional manner, the Court of Appeals construed the phrase "serious risk" to include those circumstances. *Id.*, at 701. It stated: "we read the medical emergency exception as intended by the Pennsylvania legislature to assure that compliance with its abortion regulations would not in any way pose a significant threat to the life or health of a woman." *Ibid.* As we said in *Brockett* v. *Spokane Arcades, Inc.,* 472 U.S. 491, 499-500 (1985): "Normally, . . . we defer to the construction of a state statute given it by the lower federal courts." Indeed, we have said that we will defer to lower court interpretations of state law unless they amount to "plain" error. *Palmer* v. *Hoffman*, 318 U.S. 109, 118 (1943). This "'reflect[s] our belief that district courts and courts of appeals are better schooled in and more able to interpret the laws of their respective States.'" *Frisby* v. *Schultz*, 487 U.S. 474, 482 (1988) (citation omitted). We adhere to that course today, and conclude that, as construed by the Court of Appeals, the medical emergency definition imposes no undue burden on a woman's abortion right.

We next consider the informed consent requirement. 18 Pa. Cons. Stat. Ann. § 3205. Except in a medical emergency, the statute requires that at least 24 hours before performing an abortion a physician inform the woman of the nature of the procedure, the health risks of the abortion and of childbirth, and the "probable gestational age of the unborn child." The physician or a qualified nonphysician must inform the woman of the availability of printed materials published by the State describing the fetus and providing information about medical assistance for childbirth, information about child support from the father, and a list of agencies which provide adoption and other services as alternatives to abortion. An abortion may not be performed unless the woman certifies in writing that she has been informed of the availability of these printed materials and has been provided them if she chooses to view them.

Our prior decisions establish that as with any medical procedure, the State may require a woman to give her written informed consent to an abortion. See *Planned Parenthood of Central Mo.* v. *Danforth,* 428 U. S., at 67. In this respect, the statute is unexceptional. Petitioners challenge the statute's definition of informed consent because it includes the provision of specific information by the doctor and the mandatory 24-hour waiting period. The conclusions reached by a majority of the Justices in the separate opinions filed today and the undue burden standard adopted in this opinion require us to overrule in part some of the Court's past decisions, decisions driven by the trimester framework's prohibition of all previability regulations designed to further the State's interest in fetal life.

In *Akron I,* 462 U.S. 416 (1983), we invalidated an ordinance which required that a woman seeking an abortion be provided by her physician with specific information "designed to influence the woman's informed choice between abortion or childbirth." *Id.*, at 444. As we later described the *Akron I* holding in *Thornburgh* v. *American College of Obstetricians and Gynecologists*, 476 U. S., at 762, there were two purported flaws in the Akron ordinance: the information was designed to dissuade the woman from having an abortion and the ordinance imposed "a rigid requirement that a specific body of information be given in all cases, irrespective of the particular needs of the patient. . . ." *Ibid.*

To the extent *Akron I* and *Thornburgh* find a constitutional violation when the government requires, as it does here, the giving of truthful, nonmisleading information about the nature of the procedure, the attendant health risks and those of childbirth, and the "probable gestational age" of the fetus, those cases go too far, are inconsistent with *Roe*'s acknowledgment of an important interest in potential life, and are overruled. This is clear even on the very terms of *Akron I* and *Thornburgh*. Those decisions, along with *Danforth*, recognize a substantial government interest justifying a requirement that a woman be apprised of the health risks of abortion and childbirth. *E. g., Danforth, supra*, at 66-67. It cannot be questioned that psychological well being is a facet of health. Nor can it be doubted that most women considering an abortion would deem the impact on the fetus relevant, if not dispositive, to the decision. In attempting to ensure that a woman apprehend the full consequences of her decision, the State furthers the legitimate purpose of reducing the risk that a woman may elect an abortion, only to discover later, with devastating psychological consequences, that her decision was not fully informed. If the information the State requires to be made available to the woman is truthful and not misleading, the requirement may be permissible.

We also see no reason why the State may not require doctors to inform a woman seeking an abortion of the availability of materials relating to the consequences to the fetus, even when those consequences have no direct relation to her health. An example illustrates the point. We would think it constitutional for the State to require that in order for there to be informed consent to a kidney transplant operation the recipient must be supplied with information about risks to the donor as well as risks to himself or herself. A requirement that the physician make available information similar to that mandated by the statute here was described in *Thornburgh* as "an outright attempt to wedge the Commonwealth's message discouraging abortion into the privacy of the informed consent dialogue between the woman and her physician." 476 U. S., at 762. We conclude, however, that informed choice need not be defined in such narrow terms that all considerations of the effect on the fetus are made irrelevant. As we have made clear, we depart from the holdings of *Akron I* and *Thornburgh* to the extent that we permit a State to further its legitimate goal of protecting the life of the unborn by enacting legislation aimed at ensuring a decision that is mature and informed, even when in so doing the State expresses a preference for childbirth over abortion. In short, requiring that the woman be informed of the availability of information relating to fetal development and the assistance available should she decide to carry the pregnancy to full term is a reasonable measure to insure an informed choice, one which might cause the woman to choose childbirth over abortion. This requirement cannot be considered a substantial obstacle to obtaining an abortion, and, it follows, there is no undue burden.

Our prior cases also suggest that the "straitjacket," *Thornburgh, supra*, at 762 (quoting *Danforth, supra*, at 67, n. 8), of particular information which must be given in each case interferes with a constitutional right of privacy between a pregnant woman and her physician. As a preliminary matter, it is worth noting that the statute now before us does not require a physician to comply with the informed consent provisions "if

he or she can demonstrate by a preponderance of the evidence, that he or she reasonably believed that furnishing the information would have resulted in a severely adverse effect on the physical or mental health of the patient." 18 Pa. Cons. Stat. § 3205 (1990). In this respect, the statute does not prevent the physician from exercising his or her medical judgment.

Whatever constitutional status the doctor patient relation may have as a general matter, in the present context it is derivative of the woman's position. The doctor patient relation does not underlie or override the two more general rights under which the abortion right is justified: the right to make family decisions and the right to physical autonomy. On its own, the doctor patient relation here is entitled to the same solicitude it receives in other contexts. Thus, a requirement that a doctor give a woman certain information as part of obtaining her consent to an abortion is, for constitutional purposes, no different from a requirement that a doctor give certain specific information about any medical procedure.

All that is left of petitioners' argument is an asserted First Amendment right of a physician not to provide information about the risks of abortion, and childbirth, in a manner mandated by the State. To be sure, the physician's First Amendment rights not to speak are implicated, see *Wooley* v. *Maynard*, 430 U. S. 705 (1977), but only as part of the practice of medicine, subject to reasonable licensing and regulation by the State. Cf. *Whalen* v. *Roe*, 429 U. S. 589, 603 (1977). We see no constitutional infirmity in the requirement that the physician provide the information mandated by the State here.

The Pennsylvania statute also requires us to reconsider the holding in *Akron I* that the State may not require that a physician, as opposed to a qualified assistant, provide information relevant to a woman's informed consent. 462 U. S., at 448. Since there is no evidence on this record that requiring a doctor to give the information as provided by the statute would amount in practical terms to a substantial obstacle to a woman seeking an abortion, we conclude that it is not an undue burden. Our cases reflect the fact that the Constitution gives the States broad latitude to decide that particular functions may be performed only by licensed professionals, even if an objective assessment might suggest that those same tasks could be performed by others. See *Williamson* v. *Lee Optical of Oklahoma, Inc.*, 348 U. S. 483 (1955). Thus, we uphold the provision as a reasonable means to insure that the woman's consent is informed.

Our analysis of Pennsylvania's 24-hour waiting period between the provision of the information deemed necessary to informed consent and the performance of an abortion under the undue burden standard requires us to reconsider the premise behind the decision in *Akron I* invalidating a parallel requirement. In *Akron I* we said: "Nor are we convinced that the State's legitimate concern that the woman's decision be informed is reasonably served by requiring a 24-hour delay as a matter of course." 462 U. S., at 450. We consider that conclusion to be wrong. The idea that important decisions will be more informed and deliberate if they follow some period of reflection does not strike us as unreasonable, particularly where the statute directs that important information become part of the background of the decision. The statute, as construed by the Court of Appeals, permits avoidance of the waiting period in the event of a medical emergency and the record evidence shows that in the vast majority of cases, a 24-hour delay does not create any appreciable health risk. In theory, at least, the waiting period is a reasonable measure to implement the State's interest in protecting the life of the unborn, a measure that does not amount to an undue burden.

Whether the mandatory 24-hour waiting period is nonetheless invalid because in practice it is a substantial obstacle to a woman's choice to terminate her pregnancy is a closer question. The findings of fact by the District Court indicate that because of the distances many women must travel to reach an abortion provider, the practical effect will often be a delay of much more than a day because the waiting period requires that a woman seeking an abortion make at least two visits to the doctor. The District Court also found that in many instances this will increase the exposure of women seeking abortions to "the harassment and hostility of anti abortion protestors demonstrating outside a clinic." 744 F. Supp., at 1351. As a result, the District Court found that for those women who have the fewest financial resources, those who must travel long distances, and those who have difficulty explaining their whereabouts to husbands, employers, or others, the 24-hour waiting period will be "particularly burdensome." *Id.*, at 1352.

These findings are troubling in some respects, but they do not demonstrate that the waiting period constitutes an undue burden. We do not doubt that, as the District Court held, the waiting period has the effect of "increasing the cost and risk of delay of abortions," *id.*, at 1378, but the District Court did not conclude that the increased costs and potential delays amount to substantial obstacles. Rather, applying the trimester framework's strict prohibition of all regulation designed to promote the State's interest in potential life before viability, see *id.*, at 1374, the District Court concluded that the waiting period does not further the state "interest in maternal health" and "infringes the physician's discretion to exercise sound medical judgment." *Id.*, at 1378. Yet, as we have stated, under the undue burden standard a State is permitted to enact persuasive measures which favor childbirth over abortion, even

if those measures do not further a health interest. And while the waiting period does limit a physician's discretion, that is not, standing alone, a reason to invalidate it. In light of the construction given the statute's definition of medical emergency by the Court of Appeals, and the District Court's findings, we cannot say that the waiting period imposes a real health risk.

We also disagree with the District Court's conclusion that the "particularly burdensome" effects of the waiting period on some women require its invalidation. A particular burden is not of necessity a substantial obstacle. Whether a burden falls on a particular group is a distinct inquiry from whether it is a substantial obstacle even as to the women in that group. And the District Court did not conclude that the waiting period is such an obstacle even for the women who are most burdened by it. Hence, on the record before us, and in the context of this facial challenge, we are not convinced that the 24-hour waiting period constitutes an undue burden.

We are left with the argument that the various aspects of the informed consent requirement are unconstitutional because they place barriers in the way of abortion on demand. Even the broadest reading of *Roe*, however, has not suggested that there is a constitutional right to abortion on demand. See, *e. g., Doe* v. *Bolton*, 410 U. S., at 189. Rather, the right protected by *Roe* is a right to decide to terminate a pregnancy free of undue interference by the State. Because the informed consent requirement facilitates the wise exercise of that right it cannot be classified as an interference with the right *Roe* protects. The informed consent requirement is not an undue burden on that right.

Section 3209 of Pennsylvania's abortion law provides, except in cases of medical emergency, that no physician shall perform an abortion on a married woman without receiving a signed statement from the woman that she has notified her spouse that she is about to undergo an abortion. The woman has the option of providing an alternative signed statement certifying that her husband is not the man who impregnated her; that her husband could not be located; that the pregnancy is the result of spousal sexual assault which she has reported; or that the woman believes that notifying her husband will cause him or someone else to inflict bodily injury upon her. A physician who performs an abortion on a married woman without receiving the appropriate signed statement will have his or her license revoked, and is liable to the husband for damages.

The District Court heard the testimony of numerous expert witnesses, and made detailed findings of fact regarding the effect of this statute. These included:

"273. The vast majority of women consult their husbands prior to deciding to terminate their pregnancy. . . .

"279. The 'bodily injury' exception could not be invoked by a married woman whose husband, if notified, would, in her reasonable belief, threaten to (a) publicize her intent to have an abortion to family, friends or acquaintances; (b) retaliate against her in future child custody or divorce proceedings; (c) inflict psychological intimidation or emotional harm upon her, her children or other persons; (d) inflict bodily harm on other persons such as children, family members or other loved ones; or (e) use his control over finances to deprive of necessary monies for herself or her children. . . .

"281. Studies reveal that family violence occurs in two million families in the United States. This figure, however, is a conservative one that substantially understates (because battering is usually not reported until it reaches life threatening proportions) the actual number of families affected by domestic violence. In fact, researchers estimate that one of every two women will be battered at some time in their life. . . .

"282. A wife may not elect to notify her husband of her intention to have an abortion for a variety of reasons, including the husband's illness, concern about her own health, the imminent failure of the marriage, or the husband's absolute opposition to the abortion. . . .

"283. The required filing of the spousal consent form would require plaintiff clinics to change their counseling procedures and force women to reveal their most intimate decision making on pain of criminal sanctions. The confidentiality of these revelations could not be guaranteed, since the woman's records are not immune from subpoena. . . .

"284. Women of all class levels, educational backgrounds, and racial, ethnic and religious groups are battered. . . .

"285. Wife battering or abuse can take on many physical and psychological forms. The nature and scope of the battering can cover a broad range of actions and be gruesome and torturous. . . .

"286. Married women, victims of battering, have been killed in Pennsylvania and throughout the United States. . . .

"287. Battering can often involve a substantial amount of sexual abuse, including marital rape and sexual mutilation. . . .

"288. In a domestic abuse situation, it is common for the battering husband to also abuse the children in an attempt to coerce the wife. . . .

"289. Mere notification of pregnancy is frequently a flashpoint for battering and violence within the family. The number of battering incidents is high during the pregnancy and often the worst abuse can be associated with pregnancy. . . . The battering husband may deny parentage and use the pregnancy as an excuse for abuse. . . .

"290. Secrecy typically shrouds abusive families. Family members are instructed not to tell anyone, especially police or doctors, about the abuse and violence. Battering husbands often threaten their wives or her children with further abuse if she tells an outsider of the violence and tells her that nobody will believe her. A battered woman, therefore, is highly unlikely to disclose the violence against her for fear of retaliation by the abuser. . . .

"291. Even when confronted directly by medical personnel or other helping professionals, battered women often will not admit to the battering because they have not admitted to themselves that they are battered. . . .

"294. A woman in a shelter or a safe house unknown to her husband is not 'reasonably likely' to have bodily harm inflicted upon her by her batterer, however her attempt to notify her husband pursuant to section 3209 could accidentally disclose her whereabouts to her husband. Her fear of future ramifications would be realistic under the circumstances.

"295. Marital rape is rarely discussed with others or reported to law enforcement authorities, and of those reported only few are prosecuted. . . .

"296. It is common for battered women to have sexual intercourse with their husbands to avoid being battered. While this type of coercive sexual activity would be spousal sexual assault as defined by the Act, many women may not consider it to be so and others would fear disbelief. . .

"297. The marital rape exception to section 3209 cannot be claimed by women who are victims of coercive sexual behavior other than penetration. The 90-day reporting requirement of the spousal sexual assault statute, 18 Pa. Con. Stat. Ann. § 3218(c), further narrows the class of sexually abused wives who can claim the exception, since many of these women may be psychologically unable to discuss or report the rape for several years after the incident. . . .

"298. Because of the nature of the battering relationship, battered women are unlikely to avail themselves of the exceptions to section 3209 of the Act, regardless of whether the section applies to them." 744 F. Supp., at 1360-1362.

These findings are supported by studies of domestic violence. The American Medical Association (AMA) has published a summary of the recent research in this field, which indicates that in an average 12-month period in this country, approximately two million women are the victims of severe assaults by their male partners. In a 1985 survey, women reported that nearly one of every eight husbands had assaulted their wives during the past year. The AMA views these figures as "marked underestimates," because the nature of these incidents discourages women from reporting them, and because surveys typically exclude the very poor, those who do not speak English well, and women who are homeless or in institutions or hospitals when the survey is conducted. According to the

AMA, "[r]esearchers on family violence agree that the true incidence of partner violence is probably *double* the above estimates; or four million severely assaulted women per year. Studies suggest that from one fifth to one third of all women will be physically assaulted by a partner or ex partner during their lifetime." AMA Council on Scientific Affairs, Violence Against Women 7 (1991) (emphasis in original). Thus on an average day in the United States, nearly 11,000 women are severely assaulted by their male partners. Many of these incidents involve sexual assault. *Id.,* at 3-4; Shields & Hanneke, Battered Wives' Reactions to Marital Rape, in The Dark Side of Families: Current Family Violence Research 131, 144 (D. Finkelhor, R. Gelles, G. Hataling, & M. Straus eds. 1983). In families where wife beating takes place, moreover, child abuse is often present as well. Violence Against Women, *supra,* at 12.

Other studies fill in the rest of this troubling picture. Physical violence is only the most visible form of abuse. Psychological abuse, particularly forced social and economic isolation of women, is also common. L. Walker, The Battered Woman Syndrome 27-28 (1984). Many victims of domestic violence remain with their abusers, perhaps because they perceive no superior alternative. Herbert, Silver, & Ellard, Coping with an Abusive Relationship: I. How and Why do Women Stay?, 53 J. Marriage & the Family 311 (1991). Many abused women who find temporary refuge in shelters return to their husbands, in large part because they have no other source of income. Aguirre, Why Do They Return? Abused Wives in Shelters, 30 J. Nat. Assn. of Social Workers 350, 352 (1985). Returning to one's abuser can be dangerous. Recent Federal Bureau of Investigation statistics disclose that 8.8% of all homicide victims in the United States are killed by their spouse. Mercy & Saltzman, Fatal Violence Among Spouses in the United States, 1976-85, 79 Am. J. Public Health 595 (1989). Thirty percent of female homicide victims are killed by their male partners. Domestic Violence: Terrorism in the Home, Hearing before the Subcommittee on Children, Family, Drugs and Alcoholism of the Senate Committee on Labor and Human Resources, 101st Cong., 2d Sess., 3 (1990).

The limited research that has been conducted with respect to notifying one's husband about an abortion, although involving samples too small to be representative, also supports the District Court's findings of fact. The vast majority of women notify their male partners of their decision to obtain an abortion. In many cases in which married women do not notify their husbands, the pregnancy is the result of an extramarital affair. Where the husband is the father, the primary reason women do not notify their husbands is that the husband and wife are experiencing marital difficulties, often accompanied by incidents of violence. Ryan & Plutzer, When Married

Women Have Abortions: Spousal Notification and Marital Interaction, 51 J. Marriage & the Family 41, 44 (1989).

This information and the District Court's findings reinforce what common sense would suggest. In well functioning marriages, spouses discuss important intimate decisions such as whether to bear a child. But there are millions of women in this country who are the victims of regular physical and psychological abuse at the hands of their husbands. Should these women become pregnant, they may have very good reasons for not wishing to inform their husbands of their decision to obtain an abortion. Many may have justifiable fears of physical abuse, but may be no less fearful of the consequences of reporting prior abuse to the Commonwealth of Pennsylvania. Many may have a reasonable fear that notifying their husbands will provoke further instances of child abuse; these women are not exempt from § 3209's notification requirement. Many may fear devastating forms of psychological abuse from their husbands, including verbal harassment, threats of future violence, the destruction of possessions, physical confinement to the home, the withdrawal of financial support, or the disclosure of the abortion to family and friends. These methods of psychological abuse may act as even more of a deterrent to notification than the possibility of physical violence, but women who are the victims of the abuse are not exempt from § 3209's notification requirement. And many women who are pregnant as a result of sexual assaults by their husbands will be unable to avail themselves of the exception for spousal sexual assault, § 3209(b)(3), because the exception requires that the woman have notified law enforcement authorities within 90 days of the assault, and her husband will be notified of her report once an investigation begins. § 3128(c). If anything in this field is certain, it is that victims of spousal sexual assault are extremely reluctant to report the abuse to the government; hence, a great many spousal rape victims will not be exempt from the notification requirement imposed by § 3209.

The spousal notification requirement is thus likely to prevent a significant number of women from obtaining an abortion. It does not merely make abortions a little more difficult or expensive to obtain; for many women, it will impose a substantial obstacle. We must not blind ourselves to the fact that the significant number of women who fear for their safety and the safety of their children are likely to be deterred from procuring an abortion as surely as if the Commonwealth had outlawed abortion in all cases.

Respondents attempt to avoid the conclusion that § 3209 is invalid by pointing out that it imposes almost no burden at all for the vast majority of women seeking abortions. They begin by noting that only about 20 percent of the women who obtain abortions are married. They then note that of these women about 95 percent notify their husbands of their own volition. Thus, respondents argue, the effects of § 3209 are felt by only one percent of the women who obtain abortions. Respondents argue that since some of these women will be able to notify their husbands without adverse consequences or will qualify for one of the exceptions, the statute affects fewer than one percent of women seeking abortions. For this reason, it is asserted, the statute cannot be invalid on its face. See Brief for Respondents 83-86. We disagree with respondents' basic method of analysis.

The analysis does not end with the one percent of women upon whom the statute operates; it begins there. Legislation is measured for consistency with the Constitution by its impact on those whose conduct it affects. For example, we would not say that a law which requires a newspaper to print a candidate's reply to an unfavorable editorial is valid on its face because most newspapers would adopt the policy even absent the law. See *Miami Herald Publishing Co.* v. *Tornillo*, 418 U.S. 241 (1974). The proper focus of constitutional inquiry is the group for whom the law is a restriction, not the group for whom the law is irrelevant.

Respondents' argument itself gives implicit recognition to this principle, at one of its critical points. Respondents speak of the one percent of women seeking abortions who are married and would choose not to notify their husbands of their plans. By selecting as the controlling class women who wish to obtain abortions, rather than all women or all pregnant women, respondents in effect concede that § 3209 must be judged by reference to those for whom it is an actual rather than irrelevant restriction. Of course, as we have said, § 3209's real target is narrower even than the class of women seeking abortions identified by the State: it is married women seeking abortions who do not wish to notify their husbands of their intentions and who do not qualify for one of the statutory exceptions to the notice requirement. The unfortunate yet persisting conditions we document above will mean that in a large fraction of the cases in which § 3209 is relevant, it will operate as a substantial obstacle to a woman's choice to undergo an abortion. It is an undue burden, and therefore invalid.

This conclusion is in no way inconsistent with our decisions upholding parental notification or consent requirements. See, *e. g., Akron II*, 497 U. S., at _____; *Bellotti* v. *Baird*, 443 U.S. 622 (1979) (*Bellotti II*); *Planned Parenthood of Central Mo.* v. *Danforth*, 428 U.S. at 74. Those enactments, and our judgment that they are constitutional, are based on the quite reasonable assumption that minors will benefit from consultation with their parents and that children will often not realize that their parents have their best interests at heart. We cannot adopt a parallel assumption about adult women.

We recognize that a husband has a "deep and proper concern and interest . . . in his wife's pregnancy and in the growth and development of the fetus she is carrying." *Danforth, supra,* at 69. With regard to the children he has fathered and raised, the Court has recognized his "cognizable and substantial" interest in their custody. *Stanley* v. *Illinois*, 405 U.S. 645, 651-652 (1972); see also *Quilloin* v. *Walcott*, 434 U.S. 246 (1978); *Caban* v. *Mohammed*, 441 U.S. 380 (1979); *Lehr* v. *Robertson*, 463 U.S. 248 (1983). If this case concerned a State's ability to require the mother to notify the father before taking some action with respect to a living child raised by both, therefore, it would be reasonable to conclude as a general matter that the father's interest in the welfare of the child and the mother's interest are equal.

Before birth, however, the issue takes on a very different cast. It is an inescapable biological fact that state regulation with respect to the child a woman is carrying will have a far greater impact on the mother's liberty than on the father's. The effect of state regulation on a woman's protected liberty is doubly deserving of scrutiny in such a case, as the State has touched not only upon the private sphere of the family but upon the very bodily integrity of the pregnant woman. Cf. *Cruzan* v. *Director, Missouri Dept. of Health*, 497 U. S., at 281. The Court has held that "when the wife and the husband disagree on this decision, the view of only one of the two marriage partners can prevail. Inasmuch as it is the woman who physically bears the child and who is the more directly and immediately affected by the pregnancy, as between the two, the balance weighs in her favor." *Danforth, supra,* at 71. This conclusion rests upon the basic nature of marriage and the nature of our Constitution: "[T]he marital couple is not an independent entity with a mind and heart of its own, but an association of two individuals each with a separate intellectual and emotional makeup. If the right of privacy means anything, it is the right of the *individual*, married or single, to be free from unwarranted governmental intrusion into matters so fundamentally affecting a person as the decision whether to bear or beget a child." *Eisenstadt* v. *Baird*, 405 U. S., at 453 (emphasis in original). The Constitution protects individuals, men and women alike, from unjustified state interference, even when that interference is enacted into law for the benefit of their spouses.

There was a time, not so long ago, when a different understanding of the family and of the Constitution prevailed. In *Bradwell* v. *Illinois*, 16 Wall. 130 (1873), three Members of this Court reaffirmed the common law principle that "a woman had no legal existence separate from her husband, who was regarded as her head and representative in the social state; and, notwithstanding some recent modifications of this civil status, many of the special rules of law flowing from and dependent upon this cardinal principle still exist in full force in most States." *Id.*, at 141 (Bradley J., joined by Swayne and Field, JJ., concurring in judgment). Only one generation has passed since this Court observed that "woman is still regarded as the center of home and family life," with attendant "special responsibilities" that precluded full and independent legal status under the Constitution. *Hoyt* v. *Florida*, 368 U.S. 57, 62 (1961). These views, of course, are no longer consistent with our understanding of the family, the individual, or the Constitution.

In keeping with our rejection of the common law understanding of a woman's role within the family, the Court held in *Danforth* that the Constitution does not permit a State to require a married woman to obtain her husband's consent before undergoing an abortion. 428 U. S., at 69. The principles that guided the Court in *Danforth* should be our guides today. For the great many women who are victims of abuse inflicted by their husbands, or whose children are the victims of such abuse, a spousal notice requirement enables the husband to wield an effective veto over his wife's decision. Whether the prospect of notification itself deters such women from seeking abortions, or whether the husband, through physical force or psychological pressure or economic coercion, prevents his wife from obtaining an abortion until it is too late, the notice requirement will often be tantamount to the veto found unconstitutional in *Danforth*. The women most affected by this law—those who most reasonably fear the consequences of notifying their husbands that they are pregnant—are in the gravest danger.

The husband's interest in the life of the child his wife is carrying does not permit the State to empower him with this troubling degree of authority over his wife. The contrary view leads to consequences reminiscent of the common law. A husband has no enforceable right to require a wife to advise him before she exercises her personal choices. If a husband's interest in the potential life of the child outweighs a wife's liberty, the State could require a married woman to notify her husband before she uses a postfertilization contraceptive. Perhaps next in line would be a statute requiring pregnant married women to notify their husbands before engaging in conduct causing risks to the fetus. After all, if the husband's interest in the fetus' safety is a sufficient predicate for state regulation, the State could reasonably conclude that pregnant wives should notify their husbands before drinking alcohol or smoking. Perhaps married women should notify their husbands before using contraceptives or before undergoing any type of surgery that may have complications affecting the husband's interest in his wife's reproductive organs. And if a husband's interest justifies notice in any of these cases, one might reasonably argue that it justifies exactly what the *Danforth* Court held it did not justify—a requirement of the husband's consent as well. A State may not give to a man the kind of dominion over his wife that parents exercise over their children.

Section 3209 embodies a view of marriage consonant with the common law status of married women but repugnant to our present understanding of marriage and of the nature of the rights secured by the Constitution. Women do not lose their constitutionally protected liberty when they marry. The Constitution protects all individuals, male or female, married or unmarried, from the abuse of governmental power, even where that power is employed for the supposed benefit of a member of the individual's family. These considerations confirm our conclusion that § 3209 is invalid.

We next consider the parental consent provision. Except in a medical emergency, an unemancipated young woman under 18 may not obtain an abortion unless she and one of her parents (or guardian) provides informed consent as defined above. If neither a parent nor a guardian provides consent, a court may authorize the performance of an abortion upon a determination that the young woman is mature and capable of giving informed consent and has in fact given her informed consent, or that an abortion would be in her best interests.

We have been over most of this ground before. Our cases establish, and we reaffirm today, that a State may require a minor seeking an abortion to obtain the consent of a parent or guardian, provided that there is an adequate judicial bypass procedure. See, *e. g., Akron II*, 497 U. S., at 510-519; *Hodgson*, 497 U. S., at 461; *Akron I, supra*, at 440; *Bellotti II, supra*, at 643-644 (plurality opinion). Under these precedents, in our view, the one parent consent requirement and judicial bypass procedure are constitutional.

The only argument made by petitioners respecting this provision and to which our prior decisions do not speak is the contention that the parental consent requirement is invalid because it requires informed parental consent. For the most part, petitioners' argument is a reprise of their argument with respect to the informed consent requirement in general, and we reject it for the reasons given above. Indeed, some of the provisions regarding informed consent have particular force with respect to minors: the waiting period, for example, may provide the parent or parents of a pregnant young woman the opportunity to consult with her in private, and to discuss the consequences of her decision in the context of the values and moral or religious principles of their family. See *Hodgson, supra*, at _____.

Under the recordkeeping and reporting requirements of the statute, every facility which performs abortions is required to file a report stating its name and address as well as the name and address of any related entity, such as a controlling or subsidiary organization. In the case of state funded institutions, the information becomes public.

For each abortion performed, a report must be filed identifying: the physician (and the second physician where required); the facility; the referring physician or agency; the woman's age; the number of prior pregnancies and prior abortions she has had; gestational age; the type of abortion procedure; the date of the abortion; whether there were any pre-existing medical conditions which would complicate pregnancy; medical complications with the abortion; where applicable, the basis for the determination that the abortion was medically necessary; the weight of the aborted fetus; and whether the woman was married, and if so, whether notice was provided or the basis for the failure to give notice. Every abortion facility must also file quarterly reports showing the number of abortions performed broken down by trimester. See 18 Pa. Cons. Stat. §§ 3207, 3214 (1990). In all events, the identity of each woman who has had an abortion remains confidential.

In *Danforth,* 428 U. S., at 80, we held that recordkeeping and reporting provisions "that are reasonably directed to the preservation of maternal health and that properly respect a patient's confidentiality and privacy are permissible." We think that under this standard, all the provisions at issue here except that relating to spousal notice are constitutional. Although they do not relate to the State's interest in informing the woman's choice, they do relate to health. The collection of information with respect to actual patients is a vital element of medical research, and so it cannot be said that the requirements serve no purpose other than to make abortions more difficult. Nor do we find that the requirements impose a substantial obstacle to a woman's choice. At most they might increase the cost of some abortions by a slight amount. While at some point increased cost could become a substantial obstacle, there is no such showing on the record before us.

Subsection (12) of the reporting provision requires the reporting of, among other things, a married woman's "reason for failure to provide notice" to her husband. § 3214(a)(12). This provision in effect requires women, as a condition of obtaining an abortion, to provide the Commonwealth with the precise information we have already recognized that many women have pressing reasons not to reveal. Like the spousal notice requirement itself, this provision places an undue burden on a woman's choice, and must be invalidated for that reason.

Our Constitution is a covenant running from the first generation of Americans to us and then to future generations. It is a coherent succession. Each generation must learn anew that the Constitution's written terms embody ideas and aspirations that must survive more ages than one. We accept our responsibility not to retreat from interpreting the full meaning of the covenant in light of all of our precedents. We invoke it once again to define the freedom guaranteed by the Constitution's own promise, the promise of liberty.

* * *

The judgment in No. 91-902 is affirmed. The judgment in No. 91-744 is affirmed in part and reversed in part, and the case is remanded for proceedings consistent with this opinion, including consideration of the question of severability.

It is so ordered.

[Concurring and dissenting opinions omitted.]

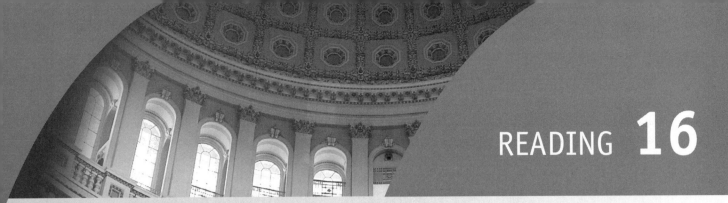

The Partial-Birth Abortion Ban Act

United States Code Title 18—Crimes and Criminal Procedure

Part I—Crimes

Chapter 74—Partial-Birth Abortion

Sec. 1531. Partial-birth abortions prohibited

(a) Any physician who, in or affecting interstate or foreign commerce, knowingly performs a partial-birth abortion and thereby kills a human fetus shall be fined under this title or imprisoned not more than 2 years, or both. This subsection does not apply to a partial-birth abortion that is necessary to save the life of a mother whose life is endangered by a physical disorder, physical illness, or physical injury, including a life-endangering physical condition caused by or arising from the pregnancy itself. This subsection takes effect 1 day after the enactment.

(b) As used in this section—

  (1) the term "partial-birth abortion" means an abortion in which the person performing the abortion—

    (A) deliberately and intentionally vaginally delivers a living fetus until, in the case of a head-first presentation, the entire fetal head is outside the body of the mother, or, in the case of breech presentation, any part of the fetal trunk past the navel is outside the body of the mother, for the purpose of performing an overt act that the person knows will kill the partially delivered living fetus; and

    (B) performs the overt act, other than completion of delivery, that kills the partially delivered living fetus; and

  (2) the term "physician" means a doctor of medicine or osteopathy legally authorized to practice medicine and surgery by the State in which the doctor performs such activity, or any other individual legally authorized by the State to perform abortions: Provided, however, That any individual who is not a physician or not otherwise legally authorized by the State to perform abortions, but who nevertheless directly performs a partial-birth abortion, shall be subject to the provisions of this section.

(c)

  (1) The father, if married to the mother at the time she receives a partial-birth abortion procedure, and if the mother has not attained the age of 18 years at the time of the abortion, the maternal grandparents of the fetus, may in a civil action obtain appropriate relief, unless the pregnancy resulted from the plaintiff's criminal conduct or the plaintiff consented to the abortion.

  (2) Such relief shall include—

    (A) money damages for all injuries, psychological and physical, occasioned by the violation of this section; and

    (B) statutory damages equal to three times the cost of the partial-birth abortion.

(d)

  (1) A defendant accused of an offense under this section may seek a hearing before the State Medical Board on whether the physician's conduct was necessary to save the life of the mother whose life was endangered

by a physical disorder, physical illness, or physical injury, including a life-endangering physical condition caused by or arising from the pregnancy itself.

(2) The findings on that issue are admissible on that issue at the trial of the defendant. Upon a motion of the defendant, the court shall delay the beginning of the trial for not more than 30 days to permit such a hearing to take place.

(e) A woman upon whom a partial-birth abortion is performed may not be prosecuted under this section, for a conspiracy to violate this section, or for an offense under section 2, 3, or 4 of this title based on a violation of this section.
(Added Pub. L. 108-105, Sec. 3(a), Nov. 5, 2003, 117 Stat. 1206.)

REFERENCES IN TEXT

The enactment, referred to in subsec. (a), probably means the date of the enactment of Pub. L. 108-105, which enacted this section and was approved Nov. 5, 2003.

Short Title

Pub. L. 108-105, Sec. 1, Nov. 5, 2003, 117 Stat. 1201, provided that: "This Act [enacting this chapter and provisions set out as a note under this section] may be cited as the 'Partial-Birth Abortion Ban Act of 2003.'"

Findings

Pub. L. 108-105, Sec. 2, Nov. 5, 2003, 117 Stat. 1201, provided that: "The Congress finds and declares the following:

"(1) A moral, medical, and ethical consensus exists that the practice of performing a partial-birth abortion—an abortion in which a physician deliberately and intentionally vaginally delivers a living, unborn child's body until either the entire baby's head is outside the body of the mother, or any part of the baby's trunk past the navel is outside the body of the mother and only the head remains inside the womb, for the purpose of performing an overt act (usually the puncturing of the back of the child's skull and removing the baby's brains) that the person knows will kill the partially delivered infant, performs this act, and then completes delivery of the dead infant—is a gruesome and inhumane procedure that is never medically necessary and should be prohibited.

"(2) Rather than being an abortion procedure that is embraced by the medical community, particularly among physicians who routinely perform other abortion procedures, partial-birth abortion remains a disfavored procedure that is not only unnecessary to preserve the health of the mother, but in fact poses serious risks to the long-term health of women and in some circumstances, their lives. As a result, at least 27 States banned the procedure as did the United States Congress which voted to ban the procedure during the 104th, 105th, and 106th Congresses.

"(3) In Stenberg v. Carhart, 530 U.S. 914, 932 (2000), the United States Supreme Court opined 'that significant medical authority supports the proposition that in some circumstances, [partial birth abortion] would be the safest procedure' for pregnant women who wish to undergo an abortion. Thus, the Court struck down the State of Nebraska's ban on partial-birth abortion procedures, concluding that it placed an 'undue burden' on women seeking abortions because it failed to include an exception for partial-birth abortions deemed necessary to preserve the 'health' of the mother.

"(4) In reaching this conclusion, the Court deferred to the Federal district court's factual findings that the partial-birth abortion procedure was statistically and medically as safe as, and in many circumstances safer than, alternative abortion procedures.

"(5) However, substantial evidence presented at the Stenberg trial and overwhelming evidence presented and compiled at extensive congressional hearings, much of which was compiled after the district court hearing in Stenberg, and thus not included in the Stenberg trial record, demonstrates that a partial-birth abortion is never necessary to preserve the health of a woman, poses significant health risks to a woman upon whom the procedure is performed and is outside the standard of medical care.

"(6) Despite the dearth of evidence in the Stenberg trial court record supporting the district court's findings, the United States Court of Appeals for the Eighth Circuit and the Supreme Court refused to set aside the district court's factual findings because, under the applicable standard of appellate review, they were not 'clearly erroneous.' A finding of fact is clearly erroneous 'when although there is evidence to support it, the reviewing court on the entire evidence is left with the definite and firm conviction that a mistake has been committed.' *Anderson v. City of Bessemer City, North Carolina,* 470 U.S. 564, 573 (1985). Under this standard, 'if the district court's account of the evidence is plausible in light of the record viewed in its entirety, the court of appeals may not reverse it even though convinced that had it been sitting as the trier of fact, it would have weighed the evidence differently.' Id. at 574.

"(7) Thus, in Stenberg, the United States Supreme Court was required to accept the very questionable findings issued by the district court judge—the effect of which was to render null and void the reasoned factual findings and policy determinations of the United States Congress and at least 27 State legislatures.

"(8) However, under well-settled Supreme Court jurisprudence, the United States Congress is not bound to accept the same factual findings that the Supreme Court was bound to accept in Stenberg under the 'clearly erroneous' standard. Rather, the United States Congress is entitled to reach its own factual findings—findings that the Supreme Court accords great deference—and to enact legislation based upon these findings so long as it seeks to pursue a legitimate interest that is within the scope of the Constitution, and draws reasonable inferences based upon substantial evidence.

"(9) In *Katzenbach v. Morgan*, 384 U.S. 641 (1966), the Supreme Court articulated its highly deferential review of congressional factual findings when it addressed the constitutionality of section 4(e) of the Voting Rights Act of 1965 [42 U.S.C. 1973b(e)]. Regarding Congress' factual determination that section 4(e) would assist the Puerto Rican community in 'gaining nondiscriminatory treatment in public services,' the Court stated that '[i]t was for Congress, as the branch that made this judgment, to assess and weigh the various conflicting considerations. It is not for us to review the congressional resolution of these factors. It is enough that we be able to perceive a basis upon which the Congress might resolve the conflict as it did. There plainly was such a basis to support section 4(e) in the application in question in this case.' Id. at 653.

"(10) Katzenbach's highly deferential review of Congress' factual conclusions was relied upon by the United States District Court for the District of Columbia when it upheld the 'bail-out' provisions of the Voting Rights Act of 1965 (42 U.S.C. 1973c), stating that 'congressional fact finding, to which we are inclined to pay great deference, strengthens the inference that, in those jurisdictions covered by the Act, state actions discriminatory in effect are discriminatory in purpose.' *City of Rome, Georgia v. U.S.*, 472 F. Supp. 221 (D.D.C. 1979) aff'd *City of Rome, Georgia v. U.S.*, 446 U.S. 156 (1980).

"(11) The Court continued its practice of deferring to congressional factual findings in reviewing the constitutional-

ity of the must-carry provisions of the Cable Television Consumer Protection and Competition Act of 1992 [Pub. L. 102-385, see Tables for classification]. See *Turner Broadcasting System, Inc. v. Federal Communications Commission*, 512 U.S. 622 (1994) (Turner I) and *Turner Broadcasting System, Inc. v. Federal Communications Commission*, 520 U.S. 180 (1997) (Turner II). At issue in the Turner cases was Congress' legislative finding that, absent mandatory carriage rules, the continued viability of local broadcast television would be 'seriously jeopardized.' The Turner I Court recognized that as an institution, 'Congress is far better equipped than the judiciary to "amass and evaluate the vast amounts of data" bearing upon an issue as complex and dynamic as that presented here,' 512 U.S. at 665–66. Although the Court recognized that 'the deference afforded to legislative findings does "not foreclose our independent judgment of the facts bearing on an issue of constitutional law,"' its 'obligation to exercise independent judgment when First Amendment rights are implicated is not a license to reweigh the evidence de novo, or to replace Congress' factual predictions with our own. Rather, it is to assure that, in formulating its judgments, Congress has drawn reasonable inferences based on substantial evidence.' Id. at 666.

"(12) Three years later in Turner II, the Court upheld the 'must-carry' provisions based upon Congress' findings, stating the Court's 'sole obligation is "to assure that, in formulating its judgments, Congress has drawn reasonable inferences based on substantial evidence." ' 520 U.S. at 195. Citing its ruling in Turner I, the Court reiterated that '[w]e owe Congress' findings deference in part because the institution "is far better equipped than the judiciary to 'amass and evaluate the vast amounts of data' bearing upon" legislative questions,' id. at 195, and added that it 'owe[d] Congress' findings an additional measure of deference out of respect for its authority to exercise the legislative power.' Id. at 196.

"(13) There exists substantial record evidence upon which Congress has reached its conclusion that a ban on partial-birth abortion is not required to contain a 'health' exception, because the facts indicate that a partial-birth abortion is never necessary to preserve the health of a woman, poses serious risks to a woman's health, and lies outside the standard of medical care. Congress was informed by extensive hearings held during the 104th, 105th, 107th, and 108th Congresses and passed a ban on partial-birth abortion in the 104th, 105th, and 106th Congresses. These findings reflect the very informed judgment of the

Congress that a partial-birth abortion is never necessary to preserve the health of a woman, poses serious risks to a woman's health, and lies outside the standard of medical care, and should, therefore, be banned.

"(14) Pursuant to the testimony received during extensive legislative hearings during the 104th, 105th, 107th, and 108th Congresses, Congress finds and declares that:

"(A) Partial-birth abortion poses serious risks to the health of a woman undergoing the procedure. Those risks include, among other things: An increase in a woman's risk of suffering from cervical incompetence, a result of cervical dilation making it difficult or impossible for a woman to successfully carry a subsequent pregnancy to term; an increased risk of uterine rupture, abruption, amniotic fluid embolus, and trauma to the uterus as a result of converting the child to a footling breech position, a procedure which, according to a leading obstetrics textbook, 'there are very few, if any, indications for * * * other than for delivery of a second twin'; and a risk of lacerations and secondary hemorrhaging due to the doctor blindly forcing a sharp instrument into the base of the unborn child's skull while he or she is lodged in the birth canal, an act which could result in severe bleeding, brings with it the threat of shock, and could ultimately result in maternal death.

"(B) There is no credible medical evidence that partial-birth abortions are safe or are safer than other abortion procedures. No controlled studies of partial-birth abortions have been conducted nor have any comparative studies been conducted to demonstrate its safety and efficacy compared to other abortion methods. Furthermore, there have been no articles published in peer-reviewed journals that establish that partial-birth abortions are superior in any way to established abortion procedures. Indeed, unlike other more commonly used abortion procedures, there are currently no medical schools that provide instruction on abortions that include the instruction in partial-birth abortions in their curriculum.

"(C) A prominent medical association has concluded that partial-birth abortion is 'not an accepted medical practice,' that it has 'never been subject to even a minimal amount of the normal medical practice development,' that 'the relative advantages and disadvantages of the procedure in specific circumstances remain unknown,' and that 'there is no consensus among obstetricians about its use.' The association has further noted that partial-birth abortion is broadly disfavored by both medical experts and the

public, is 'ethically wrong,' and 'is never the only appropriate procedure.'

"(D) Neither the plaintiff in *Stenberg v. Carhart*, nor the experts who testified on his behalf, have identified a single circumstance during which a partial-birth abortion was necessary to preserve the health of a woman.

"(E) The physician credited with developing the partial-birth abortion procedure has testified that he has never encountered a situation where a partial-birth abortion was medically necessary to achieve the desired outcome and, thus, is never medically necessary to preserve the health of a woman.

"(F) A ban on the partial-birth abortion procedure will therefore advance the health interests of pregnant women seeking to terminate a pregnancy.

"(G) In light of this overwhelming evidence, Congress and the States have a compelling interest in prohibiting partial-birth abortions. In addition to promoting maternal health, such a prohibition will draw a bright line that clearly distinguishes abortion and infanticide, that preserves the integrity of the medical profession, and promotes respect for human life.

"(H) Based upon *Roe v. Wade*, 410 U.S. 113 (1973) and *Planned Parenthood v. Casey*, 505 U.S. 833 (1992), a governmental interest in protecting the life of a child during the delivery process arises by virtue of the fact that during a partial birth abortion, labor is induced and the birth process has begun. This distinction was recognized in Roe when the Court noted, without comment, that the Texas parturition statute, which prohibited one from killing a child 'in a state of being born and before actual birth,' was not under attack. This interest becomes compelling as the child emerges from the maternal body. A child that is completely born is a full, legal person entitled to constitutional protections afforded a 'person' under the United States Constitution. Partial-birth abortions involve the killing of a child that is in the process, in fact mere inches away from, becoming a 'person.' Thus, the government has a heightened interest in protecting the life of the partially-born child.

"(I) This, too, has not gone unnoticed in the medical community, where a prominent medical association has recognized that partial-birth abortions are 'ethically different from other destructive abortion techniques because the fetus, normally twenty weeks or longer in gestation, is killed outside of the womb.' According to this medical association, the '"partial birth" gives the fetus an autonomy which separates it from the right of the woman to choose treatments for her own body.'

"(J) Partial-birth abortion also confuses the medical, legal, and ethical duties of physicians to preserve and promote life, as the physician acts directly against the physical life of a child, whom he or she had just delivered, all but the head, out of the womb, in order to end that life. Partial-birth abortion thus appropriates the terminology and techniques used by obstetricians who preserve and protect the life of the mother and the child—and instead uses those techniques to end the life of the partially-born child.

"(K) Thus, by aborting a child in the manner that purposefully seeks to kill the child after he or she has begun the process of birth, partial-birth abortion undermines the public's perception of the appropriate role of a physician during the delivery process, and perverts a process during which life is brought into the world, in order to destroy a partially-born child.

"(L) The gruesome and inhumane nature of the partial-birth abortion procedure and its disturbing similarity to the killing of a newborn infant promotes a complete disregard for infant human life that can only be counted by a prohibition of the procedure.

"(M) The vast majority of babies killed during partial-birth abortions are alive until the end of the procedure. It is a medical fact, however, that unborn infants at this stage can feel pain when subjected to painful stimuli and that their perception of this pain is even more intense than that of newborn infants and older children when subjected to the same stimuli. Thus, during a partial-birth abortion procedure, the child will fully experience the pain associated with piercing his or her skull and sucking out his or her brain.

"(N) Implicitly approving such a brutal and inhumane procedure by choosing not to prohibit it will further coarsen society to the humanity of not only newborns, but all vulnerable and innocent human life, making it increasingly difficult to protect such life. Thus, Congress has a compelling interest in acting—indeed it must act—to prohibit this inhumane procedure.

"(O) For these reasons, Congress finds that partial-birth abortion is never medically indicated to preserve the health of the mother; is in fact unrecognized as a valid abortion procedure by the mainstream medical community; poses additional health risks to the mother; blurs the line between abortion and infanticide in the killing of a

partially-born child just inches from birth; and confuses the role of the physician in childbirth and should, there, be banned."

SEC. 3. PROHIBITION ON PARTIAL-BIRTH ABORTIONS.

(a) IN GENERAL.—Title 18, United States Code, is amended by inserting after chapter 73 the following:
"CHAPTER 74—PARTIAL-BIRTH ABORTIONS
"Sec. "1531. Partial-birth abortions prohibited.
"§ 1531. Partial-birth abortions prohibited
"(a) Any physician who, in or affecting interstate or foreign commerce, knowingly performs a partial-birth abortion and thereby kills a human fetus shall be fined under this title or imprisoned not more than 2 years, or both. This subsection does not apply to a partial-birth abortion that is necessary to save the life of a mother whose life is endangered by a physical disorder, physical illness, or physical injury, including a life-endangering physical condition caused by or arising from the pregnancy itself. This subsection takes effect 1 day after the enactment.
"(b) As used in this section—
   "(1) the term 'partial-birth abortion' means an abortion in which the person performing the abortion—
      "(A) deliberately and intentionally vaginally delivers a living fetus until, in the case of a head-first presentation, the entire fetal head is outside the body of the mother, or, in the case of breech presentation, any part of the fetal trunk past the navel is outside the body of the mother, for the purpose of performing an overt act that the person knows will kill the partially delivered living fetus; and
      "(B) performs the overt act, other than completion of delivery, that kills the partially delivered living fetus; and
   "(2) the term 'physician' means a doctor of medicine or osteopathy legally authorized to practice medicine and surgery by the State in which the doctor performs such activity, or any other individual legally authorized by the State to perform abortions: *Provided, however,* That any individual who is not a physician or not otherwise legally authorized by the State to perform abortions, but who nevertheless directly performs a partial-birth abortion, shall be subject to the provisions of this section.

"(c)(1) The father, if married to the mother at the time she receives a partial-birth abortion procedure, and if the mother has not attained the age of 18 years at the time of the abortion, the maternal grandparents of the fetus, may in a civil action obtain appropriate relief, unless the pregnancy resulted from the plaintiff's criminal conduct or the plaintiff consented to the abortion.

"(2) Such relief shall include—

"(A) money damages for all injuries, psychological and physical, occasioned by the violation of this section; and

"(B) statutory damages equal to three times the cost of the partial-birth abortion.

"(d)(1) A defendant accused of an offense under this section may seek a hearing before the State Medical Board on whether the physician's conduct was necessary to save the life of the mother whose life was endangered by a physical disorder, physical illness, or physical injury, including a life-endangering physical condition caused by or arising from the pregnancy itself.

"(2) The findings on that issue are admissible on that issue at the trial of the defendant. Upon a motion of the defendant, the court shall delay the beginning of the trial for not more than 30 days to permit such a hearing to take place.

"(e) A woman upon whom a partial-birth abortion is performed may not be prosecuted under this section, for a conspiracy to violate this section, or for an offense under section 2, 3, or 4 of this title based on a violation of this section.".

(b) CLERICAL AMENDMENT.—The table of chapters for part I of title 18, United States Code, is amended by inserting after the item relating to chapter 73 the following new item:

"74. Partial-birth abortions .... 1531".

Approved November 5, 2003.

Case Law: *Gonzales v. Carhart* (Constitutionality of the Partial Birth Abortion Ban Act)

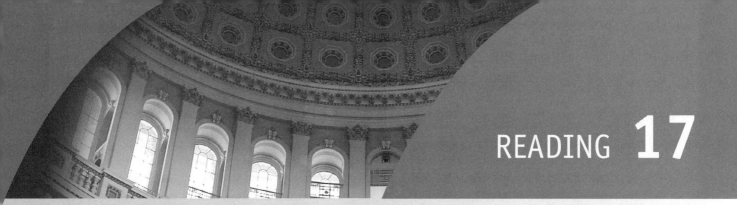

SUPREME COURT OF THE UNITED STATES

GONZALES, ATTORNEY GENERAL v. CARHART ET AL.

CERTIORARI TO THE UNITED STATES COURT OF APPEALS FOR THE EIGHTH CIRCUIT

No. 05–380. Argued November 8, 2006—Decided April 18, 2007

Opinion of the Court

JUSTICE KENNEDY delivered the opinion of the Court.

These cases require us to consider the validity of the Partial-Birth Abortion Ban Act of 2003 (Act), 18 U. S. C. §1531 (2000 ed., Supp. IV), a federal statute regulating abortion procedures. In recitations preceding its operative provisions the Act refers to the Court's opinion in *Stenberg* v. *Carhart*, 530 U. S. 914 (2000), which also addressed the subject of abortion procedures used in the later stages of pregnancy. Compared to the state statute at issue in *Stenberg*, the Act is more specific concerning the instances to which it applies and in this respect more precise in its coverage. We conclude the Act should be sustained against the objections lodged by the broad, facial attack brought against it.

In No. 05–380 *(Carhart)* respondents are LeRoy Carhart, William G. Fitzhugh, William H. Knorr, and Jill L. Vibhakar, doctors who perform second-trimester abortions. These doctors filed their complaint against the Attorney General of the United States in the United States District Court for the District of Nebraska. They challenged the constitutionality of the Act and sought a permanent injunction against its enforcement. *Carhart* v. *Ashcroft*, 331 F. Supp. 2d 805 (2004). In 2004, after a 2-week trial, the District Court granted a permanent injunction that prohibited the Attorney General from enforcing the Act

in all cases but those in which there was no dispute the fetus was viable. *Id.*, at 1048. The Court of Appeals for the Eighth Circuit affirmed. 413 F. 3d 791 (2005). We granted certiorari. 546 U. S. 1169 (2006).

In No. 05–1382 *(Planned Parenthood)* respondents are Planned Parenthood Federation of America, Inc., Planned Parenthood Golden Gate, and the City and County of San Francisco. The Planned Parenthood entities sought to enjoin enforcement of the Act in a suit filed in the United States District Court for the Northern District of California. *Planned Parenthood Federation of Am.* v. *Ashcroft*, 320 F. Supp. 2d 957 (2004). The City and County of San Francisco intervened as a plaintiff. In 2004, the District Court held a trial spanning a period just short of three weeks, and it, too, enjoined the Attorney General from enforcing the Act. *Id.*, at 1035. The Court of Appeals for the Ninth Circuit affirmed. 435 F. 3d 1163 (2006). We granted certiorari. 547 U.S. ____ (2006).

I

A

The Act proscribes a particular manner of ending fetal life, so it is necessary here, as it was in *Stenberg*, to discuss abortion procedures in some detail. Three United States District Courts heard extensive evidence describing the procedures. In addition to the two courts involved in the instant cases the District Court for the Southern District of New York also considered the constitutionality of the Act. *Nat. Abortion Federation* v. *Ashcroft*, 330 F. Supp. 2d 436 (2004). It found the Act unconstitutional, *id.*, at 493, and the Court of Appeals for the Second Circuit affirmed, *Nat. Abortion Federation* v. *Gonzales*, 437 F. 3d 278 (2006). The three District Courts relied on similar medical evidence; indeed, much of the evidence submitted to the *Carhart* court previously had been submitted to the other two courts. 331 F. Supp. 2d, at 809–810. We refer to the District Courts' exhaustive opinions in our own discussion of abortion procedures.

Abortion methods vary depending to some extent on the preferences of the physician and, of course, on the term of the pregnancy and the resulting stage of the unborn child's development. Between 85 and 90 percent of the approximately 1.3 million abortions performed each year in the United States take place in the first three months of pregnancy, which is to say in the first trimester. *Planned Parenthood*, 320 F. Supp. 2d, at 960, and n. 4; App. in No. 05–1382, pp. 45–48. The most common first-trimester abortion method is vacuum aspiration (otherwise known as suction curettage) in which the physician vacuums out the embryonic tissue. Early in this trimester an alternative is to use medication, such as mifepristone (commonly known as RU–486), to terminate the pregnancy. *Nat. Abortion Federation, supra*, at 464, n. 20. The Act does not regulate these procedures.

Of the remaining abortions that take place each year, most occur in the second trimester. The surgical procedure referred to as "dilation and evacuation" or "D&E" is the usual abortion method in this trimester. *Planned Parenthood*, 320 F. Supp. 2d, at 960–961. Although individual techniques for performing D&E differ, the general steps are the same.

A doctor must first dilate the cervix at least to the extent needed to insert surgical instruments into the uterus and to maneuver them to evacuate the fetus. *Nat. Abortion Federation, supra*, at 465; App. in No. 05–1382, at 61. The steps taken to cause dilation differ by physician and gestational age of the fetus. See, *e.g., Carhart*, 331 F. Supp. 2d, at 852, 856, 859, 862–865, 868, 870, 873–874, 876–877, 880, 883, 886. A doctor often begins the dilation process by inserting osmotic dilators, such as laminaria (sticks of seaweed), into the cervix. The dilators can be used in combination with drugs, such as misoprostol, that increase dilation. The resulting amount of dilation is not uniform, and a doctor does not know in advance how an individual patient will respond. In general the longer dilators remain in the cervix, the more it will dilate. Yet the length of time doctors employ osmotic dilators varies. Some may keep dilators in the cervix for two days, while others use dilators for a day or less. *Nat. Abortion Federation, supra*, at 464–465; *Planned Parenthood, supra*, at 961.

After sufficient dilation the surgical operation can commence. The woman is placed under general anesthesia or conscious sedation. The doctor, often guided by ultrasound, inserts grasping forceps through the woman's cervix and into the uterus to grab the fetus. The doctor grips a fetal part with the forceps and pulls it back through the cervix and vagina, continuing to pull even after meeting resistance from the cervix. The friction causes the fetus to tear apart. For example, a leg might be ripped off the fetus as it is pulled through the cervix and out of the woman. The process of evacuating the fetus piece by piece continues until it has been completely removed. A doctor may make 10 to 15 passes with the forceps to evacuate the fetus in its entirety, though sometimes removal is completed with fewer passes. Once the fetus has been evacuated, the placenta and any remaining fetal material are suctioned or scraped out of the uterus. The doctor examines the different parts to ensure the entire fetal body has been removed. See, *e.g., Nat. Abortion Federation, supra*, at 465; *Planned Parenthood, supra*, at 962.

Some doctors, especially later in the second trimester, may kill the fetus a day or two before performing the surgical evacuation. They inject digoxin or potassium chloride into the fetus, the umbilical cord, or the amniotic fluid. Fetal demise may cause contractions and make greater dilation possible. Once dead, moreover, the fetus' body will soften, and its removal will be easier. Other doctors refrain from injecting chemical agents, believing it adds risk with little or no medical benefit. *Carhart, supra*, at 907–912; *Nat. Abortion Federation, supra*, at 474–475.

The abortion procedure that was the impetus for the numerous bans on "partial-birth abortion," including the Act, is a variation of this standard D&E. See M. Haskell, Dilation and Extraction for Late Second Trimester Abortion (1992), 1 Appellant's App. in No. 04–3379 (CA8), p. 109 (hereinafter Dilation and Extraction). The medical community has not reached unanimity on the appropriate name for this D&E variation. It has been referred to as "intact D&E," "dilation and extraction" (D&X), and "intact D&X." *Nat. Abortion Federation, supra*, at 440, n. 2; see also F. Cunningham et al., Williams Obstetrics 243 (22d ed. 2005) (identifying the procedure as D&X); Danforth's Obstetrics and Gynecology 567 (J. Scott, R. Gibbs, B. Karlan, & A. Haney eds. 9th ed. 2003) (identifying the procedure as intact D&X); M. Paul, E. Lichtenberg, L. Borgatta, D. Grimes, & P. Stubblefield, A Clinician's Guide to Medical and Surgical Abortion 136 (1999) (identifying the procedure as intact D&E). For discussion purposes this D&E variation will be referred to as intact D&E. The main difference between the two procedures is that in intact D&E a doctor extracts the fetus intact or largely intact with only a few passes. There are no comprehensive statistics indicating what percentage of all D&Es are performed in this manner.

Intact D&E, like regular D&E, begins with dilation of the cervix. Sufficient dilation is essential for the procedure. To achieve intact extraction some doctors thus may attempt to dilate the cervix to a greater degree. This approach has been called "serial" dilation. *Carhart, supra*, at 856, 870, 873; *Planned Parenthood, supra*, at 965. Doctors who attempt at the outset to perform intact D&E may dilate for two full days or use up to 25 osmotic dilators. See, *e.g.*, Dilation and Extraction 110; *Carhart, supra*, at 865, 868, 876, 886.

In an intact D&E procedure the doctor extracts the fetus in a way conducive to pulling out its entire body, instead of ripping it apart. One doctor, for example, testified:

> "If I know I have good dilation and I reach in and the fetus starts to come out and I think I can accomplish it, the abortion with an intact delivery, then I use my forceps a little bit differently. I don't close them quite so much, and I just gently draw the tissue out attempting to have an intact delivery, if possible." App. in No. 05–1382, at 74.

Rotating the fetus as it is being pulled decreases the odds of dismemberment. *Carhart, supra*, at 868–869; App. In No. 05–380, pp. 40–41; 5 Appellant's App. in No. 04–3379 (CA8), p. 1469. A doctor also "may use forceps to grasp a fetal part, pull it down, and re-grasp the fetus at a higher level—sometimes using both his hand and a forceps—to exert traction to retrieve the fetus intact until the head is lodged in the [cervix]." *Carhart*, 331 F. Supp. 2d, at 886–887.

Intact D&E gained public notoriety when, in 1992, Dr. Martin Haskell gave a presentation describing his method of performing the operation. Dilation and Extraction 110–111. In the usual intact D&E the fetus' head lodges in the cervix, and dilation is insufficient to allow it to pass. See, *e.g., ibid.;* App. in No. 05–380, at 577; App. in No. 05–1382, at 74, 282. Haskell explained the next step as follows:

> " 'At this point, the right-handed surgeon slides the fingers of the left [hand] along the back of the fetus and "hooks" the shoulders of the fetus with the index and ring fingers (palm down).
> " 'While maintaining this tension, lifting the cervix and applying traction to the shoulders with the fingers of the left hand, the surgeon takes a pair of blunt curved Metzenbaum scissors in the right hand. He carefully advances the tip, curved down, along the spine and under his middle finger until he feels it contact the base of the skull under the tip of his middle finger.
> " '[T]he surgeon then forces the scissors into the base of the skull or into the foramen magnum. Having safely entered the skull, he spreads the scissors to enlarge the opening.

> " 'The surgeon removes the scissors and introduces a suction catheter into this hole and evacuates the skull contents. With the catheter still in place, he applies traction to the fetus, removing it completely from the patient.' " H. R. Rep. No. 108–58, p. 3 (2003).

This is an abortion doctor's clinical description. Here is another description from a nurse who witnessed the same method performed on a 26½-week fetus and who testified before the Senate Judiciary Committee:

> " 'Dr. Haskell went in with forceps and grabbed the baby's legs and pulled them down into the birth canal. Then he delivered the baby's body and the arms—everything but the head. The doctor kept the head right inside the uterus. . . .
> " 'The baby's little fingers were clasping and unclasping, and his little feet were kicking. Then the doctor stuck the scissors in the back of his head, and the baby's arms jerked out, like a startle reaction, like a flinch, like a baby does when he thinks he is going to fall.
> " 'The doctor opened up the scissors, stuck a high-powered suction tube into the opening, and sucked the baby's brains out. Now the baby went completely limp. . . .
> " 'He cut the umbilical cord and delivered the placenta. He threw the baby in a pan, along with the placenta and the instruments he had just used.' " *Ibid.*

Dr. Haskell's approach is not the only method of killing the fetus once its head lodges in the cervix, and "the process has evolved" since his presentation. *Planned Parenthood*, 320 F. Supp. 2d, at 965. Another doctor, for example, squeezes the skull after it has been pierced "so that enough brain tissue exudes to allow the head to pass through." App. in No. 05–380, at 41; see also *Carhart, supra,* at 866–867, 874. Still other physicians reach into the cervix with their forceps and crush the fetus' skull. *Carhart, supra,* at 858, 881. Others continue to pull the fetus out of the woman until it disarticulates at the neck, in effect decapitating it. These doctors then grasp the head with forceps, crush it, and remove it. *Id.,* at 864, 878; see also *Planned Parenthood, supra,* at 965.

Some doctors performing an intact D&E attempt to remove the fetus without collapsing the skull. See *Carhart, supra,* at 866, 869. Yet one doctor would not allow delivery of a live fetus younger than 24 weeks because "the objective of [his] procedure is to perform an abortion," not a birth. App. in No. 05–1382, at

408–409. The doctor thus answered in the affirmative when asked whether he would "hold the fetus' head on the internal side of the [cervix] in order to collapse the skull" and kill the fetus before it is born. *Id.,* at 409; see also *Carhart, supra,* at 862, 878. Another doctor testified he crushes a fetus' skull not only to reduce its size but also to ensure the fetus is dead before it is removed. For the staff to have to deal with a fetus that has "some viability to it, some movement of limbs," according to this doctor, "[is] always a difficult situation." App. in No. 05–380, at 94; see *Carhart, supra,* at 858.

D&E and intact D&E are not the only second-trimester abortion methods. Doctors also may abort a fetus through medical induction. The doctor medicates the woman to induce labor, and contractions occur to deliver the fetus. Induction, which unlike D&E should occur in a hospital, can last as little as 6 hours but can take longer than 48. It accounts for about five percent of second-trimester abortions before 20 weeks of gestation and 15 percent of those after 20 weeks. Doctors turn to two other methods of second-trimester abortion, hysterotomy and hysterectomy, only in emergency situations because they carry increased risk of complications. In a hysterotomy, as in a cesarean section, the doctor removes the fetus by making an incision through the abdomen and uterine wall to gain access to the uterine cavity. A hysterectomy requires the removal of the entire uterus. These two procedures represent about .07% of second-trimester abortions. *Nat. Abortion Federation,* 330 F. Supp. 2d, at 467; *Planned Parenthood, supra,* at 962–963.

B

After Dr. Haskell's procedure received public attention, with ensuing and increasing public concern, bans on "'partial birth abortion'" proliferated. By the time of the *Stenberg* decision, about 30 States had enacted bans designed to prohibit the procedure. 530 U. S., at 995–996, and nn. 12–13 (THOMAS, J., dissenting); see also H. R. Rep. No. 108–58, at 4–5. In 1996, Congress also acted to ban partial-birth abortion. President Clinton vetoed the congressional legislation, and the Senate failed to override the veto. Congress approved another bill banning the procedure in 1997, but President Clinton again vetoed it. In 2003, after this Court's decision in *Stenberg,* Congress passed the Act at issue here. H. R. Rep. No. 108–58, at 12–14. On November 5, 2003, President Bush signed the Act into law. It was to take effect the following day. 18 U. S. C. §1531(a) (2000 ed., Supp. IV).

The Act responded to *Stenberg* in two ways. First, Congress made factual findings. Congress determined that this Court in *Stenberg* "was required to accept the very questionable findings issued by the district court judge," §2(7), 117 Stat. 1202, notes following 18 U. S. C. §1531 (2000 ed., Supp. IV), p. 768,

¶(7) (Congressional Findings), but that Congress was "not bound to accept the same factual findings," *ibid.,* ¶(8). Congress found, among other things, that "[a] moral, medical, and ethical consensus exists that the practice of performing a partial-birth abortion . . . is a gruesome and inhumane procedure that is never medically necessary and should be prohibited." *Id.,* at 767, ¶(1).

Second, and more relevant here, the Act's language differs from that of the Nebraska statute struck down in *Stenberg.* See 530 U. S., at 921–922 (quoting Neb. Rev. Stat. Ann. §§28–328(1), 28–326(9) (Supp. 1999)). The operative provisions of the Act provide in relevant part:

> "(a) Any physician who, in or affecting interstate or foreign commerce, knowingly performs a partial-birth abortion and thereby kills a human fetus shall be fined under this title or imprisoned not more than 2 years, or both. This subsection does not apply to a partial-birth abortion that is necessary to save the life of a mother whose life is endangered by a physical disorder, physical illness, or physical injury, including a life-endangering physical condition caused by or arising from the pregnancy itself. This subsection takes effect 1 day after the enactment.

> "(b) As used in this section—

> "(1) the term 'partial-birth abortion' means an abortion in which the person performing the abortion—

> "(A) deliberately and intentionally vaginally delivers a living fetus until, in the case of a head-first presentation, the entire fetal head is outside the body of the mother, or, in the case of breech presentation, any part of the fetal trunk past the navel is outside the body of the mother, for the purpose of performing an overt act that the person knows will kill the partially delivered living fetus; and

> "(B) performs the overt act, other than completion of delivery, that kills the partially delivered living fetus; and

> "(2) the term 'physician' means a doctor of medicine or osteopathy legally authorized to practice medicine and surgery by the State in which the doctor performs such activity, or any other individual legally authorized by the State to perform abortions: *Provided, however,* That any

individual who is not a physician or not otherwise legally authorized by the State to perform abortions, but who nevertheless directly performs a partial-birth abortion, shall be subject to the provisions of this section.

"(d)(1) A defendant accused of an offense under this section may seek a hearing before the State Medical Board on whether the physician's conduct was necessary to save the life of the mother whose life was endangered by a physical disorder, physical illness, or physical injury, including a life-endangering physical condition caused by or arising from the pregnancy itself.

"(2) The findings on that issue are admissible on that issue at the trial of the defendant. Upon a motion of the defendant, the court shall delay the beginning of the trial for not more than 30 days to permit such a hearing to take place.

"(e) A woman upon whom a partial-birth abortion is performed may not be prosecuted under this section, for a conspiracy to violate this section, or for an offense under section 2, 3, or 4 of this title based on a violation of this section." 18 U. S. C. §1531 (2000 ed., Supp. IV).

The Act also includes a provision authorizing civil actions that is not of relevance here. §1531(c).

C

The District Court in *Carhart* concluded the Act was unconstitutional for two reasons. First, it determined the Act was unconstitutional because it lacked an exception allowing the procedure where necessary for the health of the mother. 331 F. Supp. 2d, at 1004–1030. Second, the District Court found the Act deficient because it covered not merely intact D&E but also certain other D&Es. *Id.*, at 1030–1037.

The Court of Appeals for the Eighth Circuit addressed only the lack of a health exception. 413 F. 3d, at 803–804. The court began its analysis with what it saw as the appropriate question—"whether 'substantial medical authority' supports the medical necessity of the banned procedure." *Id.*, at 796 (quoting *Stenberg*, 530 U. S., at 938). This was the proper framework, according to the Court of Appeals, because "when a lack of consensus exists in the medical community, the Constitution requires legislatures to err on the side of protecting women's health by including a health exception." 413 F. 3d, at 796. The court rejected the Attorney General's attempt to demonstrate changed evidentiary circumstances since *Stenberg*

and considered itself bound by *Stenberg*'s conclusion that a health exception was required. 413 F. 3d, at 803 (explaining "[t]he record in [the] case and the record in *Stenberg* [were] similar in all significant respects"). It invalidated the Act. *Ibid.*

D

The District Court in *Planned Parenthood* concluded the Act was unconstitutional "because it (1) pose[d] an undue burden on a woman's ability to choose a second trimester abortion; (2) [was] unconstitutionally vague; and (3) require[d] a health exception as set forth by . . . *Stenberg*." 320 F. Supp. 2d, at 1034–1035.

The Court of Appeals for the Ninth Circuit agreed. Like the Court of Appeals for the Eighth Circuit, it concluded the absence of a health exception rendered the Act unconstitutional. The court interpreted *Stenberg* to require a health exception unless "there is *consensus in the medical community* that the banned procedure is never medically necessary to preserve the health of women." 435 F. 3d, at 1173. Even after applying a deferential standard of review to Congress' factual findings, the Court of Appeals determined "substantial disagreement exists in the medical community regarding whether" the procedures prohibited by the Act are ever necessary to preserve a woman's health. *Id.*, at 1175–1176.

The Court of Appeals concluded further that the Act placed an undue burden on a woman's ability to obtain a second-trimester abortion. The court found the textual differences between the Act and the Nebraska statute struck down in *Stenberg* insufficient to distinguish D&E and intact D&E. 435 F. 3d, at 1178–1180. As a result, according to the Court of Appeals, the Act imposed an undue burden because it prohibited D&E. *Id.*, at 1180–1181.

Finally, the Court of Appeals found the Act void for vagueness. *Id.*, at 1181. Abortion doctors testified they were uncertain which procedures the Act made criminal. The court thus concluded the Act did not offer physicians clear warning of its regulatory reach. *Id.*, at 1181–1184. Resting on its understanding of the remedial framework established by this Court in *Ayotte* v. *Planned Parenthood of Northern New Eng.*, 546 U. S. 320, 328–330 (2006), the Court of Appeals held the Act was unconstitutional on its face and should be permanently enjoined. 435 F. 3d, at 1184–1191.

II

The principles set forth in the joint opinion in *Planned Parenthood of Southeastern Pa.* v. *Casey*, 505 U. S. 833 (1992), did not find support from all those who join the instant opinion. See *id.*, at 979–1002 (SCALIA, J., joined by THOMAS, J., *inter alios*, concurring in judgment in part and dissenting in part). Whatever one's views concerning the *Casey* joint opinion, it is evident a premise central to its conclusion—that the government has a legitimate and substantial interest in preserving and promoting fetal life—would be repudiated were the Court now to affirm the judgments of the Courts of Appeals.

Casey involved a challenge to *Roe* v. *Wade*, 410 U. S. 113 (1973). The opinion contains this summary:

> "It must be stated at the outset and with clarity that *Roe*'s essential holding, the holding we reaffirm, has three parts. First is a recognition of the right of the woman to choose to have an abortion before viability and to obtain it without undue interference from the State. Before viability, the State's interests are not strong enough to support a prohibition of abortion or the imposition of a substantial obstacle to the woman's effective right to elect the procedure. Second is a confirmation of the State's power to restrict abortions after fetal viability, if the law contains exceptions for pregnancies which endanger the woman's life or health. And third is the principle that the State has legitimate interests from the outset of the pregnancy in protecting the health of the woman and the life of the fetus that may become a child. These principles do not contradict one another; and we adhere to each." 505 U. S., at 846 (opinion of the Court).

Though all three holdings are implicated in the instant cases, it is the third that requires the most extended discussion; for we must determine whether the Act furthers the legitimate interest of the Government in protecting the life of the fetus that may become a child.

To implement its holding, *Casey* rejected both *Roe*'s rigid trimester framework and the interpretation of *Roe* that considered all previability regulations of abortion unwarranted. 505 U. S., at 875–876, 878 (plurality opinion). On this point *Casey* overruled the holdings in two cases because they undervalued the State's interest in potential life. See *id.*, at 881–883 (joint opinion) (overruling *Thornburgh* v. *American College of Obstetricians and Gynecologists*, 476 U. S. 747 (1986) and *Akron* v. *Akron Center for Reproductive Health, Inc.*, 462 U. S. 416 (1983)).

We assume the following principles for the purposes of this opinion. Before viability, a State "may not prohibit any woman from making the ultimate decision to terminate her pregnancy." 505 U. S., at 879 (plurality opinion). It also may not impose upon this right an undue burden, which exists if a reg-

ulation's "purpose or effect is to place a substantial obstacle in the path of a woman seeking an abortion before the fetus attains viability." *Id.*, at 878. On the other hand, "[r]egulations which do no more than create a structural mechanism by which the State, or the parent or guardian of a minor, may express profound respect for the life of the unborn are permitted, if they are not a substantial obstacle to the woman's exercise of the right to choose." *Id.*, at 877. *Casey*, in short, struck a balance. The balance was central to its holding. We now apply its standard to the cases at bar.

III

We begin with a determination of the Act's operation and effect. A straightforward reading of the Act's text demonstrates its purpose and the scope of its provisions: It regulates and proscribes, with exceptions or qualifications to be discussed, performing the intact D&E procedure.

Respondents agree the Act encompasses intact D&E, but they contend its additional reach is both unclear and excessive. Respondents assert that, at the least, the Act is void for vagueness because its scope is indefinite. In the alternative, respondents argue the Act's text proscribes all D&Es. Because D&E is the most common second-trimester abortion method, respondents suggest the Act imposes an undue burden. In this litigation the Attorney General does not dispute that the Act would impose an undue burden if it covered standard D&E.

We conclude that the Act is not void for vagueness, does not impose an undue burden from any overbreadth, and is not invalid on its face.

A

The Act punishes "knowingly perform[ing]" a "partial birth abortion." §1531(a) (2000 ed., Supp. IV). It defines the unlawful abortion in explicit terms. §1531(b)(1).

First, the person performing the abortion must "vaginally delive[r] a living fetus." §1531(b)(1)(A). The Act does not restrict an abortion procedure involving the delivery of an expired fetus. The Act, furthermore, is inapplicable to abortions that do not involve vaginal delivery (for instance, hysterotomy or hysterectomy). The Act does apply both previability and postviability because, by common understanding and scientific terminology, a fetus is a living organism while within the womb, whether or not it is viable outside the womb. See, *e.g.*, *Planned Parenthood*, 320 F. Supp. 2d, at 971–972. We do not understand this point to be contested by the parties.

Second, the Act's definition of partial-birth abortion requires the fetus to be delivered "until, in the case of a head-first presentation, the entire fetal head is outside the body of the mother, or, in the case of breech presentation, any part of the fetal trunk past the navel is outside the body of the mother." §1531(b)(1)(A) (2000 ed., Supp. IV). The Attorney General concedes, and we agree, that if an abortion procedure does not involve the delivery of a living fetus to one of these "anatomical 'landmarks'"—where, depending on the presentation, either the fetal head or the fetal trunk past the navel is outside the body of the mother—the prohibitions of the Act do not apply. Brief for Petitioner in No. 05–380, p. 46.

Third, to fall within the Act, a doctor must perform an "overt act, other than completion of delivery, that kills the partially delivered living fetus." §1531(b)(1)(B) (2000 ed., Supp. IV). For purposes of criminal liability, the overt act causing the fetus' death must be separate from delivery. And the overt act must occur after the delivery to an anatomical landmark. This is because the Act proscribes killing "the partially delivered" fetus, which, when read in context, refers to a fetus that has been delivered to an anatomical landmark. *Ibid.*

Fourth, the Act contains scienter requirements concerning all the actions involved in the prohibited abortion. To begin with, the physician must have "deliberately and intentionally" delivered the fetus to one of the Act's anatomical landmarks. §1531(b)(1)(A). If a living fetus is delivered past the critical point by accident or inadvertence, the Act is inapplicable. In addition, the fetus must have been delivered "for the purpose of performing an overt act that the [doctor] knows will kill [it]." *Ibid.* If either intent is absent, no crime has occurred. This follows from the general principle that where scienter is required no crime is committed absent the requisite state of mind. See generally 1 W. LaFave, Substantive Criminal Law §5.1 (2d ed. 2003) (hereinafter LaFave); 1 C. Torcia, Wharton's Criminal Law §27 (15th ed. 1993).

B

Respondents contend the language described above is indeterminate, and they thus argue the Act is unconstitutionally vague on its face. "As generally stated, the void-for-vagueness doctrine requires that a penal statute define the criminal offense with sufficient definiteness that ordinary people can understand what conduct is prohibited and in a manner that does not encourage arbitrary and discriminatory enforcement." *Kolender* v. *Lawson*, 461 U. S. 352, 357 (1983); *Posters 'N' Things, Ltd.* v. *United States*, 511 U. S. 513, 525 (1994). The Act satisfies both requirements.

The Act provides doctors "of ordinary intelligence a reasonable opportunity to know what is prohibited." *Grayned* v. *City of Rockford*, 408 U. S. 104, 108 (1972). Indeed, it sets forth "relatively clear guidelines as to prohibited conduct" and provides "objective criteria" to evaluate whether a doctor has performed a prohibited procedure. *Posters 'N' Things, supra*, at

525–526. Unlike the statutory language in *Stenberg* that prohibited the delivery of a "'substantial portion'" of the fetus—where a doctor might question how much of the fetus is a substantial portion—the Act defines the line between potentially criminal conduct on the one hand and lawful abortion on the other. *Stenberg*, 530 U. S., at 922 (quoting Neb. Rev. Stat. Ann. §28–326(9) (Supp. 1999)). Doctors performing D&E will know that if they do not deliver a living fetus to an anatomical landmark they will not face criminal liability.

This conclusion is buttressed by the intent that must be proved to impose liability. The Court has made clear that scienter requirements alleviate vagueness concerns. *Posters 'N' Things, supra*, at 526; see also *Colautti* v. *Franklin*, 439 U. S. 379, 395 (1979) ("This Court has long recognized that the constitutionality of a vague statutory standard is closely related to whether that standard incorporates a requirement of *mens rea*"). The Act requires the doctor deliberately to have delivered the fetus to an anatomical landmark. §1531(b)(1)(A) (2000 ed., Supp. IV). Because a doctor performing a D&E will not face criminal liability if he or she delivers a fetus beyond the prohibited point by mistake, the Act cannot be described as "a trap for those who act in good faith." *Colautti, supra*, at 395 (internal quotation marks omitted).

Respondents likewise have failed to show that the Act should be invalidated on its face because it encourages arbitrary or discriminatory enforcement. *Kolender, supra*, at 357. Just as the Act's anatomical landmarks provide doctors with objective standards, they also "establish minimal guidelines to govern law enforcement." *Smith* v. *Goguen*, 415 U. S. 566, 574 (1974). The scienter requirements narrow the scope of the Act's prohibition and limit prosecutorial discretion. It cannot be said that the Act "vests virtually complete discretion in the hands of [law enforcement] to determine whether the [doctor] has satisfied [its provisions]." *Kolender, supra*, at 358 (invalidating a statute regulating loitering). Respondents' arguments concerning arbitrary enforcement, furthermore, are somewhat speculative. This is a preenforcement challenge, where "no evidence has been, or could be, introduced to indicate whether the [Act] has been enforced in a discriminatory manner or with the aim of inhibiting [constitutionally protected conduct]." *Hoffman Estates* v. *Flipside, Hoffman Estates, Inc.*, 455 U. S. 489, 503 (1982). The Act is not vague.

C

We next determine whether the Act imposes an undue burden, as a facial matter, because its restrictions on second-trimester abortions are too broad. A review of the statutory text discloses the limits of its reach. The Act prohibits intact D&E; and, notwithstanding respondents' arguments, it does not prohibit the D&E procedure in which the fetus is removed in parts.

1

The Act prohibits a doctor from intentionally performing an intact D&E. The dual prohibitions of the Act, both of which are necessary for criminal liability, correspond with the steps generally undertaken during this type of procedure. First, a doctor delivers the fetus until its head lodges in the cervix, which is usually past the anatomical landmark for a breech presentation. See 18 U. S. C. §1531(b)(1)(A) (2000 ed., Supp. IV). Second, the doctor proceeds to pierce the fetal skull with scissors or crush it with forceps. This step satisfies the overt-act requirement because it kills the fetus and is distinct from delivery. See §1531(b)(1)(B). The Act's intent requirements, however, limit its reach to those physicians who carry out the intact D&E after intending to undertake both steps at the outset.

The Act excludes most D&Es in which the fetus is removed in pieces, not intact. If the doctor intends to remove the fetus in parts from the outset, the doctor will not have the requisite intent to incur criminal liability. A doctor performing a standard D&E procedure can often "tak[e] about 10–15 'passes' through the uterus to remove the entire fetus." *Planned Parenthood*, 320 F. Supp. 2d, at 962. Removing the fetus in this manner does not violate the Act because the doctor will not have delivered the living fetus to one of the anatomical landmarks or committed an additional overt act that kills the fetus after partial delivery. §1531(b)(1) (2000 ed., Supp. IV).

A comparison of the Act with the Nebraska statute struck down in *Stenberg* confirms this point. The statute in *Stenberg* prohibited "'deliberately and intentionally delivering into the vagina a living unborn child, or a substantial portion thereof, for the purpose of performing a procedure that the person performing such procedure knows will kill the unborn child and does kill the unborn child.'" 530 U. S., at 922 (quoting Neb. Rev. Stat. Ann. §28–326(9) (Supp. 1999)). The Court concluded that this statute encompassed D&E because "D&E will often involve a physician pulling a 'substantial portion' of a still living fetus, say, an arm or leg, into the vagina prior to the death of the fetus." 530 U. S., at 939. The Court also rejected the limiting interpretation urged by Nebraska's Attorney General that the statute's reference to a "procedure" that "'kill[s] the unborn child'" was to a distinct procedure, not to the abortion procedure as a whole. *Id.*, at 943.

Congress, it is apparent, responded to these concerns because the Act departs in material ways from the statute in *Stenberg*. It adopts the phrase "delivers a living fetus," §1531(b)(1)(A) (2000 ed., Supp. IV), instead of "'delivering . . . a living unborn child, or a substantial portion thereof,'" 530 U. S., at 938 (quoting Neb. Rev. Stat. Ann. §28–326(9) (Supp.

1999)). The Act's language, unlike the statute in *Stenberg*, expresses the usual meaning of "deliver" when used in connection with "fetus," namely, extraction of an entire fetus rather than removal of fetal pieces. See Stedman's Medical Dictionary 470 (27th ed. 2000) (defining deliver as "[t]o assist a woman in childbirth" and "[t]o extract from an enclosed place, as the fetus from the womb, an object or foreign body"); see also I. Dox, B. Melloni, G. Eisner, & J. Melloni, The HarperCollins Illustrated Medical Dictionary 160 (4th ed. 2001); Merriam Webster's Collegiate Dictionary 306 (10th ed. 1997). The Act thus displaces the interpretation of "delivering" dictated by the Nebraska statute's reference to a "substantial portion" of the fetus. *Stenberg, supra,* at 944 (indicating that the Nebraska "statute itself specifies that it applies *both* to delivering 'an intact unborn child' *or* 'a substantial portion thereof'"). In interpreting statutory texts courts use the ordinary meaning of terms unless context requires a different result. See, *e.g.,* 2A N. Singer, Sutherland on Statutes and Statutory Construction §47:28 (rev. 6th ed. 2000). Here, unlike in *Stenberg*, the language does not require a departure from the ordinary meaning. D&E does not involve the delivery of a fetus because it requires the removal of fetal parts that are ripped from the fetus as they are pulled through the cervix.

The identification of specific anatomical landmarks to which the fetus must be partially delivered also differentiates the Act from the statute at issue in *Stenberg*. §1531(b)(1)(A) (2000 ed., Supp. IV). The Court in *Stenberg* interpreted "'substantial portion'" of the fetus to include an arm or a leg. 530 U. S., at 939. The Act's anatomical landmarks, by contrast, clarify that the removal of a small portion of the fetus is not prohibited. The landmarks also require the fetus to be delivered so that it is partially "outside the body of the mother." §1531(b)(1)(A). To come within the ambit of the Nebraska statute, on the other hand, a substantial portion of the fetus only had to be delivered into the vagina; no part of the fetus had to be outside the body of the mother before a doctor could face criminal sanctions. *Id.,* at 938–939.

By adding an overt-act requirement Congress sought further to meet the Court's objections to the state statute considered in *Stenberg*. Compare 18 U. S. C. §1531(b)(1) (2000 ed., Supp. IV) with Neb. Rev. Stat. Ann. §28–326(9) (Supp. 1999). The Act makes the distinction the Nebraska statute failed to draw (but the Nebraska Attorney General advanced) by differentiating between the overall partial birth abortion and the distinct overt act that kills the fetus. See *Stenberg*, 530 U. S., at 943–944. The fatal overt act must occur after delivery to an anatomical landmark, and it must be something "other than [the] completion of delivery." §1531(b)(1)(B). This distinction matters because, unlike intact D&E, standard D&E does not involve a delivery followed by a fatal act.

The canon of constitutional avoidance, finally, extinguishes any lingering doubt as to whether the Act covers the prototypical D&E procedure. " '[T]he elementary rule is that every reasonable construction must be resorted to, in order to save a statute from unconstitutionality.' " *Edward J. DeBartolo Corp.* v. *Florida Gulf Coast Building & Constr. Trades Council,* 485 U. S. 568, 575 (1988) (quoting *Hooper* v. *California,* 155 U. S. 648, 657 (1895)). It is true this longstanding maxim of statutory interpretation has, in the past, fallen by the wayside when the Court confronted a statute regulating abortion. The Court at times employed an antagonistic " 'canon of construction under which in cases involving abortion, a permissible reading of a statute [was] to be avoided at all costs.' " *Stenberg, supra,* at 977 (KENNEDY, J., dissenting) (quoting *Thornburgh,* 476 U. S., at 829 (O'Connor, J., dissenting)). *Casey* put this novel statutory approach to rest. *Stenberg, supra,* at 977 (KENNEDY, J., dissenting). *Stenberg* need not be interpreted to have revived it. We read that decision instead to stand for the uncontroversial proposition that the canon of constitutional avoidance does not apply if a statute is not "genuinely susceptible to two constructions." *Almendarez-Torres* v. *United States,* 523 U. S. 224, 238 (1998); see also *Clark* v. *Martinez,* 543 U. S. 371, 385 (2005). In *Stenberg* the Court found the statute covered D&E. 530 U. S., at 938–945. Here, by contrast, interpreting the Act so that it does not prohibit standard D&E is the most reasonable reading and understanding of its terms.

2

Contrary arguments by the respondents are unavailing. Respondents look to situations that might arise during D&E, situations not examined in *Stenberg.* They contend—relying on the testimony of numerous abortion doctors—that D&E may result in the delivery of a living fetus beyond the Act's anatomical landmarks in a significant fraction of cases. This is so, respondents say, because doctors cannot predict the amount the cervix will dilate before the abortion procedure. It might dilate to a degree that the fetus will be removed largely intact. To complete the abortion, doctors will commit an overt act that kills the partially delivered fetus. Respondents thus posit that any D&E has the potential to violate the Act, and that a physician will not know beforehand whether the abortion will proceed in a prohibited manner. Brief for Respondent Planned Parenthood et al. in No. 05–1382, p. 38.

This reasoning, however, does not take account of the Act's intent requirements, which preclude liability from attaching to an accidental intact D&E. If a doctor's intent at the outset is to perform a D&E in which the fetus would not be delivered to either of the Act's anatomical landmarks, but the fetus nonetheless is delivered past one of those points, the requisite and prohibited scienter is not present. 18 U. S. C. §1531(b)

(1)(A) (2000 ed., Supp. IV). When a doctor in that situation completes an abortion by performing an intact D&E, the doctor does not violate the Act. It is true that intent to cause a result may sometimes be inferred if a person "knows that that result is practically certain to follow from his conduct." 1 LaFave §5.2(a), at 341. Yet abortion doctors intending at the outset to perform a standard D&E procedure will not know that a prohibited abortion "is practically certain to follow from" their conduct. *Ibid.* A fetus is only delivered largely intact in a small fraction of the overall number of D&E abortions. *Planned Parenthood,* 320 F. Supp. 2d, at 965.

The evidence also supports a legislative determination that an intact delivery is almost always a conscious choice rather than a happenstance. Doctors, for example, may remove the fetus in a manner that will increase the chances of an intact delivery. See, *e.g.,* App. in No. 05–1382, at 74, 452. And intact D&E is usually described as involving some manner of serial dilation. See, *e.g.,* Dilation and Extraction 110. Doctors who do not seek to obtain this serial dilation perform an intact D&E on far fewer occasions. See, *e.g., Carhart,* 331 F. Supp. 2d, at 857–858 ("In order for intact removal to occur on a regular basis, Dr. Fitzhugh would have to dilate his patients with a second round of laminaria"). This evidence belies any claim that a standard D&E cannot be performed without intending or foreseeing an intact D&E.

Many doctors who testified on behalf of respondents, and who objected to the Act, do not perform an intact D&E by accident. On the contrary, they begin every D&E abortion with the objective of removing the fetus as intact as possible. See, *e.g., id.,* at 869 ("Since Dr. Chasen believes that the intact D & E is safer than the dismemberment D & E, Dr. Chasen's goal is to perform an intact D & E every time"); see also *id.,* at 873, 886. This does not prove, as respondents suggest, that every D&E might violate the Act and that the Act therefore imposes an undue burden. It demonstrates only that those doctors who intend to perform a D&E that would involve delivery of a living fetus to one of the Act's anatomical landmarks must adjust their conduct to the law by not attempting to deliver the fetus to either of those points. Respondents have not shown that requiring doctors to intend dismemberment before delivery to an anatomical landmark will prohibit the vast majority of D&E abortions. The Act, then, cannot be held invalid on its face on these grounds.

IV

Under the principles accepted as controlling here, the Act, as we have interpreted it, would be unconstitutional "if its purpose or effect is to place a substantial obstacle in the path of a woman seeking an abortion before the fetus attains viability." *Casey,* 505 U. S., at 878 (plurality pinion). The abortions affected by the Act's regulations take place both previability and postviability; so the quoted language and the undue burden analysis it relies upon are applicable. The question is whether the Act, measured by its text in this facial attack, imposes a substantial obstacle to late-term, but previability, abortions. The Act does not on its face impose a substantial obstacle, and we reject this further facial challenge to its validity.

A

The Act's purposes are set forth in recitals preceding its operative provisions. A description of the prohibited abortion procedure demonstrates the rationale for the congressional enactment. The Act proscribes a method of abortion in which a fetus is killed just inches before completion of the birth process. Congress stated as follows: "Implicitly approving such a brutal and inhumane procedure by choosing not to prohibit it will further coarsen society to the humanity of not only newborns, but all vulnerable and innocent human life, making it increasingly difficult to protect such life." Congressional Findings (14)(N), in notes following 18 U. S. C. §1531 (2000 ed., Supp. IV), p. 769. The Act expresses respect for the dignity of human life.

Congress was concerned, furthermore, with the effects on the medical community and on its reputation caused by the practice of partial-birth abortion. The findings in the Act explain:

> "Partial-birth abortion . . . confuses the medical, legal, and ethical duties of physicians to preserve and promote life, as the physician acts directly against the physical life of a child, whom he or she had just delivered, all but the head, out of the womb, in order to end that life." Congressional Findings (14)(J), *ibid.*

There can be no doubt the government "has an interest in protecting the integrity and ethics of the medical profession." *Washington* v. *Glucksberg*, 521 U. S. 702, 731 (1997); see also *Barsky* v. *Board of Regents of Univ. of N. Y.*, 347 U. S. 442, 451 (1954) (indicating the State has "legitimate concern for maintaining high standards of professional conduct" in the practice of medicine). Under our precedents it is clear the State has a significant role to play in regulating the medical profession.

Casey reaffirmed these governmental objectives. The government may use its voice and its regulatory authority to show its profound respect for the life within the woman. A central premise of the opinion was that the Court's precedents after *Roe* had "undervalue[d] the State's interest in potential life." 505 U. S., at 873 (plurality opinion); see also *id.*, at 871. The plurality opinion indicated "[t]he fact that a law which serves a valid purpose, one not designed to strike at the right itself, has

the incidental effect of making it more difficult or more expensive to procure an abortion cannot be enough to invalidate it." *Id.*, at 874. This was not an idle assertion. The three premises of *Casey* must coexist. See *id.*, at 846 (opinion of the Court). The third premise, that the State, from the inception of the pregnancy, maintains its own regulatory interest in protecting the life of the fetus that may become a child, cannot be set at naught by interpreting *Casey*'s requirement of a health exception so it becomes tantamount to allowing a doctor to choose the abortion method he or she might prefer. Where it has a rational basis to act, and it does not impose an undue burden, the State may use its regulatory power to bar certain procedures and substitute others, all in furtherance of its legitimate interests in regulating the medical profession in order to promote respect for life, including life of the unborn.

The Act's ban on abortions that involve partial delivery of a living fetus furthers the Government's objectives. No one would dispute that, for many, D&E is a procedure itself laden with the power to devalue human life. Congress could nonetheless conclude that the type of abortion proscribed by the Act requires specific regulation because it implicates additional ethical and moral concerns that justify a special prohibition. Congress determined that the abortion methods it proscribed had a "disturbing similarity to the killing of a newborn infant," Congressional Findings (14)(L), in notes following 18 U. S. C. §1531 (2000 ed., Supp. IV), p. 769, and thus it was concerned with "draw[ing] a bright line that clearly distinguishes abortion and infanticide." Congressional Findings (14)(G), *ibid.* The Court has in the past confirmed the validity of drawing boundaries to prevent certain practices that extinguish life and are close to actions that are condemned. *Glucksberg* found reasonable the State's "fear that permitting assisted suicide will start it down the path to voluntary and perhaps even involuntary euthanasia." 521 U. S., at 732–735, and n. 23.

Respect for human life finds an ultimate expression in the bond of love the mother has for her child. The Act recognizes this reality as well. Whether to have an abortion requires a difficult and painful moral decision. *Casey, supra,* at 852–853 (opinion of the Court). While we find no reliable data to measure the phenomenon, it seems unexceptionable to conclude some women come to regret their choice to abort the infant life they once created and sustained. See Brief for Sandra Cano et al. as *Amici Curiae* in No. 05–380, pp. 22–24. Severe depression and loss of esteem can follow. See *ibid.*

In a decision so fraught with emotional consequence some doctors may prefer not to disclose precise details of the means that will be used, confining themselves to the required statement of risks the procedure entails. From one standpoint this ought not to be surprising. Any number of patients facing imminent surgical procedures would prefer not to hear all details, lest the usual anxiety preceding invasive medical procedures become the more intense. This is likely the case with the abortion procedures here in issue. See, *e.g., Nat. Abortion Federation*, 330 F. Supp. 2d, at 466, n. 22 ("Most of [the plaintiffs'] experts acknowledged that they do not describe to their patients what [the D&E and intact D&E] procedures entail in clear and precise terms"); see also *id.,* at 479.

It is, however, precisely this lack of information concerning the way in which the fetus will be killed that is of legitimate concern to the State. *Casey, supra,* at 873 (plurality opinion) ("States are free to enact laws to provide a reasonable framework for a woman to make a decision that has such profound and lasting meaning"). The State has an interest in ensuring so grave a choice is well informed. It is self-evident that a mother who comes to regret her choice to abort must struggle with grief more anguished and sorrow more profound when she learns, only after the event, what she once did not know: that she allowed a doctor to pierce the skull and vacuum the fast-developing brain of her unborn child, a child assuming the human form.

It is a reasonable inference that a necessary effect of the regulation and the knowledge it conveys will be to encourage some women to carry the infant to full term, thus reducing the absolute number of late-term abortions. The medical profession, furthermore, may find different and less shocking methods to abort the fetus in the second trimester, thereby accommodating legislative demand. The State's interest in respect for life is advanced by the dialogue that better informs the political and legal systems, the medical profession, expectant mothers, and society as a whole of the consequences that follow from a decision to elect a late-term abortion.

It is objected that the standard D&E is in some respects as brutal, if not more, than the intact D&E, so that the legislation accomplishes little. What we have already said, however, shows ample justification for the regulation. Partial-birth abortion, as defined by the Act, differs from a standard D&E because the former occurs when the fetus is partially outside the mother to the point of one of the Act's anatomical landmarks. It was reasonable for Congress to think that partial-birth abortion, more than standard D&E, "undermines the public's perception of the appropriate role of a physician during the delivery process, and perverts a process during which life is brought into the world." Congressional Findings (14)(K), in notes following 18 U. S. C. §1531 (2000 ed., Supp. IV), p. 769. There would be a flaw in this Court's logic, and an irony in its jurisprudence, were we first to conclude a ban on both D&E and intact D&E was overbroad and then to say it is irrational to ban only intact D&E because that does not proscribe both procedures. In sum, we reject

the contention that the congressional purpose of the Act was "to place a substantial obstacle in the path of a woman seeking an abortion." 505 U. S., at 878 (plurality opinion).

B

The Act's furtherance of legitimate government interests bears upon, but does not resolve, the next question: whether the Act has the effect of imposing an unconstitutional burden on the abortion right because it does not allow use of the barred procedure where " 'necessary, in appropriate medical judgment, for [the] preservation of the . . . health of the mother.'" *Ayotte,* 546 U. S., at 327–328 (quoting *Casey, supra,* at 879 (plurality opinion)). The prohibition in the Act would be unconstitutional, under precedents we here assume to be controlling, if it "subject[ed] [women] to significant health risks." *Ayotte, supra,* at 328; see also *Casey, supra,* at 880 (opinion of the Court). In *Ayotte* the parties agreed a health exception to the challenged parental-involvement statute was necessary "to avert serious and often irreversible damage to [a pregnant minor's] health." 546 U. S., at 328. Here, by contrast, whether the Act creates significant health risks for women has been a contested factual question. The evidence presented in the trial courts and before Congress demonstrates both sides have medical support for their position.

Respondents presented evidence that intact D&E may be the safest method of abortion, for reasons similar to those adduced in *Stenberg.* See 530 U. S., at 932. Abortion doctors testified, for example, that intact D&E decreases the risk of cervical laceration or uterine perforation because it requires fewer passes into the uterus with surgical instruments and does not require the removal of bony fragments of the dismembered fetus, fragments that may be sharp. Respondents also presented evidence that intact D&E was safer both because it reduces the risks that fetal parts will remain in the uterus and because it takes less time to complete. Respondents, in addition, proffered evidence that intact D&E was safer for women with certain medical conditions or women with fetuses that had certain anomalies. See, *e.g., Carhart,* 331 F. Supp. 2d, at 923–929; *Nat. Abortion Federation, supra,* at 470–474; *Planned Parenthood,* 320 F. Supp. 2d, at 982–983.

These contentions were contradicted by other doctors who testified in the District Courts and before Congress. They concluded that the alleged health advantages were based on speculation without scientific studies to support them. They considered D&E always to be a safe alternative. See, *e.g., Carhart, supra,* at 930–940; *Nat. Abortion Federation,* 330 F. Supp. 2d, at 470–474; *Planned Parenthood,* 320 F. Supp. 2d, at 983.

There is documented medical disagreement whether the Act's prohibition would ever impose significant health risks on women. See, *e.g., id.*, at 1033 ("[T]here continues to be a division of opinion among highly qualified experts regarding the necessity or safety of intact D & E"); see also *Nat. Abortion Federation, supra*, at 482. The three District Courts that considered the Act's constitutionality appeared to be in some disagreement on this central factual question. The District Court for the District of Nebraska concluded "the banned procedure is, sometimes, the safest abortion procedure to preserve the health of women." *Carhart, supra*, at 1017. The District Court for the Northern District of California reached a similar conclusion. *Planned Parenthood, supra*, at 1002 (finding intact D&E was "under certain circumstances . . . significantly safer than D & E by disarticulation"). The District Court for the Southern District of New York was more skeptical of the purported health benefits of intact D&E. It found the Attorney General's "expert witnesses reasonably and effectively refuted [the plaintiffs'] proffered bases for the opinion that [intact D&E] has safety advantages over other second-trimester abortion procedures." *Nat. Abortion Federation*, 330 F. Supp. 2d, at 479. In addition it did "not believe that many of [the plaintiffs'] purported reasons for why [intact D&E] is medically necessary [were] credible; rather [it found them to be] theoretical or false." *Id.*, at 480. The court nonetheless invalidated the Act because it determined "a significant body of medical opinion . . . holds that D & E has safety advantages over induction and that [intact D&E] has some safety advantages (however hypothetical and unsubstantiated by scientific evidence) over D & E for some women in some circumstances." *Ibid.*

The question becomes whether the Act can stand when this medical uncertainty persists. The Court's precedents instruct that the Act can survive this facial attack. The Court has given state and federal legislatures wide discretion to pass legislation in areas where there is medical and scientific uncertainty. See *Kansas v. Hendricks*, 521 U. S. 346, 360, n. 3 (1997); *Jones v. United States*, 463 U. S. 354, 364–365, n. 13, 370 (1983); *Lambert v. Yellowley*, 272 U. S. 581, 597 (1926); *Collins v. Texas*, 223 U. S. 288, 297–298 (1912); *Jacobson v. Massachusetts*, 197 U. S. 11, 30–31 (1905); see also *Stenberg, supra*, at 969–972 (KENNEDY, J., dissenting); *Marshall v. United States*, 414 U. S. 417, 427 (1974) ("When Congress undertakes to act in areas fraught with medical and scientific uncertainties, legislative options must be especially broad").

This traditional rule is consistent with *Casey*, which confirms the State's interest in promoting respect for human life at all stages in the pregnancy. Physicians are not entitled to ignore regulations that direct them to use reasonable alternative procedures. The law need not give abortion doctors unfettered choice in the course of their medical practice, nor should it el-

evate their status above other physicians in the medical community. In *Casey* the controlling opinion held an informed-consent requirement in the abortion context was "no different from a requirement that a doctor give certain specific information about any medical procedure." 505 U. S., at 884 (joint opinion). The opinion stated "the doctor-patient relation here is entitled to the same solicitude it receives in other contexts." *Ibid.*; see also *Webster v. Reproductive Health Services*, 492 U. S. 490, 518–519 (1989) (plurality opinion) (criticizing *Roe's* trimester framework because, *inter alia*, it "left this Court to serve as the country's *ex officio* medical board with powers to approve or disapprove medical and operative practices and standards throughout the United States" (internal quotation marks omitted)); *Mazurek v. Armstrong*, 520 U. S. 968, 973 (1997) *(per curiam)* (upholding a restriction on the performance of abortions to licensed physicians despite the respondents' contention "all health evidence contradicts the claim that there is any health basis for the law" (internal quotation marks omitted)).

Medical uncertainty does not foreclose the exercise of legislative power in the abortion context any more than it does in other contexts. See *Hendricks, supra*, at 360, n. 3. The medical uncertainty over whether the Act's prohibition creates significant health risks provides a sufficient basis to conclude in this facial attack that the Act does not impose an undue burden.

The conclusion that the Act does not impose an undue burden is supported by other considerations. Alternatives are available to the prohibited procedure. As we have noted, the Act does not proscribe D&E. One District Court found D&E to have extremely low rates of medical complications. *Planned Parenthood, supra*, at 1000. Another indicated D&E was "generally the safest method of abortion during the second trimester." *Carhart*, 331 F. Supp. 2d, at 1031; see also *Nat. Abortion Federation, supra*, at 467–468 (explaining that "[e]xperts testifying for both sides" agreed D&E was safe). In addition the Act's prohibition only applies to the delivery of "a living fetus." 18 U. S. C. §1531(b)(1)(A) (2000 ed., Supp. IV). If the intact D&E procedure is truly necessary in some circumstances, it appears likely an injection that kills the fetus is an alternative under the Act that allows the doctor to perform the procedure.

The instant cases, then, are different from *Planned Parenthood of Central Mo. v. Danforth*, 428 U. S. 52, 77–79 (1976), in which the Court invalidated a ban on saline amniocentesis, the then-dominant second-trimester abortion method. The Court found the ban in *Danforth* to be "an unreasonable or arbitrary regulation designed to inhibit, and having the effect of inhibiting, the vast majority of abortions after the first 12 weeks." *Id.*, at 79. Here the Act allows, among other means, a commonly used and generally accepted method, so it does not construct a substantial obstacle to the abortion right.

In reaching the conclusion the Act does not require a health exception we reject certain arguments made by the parties on both sides of these cases. On the one hand, the Attorney General urges us to uphold the Act on the basis of the congressional findings alone. Brief for Petitioner in No. 05–380, at 23. Although we review congressional fact finding under a deferential standard, we do not in the circumstances here place dispositive weight on Congress' findings. The Court retains an independent constitutional duty to review factual findings where constitutional rights are at stake. See *Crowell* v. *Benson*, 285 U. S. 22, 60 (1932) ("In cases brought to enforce constitutional rights, the judicial power of the United States necessarily extends to the independent determination of all questions, both of fact and law, necessary to the performance of that supreme function").

As respondents have noted, and the District Courts recognized, some recitations in the Act are factually incorrect. See *Nat. Abortion Federation*, 330 F. Supp. 2d, at 482, 488–491. Whether or not accurate at the time, some of the important findings have been superseded. Two examples suffice. Congress determined no medical schools provide instruction on the prohibited procedure. Congressional Findings (14)(B), in notes following 18 U. S. C. §1531 (2000 ed., Supp. IV), p. 769. The testimony in the District Courts, however, demonstrated intact D&E is taught at medical schools. *Nat. Abortion Federation*, *supra*, at 490; *Planned Parenthood*, 320 F. Supp. 2d, at 1029. Congress also found there existed a medical consensus that the prohibited procedure is never medically necessary. Congressional Findings (1), in notes following 18 U. S. C. §1531 (2000 ed., Supp. IV), p. 767. The evidence presented in the District Courts contradicts that conclusion. See, *e.g.*, *Carhart*, *supra*, at 1012–1015; *Nat. Abortion Federation*, *supra*, at 488–489; *Planned Parenthood*, *supra*, at 1025–1026. Uncritical deference to Congress' factual findings in these cases is inappropriate.

On the other hand, relying on the Court's opinion in *Stenberg*, respondents contend that an abortion regulation must contain a health exception "if 'substantial medical authority supports the proposition that banning a particular procedure could endanger women's health.'" Brief for Respondents in No. 05–380, p. 19 (quoting 530 U. S., at 938); see also Brief for Respondent Planned Parenthood et al. in No. 05–1382, at 12 (same). As illustrated by respondents' arguments and the decisions of the Courts of Appeals, *Stenberg* has been interpreted to leave no margin of error for legislatures to act in the face of medical uncertainty. *Carhart*, 413 F. 3d, at 796; *Planned*

Parenthood, 435 F. 3d, at 1173; see also *Nat. Abortion Federation*, 437 F. 3d, at 296 (Walker, C. J., concurring) (explaining the standard under *Stenberg* "is a virtually insurmountable evidentiary hurdle").

A zero tolerance policy would strike down legitimate abortion regulations, like the present one, if some part of the medical community were disinclined to follow the proscription. This is too exacting a standard to impose on the legislative power, exercised in this instance under the Commerce Clause, to regulate the medical profession. Considerations of marginal safety, including the balance of risks, are within the legislative competence when the regulation is rational and in pursuit of legitimate ends. When standard medical options are available, mere convenience does not suffice to displace them; and if some procedures have different risks than others, it does not follow that the State is altogether barred from imposing reasonable regulations. The Act is not invalid on its face where there is uncertainty over whether the barred procedure is ever necessary to preserve a woman's health, given the availability of other abortion procedures that are considered to be safe alternatives.

V

The considerations we have discussed support our further determination that these facial attacks should not have been entertained in the first instance. In these circumstances the proper means to consider exceptions is by as-applied challenge. The Government has acknowledged that preenforcement, as-applied challenges to the Act can be maintained. Tr. of Oral Arg. in No. 05–380, pp. 21–23. This is the proper manner to protect the health of the woman if it can be shown that in discrete and well-defined instances a particular condition has or is likely to occur in which the procedure prohibited by the Act must be used. In an as-applied challenge the nature of the medical risk can be better quantified and balanced than in a facial attack.

The latitude given facial challenges in the First Amendment context is inapplicable here. Broad challenges of this type impose "a heavy burden" upon the parties maintaining the suit. *Rust* v. *Sullivan*, 500 U. S. 173, 183 (1991). What that burden consists of in the specific context of abortion statutes has been a subject of some question. Compare *Ohio* v. *Akron Center for Reproductive Health*, 497 U. S. 502, 514 (1990) ("[B]ecause appellees are making a facial challenge to a statute, they must show that no set of circumstances exists under which the Act would be valid" (internal quotation marks omitted)), with *Casey*, 505 U. S., at 895 (opinion of the Court) (indicating a spousal-notification statute would impose an undue burden "in a large fraction of the cases in which [it] is relevant" and holding the statutory provision facially invalid). See also

Janklow v. *Planned Parenthood, Sioux Falls Clinic*, 517 U. S. 1174 (1996). We need not resolve that debate.

As the previous sections of this opinion explain, respondents have not demonstrated that the Act would be unconstitutional in a large fraction of relevant cases. *Casey, supra,* at 895 (opinion of the Court). We note that the statute here applies to all instances in which the doctor proposes to use the prohibited procedure, not merely those in which the woman suffers from medical complications. It is neither our obligation nor within our traditional institutional role to resolve questions of constitutionality with respect to each potential situation that might develop. "[I]t would indeed be undesirable for this Court to consider every conceivable situation which might possibly arise in the application of complex and comprehensive legislation." *United States* v. *Raines,* 362 U. S. 17, 21 (1960) (internal quotation marks omitted). For this reason, "[a]s-applied challenges are the basic building blocks of constitutional adjudication." Fallon, As-Applied and Facial Challenges and Third-Party Standing, 113 Harv. L. Rev. 1321, 1328 (2000).

The Act is open to a proper as-applied challenge in a discrete case. Cf. *Wisconsin Right to Life, Inc.* v. *Federal Election Comm'n,* 546 U. S. 410, 411–412 (2006) *(per curiam).* No as-applied challenge need be brought if the prohibition in the Act threatens a woman's life because the Act already contains a life exception. 18 U. S. C. §1531(a) (2000 ed., Supp. IV).

Respondents have not demonstrated that the Act, as a facial matter, is void for vagueness, or that it imposes an undue burden on a woman's right to abortion based on its overbreadth or lack of a health exception. For these reasons the judgments of the Courts of Appeals for the Eighth and Ninth Circuits are reversed.

It is so ordered.

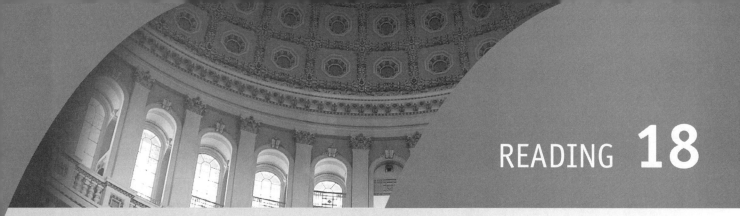

Case Law: *Cruzan v. Director, Missouri Department of Health* (Constitutional Right to Withdraw Life-Sustaining Treatment)

CRUZAN v. DIRECTOR, MDH, 497 U.S. 261 (1990)

CRUZAN, BY HER PARENTS AND CO-GUARDIANS CRUZAN ET UX. v. DIRECTOR, MISSOURI DEPARTMENT OF HEALTH, ET AL.

CERTIORARI TO THE SUPREME COURT OF MISSOURI

No. 88-1503.

Argued December 6, 1989

Decided June 25, 1990

REHNQUIST, C.J., delivered the opinion of the Court, in which WHITE, O'CONNOR, SCALIA, and KENNEDY, JJ., joined. O'CONNOR, J., post, p. 287, and SCALIA, J., post, p. 292, filed concurring opinions. BRENNAN, J., filed a dissenting opinion, in which MARSHALL and BLACKMUN, JJ., joined, post, p. 301. STEVENS, J., filed a dissenting opinion, post, p. 330.

CHIEF JUSTICE REHNQUIST delivered the opinion of the Court.

Petitioner Nancy Beth Cruzan was rendered incompetent as a result of severe injuries sustained during an automobile accident. Copetitioners Lester and Joyce Cruzan, Nancy's parents and coguardians, sought a court order directing the withdrawal of their daughter's artificial feeding and hydration equipment after it became apparent that she had virtually no chance of recovering her cognitive faculties. The Supreme Court of Missouri held that, because there was no clear and convincing evidence of Nancy's desire to have life-sustaining treatment withdrawn under such circumstances, her parents lacked authority to effectuate such a request. We granted certiorari, 492 U.S. 917 (1989), and now affirm.

On the night of January 11, 1983, Nancy Cruzan lost control of her car as she traveled down Elm Road in Jasper County, Missouri. The vehicle overturned, and Cruzan was discovered lying face down in a ditch without detectable respiratory or cardiac function. Paramedics were able to restore her breathing and heartbeat at the accident site, and she was transported to a hospital in an unconscious state. An attending neurosurgeon diagnosed her as having sustained probable cerebral contusions compounded by significant anoxia (lack of oxygen). The Missouri trial court in this case found that permanent brain damage generally results after 6 minutes in an anoxic state; it was estimated that Cruzan was deprived of oxygen from 12 to 14 minutes. She remained in a coma for approximately three weeks, and then progressed to an unconscious state in which she was able to orally ingest some nutrition. In order to ease feeding and further the recovery, surgeons implanted a gastrostomy feeding and hydration tube in Cruzan with the consent of her then husband. Subsequent rehabilitative efforts proved unavailing. She now lies in a Missouri state hospital in what is commonly referred to as a persistent vegetative state: generally, a condition in which a person exhibits motor reflexes but evinces no indications of significant cognitive function. [1] The State of Missouri is bearing the cost of her care. After it had become apparent that Nancy Cruzan had virtually no chance of regaining her mental faculties, her parents

---

[1] The State Supreme Court, adopting much of the trial court's findings, described Nancy Cruzan's medical condition as follows:

"... (1) [H]er respiration and circulation are not artificially maintained and are within the normal limits of a thirty-year-old female; (2) she is oblivious to her environment except

asked hospital employees to terminate the artificial nutrition and hydration procedures. All agree that such a removal would cause her death. The employees refused to honor the request without court approval. The parents then sought and received authorization from the state trial court for termination. The court found that a person in Nancy's condition had a fundamental right under the State and Federal Constitutions to refuse or direct the withdrawal of "death prolonging procedures." App. to Pet. for Cert. A99. The court also found that Nancy's "expressed thoughts at age twenty-five in somewhat serious conversation with a housemate friend that, if sick or injured, she would not wish to continue her life unless she could live at least halfway normally suggests that, given her present condition, she would not wish to continue on with her nutrition and hydration." *Id.*, at A97–A98.

---

for reflexive responses to sound and perhaps painful stimuli; (3) she suffered anoxia of the brain, resulting in a massive enlargement of the ventricles filling with cerebrospinal fluid in the area where the brain has degenerated and [her] cerebral cortical atrophy is irreversible, permanent, progressive and ongoing; (4) her highest cognitive brain function is exhibited by her grimacing perhaps in recognition of ordinarily painful stimuli, indicating the experience of pain and apparent response to sound; (5) she is a spastic quadriplegic; (6) her four extremities are contracted with irreversible muscular and tendon damage to all extremities; (7) she has no cognitive or reflexive ability to swallow food or water to maintain her daily essential needs and . . . she will never recover her ability to swallow sufficient [sic] to satisfy her needs. In sum, Nancy is diagnosed as in a persistent vegetative state. She is not dead. She is not terminally ill. Medical experts testified that she could live another thirty years." *Cruzan v. Harmon*, 760 S.W.2d 408, 411 (Mo. 1988) (en banc) (quotations omitted; footnote omitted).

In observing that Cruzan was not dead, the court referred to the following Missouri statute:

"For all legal purposes, the occurrence of human death shall be determined in accordance with the usual and customary standards of medical practice, provided that death shall not be determined to have occurred unless the following minimal conditions have been met:

"(1) When respiration and circulation are not artificially maintained, there is an irreversible cessation of spontaneous respiration and circulation; or

"(2) When respiration and circulation are artificially maintained, and there is total and irreversible cessation of all brain function, including the brain stem and that such determination is made by a licensed physician." Mo.Rev.Stat. 194.005 (1986).

Since Cruzan's respiration and circulation were not being artificially maintained, she obviously fit within the first proviso of the statute.

Dr. Fred Plum, the creator of the term "persistent vegetative state" and a renowned expert on the subject, has described the "vegetative state" in the following terms:

"'Vegetative state describes a body which is functioning entirely in terms of its internal controls. It maintains temperature. It maintains heart beat and pulmonary ventilation. It maintains digestive activity. It maintains reflex activity of muscles and nerves for low level conditioned responses. But there is no behavioral evidence of either self-awareness or awareness of the surroundings in a learned manner.'" *In re Jobes*, 108 N.J. 394, 403, 529 A.2d 434, 438 (1987).

See also Brief for American Medical Association et al., as Amici Curiae 6 ("The persistent vegetative state can best be understood as one of the conditions in which patients have suffered a loss of consciousness").

The Supreme Court of Missouri reversed by a divided vote. The court recognized a right to refuse treatment embodied in the common law doctrine of informed consent, but expressed skepticism about the application of that doctrine in the circumstances of this case. *Cruzan v. Harmon*, 760 S.W.2d 408, 416–417 (1988) (en banc). The court also declined to read a broad right of privacy into the State Constitution which would "support the right of a person to refuse medical treatment in every circumstance," and expressed doubt as to whether such a right existed under the United States Constitution. *Id.*, at 417–418. It then decided that the Missouri Living Will statute, Mo.Rev.Stat. 459.010 *et seq.* (1986), embodied a state policy strongly favoring the preservation of life. 760 S.W.2d, at 419–420. The court found that Cruzan's statements to her roommate regarding her desire to live or die under certain conditions were "unreliable for the purpose of determining her intent," *id.*, at 424, "and thus insufficient to support the coguardians['] claim to exercise substituted judgment on Nancy's behalf." *Id.*, at 426. It rejected the argument that Cruzan's parents were entitled to order the termination of her medical treatment, concluding that "no person can assume that choice for an incompetent in the absence of the formalities required under Missouri's Living Will statutes or the clear and convincing, inherently reliable evidence absent here." *Id.*, at 425. The court also expressed its view that "[b]road policy questions bearing on life and death are more properly addressed by representative assemblies" than judicial bodies. *Id.*, at 426.

We granted certiorari to consider the question of whether Cruzan has a right under the United States Constitution which would require the hospital to withdraw life-sustaining treatment from her under these circumstances.

At common law, even the touching of one person by another without consent and without legal justification was a battery. See W. Keeton, D. Dobbs, R. Keeton, & D. Owen, Prosser and Keeton on Law of Torts 9, pp. 39–42 (5th ed. 1984). Before the turn of the century, this Court observed that "[n]o right is held more sacred, or is more carefully guarded by the common law, than the right of every individual to the possession and control of his own person, free from all restraint or interference of others, unless by clear and unquestionable authority of law." *Union Pacific R. Co. v. Botsford*, 141 U.S. 250, 251 (1891). This notion of bodily integrity has been embodied in the requirement that informed consent is generally required for medical treatment. Justice Cardozo, while on the Court of Appeals of New York, aptly described this doctrine: "Every human being of adult years and sound mind has a right to determine what shall be done with his own body, and a surgeon who performs an operation without his patient's consent commits an assault, for which he is liable in damages." *Schloendorff v. Society of New York Hospital*, 211 N.Y. 125, 129–30, 105 N.E. 92, 93 (1914). The informed consent doctrine has become firmly entrenched in American tort law. See Dobbs, Keeton, & Owen, *supra*, 32, pp. 189–192; F. Rozovsky, Consent to Treatment, A Practical Guide 1–98 (2d ed. 1990).

The logical corollary of the doctrine of informed consent is that the patient generally possesses the right not to consent, that is, to refuse treatment. Until about 15 years ago and the seminal decision in *In re Quinlan*, 70 N.J. 10, 355 A.2d 647, cert. denied *sub nom. Garger v. New Jersey*, 429 U.S. 922 (1976), the number of right-to-refuse-treatment decisions were relatively few. [2] Most of the earlier cases involved patients who refused medical treatment forbidden by their religious beliefs, thus implicating First Amendment rights as well as common law rights of self-determination. [3] More recently, however, with the advance of medical technology capable of sustaining life well past the point where natural forces would have brought certain death in earlier times, cases involving the right to refuse life-sustaining treatment have burgeoned. See 760 S.W.2d at 412, n. 4 (collecting 54 reported decisions from 1976 through 1988).

In the *Quinlan* case, young Karen Quinlan suffered severe brain damage as the result of anoxia, and entered a persistent vegetative state. Karen's father sought judicial approval to disconnect his daughter's respirator. The New Jersey Supreme Court granted the relief, holding that Karen had a right of privacy grounded in the Federal Constitution to terminate treatment. *In re Quinlan*, 70 N.J. at 38–42, 355 A.2d at 662–664. Recognizing that this right was not absolute, however, the court balanced it against asserted state interests. Noting that the State's interest "weakens and the individual's right to privacy grows as the degree of bodily invasion increases and the prognosis dims," the court concluded that the state interests had to give way in that case. *Id.*, at 41, 355 A.2d at 664. The court also concluded that the "only practical way" to prevent the loss of Karen's privacy right due to her incompetence was to allow her guardian and family to decide "whether she would exercise it in these circumstances." *Ibid.*

After *Quinlan*, however, most courts have based a right to refuse treatment either solely on the common law right to informed consent or on both the common law right and a constitutional privacy right. See L. Tribe, American Constitutional Law 15–11, p. 1365 (2d ed. 1988). In *Superintendent of Belchertown State School v. Saikewicz*, 373 Mass. 728, 370 N.E.2d 417 (1977), the Supreme Judicial Court of Massachusetts relied on both the right of privacy and the right of informed consent to permit the withholding of chemotherapy from a profoundly-retarded 67-year-old man suffering from leukemia. *Id.*, at 737–738, 370 N.E.2d at 424. Reasoning that an incompetent person retains the same rights as a competent individual "because the value of human dignity extends to both," the court adopted a "substituted judgment" standard whereby courts were to determine what an incompetent individual's decision would have been under the circumstances. *Id.*, at 745, 752–753, 757–758, 370 N.E.2d at 427, 431, 434. Distilling certain state interests from prior case law—the preservation of life, the protection of the interests of innocent third parties, the prevention of suicide, and the maintenance of the ethical integrity of the medical profession—the court recognized the first interest as paramount and noted it was greatest when an affliction was curable, "as opposed to the State interest where, as here, the issue is not whether, but when, for how long, and at what cost to the individual [a] life may be briefly extended." *Id.*, at 742, 370 N.E.2d at 426.

In *In re Storar*, 52 N.Y.2d 363, 438 N.Y.S.2d 266, 420 N.E.2d 64, cert. denied, 454 U.S. 858 (1981), the New York Court of Appeals declined to base a right to refuse treatment on a constitutional privacy right. Instead, it found such a right "adequately supported" by the informed consent doctrine. *Id.*, at 376–377, 420 N.E.2d at 70. In *In re Eichner* (decided with *In re Storar*, *supra*), an 83-year-old man who had suffered brain damage from anoxia entered a vegetative state and was thus incompetent to consent to the removal of his respirator. The court, however, found it unnecessary to reach the question of whether his rights could be exercised by others, since it found the evidence clear and convincing from statements made by the patient when competent that he "did not want to be maintained in a vegetative coma by use of a respirator." *Id.*, at 380, 420 N.E.2d at 72. In the companion Storar case, a 52-year-old man suffering from bladder cancer had been profoundly retarded during most of his life. Implicitly rejecting the approach taken in Saikewicz, *supra*, the court reasoned that, due to such lifelong incompetency, "it is unrealistic to attempt to determine whether he would want to continue potentially life-prolonging treatment if he were competent." 52 N.Y.2d at 380, 420 N.E.2d at 72. As the evidence showed that the patient's required blood transfusions did not involve excessive pain and, without them, his mental and physical abilities would deteriorate, the court concluded that it should not "allow an incompetent patient to bleed to death because someone, even someone as close as a

---

[2]See generally Karnezis, Patient's Right to Refuse Treatment Allegedly Necessary to Sustain Life, 93 A.L.R.3d 67 (1979) (collecting cases); Cantor, A Patient's Decision to Decline Life-Saving Medical Treatment: Bodily Integrity Versus the Preservation of Life, 26 Rutgers L.Rev. 228, 229, and n. 5 (1973) (noting paucity of cases).

[3]See Chapman, The Uniform Rights of the Terminally Ill Act: Too Little, Too Late?, 42 Ark.L.Rev. 319, 324, n. 15 (1989); see also F. Rozovsky, Consent to Treatment, A Practical Guide 415–423 (2d ed. 1984).

parent or sibling, feels that this is best for one with an incurable disease." *Id.*, at 382, 420 N.E.2d, at 73.

Many of the later cases build on the principles established in Quinlan, Saikewicz and Storar/Eichner. For instance, in *In re Conroy*, 98 N.J. 321, 486 A.2d 1209 (1985), the same court that decided Quinlan considered whether a nasogastric feeding tube could be removed from an 84-year-old incompetent nursing-home resident suffering irreversible mental and physical ailments. While recognizing that a federal right of privacy might apply in the case, the court, contrary to its approach in Quinlan, decided to base its decision on the common law right to self-determination and informed consent. 98 N.J. at 348, 486 A.2d at 1223. "On balance, the right to self-determination ordinarily outweighs any countervailing state interests, and competent persons generally are permitted to refuse medical treatment, even at the risk of death. Most of the cases that have held otherwise, unless they involved the interest in protecting innocent third parties, have concerned the patient's competency to make a rational and considered choice." *Id.*, at 353–354, 486 A.2d at 1225.

Reasoning that the right of self-determination should not be lost merely because an individual is unable to sense a violation of it, the court held that incompetent individuals retain a right to refuse treatment. It also held that such a right could be exercised by a surrogate decision maker using a "subjective" standard when there was clear evidence that the incompetent person would have exercised it. Where such evidence was lacking, the court held that an individual's right could still be invoked in certain circumstances under objective "best interest" standards. *Id.*, at 361–368, 486 A.2d at 1229–1233. Thus, if some trustworthy evidence existed that the individual would have wanted to terminate treatment, but not enough to clearly establish a person's wishes for purposes of the subjective standard, and the burden of a prolonged life from the experience of pain and suffering markedly outweighed its satisfactions, treatment could be terminated under a "limited-objective" standard. Where no trustworthy evidence existed, and a person's suffering would make the administration of life-sustaining treatment inhumane, a "pure-objective" standard could be used to terminate treatment. If none of these conditions obtained, the court held it was best to err in favor of preserving life. *Id.*, at 364–368, 486 A.2d at 1231–1233.

The court also rejected certain categorical distinctions that had been drawn in prior refusal-of-treatment cases as lacking substance for decision purposes: the distinction between actively hastening death by terminating treatment and passively allowing a person to die of a disease; between treating individuals as an initial matter versus withdrawing treatment afterwards; between ordinary versus extraordinary

treatment; and between treatment by artificial feeding versus other forms of life-sustaining medical procedures. *Id.*, at 369–374, 486 A.2d at 1233–1237. As to the last item, the court acknowledged the "emotional significance" of food, but noted that feeding by implanted tubes is a "medical procedur[e] with inherent risks and possible side effects, instituted by skilled healthcare providers to compensate for impaired physical functioning" which analytically was equivalent to artificial breathing using a respirator. *Id.*, at 373, 486 A.2d at 1236. [4]

In contrast to Conroy, the Court of Appeals of New York recently refused to accept less than the clearly expressed wishes of a patient before permitting the exercise of her right to refuse treatment by a surrogate decision maker. *In re Westchester County Medical Center on behalf of O'Connor*, 72 N.Y.2d 517, 534 N.Y.S.2d 886, 531 N.E.2d 607 (1988) (*O'Connor*). There, the court, over the objection of the patient's family members, granted an order to insert a feeding tube into a 77-year-old woman rendered incompetent as a result of several strokes. While continuing to recognize a common law right to refuse treatment, the court rejected the substituted judgment approach for asserting it "because it is inconsistent with our fundamental commitment to the notion that no person or court should substitute its judgment as to what would be an acceptable quality of life for another. Consequently, we adhere to the view that, despite its pitfalls and inevitable uncertainties, the inquiry must always be narrowed to the patient's expressed intent, with every effort made to minimize the opportunity for error." *Id.*, at 530, 531 N.E.2d, at 613 (citation omitted). The court held that the record lacked the requisite clear and convincing evidence of the patient's expressed intent to withhold life-sustaining treatment. *Id.*, at 531–534, 531 N.E.2d, at 613–615.

Other courts have found state statutory law relevant to the resolution of these issues. In *Conservatorship of Drabick*, 200 Cal.App. 3d 185, 245 Cal.Rptr. 840, cert. denied, 488 U.S.

---

[4] In a later trilogy of cases, the New Jersey Supreme Court stressed that the analytic framework adopted in Conroy was limited to elderly, incompetent patients with shortened life expectancies, and established alternative approaches to deal with a different set of situations. See *In re Farrell*, 108 N.J. 335, 529 A.2d 404 (1987) (37-year-old competent mother with terminal illness had right to removal of respirator based on common law and constitutional principles which overrode competing state interests); *In re Peter*, 108 N.J. 365, 529 A.2d 419 (1987) (65-year-old woman in persistent vegetative state had right to removal of nasogastric feeding tube—under Conroy subjective test, power of attorney and hearsay testimony constituted clear and convincing proof of patient's intent to have treatment withdrawn); *In re Jobes*, 108 N.J. 394, 529 A.2d 434 (1987) (31-year-old woman in persistent vegetative state entitled to removal of jejunostomy feeding tube—even though hearsay testimony regarding patient's intent insufficient to meet clear and convincing standard of proof, under Quinlan, family or close friends entitled to make a substituted judgment for patient).

958 (1988), the California Court of Appeal authorized the removal of a nasogastric feeding tube from a 44-year-old man who was in a persistent vegetative state as a result of an auto accident. Noting that the right to refuse treatment was grounded in both the common law and a constitutional right of privacy, the court held that a state probate statute authorized the patient's conservator to order the withdrawal of life-sustaining treatment when such a decision was made in good faith based on medical advice and the conservatee's best interests. While acknowledging that "to claim that [a patient's] 'right to choose' survives incompetence is a legal fiction at best," the court reasoned that the respect society accords to persons as individuals is not lost upon incompetence, and is best preserved by allowing others "to make a decision that reflects [a patient's] interests more closely than would a purely technological decision to do whatever is possible."[5] *Id.*, at 208, 245 Cal. Rptr., at 854–855. See also In re Conservatorship of Torres, 357 N.W.2d 332 (Minn. 1984) (Minnesota court had constitutional and statutory authority to authorize a conservator to order the removal of an incompetent individual's respirator since in patient's best interests).

In *In re Estate of Longeway*, 133 Ill.2d 33, 549 N.E.2d 292 (1989), the Supreme Court of Illinois considered whether a 76-year-old woman rendered incompetent from a series of strokes had a right to the discontinuance of artificial nutrition and hydration. Noting that the boundaries of a federal right of privacy were uncertain, the court found a right to refuse treatment in the doctrine of informed consent. *Id.*, at 43–45, 549 N.E.2d at 296–297. The court further held that the State Probate Act impliedly authorized a guardian to exercise a ward's right to refuse artificial sustenance in the event that the ward was terminally ill and irreversibly comatose. *Id.*, at 45-47, 549 N.E.2d at 298. Declining to adopt a best interests standard for deciding when it would be appropriate to exercise a ward's right because it "lets another make a determination of a patient's quality of life," the court opted instead for a substituted judgment standard. *Id.*, at 49, 549 N.E.2d at 299. Finding the "expressed intent" standard utilized in O'Connor, *supra*, too rigid, the court noted that other clear and convincing evidence of the patient's intent could be considered. 133 Ill.2d, at 50-51,

549 N.E.2d, at 300. The court also adopted the "consensus opinion [that] treats artificial nutrition and hydration as medical treatment." *Id.*, at 42, 549 N.E.2d at 296. Cf. *McConnell v. Beverly Enterprises-Connecticut, Inc.*, 209 Conn. 692, 705, 553 A.2d 596, 603 (1989) (right to withdraw artificial nutrition and hydration found in the Connecticut Removal of Life Support Systems Act, which "provid[es] functional guidelines for the exercise of the common law and constitutional rights of self-determination"; attending physician authorized to remove treatment after finding that patient is in a terminal condition, obtaining consent of family, and considering expressed wishes of patient).[6]

As these cases demonstrate, the common law doctrine of informed consent is viewed as generally encompassing the right of a competent individual to refuse medical treatment. Beyond that, these decisions demonstrate both similarity and diversity in their approach to decision of what all agree is a perplexing question with unusually strong moral and ethical overtones. State courts have available to them for decision a number of sources—state constitutions, statutes, and common law—which are not available to us. In this Court, the question is simply and starkly whether the United States Constitution prohibits Missouri from choosing the rule of decision which it did. This is the first case in which we have been squarely presented with the issue of whether the United States Constitution grants what is in common parlance referred to as a "right to die." We follow the judicious counsel of our decision in *Twin City Bank v. Nebeker*, 167 U.S. 196, 202 (1897), where we said that, in deciding "a question of such magnitude and importance . . . it is the [better] part of wisdom not to attempt, by any general statement, to cover every possible phase of the subject."

The Fourteenth Amendment provides that no State shall "deprive any person of life, liberty, or property, without due process of law." The principle that a competent person has a constitutionally protected liberty interest in refusing unwanted medical treatment may be inferred from our prior decisions. In *Jacobson v. Massachusetts*, 197 U.S. 11, 24–30 (1905), for instance, the Court balanced an individual's liberty interest in declining

---

[5]The Drabick court drew support for its analysis from earlier, influential decisions rendered by California courts of appeal. See *Bouvia v. Superior Court*, 179 Cal.App. 3d 1127, 225 Cal. Rptr. 297 (1986) (competent 28-year-old quadriplegic had right to removal of nasogastric feeding tube inserted against her will); *Bartling v. Superior Court*, 163 Cal.App. 3d 186, 209 Cal. Rptr. 220 (1984) (competent 70-year-old, seriously-ill man had right to the removal of respirator); *Barber v. Superior Court*, 147 Cal.App. 3d 1006, 195 Cal.Rptr. 484 (1983) (physicians could not be prosecuted for homicide on account of removing respirator and intravenous feeding tubes of patient in persistent vegetative state).

[6]Besides the Missouri Supreme Court in Cruzan and the courts in McConnell, Longeway, Drabick, Bouvia, Barber, O'Connor, Conroy, Jobes, and Peter, appellate courts of at least four other States and one Federal District Court have specifically considered and discussed the issue of withholding or withdrawing artificial nutrition and hydration from incompetent individuals. See *Gray v. Romeo*, 697 F.Supp. 580 (RI 1988); *In re Gardner*, 534 A.2d 947 (Me. 1987); *In re Grant*, 109 Wash.2d 545, 747 P.2d 445 (1987); *Brophy v. New England Sinai Hospital, Inc.*, 398 Mass. 417, 497 N.E.2d 626 (1986); *Corbett v. D'Alessandro*, 487 So.2d 368 (Fla.App. 1986). All of these courts permitted or would permit the termination of such measures based on rights grounded in the common law, or in the State or Federal Constitution.

an unwanted smallpox vaccine against the State's interest in preventing disease. Decisions prior to the incorporation of the Fourth Amendment into the Fourteenth Amendment analyzed searches and seizures involving the body under the Due Process Clause and were thought to implicate substantial liberty interests. See, e.g., *Breithaupt v. Abram*, 352 U.S. 432, 439 (1957) ("As against the right of an individual that his person be held inviolable . . . must be set the interests of society. . . .")

Just this Term, in the course of holding that a State's procedures for administering antipsychotic medication to prisoners were sufficient to satisfy due process concerns, we recognized that prisoners possess "a significant liberty interest in avoiding the unwanted administration of antipsychotic drugs under the Due Process Clause of the Fourteenth Amendment." *Washington v. Harper*, 494 U.S. 210, 221–222 (1990); see also *id.*, at 229 ("The forcible injection of medication into a nonconsenting person's body represents a substantial interference with that person's liberty"). Still other cases support the recognition of a general liberty interest in refusing medical treatment. *Vitek v. Jones*, 445 U.S. 480, 494 (1980) (transfer to mental hospital coupled with mandatory behavior modification treatment implicated liberty interests); *Parham v. J.R.*, 442 U.S. 584, 600 (1979) ("a child, in common with adults, has a substantial liberty interest in not being confined unnecessarily for medical treatment").

But determining that a person has a "liberty interest" under the Due Process Clause does not end the inquiry;[7] "whether respondent's constitutional rights have been violated must be determined by balancing his liberty interests against the relevant state interests." *Youngberg v. Romeo*, 457 U.S. 307, 321 (1982). See also *Mills v. Rogers*, 457 U.S. 291, 299 (1982).

Petitioners insist that, under the general holdings of our cases, the forced administration of life-sustaining medical treatment, and even of artificially-delivered food and water essential to life, would implicate a competent person's liberty interest. Although we think the logic of the cases discussed above would embrace such a liberty interest, the dramatic consequences involved in refusal of such treatment would inform the inquiry as to whether the deprivation of that interest is constitutionally permissible. But for purposes of this case, we assume that the United States Constitution would grant a competent person a constitutionally protected right to refuse lifesaving hydration and nutrition.

Petitioners go on to assert that an incompetent person should possess the same right in this respect as is possessed by a competent person. They rely primarily on our decisions in *Parham v. J.R., supra*, and *Youngberg v. Romeo, supra*. In *Parham*, we held that a mentally disturbed minor child had a liberty interest in "not being confined unnecessarily for medical treatment," 442 U.S., at 600, but we certainly did not intimate that such a minor child, after commitment, would have a liberty interest in refusing treatment. In *Youngberg*, we held that a seriously retarded adult had a liberty interest in safety and freedom from bodily restraint, 457 U.S., at 320. *Youngberg*, however, did not deal with decisions to administer or withhold medical treatment.

The difficulty with petitioners' claim is that, in a sense, it begs the question: an incompetent person is not able to make an informed and voluntary choice to exercise a hypothetical right to refuse treatment or any other right. Such a "right" must be exercised for her, if at all, by some sort of surrogate. Here, Missouri has in effect recognized that, under certain circumstances, a surrogate may act for the patient in electing to have hydration and nutrition withdrawn in such a way as to cause death, but it has established a procedural safeguard to assure that the action of the surrogate conforms as best it may to the wishes expressed by the patient while competent. Missouri requires that evidence of the incompetent's wishes as to the withdrawal of treatment be proved by clear and convincing evidence. The question, then, is whether the United States Constitution forbids the establishment of this procedural requirement by the State. We hold that it does not.

Whether or not Missouri's clear and convincing evidence requirement comports with the United States Constitution depends in part on what interests the State may properly seek to protect in this situation. Missouri relies on its interest in the protection and preservation of human life, and there can be no gainsaying this interest. As a general matter, the States—indeed, all civilized nations—demonstrate their commitment to life by treating homicide as serious crime. Moreover, the majority of States in this country have laws imposing criminal penalties on one who assists another to commit suicide.[8] We do not think a State is required to remain neutral in the face of an informed and voluntary decision by a physically able adult to starve to death.

But in the context presented here, a State has more particular interests at stake. The choice between life and death is a deeply personal decision of obvious and overwhelming finality.

---

[7]Although many state courts have held that a right to refuse treatment is encompassed by a generalized constitutional right of privacy, we have never so held. We believe this issue is more properly analyzed in terms of a Fourteenth Amendment liberty interest. See *Bowers v. Hardwick*, 478 U.S. 186, 194–195 (1986).

[8]See Smith, All's Well That Ends Well: Toward a Policy of Assisted Rational Suicide or Merely Enlightened Self-Determination?, 22 U.C. D. L.Rev. 275, 290–291, n. 106 (1989) (compiling statutes).

We believe Missouri may legitimately seek to safeguard the personal element of this choice through the imposition of heightened evidentiary requirements. It cannot be disputed that the Due Process Clause protects an interest in life as well as an interest in refusing life-sustaining medical treatment. Not all incompetent patients will have loved ones available to serve as surrogate decision makers. And even where family members are present, "[t]here will, of course, be some unfortunate situations in which family members will not act to protect a patient." *In re Jobes*, 108 N.J. 394, 419, 529 A.2d 434, 477 (1987). A State is entitled to guard against potential abuses in such situations. Similarly, a State is entitled to consider that a judicial proceeding to make a determination regarding an incompetent's wishes may very well not be an adversarial one, with the added guarantee of accurate factfinding that the adversary process brings with it.[9] See *Ohio v. Akron Center for Reproductive Health*, post, at 515–516 (1990). Finally, we think a State may properly decline to make judgments about the "quality" of life that a particular individual may enjoy, and simply assert an unqualified interest in the preservation of human life to be weighed against the constitutionally protected interests of the individual.

In our view, Missouri has permissibly sought to advance these interests through the adoption of a "clear and convincing" standard of proof to govern such proceedings. "The function of a standard of proof, as that concept is embodied in the Due Process Clause and in the realm of fact finding, is to 'instruct the factfinder concerning the degree of confidence our society thinks he should have in the correctness of factual conclusions for a particular type of adjudication.'" *Addington v. Texas*, 441 U.S. 418, 423 (1979) (quoting *In re Winship*, 397 U.S. 358, 370 (1970) (Harlan, J., concurring)). "This Court has mandated an intermediate standard of proof—'clear and convincing evidence'—when the individual interests at stake in a state proceeding are both 'particularly important' and 'more

substantial than mere loss of money.'" *Santosky v. Kramer*, 455 U.S. 745, 756 (1982) (quoting *Addington, supra*, at 424). Thus, such a standard has been required in deportation proceedings, *Woodby v. INS*, 385 U.S. 276 (1966), in denaturalization proceedings, *Schneiderman v. United States*, 320 U.S. 118 (1943), in civil commitment proceedings, *Addington, supra*, and in proceedings for the termination of parental rights. *Santosky, supra.*[10] Further, this level of proof, "or an even higher one, has traditionally been imposed in cases involving allegations of civil fraud, and in a variety of other kinds of civil cases involving such issues as . . . lost wills, oral contracts to make bequests, and the like." *Woodby, supra*, at 285, n. 18.

We think it self-evident that the interests at stake in the instant proceedings are more substantial, both on an individual and societal level, than those involved in a run-of-the-mine civil dispute. But not only does the standard of proof reflect the importance of a particular adjudication, it also serves as "a societal judgment about how the risk of error should be distributed between the litigants." *Santosky, supra*, at 755; *Addington, supra*, at 423. The more stringent the burden of proof a party must bear, the more that party bears the risk of an erroneous decision. We believe that Missouri may permissibly place an increased risk of an erroneous decision on those seeking to terminate an incompetent individual's life-sustaining treatment. An erroneous decision not to terminate results in a maintenance of the status quo; the possibility of subsequent developments such as advancements in medical science, the discovery of new evidence regarding the patient's intent, changes in the law, or simply the unexpected death of the patient despite the administration of life-sustaining treatment, at least create the potential that a wrong decision will eventually be corrected or its impact mitigated. An erroneous decision to withdraw life-sustaining treatment, however, is not susceptible of correction. In *Santosky*, one of the factors which led the Court to require proof by clear and convincing evidence in a proceeding to terminate parental rights was that a decision in such a case was final and irrevocable. *Santosky, supra*, at 759. The same must surely be said of the decision to discontinue hydration and nutrition of a patient such as Nancy Cruzan, which all agree will result in her death.

---

[9]Since Cruzan was a patient at a state hospital when this litigation commenced, the State has been involved as an adversary from the beginning. However, it can be expected that many of these types of disputes will arise in private institutions, where a guardian *ad litem* or similar party will have been appointed as the sole representative of the incompetent individual in the litigation. In such cases, a guardian may act in entire good faith, and yet not maintain a position truly adversarial to that of the family. Indeed, as noted by the court below, "[t]he guardian *ad litem* [in this case] finds himself in the predicament of believing that it is in Nancy's 'best interest to have the tube feeding discontinued,' but 'feeling that an appeal should be made because our responsibility to her as attorneys and guardians *ad litem* was to pursue this matter to the highest court in the state in view of the fact that this is a case of first impression in the State of Missouri.'" 760 S.W.2d at 410, n. 1. Cruzan's guardian *ad litem* has also filed a brief in this Court urging reversal of the Missouri Supreme Court's decision. None of this is intended to suggest that the guardian acted the least bit improperly in this proceeding. It is only meant to illustrate the limits which may obtain on the adversarial nature of this type of litigation.

[10]We recognize that these cases involved instances where the government sought to take action against an individual. See *Price Waterhouse v. Hopkins*, 490 U.S. 228, 253 (1989) (plurality opinion). Here, by contrast, the government seeks to protect the interests of an individual as well as its own institutional interests, in life. We do not see any reason why important individual interests should be afforded less protection simply because the government finds itself in the position of defending them. "[W]e find it significant that . . . the defendant rather than the plaintiff seeks the clear and convincing standard of proof—suggesting that this standard ordinarily serves as a shield rather than . . . a sword." *Id.*, at 253. That it is the government that has picked up the shield should be of no moment.

It is also worth noting that most, if not all, States simply forbid oral testimony entirely in determining the wishes of parties in transactions which, while important, simply do not have the consequences that a decision to terminate a person's life does. At common law and by statute in most States, the parol evidence rule prevents the variations of the terms of a written contract by oral testimony. The statute of frauds makes unenforceable oral contracts to leave property by will, and statutes regulating the making of wills universally require that those instruments be in writing. See 2 A. Corbin, Contracts 398, pp. 360–361 (1950); 2 W. Page, Law of Wills 19.3–19.5, pp. 61–71 (1960). There is no doubt that statutes requiring wills to be in writing, and statutes of frauds which require that a contract to make a will be in writing, on occasion frustrate the effectuation of the intent of a particular decedent, just as Missouri's requirement of proof in this case may have frustrated the effectuation of the not-fully-expressed desires of Nancy Cruzan. But the Constitution does not require general rules to work faultlessly; no general rule can.

In sum, we conclude that a State may apply a clear and convincing evidence standard in proceedings where a guardian seeks to discontinue nutrition and hydration of a person diagnosed to be in a persistent vegetative state. We note that many courts which have adopted some sort of substituted judgment procedure in situations like this, whether they limit consideration of evidence to the prior expressed wishes of the incompetent individual, or whether they allow more general proof of what the individual's decision would have been, require a clear and convincing standard of proof for such evidence. See, e.g., *Longeway*, 133 Ill.2d at 50–51, 549 N.E.2d at 300; *McConnell*, 209 Conn., at 707–710, 553 A.2d at 604–605; *O'Connor*, 72 N.Y.2d at 529–530, 531 N.E.2d at 613; *In re Gardner*, 534 A.2d 947, 952–953 (Me. 1987); *In re Jobes*, 108 N.J. at 412–413, 529 A.2d at 443; *Leach v. Akron General Medical Center*, 68 Ohio Misc. 1, 11, 426 N.E.2d 809, 815 (1980).

The Supreme Court of Missouri held that, in this case, the testimony adduced at trial did not amount to clear and convincing proof of the patient's desire to have hydration and nutrition withdrawn. In so doing, it reversed a decision of the Missouri trial court, which had found that the evidence "sug-gest[ed]" Nancy Cruzan would not have desired to continue such measures, App. to Pet. for Cert. A98, but which had not adopted the standard of "clear and convincing evidence" enunciated by the Supreme Court. The testimony adduced at trial consisted primarily of Nancy Cruzan's statements, made to a housemate about a year before her accident, that she would not want to live should she face life as a "vegetable," and other observations to the same effect. The observations did not deal in terms with withdrawal of medical treatment or of hydration

and nutrition. We cannot say that the Supreme Court of Missouri committed constitutional error in reaching the conclusion that it did.[11]

Petitioners alternatively contend that Missouri must accept the "substituted judgment" of close family members even in the absence of substantial proof that their views reflect the views of the patient. They rely primarily upon our decisions in *Michael H. v. Gerald D.*, 491 U.S. 110 (1989), and *Parham v. J.R.*, 442 U.S. 584 (1979). But we do not think these cases support their claim. In *Michael H.*, we upheld the constitutionality of California's favored treatment of traditional family relationships; such a holding may not be turned around into a constitutional requirement that a State must recognize the primacy of those relationships in a situation like this. And in Parham, where the patient was a minor, we also upheld the constitutionality of a state scheme in which parents made certain decisions for mentally ill minors. Here again, petitioners would seek to turn a decision which allowed a State to rely on family decision-making into a constitutional requirement that the State recognize such decision-making. But constitutional law does not work that way.

No doubt is engendered by anything in this record but that Nancy Cruzan's mother and father are loving and caring parents. If the State were required by the United States Constitution to repose a right of "substituted judgment" with anyone, the Cruzans would surely qualify. But we do not think the Due Process Clause requires the State to repose judgment on these matters with anyone but the patient herself. Close family members may have a strong feeling—a feeling not at all ignoble or unworthy, but not entirely disinterested, either—that they do not wish to witness the continuation of the life of a loved one which they regard as hopeless, meaningless, and even degrading. But there is no automatic assurance that the view of close family members will necessarily be the same as the patient's would have been had she been confronted with the prospect of her situation while competent. All of the reasons

---

[11]The clear and convincing standard of proof has been variously defined in this context as "proof sufficient to persuade the trier of fact that the patient held a firm and settled commitment to the termination of life supports under the circumstances like those presented," *In re Westchester County Medical Center on behalf of O'Connor*, 72 N.Y.2d 517, 534 N.Y.S.2d 886, 892, 531 N.E.2d 607, 613 (1988) (*O'Connor*), and as evidence which "produces in the mind of the trier of fact a firm belief or conviction as to the truth of the allegations sought to be established, evidence so clear, direct and weighty and convincing as to enable [the fact finder] to come to a clear conviction, without hesitancy, of the truth of the precise facts in issue." *In re Jobes*, 108 N.J. at 407–408, 529 A.2d at 441 (quotation omitted). In both of these cases, the evidence of the patient's intent to refuse medical treatment was arguably stronger than that presented here. The New York Court of Appeals and the Supreme Court of New Jersey, respectively, held that the proof failed to meet a clear and convincing threshold. See *O'Connor*, supra, at 526–534, 534 531 N.E.2d at 610–615; *Jobes*, supra, at 442–443.

previously discussed for allowing Missouri to require clear and convincing evidence of the patient's wishes lead us to conclude that the State may choose to defer only to those wishes, rather than confide the decision to close family members. [12]

The judgment of the Supreme Court of Missouri is Affirmed.

[Concurring opinions omitted.]

JUSTICE BRENNAN, with whom JUSTICE MARSHALL and JUSTICE BLACKMUN join, dissenting.

"Medical technology has effectively created a twilight zone of suspended animation where death commences while life, in some form, continues. Some patients, however, want no part of a life sustained only by medical technology. Instead, they prefer a plan of medical treatment that allows nature to take its course and permits them to die with dignity."[1]

Nancy Cruzan has dwelt in that twilight zone for six years. She is oblivious to her surroundings and will remain so. *Cruzan v. Harmon*, 760 S.W.2d 408, 411 (Mo. 1988). Her body twitches only reflexively, without consciousness. *Ibid.* The areas of her brain that once thought, felt, and experienced sensations have degenerated badly, and are continuing to do so. The cavities remaining are filling with cerebrospinal fluid. The " 'cerebral cortical atrophy is irreversible, permanent, progressive and ongoing.' " *Ibid.* "Nancy will never interact meaningfully with her environment again. She will remain in a persistent vegetative state until her death." *Id.*, at 422.2. Because she cannot swallow, her nutrition and hydration are delivered through a tube surgically implanted in her stomach.

A grown woman at the time of the accident, Nancy had previously expressed her wish to forgo continuing medical care under circumstances such as these. Her family and her friends are convinced that this is what she would want. See n. 20, *infra*. A guardian *ad litem* appointed by the trial court is also convinced that this is what Nancy would want. See 760 S.W.2d at 444 (Higgins, J., dissenting from denial of rehearing). Yet the Missouri Supreme Court, alone among state courts deciding

such a question, has determined that an irreversibly vegetative patient will remain a passive prisoner of medical technology—for Nancy, perhaps for the next 30 years. See *id.*, at 424, 427.[2]

Today the Court, while tentatively accepting that there is some degree of constitutionally protected liberty interest in avoiding unwanted medical treatment, including life-sustaining medical treatment such as artificial nutrition and hydration, affirms the decision of the Missouri Supreme Court. The majority opinion, as I read it, would affirm that decision on the ground that a State may require "clear and convincing" evidence of Nancy Cruzan's prior decision to forgo life-sustaining treatment under circumstances such as hers in order to ensure that her actual wishes are honored. See *ante* at 282–283, 286–287. Because I believe that Nancy Cruzan has a fundamental right to be free of unwanted artificial nutrition and hydration, which right is not outweighed by any interests of the State, and because I find that the improperly biased procedural obstacles imposed by the Missouri Supreme Court impermissibly burden that right, I respectfully dissent. Nancy Cruzan is entitled to choose to die with dignity.

I

A

"[T]he timing of death—once a matter of fate—is now a matter of human choice." Office of Technology Assessment Task Force, Life Sustaining Technologies and the Elderly 41 (1988). Of the approximately two million people who die each year, 80% die in hospitals and long-term care institutions,[3] Page 497 U.S. 261, 303 and perhaps 70% of those after a decision to forgo life-sustaining treatment has been made.[4] Nearly every death involves a decision whether to undertake some medical procedure that could prolong the process of dying. Such decisions are difficult and personal. They must be made on the basis of individual values, informed by medical realities, yet within a framework governed by law. The role of the courts is confined to defining that framework, delineating the ways in which government may and may not participate in such decisions.

The question before this Court is a relatively narrow one: whether the Due Process Clause allows Missouri to require a

---

[12]We are not faced in this case with the question of whether a State might be required to defer to the decision of a surrogate if competent and probative evidence established that the patient herself had expressed a desire that the decision to terminate life sustaining treatment be made for her by that individual.

Petitioners also adumbrate in their brief a claim based on the Equal Protection Clause of the Fourteenth Amendment to the effect that Missouri has impermissibly treated incompetent patients differently from competent ones, citing the statement in *Cleburne v. Cleburne Living Center, Inc.*, 473 U.S. 432, 439 (1985), that the clause is "essentially a direction that all persons similarly situated should be treated alike." The differences between the choice made by a competent person to refuse medical treatment and the choice made for an incompetent person by someone else to refuse medical treatment are so obviously different that the State is warranted in establishing rigorous procedures for the latter class of cases which do not apply to the former class.

[1]*Rasmussen v. Fleming*, 154 Ariz. 207, 211, 741 P.2d 674, 678 (1987) (en banc).

---

[2]Vegetative state patients may react reflexively to sounds, movements and normally painful stimuli, but they do not feel any pain or sense anybody or anything. Vegetative state patients may appear awake, but are completely unaware. See Cranford, The Persistent Vegetative State: The Medical Reality, 18 Hastings Ctr.Rep. 27, 28, 31 (1988).

[3]See President's Commission for the Study of Ethical Problems in Medicine and Biomedical and Behavioral Research, Deciding to Forego Life Sustaining Treatment 15, n. 1, and 17–18 (1983) (hereafter President's Commission).

[4]See Lipton, Do-Not-Resuscitate Decisions in a Community Hospital: Incidence, Implications and Outcomes, 256 JAMA 1164, 1168 (1986).

now-incompetent patient in an irreversible persistent vegetative state to remain on life-support absent rigorously clear and convincing evidence that avoiding the treatment represents the patient's prior, express. choice. See *ante* at 277–278. If a fundamental right is at issue, Missouri's rule of decision must be scrutinized under the standards this Court has always applied in such circumstances. As we said in *Zablocki v. Redhail*, 434 U.S. 374, 388 (1978), if a requirement imposed by a State "significantly interferes with the exercise of a fundamental right, it cannot be upheld unless it is supported by sufficiently important state interests and is closely tailored to effectuate only those interests." The Constitution imposes on this Court the obligation to "examine carefully . . . the extent to which [the legitimate government interests advanced] are served by the challenged regulation." *Moore v. East Cleveland*, 431 U.S. 494, 499 (1977). See also *Carey v. Population Services International*, 431 U.S. 678, 690 (1977) (invalidating a requirement that bore "no relation to the State's interest"). An evidentiary rule, just as a substantive prohibition, must meet these standards if it significantly burdens a fundamental liberty interest. Fundamental rights "are protected not only against heavy-handed frontal attack, but also from being stifled by more subtle governmental interference." *Bates v. Little Rock*, 361 U.S. 516, 523 (1960).

B

The starting point for our legal analysis must be whether a competent person has a constitutional right to avoid unwanted medical care. Earlier this Term, this Court held that the Due Process Clause of the Fourteenth Amendment confers a significant liberty interest in avoiding unwanted medical treatment. *Washington v. Harper*, 494 U.S. 210, 221–222 (1990). Today, the Court concedes that our prior decisions "support the recognition of a general liberty interest in refusing medical treatment." See *ante* at 278. The Court, however, avoids discussing either the measure of that liberty interest or its application by assuming, for purposes of this case only, that a competent person has a constitutionally protected liberty interest in being free of unwanted artificial nutrition and hydration. See *ante* at 279. JUSTICE O'CONNOR's opinion is less parsimonious. She openly affirms that "the Court has often deemed state incursions into the body repugnant to the interests protected by the Due Process Clause," that there is a liberty interest in avoiding unwanted medical treatment, and that it encompasses the right to be free of "artificially delivered food and water." See *ante* at 287.

But if a competent person has a liberty interest to be free of unwanted medical treatment, as both the majority and JUSTICE O'CONNOR concede, it must be fundamental. "We are dealing here with [a decision] which involves one of the basic

civil rights of man." *Skinner v. Oklahoma ex rel. Williamson*, 316 U.S. 535, 541 (1942) (invalidating a statute authorizing sterilization of certain felons). Whatever other liberties protected by the Due Process Clause are fundamental, "those liberties that are 'deeply rooted in this Nation's history and tradition'" are among them. *Bowers v. Hardwick*, 478 U.S. 186, 192 (1986) (quoting *Moore v. East Cleveland, supra*, at 503 (plurality opinion)). "Such a tradition commands respect in part because the Constitution carries the gloss of history." *Richmond Newspapers, Inc. v. Virginia*, 448 U.S. 555, 589 (1980) (BRENNAN, J., concurring in judgment).

The right to be free from medical attention without consent, to determine what shall be done with one's own body, is deeply rooted in this Nation's traditions, as the majority acknowledges. See *ante* at 270. This right has long been "firmly entrenched in American tort law" and is securely grounded in the earliest common law. *Ante*, at 269. See also *Mills v. Rogers*, 457 U.S. 291, 294, n. 4 (1982) ("[T]he right to refuse any medical treatment emerged from the doctrines of trespass and battery, which were applied to unauthorized touchings by a physician"). "Anglo-American law starts with the premise of thorough-going self-determination. It follows that each man is considered to be master of his own body, and he may, if he be of sound mind, expressly prohibit the performance of lifesaving surgery or other medical treatment." *Natanson v. Kline*, 186 Kan. 393, 406–407, 350 P.2d 1093, 1104 (1960). "The inviolability of the person" has been held as "sacred" and "carefully guarded" as any common law right. *Union Pacific R. Co. v. Botsford*, 141 U.S. 250, 251–252 (1891). Thus, freedom from unwanted medical attention is unquestionably among those principles "so rooted in the traditions and conscience of our people as to be ranked as fundamental." *Snyder v. Massachusetts*, 291 U.S. 97, 105 (1934).[5]

That there may be serious consequences involved in refusal of the medical treatment at issue here does not vitiate the right under our common law tradition of medical self-determination. It is "a well-established rule of general law . . . that it is the patient, not the physician, who ultimately decides if treatment—any treatment—is to be given at all. . . . The rule has never been qualified in its application by either the nature or purpose of the treatment, or the gravity of the consequences

---

[5]See e.g., *Canterbury v. Spence*, 150 U.S. App. D.C. 263, 271, 464 F.2d 772, 780, cert. denied, 409 U.S. 1064 (1972) ("The root premise" of informed consent "is the concept, fundamental in American jurisprudence, that '[e]very human being of adult years and sound mind has a right to determine what shall be done with his own body'") (quoting *Schloendorff v. Society of New York Hospital*, 211 N.Y. 125, 129–130, 105 N.E. 92, 93 (1914) (Cardozo, J.)). See generally *Washington v. Harper*, 494 U.S. 210, 241 (1990) (STEVENS, J., dissenting) ("There is no doubt . . . that a competent individual's right to refuse [psychotropic] medication is a fundamental liberty interest deserving the highest order of protection").

of acceding to or foregoing it." *Tune v. Walter Reed Army Medical Hospital*, 602 F.Supp. 1452, 1455 (DC 1985). See also *Downer v. Veilleux*, 322 A.2d 82, 91 (Me. 1974) ("The rationale of this rule lies in the fact that every competent adult has the right to forego treatment, or even cure, if it entails what for him are intolerable consequences or risks, however unwise his sense of values may be to others").[6]

No material distinction can be drawn between the treatment to which Nancy Cruzan continues to be subject—artificial nutrition and hydration—and any other medical treatment. See *ante* at 288–289 (O'CONNOR, J., concurring). The artificial delivery of nutrition and hydration is undoubtedly medical treatment. The technique to which Nancy Cruzan is subject—artificial feeding through a gastrostomy tube—involves a tube implanted surgically into her stomach through incisions in her abdominal wall. It may obstruct the intestinal tract, erode and pierce the stomach wall, or cause leakage of the stomach's contents into the abdominal cavity. See Page, Andrassy, & Sandler, Techniques in Delivery of Liquid Diets, in Nutrition in Clinical Surgery 66–67 (M. Deitel 2d ed. 1985). The tube can cause pneumonia from reflux of the stomach's contents into the lung. See Bernard & Forlaw, Complications and Their Prevention, in Enteral and Tube Feeding 553 (J. Rombeau & M. Caldwell eds. 1984). Typically, and in this case (see Tr. 377), commercially prepared formulas are used, rather than fresh food. See Matarese, Enteral Alimentation, in Surgical Nutrition 726 (J. Fischer ed. 1983). The type of formula and method of administration must be experimented with to avoid gastrointestinal problems. *Id.*, at 748. The patient must be monitored daily by medical personnel as to weight, fluid intake and fluid output; blood tests must be done weekly. *Id.*, at 749, 751.

Artificial delivery of food and water is regarded as medical treatment by the medical profession and the Federal Government.[7] According to the American Academy of Neurology:

> "The artificial provision of nutrition and hydration is a form of medical treatment . . . analogous to other forms of life-sustaining treatment, such as the use of the respirator. When a patient is unconscious, both a respirator and an artificial feeding device serve to support or replace normal bodily functions that are compromised as a result of the patient's illness."

Position of the American Academy of Neurology on Certain Aspects of the Care and Management of the Persistent Vegetative State Patient, 39 Neurology 125 (Jan. 1989). See also Council on Ethical and Judicial Affairs of the American Medical Association, Current Opinions, Opinion 2.20 (1989) ("Life-prolonging medical treatment includes medication and artificially or technologically supplied respiration, nutrition or hydration"); President's Commission 88 (life-sustaining treatment includes respirators, kidney dialysis machines, special feeding procedures). The Federal Government permits the cost of the medical devices and formulas used in enteral feeding to be reimbursed under Medicare. See Pub.L. 99–509, 9340, note following 42 U.S.C. 1395u, p. 592 (1982 ed., Supp. V). The formulas are regulated by the Federal Drug Administration as "medical foods," see 21 U.S.C. 360ee, and the feeding tubes are regulated as medical devices, 21 CFR 876.5980 (1989).

Nor does the fact that Nancy Cruzan is now incompetent deprive her of her fundamental rights. See *Youngberg v. Romeo*, 457 U.S. 307, 315, 316, 319 (1982) (holding that severely retarded man's liberty interests in safety, freedom from bodily restraint and reasonable training survive involuntary commitment); *Parham v. J.R.*, 442 U.S. 584, 600 (1979) (recognizing a child's substantial liberty interest in not being confined unnecessarily for medical treatment); *Jackson v. Indiana*, 406 U.S. 715, 730, 738 (1972) (holding that Indiana could not violate the due process and equal protection rights of a mentally retarded deaf mute by committing him for an indefinite amount of time simply because he was incompetent to stand trial on the criminal charges filed against him). As the majority

---

[6]Under traditional tort law, exceptions have been found only to protect dependent children. See *Cruzan v. Harmon*, 760 S.W.2d 408, 422, n. 17 (Mo. 1988) (citing cases where Missouri courts have ordered blood transfusions for children over the religious objection of parents); see also *Winthrop University Hospital v. Hess*, 128 Misc.2d 804, 490 N.Y.S.2d 996 (Sup.Ct. Nassau Co. 1985) (court ordered blood transfusion for religious objector because she was the mother of an infant and had explained that her objection was to the signing of the consent, not the transfusion itself); Application of President & Directors of Georgetown College, Inc., 118 U.S. App. D.C. 80, 88, 331 F.2d 1000, 1008, cert. denied, 377 U.S. 978 (1964) (blood transfusion ordered for mother of infant). Cf. *In re Estate of Brooks*, 32 Ill.2d 361, 373, 205 N.E.2d 435, 441–442 (1965) (finding that lower court erred in ordering a blood transfusion for a woman—whose children were grown—and concluding: "Even though we may consider appellant's beliefs unwise, foolish or ridiculous, in the absence of an overriding danger to society we may not permit interference therewith in the form of a conservatorship established in the waning hours of her life for the sole purpose of compelling her to accept medical treatment forbidden by her religious principles, and previously refused by her with full knowledge of the probable consequences").

[7]The Missouri court appears to be alone among state courts to suggest otherwise, 760 S.W.2d at 419 and 423, although the court did not rely on a distinction between artificial feeding and other forms of medical treatment. *Id.*, at 423. See, e.g., *Delio v. Westchester County Medical Center*, 129 App. Div.2d 1, 19, 516 N.Y.S.2d 677, 689 (1987) ("review of the decisions in other jurisdictions . . . failed to uncover a single case in which a court confronted with an application to discontinue feeding by artificial means has evaluated medical procedures to provide nutrition and hydration differently from other types of life-sustaining procedures").

recognizes, *ante* at 280, the question is not whether an incompetent has constitutional rights, but how such rights may be exercised. As we explained in *Thompson v. Oklahoma*, 487 U.S. 815 (1988), "[t]he law must often adjust the manner in which it affords rights to those whose status renders them unable to exercise choice freely and rationally. Children, the insane, and those who are irreversibly ill with loss of brain function, for instance, all retain 'rights,' to be sure, but often such rights are only meaningful as they are exercised by agents acting with the best interests of their principals in mind." *Id.*, at 825, n. 23 (emphasis added). "To deny [its] exercise because the patient is unconscious or incompetent would be to deny the right." *Foody v. Manchester Memorial Hospital*, 40 Conn.Supp. 127, 133, 482 A.2d 713, 718 (1984).

II

A

The right to be free from unwanted medical attention is a right to evaluate the potential benefit of treatment and its possible consequences according to one's own values and to make a personal decision whether to subject oneself to the intrusion. For a patient like Nancy Cruzan, the sole benefit of medical treatment is being kept metabolically alive. Neither artificial nutrition nor any other form of medical treatment available today can cure or in any way ameliorate her condition.[8] Irreversibly vegetative patients are devoid of thought, emotion and sensation; they are permanently and completely unconscious. See n. 2, *supra*.[9] As the President's Commission con-

cluded in approving the withdrawal of life support equipment from irreversibly vegetative patients:

> "[T]reatment ordinarily aims to benefit a patient through preserving life, relieving pain and suffering, protecting against disability, and returning maximally effective functioning. If a prognosis of permanent unconsciousness is correct, however, continued treatment cannot confer such benefits. Pain and suffering are absent, as are joy, satisfaction, and pleasure. Disability is total, and no return to an even minimal level of social or human functioning is possible." President's Commission 181–182.

There are also affirmative reasons why someone like Nancy might choose to forgo artificial nutrition and hydration under these circumstances. Dying is personal. And it is profound. For many, the thought of an ignoble end, steeped in decay, is abhorrent. A quiet, proud death, bodily integrity intact, is a matter of extreme consequence. "In certain, thankfully rare, circumstances the burden of maintaining the corporeal existence degrades the very humanity it was meant to serve." *Brophy v. New England Sinai Hospital, Inc.*, 398 Mass. 417, 434, 497 N.E.2d 626, 635–636 (1986) (finding the subject of the proceeding "in a condition which [he] has indicated he would consider to be degrading and without human dignity" and holding that "[t]he duty of the State to preserve life must encompass a recognition of an individual's right to avoid circumstances in which the individual himself would feel that efforts to sustain life demean or degrade his humanity"). Another court, hearing a similar case, noted:

> "It is apparent from the testimony that what was on [the patient's] mind was not only the invasiveness of life-sustaining systems, such as the [nasogastric] tube, upon the integrity of his body. It was also the utter helplessness of the permanently comatose person, the wasting of a once strong body, and the submission of the most private bodily functions to the attention of others." *In re Gardner*, 534 A.2d 947, 953 (Me. 1987).

Such conditions are, for many, humiliating to contemplate,[10] as is visiting a prolonged and anguished vigil on one's

---

[8]While brain stem cells can survive 15 to 20 minutes without oxygen, cells in the cerebral hemispheres are destroyed if they are deprived of oxygen for as few as 4 to 6 minutes. See Cranford & Smith, Some Critical Distinctions Between Brain Death and the Persistent Vegetative State, 6 Ethics Sci. & Med. 199, 203 (1979). It is estimated that Nancy's brain was deprived of oxygen from 12 to 14 minutes. See *ante* at 266. Out of the 100,000 patients who, like Nancy, have fallen into persistent vegetative states in the past 20 years due to loss of oxygen to the brain, there have been only three even partial recoveries documented in the medical literature. Brief for American Medical Association et al. as Amici Curiae 11–12. The longest any person has ever been in a persistent vegetative state and recovered was 22 months. See Snyder, Cranford, Rubens, Bundlic, & Rockswold, Delayed Recovery from Postanoxic Persistent Vegetative State, 14 Annals Neurol. 156 (1983). Nancy has been in this state for seven years.

[9]The American Academy of Neurology offers three independent bases on which the medical profession rests these neurological conclusions:

"First, direct clinical experience with these patients demonstrates that there is no behavioral indication of any awareness of pain or suffering.

"Second, in all persistent vegetative state patients studied to date, postmortem examination reveals overwhelming bilateral damage to the cerebral hemispheres to a degree incompatible with consciousness....

"Third, recent data utilizing positron emission tomography indicates that the metabolic rate for glucose in the cerebral cortex is greatly reduced in persistent vegetative state patients, to a degree incompatible with consciousness."

Position of the American Academy of Neurology on Certain Aspects of the Care and Management of the Persistent Vegetative State Patient, 39 Neurology 125 (Jan. 1989).

---

[10]Nancy Cruzan, for instance, is totally and permanently disabled. All four of her limbs are severely contracted; her fingernails cut into her wrists. App. to Pet. for Cert. A93. She is incontinent of bowel and bladder. The most intimate aspects of her existence are exposed to and controlled by strangers. Brief for Respondent Guardian Ad Litem 2. Her family is convinced that Nancy would find this state degrading. See n. 20, infra.

parents, spouse, and children. A long, drawn-out death can have a debilitating effect on family members. See Carnwath & Johnson, Psychiatric Morbidity Among Spouses of Patients With Stroke, 294 Brit.Med.J. 409 (1987); Livingston, Families Who Care, 291 Brit.Med.J. 919 (1985). For some, the idea of being remembered in their persistent vegetative states, rather than as they were before their illness or accident, may be very disturbing.[11]

B

Although the right to be free of unwanted medical intervention, like other constitutionally protected interests, may not be absolute,[12] no State interest could outweigh the rights of an individual in Nancy Cruzan's position. Whatever a State's possible interests in mandating life-support treatment under other circumstances, there is no good to be obtained here by Missouri's insistence that Nancy Cruzan remain on life-support systems if it is indeed her wish not to do so. Missouri does not claim, nor could it, that society as a whole will be benefited by Nancy's receiving medical treatment. No third party's situation will be improved, and no harm to others will be averted. Cf. nn. 6 and 8, *supra*.[13]

The only state interest asserted here is a general interest in the preservation of life.[14] But the State has no legitimate general interest in someone's life, completely abstracted from the interest of the person living that life, that could outweigh the person's choice to avoid medical treatment. "[T]he regulation of constitutionally protected decisions . . . must be predicated on legitimate state concerns other than disagreement with the choice the individual has made. . . . Otherwise, the interest in liberty protected by the Due Process Clause would be a nullity." *Hodgson v. Minnesota*, post, at 435 (1990) (Opinion of STEVENS, J.) (emphasis added). Thus, the State's general interest in life must accede to Nancy Cruzan's particularized and intense interest in self-determination in her choice of medical treatment. There is simply nothing legitimately within the State's purview to be gained by superseding her decision.

Moreover, there may be considerable danger that Missouri's rule of decision would impair rather than serve any interest the State does have in sustaining life. Current medical practice recommends use of heroic measures if there is a scintilla of a chance that the patient will recover, on the assumption that the measures will be discontinued should the patient improve. When the President's Commission in 1982 approved the withdrawal of life support equipment from irreversibly vegetative patients, it explained that "[a]n even more troubling wrong occurs when a treatment that might save life or improve health is not started because the health care personnel are afraid that they will find it very difficult to stop the treatment if, as is fairly likely, it proves to be of little benefit and greatly burdens the patient." President's Commission 75. A New Jersey court recognized that families as well as doctors might be discouraged by an inability to stop life-support measures from "even attempting certain types of care [which] could thereby force them into hasty and premature decisions to allow a patient to die." *In re Conroy*, 98 N.J. 321, 370, 486 A.2d 1209, 1234

---

[11]What general information exists about what most people would choose or would prefer to have chosen for them under these circumstances also indicates the importance of ensuring a means for now-incompetent patients to exercise their right to avoid unwanted medical treatment. A 1988 poll conducted by the American Medical Association found that 80% of those surveyed favored withdrawal of life support systems from hopelessly ill or irreversibly comatose patients if they or their families requested it. New York Times, June 5, 1988, p. 14, col. 4 (citing American Medical News, June 3, 1988, p. 9, col. 1). Another 1988 poll conducted by the Colorado University Graduate School of Public Affairs showed that 85% of those questioned would not want to have their own lives maintained with artificial nutrition and hydration if they became permanently unconscious. The Coloradoan, Sept. 29, 1988, p. 1.

Such attitudes have been translated into considerable political action. Since 1976, 40 States and the District of Columbia have enacted natural death acts, expressly providing for self-determination under some or all of these situations. See Brief for Society for the Right to Die, Inc. as Amicus Curiae 8; Weiner, Privacy Family, and Medical Decision Making for Persistent Vegetative Patients, 11 Cardozo L.Rev. 713, 720 (1990). Thirteen States and the District of Columbia have enacted statutes authorizing the appointment of proxies for making health care decisions. See ante at 290, n. 2 (O'CONNOR, J., concurring).

[12]See *Jacobson v. Massachusetts*, 197 U.S. 11, 26–27 (1905) (upholding a Massachusetts law imposing fines or imprisonment on those refusing to be vaccinated as "of paramount necessity" to that State's fight against a smallpox epidemic).

[13]Were such interests at stake, however, I would find that the Due Process Clause places limits on what invasive medical procedures could be forced on an unwilling comatose patient in pursuit of the interests of a third party. If Missouri were correct that its interests outweigh Nancy's interest in avoiding medical procedures as long as she is free of pain and physical discomfort, see 760 S.W.2d at 424, it is not apparent why a State could not choose to remove one of her kidneys without consent on the ground that society would be better off if the recipient of that kidney were saved from renal poisoning. Nancy cannot feel surgical pain. See n. 2, *supra*. Nor would removal of one kidney be

expected to shorten her life expectancy. See The American Medical Association Family Medical Guide 506 (J. Kunz ed. 1982). Patches of her skin could also be removed to provide grafts for burn victims, and scrapings of bone marrow to provide grafts for someone with leukemia. Perhaps the State could lawfully remove more vital organs for transplanting into others who would then be cured of their ailments, provided the State placed Nancy on some other life-support equipment to replace the lost function. Indeed, why could the State not perform medical experiments on her body, experiments that might save countless lives, and would cause her no greater burden than she already bears by being fed through the gastrostomy tube? This would be too brave a new world for me and, I submit, for our Constitution.

[14]The Missouri Supreme Court reviewed the state interests that had been identified by other courts as potentially relevant—prevention of homicide and suicide, protection of interests of innocent third parties, maintenance of the ethical integrity of the medical profession, and preservation of life—and concluded that: "In this case, only the state's interest in the preservation of life is implicated." 760 S.W.2d at 419.

(1985). See also Brief for American Academy of Neurology as Amicus Curiae 9 (expressing same concern).[15]

III

This is not to say that the State has no legitimate interests to assert here. As the majority recognizes, *ante* at 281–282, Missouri has a *parens patriae* interest in providing Nancy Cruzan, now incompetent, with as accurate as possible a determination of how she would exercise her rights under these circumstances. Second, if and when it is determined that Nancy Cruzan would want to continue treatment, the State may legitimately assert an interest in providing that treatment. But until Nancy's wishes have been determined, the only state interest that may be asserted is an interest in safe-guarding the accuracy of that determination.

Accuracy, therefore, must be our touchstone. Missouri may constitutionally impose only those procedural requirements that serve to enhance the accuracy of a determination of Nancy Cruzan's wishes or are at least consistent with an accurate determination. The Missouri "safeguard" that the Court upholds today does not meet that standard. The determination needed in this context is whether the incompetent person would choose to live in a persistent vegetative state on life-support or to avoid this medical treatment. Missouri's rule of decision imposes a markedly asymmetrical evidentiary burden. Only evidence of specific statements of treatment choice made by the patient when competent is admissible to support a finding that the patient, now in a persistent vegetative state, would wish to avoid further medical treatment. Moreover, this evidence must be clear and convincing. No proof is required to support a finding that the incompetent person would wish to continue treatment.

A

The majority offers several justifications for Missouri's heightened evidentiary standard. First, the majority explains that the State may constitutionally adopt this rule to govern determinations of an incompetent's wishes in order to advance the State's substantive interests, including its unqualified interest in the preservation of human life. See *ante* at 282–283 and n. 10. Missouri's evidentiary standard, however, cannot rest on the State's own interest in a particular substantive result. To be sure, courts have long erected clear and convincing evidence standards to place the greater risk of erroneous decisions on those bringing disfavored claims.[16] In such cases, however, the choice to discourage certain claims was a legitimate, constitutional policy choice. In contrast, Missouri has no such power to disfavor a choice by Nancy Cruzan to avoid medical treatment, because Missouri has no legitimate interest in providing Nancy with treatment until it is established that this represents her choice. See *supra* at 312–314. Just as a State may not override Nancy's choice directly, it may not do so indirectly through the imposition of a procedural rule.

Second, the majority offers two explanations for why Missouri's clear and convincing evidence standard is a means of enhancing accuracy, but neither is persuasive. The majority initially argues that a clear and convincing evidence standard is necessary to compensate for the possibility that such proceedings will lack the "guarantee of accurate fact-finding that the adversary process brings with it," citing *Ohio v. Akron Center for*

---

[15]In any event, the State interest identified by the Missouri Supreme Court—a comprehensive and "unqualified" interest in preserving life, *id.*, at 420, 424 is not even well supported by that State's own enactments. In the first place, Missouri has no law requiring every person to procure any needed medical care nor a state health insurance program to underwrite such care. *Id.*, at 429 (Blackmar, J., dissenting). Second, as the state court admitted, Missouri has a living will statute which specifically "allows and encourages the pre-planned termination of life." *Ibid.*; see Mo.Rev.Stat. 459.015.1 (1986). The fact that Missouri actively provides for its citizens to choose a natural death under certain circumstances suggests that the State's interest in life is not so unqualified as the court below suggests. It is true that this particular statute does not apply to nonterminal patients and does not include artificial nutrition and hydration as one of the measures that may be declined. Nonetheless, Missouri has also not chosen to require court review of every decision to withhold or withdraw life-support made on behalf of an incompetent patient. Such decisions are made every day, without state participation. See 760 S.W.2d at 428 (Blackmar, J., dissenting).

In addition, precisely what implication can be drawn from the statute's limitations is unclear, given the inclusion of a series of "interpretive" provisions in the Act. The first such provision explains that the Act is to be interpreted consistently with the following: "Each person has the primary right to request or refuse medical treatment subject to the state's interest in protecting innocent third parties, preventing homicide and suicide and preserving good ethical standards in the medical profession." Mo.Rev.Stat. 459.055(1) (1986). The second of these subsections explains that the Act's provisions are cumulative, and not intended to increase or decrease the right of a patient to make decisions or lawfully effect the withholding or withdrawal of medical care. 459.055(2). The third subsection provides that "no presumption concerning the intention of an individual who has not executed a declaration to consent to the use or withholding of medical procedures" shall be created. 459.055(3).

Thus, even if it were conceivable that a State could assert an interest sufficiently compelling to overcome Nancy Cruzan's constitutional right, Missouri law demonstrates a more modest interest at best. See generally *Capital Cities Cable, Inc. v. Crisp*, 467 U.S. 691, 715 (1984) (finding that state regulations narrow in scope indicated that State had only a moderate interest in its professed goal).

[16]See *Colorado v. New Mexico*, 467 U.S. 310 (1984) (requiring clear and convincing evidence before one State is permitted to divert water from another to accommodate society's interests in stable property rights and efficient use of resources); *New York v. New Jersey*, 256 U.S. 296 (1921) (promoting federalism by requiring clear and convincing evidence before using Court's power to control the conduct of one State at the behest of another); Maxwell Land-Grant Case, 121 U.S. 325 (1887) (requiring clear, unequivocal, and convincing evidence to set aside, annul or correct a patent or other title to property issued by the Government in order to secure settled expectations concerning property rights); *Marcum v. Zaring*, 406 P.2d 970 (Okla. 1965) (promoting stability of marriage by requiring clear and convincing evidence to prove its invalidity); *Stevenson v. Stein*, 412 Pa. 478, 195 A.2d 268 (1963) (promoting settled expectations concerning property rights by requiring clear and convincing evidence to prove adverse possession).

Reproductive Health, post at 515–516 (upholding a clear and convincing evidence standard for an ex parte proceeding). Ante, at 281–282. Without supporting the Court's decision in that case, I note that the proceeding to determine an incompetent's wishes is quite different from a proceeding to determine whether a minor may bypass notifying her parents before undergoing an abortion on the ground that she is mature enough to make the decision or that the abortion is in her best interest.

An adversarial proceeding is of particular importance when one side has a strong personal interest which needs to be counterbalanced to assure the court that the questions will be fully explored. A minor who has a strong interest in obtaining permission for an abortion without notifying her parents may come forward whether or not society would be satisfied that she has made the decision with the seasoned judgment of an adult. The proceeding here is of a different nature. Barring venal motives, which a trial court has the means of ferreting out, the decision to come forward to request a judicial order to stop treatment represents a slowly and carefully considered resolution by at least one adult and more frequently several adults that discontinuation of treatment is the patient's wish.

In addition, the bypass procedure at issue in Akron, *supra,* is *ex parte* and secret. The court may not notify the minor's parents, siblings or friends. No one may be present to submit evidence unless brought forward by the minor herself. In contrast, the proceeding to determine Nancy Cruzan's wishes was neither *ex parte* nor secret. In a hearing to determine the treatment preferences of an incompetent person, a court is not limited to adjusting burdens of proof as its only means of protecting against a possible imbalance. Indeed, any concern that those who come forward will present a one-sided view would be better addressed by appointing a guardian ad litem, who could use the State's powers of discovery to gather and present evidence regarding the patient's wishes. A guardian *ad litem*'s task is to uncover any conflicts of interest and ensure that each party likely to have relevant evidence is consulted and brought forward—for example, other members of the family, friends, clergy, and doctors. See, e.g., *In re Colyer,* 99 Wash.2d 114, 133, 660 P.2d 738, 748–749 (1983). Missouri's heightened evidentiary standard attempts to achieve balance by discounting evidence; the guardian ad litem technique achieves balance by probing for additional evidence. Where, as here, the family members, friends, doctors and guardian ad litem agree, it is not because the process has failed, as the majority suggests. See *ante* at 281, n. 9. It is because there is no genuine dispute as to Nancy's preference.

The majority next argues that where, as here, important individual rights are at stake, a clear and convincing evidence standard has long been held to be an appropriate means of en-

hancing accuracy, citing decisions concerning what process an individual is due before he can be deprived of a liberty interest. See *ante,* at 283. In those cases, however, this Court imposed a clear and convincing standard as a constitutional minimum on the basis of its evaluation that one side's interests clearly outweighed the second side's interests, and therefore the second side should bear the risk of error. See *Santosky v. Kramer,* 455 U.S. 745, 753, 766–767 (1982) (requiring a clear and convincing evidence standard for termination of parental rights because the parent's interest is fundamental, but the State has no legitimate interest in termination unless the parent is unfit, and finding that the State's interest in finding the best home for the child does not arise until the parent has been found unfit); *Addington v. Texas,* 441 U.S. 418, 426–427 (1979) (requiring clear and convincing evidence in an involuntary commitment hearing because the interest of the individual far outweighs that of a State, which has no legitimate interest in confining individuals who are not mentally ill and do not pose a danger to themselves or others). Moreover, we have always recognized that shifting the risk of error reduces the likelihood of errors in one direction at the cost of increasing the likelihood of errors in the other. See *Addington, supra,* at 423 (contrasting heightened standards of proof to a preponderance standard in which the two sides "share the risk of error in roughly equal fashion" because society does not favor one outcome over the other). In the cases cited by the majority, the imbalance imposed by a heightened evidentiary standard was not only acceptable, but required because the standard was deployed to protect an individual's exercise of a fundamental right, as the majority admits, *ante* at 282–283, n. 10. In contrast, the Missouri court imposed a clear and convincing standard as an obstacle to the exercise of a fundamental right.

The majority claims that the allocation of the risk of error is justified because it is more important not to terminate life-support for someone who would wish it continued than to honor the wishes of someone who would not. An erroneous decision to terminate life-support is irrevocable, says the majority, while an erroneous decision not to terminate "results in a maintenance of the status quo." See *ante* at 283.[17] But, from

---

[17]The majority's definition of the "status quo," of course, begs the question. Artificial delivery of nutrition and hydration represents the "status quo" only if the State has chosen to permit doctors and hospitals to keep a patient on life-support systems over the protests of his family or guardian. The "status quo" absent that state interference would be the natural result of his accident or illness (and the family's decision). The majority's definition of status quo, however, is "to a large extent a predictable, yet accidental confluence of technology, psyche, and inertia. The general citizenry . . . never said that it favored the creation of coma wards where permanently unconscious patients would be tended for years and years. Nor did the populace as a whole authorize the preeminence of doctors over families in making treatment decisions for incompetent patients." Rhoden, Litigating Life and Death, 102 Harv.L.Rev. 375, 433–434 (1988).

the point of view of the patient, an erroneous decision in either direction is irrevocable. An erroneous decision to terminate artificial nutrition and hydration, to be sure, will lead to failure of that last remnant of physiological life, the brain stem, and result in complete brain death. An erroneous decision not to terminate life-support, however, robs a patient of the very qualities protected by the right to avoid unwanted medical treatment. His own degraded existence is perpetuated; his family's suffering is protracted; the memory he leaves behind becomes more and more distorted.

Even a later decision to grant him his wish cannot undo the intervening harm. But a later decision is unlikely in any event. "[T]he discovery of new evidence," to which the majority refers, *ibid.*, is more hypothetical than plausible. The majority also misconceives the relevance of the possibility of "advancements in medical science," *ibid.*, by treating it as a reason to force someone to continue medical treatment against his will. The possibility of a medical miracle is indeed part of the calculus, but it is a part of the patient's calculus. If current research suggests that some hope for cure or even moderate improvement is possible within the life-span projected, this is a factor that should be and would be accorded significant weight in assessing what the patient himself would choose.[18]

B

Even more than its heightened evidentiary standard, the Missouri court's categorical exclusion of relevant evidence dispenses with any semblance of accurate fact finding. The court adverted to no evidence supporting its decision, but held that no clear and convincing, inherently reliable evidence had been presented to show that Nancy would want to avoid further treatment. In doing so, the court failed to consider statements Nancy had made to family members and a close friend.[19] The court also failed to consider testimony from Nancy's mother

and sister that they were certain that Nancy would want to discontinue artificial nutrition and hydration,[20] even after the court found that Nancy's family was loving and without malignant motive. See 760 S.W.2d at 412. The court also failed to consider the conclusions of the guardian ad litem, appointed by the trial court, that there was clear and convincing evidence that Nancy would want to discontinue medical treatment and that this was in her best interests. *Id.*, at 444 (Higgins, J., dissenting from denial of rehearing); Brief for Respondent Guardian *Ad Litem* 2–3. The court did not specifically define what kind of evidence it would consider clear and convincing, but its general discussion suggests that only a living will or equivalently formal directive from the patient when competent would meet this standard. See 760 S.W.2d at 424–425.

Too few people execute living wills or equivalently formal directives for such an evidentiary rule to ensure adequately that the wishes of incompetent persons will be honored.[21] While it might be a wise social policy to encourage people to

---

[18]For Nancy Cruzan, no such cure or improvement is in view. So much of her brain has deteriorated and been replaced by fluid, see App. to Pet. for Cert. A94, that apparently the only medical advance that could restore consciousness to her body would be a brain transplant. Cf. n. 22, infra.

[19]The trial court had relied on the testimony of Athena Comer, a long-time friend, coworker and a housemate for several months, as sufficient to show that Nancy Cruzan would wish to be free of medical treatment under her present circumstances. App. to Pet. for Cert. A94. Ms. Comer described a conversation she and Nancy had while living together concerning Ms. Comer's sister, who had become ill suddenly and died during the night. The Comer family had been told that, if she had lived through the night, she would have been in a vegetative state. Nancy had lost a grandmother a few months before. Ms. Comer testified that: "Nancy said she would never want to live [as a vegetative state] because if she couldn't be normal or even, you know, like half way, and do things for yourself, because Nancy always did, that she didn't want to live . . . and we talked about it a lot." Tr. 388–389. She said "several times" that "she wouldn't want to live that way because if she was going to live, she wanted to be able to live, not to just lay in a bed and not be able to move because you can't

do anything for yourself." *Id.*, at 390, 396. "[S]he said that she hoped that [all the] people in her family knew that she wouldn't want to live [in a vegetative state] because she knew it was usually up to the family whether you lived that way or not." *Id.*, at 399.

The conversation took place approximately a year before Nancy's accident, and was described by Ms. Comer as a "very serious" conversation that continued for approximately half an hour without interruption. *Id.*, at 390. The Missouri Supreme Court dismissed Nancy's statement as "unreliable" on the ground that it was an informally expressed reaction to other people's medical conditions. 760 S.W.2d at 424.

The Missouri Supreme Court did not refer to other evidence of Nancy's wishes or explain why it was rejected. Nancy's sister Christy, to whom she was very close, testified that she and Nancy had had two very serious conversations about a year and a half before the accident. A day or two after their niece was stillborn (but would have been badly damaged if she had lived), Nancy had said that maybe it was part of a "greater plan" that the baby had been stillborn and did not have to face "the possible life of mere existence." Tr. 537. A month later, after their grandmother had died after a long battle with heart problems, Nancy said that "it was better for my grandmother not to be kind of brought back and forth [by] medical [treatment], brought back from a critical near point of death. . . ." *Id.*, at 541.

[20]Nancy's sister Christy, Nancy's mother, and another of Nancy's friends testified that Nancy would want to discontinue the hydration and nutrition. Christy said that "Nancy would be horrified at the state she is in." *Id.*, at 535. She would also "want to take that burden away from [her family]." *Id.*, at 544. Based on "a lifetime of experience, [I know Nancy's wishes] are to discontinue the hydration and the nutrition." *Id.*, at 542. Nancy's mother testified: "Nancy would not want to be like she is now. [I]f it were me up there or Christy or any of us, she would be doing for us what we are trying to do for her. I know she would, . . . as her mother." *Id.*, at 526.

[21]Surveys show that the overwhelming majority of Americans have not executed such written instructions. See Emmanuel & Emmanuel, The Medical Directive: A New Comprehensive Advance Care Document, 261 JAMA 3288 (1989) (only 9% of Americans execute advance directives about how they would wish treatment decisions to be handled if they became incompetent); American Medical Association Surveys of Physician and Public Opinion on Health Care Issues 29–30 (1988) (only 15% of those surveyed had executed living wills); 2 President's Commission for the Study of Ethical Problems in Medicine and Biomedical and Behavioral Research, Making Health Care Decisions 241–242 (1982) (23% of those surveyed said that they had put treatment instructions in writing).

furnish such instructions, no general conclusion about a patient's choice can be drawn from the absence of formalities. The probability of becoming irreversibly vegetative is so low that many people may not feel an urgency to marshal formal evidence of their preferences. Some may not wish to dwell on their own physical deterioration and mortality. Even someone with a resolute determination to avoid life-support under circumstances such as Nancy's would still need to know that such things as living wills exist and how to execute one. Often legal help would be necessary, especially given the majority's apparent willingness to permit States to insist that a person's wishes are not truly known unless the particular medical treatment is specified. See *ante* at 285.

As a California appellate court observed:

> "The lack of generalized public awareness of the statutory scheme and the typically human characteristics of procrastination and reluctance to contemplate the need for such arrangements however makes this a tool which will all too often go unused by those who might desire it."

Barber v. Superior Court, 147 Cal.App. 3d 1006, 1015, 195 Cal.Rptr. 484, 489 (1983). When a person tells family or close friends that she does not want her life sustained artificially, she is "express[ing] her wishes in the only terms familiar to her, and . . . as clearly as a lay person should be asked to express them. To require more is unrealistic, and for all practical purposes, it precludes the rights of patients to forego life-sustaining treatment." *In re O'Connor*, 72 N.Y.2d 517, 551, 534 N.Y.S.2d 886, 905, 531 N.E.2d 607, 626 (1988) (Simons, J., dissenting).[22] When Missouri enacted a living will statute, it specifically provided that the absence of a living will does not warrant a presumption that a patient wishes continued medical treatment.

See n. 15, *supra*. Thus, apparently not even Missouri's own legislature believes that a person who does not execute a living will fails to do so because he wishes continuous medical treatment under all circumstances.

The testimony of close friends and family members, on the other hand, may often be the best evidence available of what the patient's choice would be. It is they with whom the patient most likely will have discussed such questions and they who know the patient best. "Family members have a unique knowledge of the patient which is vital to any decision on his or her behalf." Newman, Treatment Refusals for the Critically and Terminally Ill: Proposed Rules for the Family, the Physician, and the State, 3 N.Y.L.S. Human Rights Annual 35, 46 (1985). The Missouri court's decision to ignore this whole category of testimony is also at odds with the practices of other States. See, e.g., *In re Peter*, 108 N.J. 365, 529 A.2d 419 (1987); *Brophy v. New England Sinai Hospital, Inc.*, 398 Mass. 417, 497 N.E.2d 626 (1986); *In re Severns*, 425 A.2d 156 (Del.Ch. 1980).

The Missouri court's disdain for Nancy's statements in serious conversations not long before her accident, for the opinions of Nancy's family and friends as to her values, beliefs and certain choice, and even for the opinion of an outside objective factfinder appointed by the State, evinces a disdain for Nancy Cruzan's own right to choose. The rules by which an incompetent person's wishes are determined must represent every effort to determine those wishes. The rule that the Missouri court adopted and that this Court upholds, however, skews the result away from a determination that as accurately as possible reflects the individual's own preferences and beliefs. It is a rule that transforms human beings into passive subjects of medical technology.

> "[M]edical care decisions must be guided by the individual patient's interests and values. Allowing persons to determine their own medical treatment is an important way in which society respects persons as individuals. Moreover, the respect due to persons as individuals does not diminish simply because they have become incapable of participating in treatment decisions. . . . [I]t is still possible for others to make a decision that reflects [the patient's] interests more closely than would a purely technological decision to do whatever is possible. Lacking the ability to decide, [a patient] has a right to a decision that takes his interests into account."

Conservatorship of Drabick, 200 Cal.App. 3d 185, 208, 245 Cal.Rptr. 840, 854–855, cert. denied, 488 U.S. 958 (1988).

---

[22]New York is the only State besides Missouri to deny a request to terminate life support on the ground that clear and convincing evidence of prior, expressed intent was absent, although New York did so in the context of very different situations. Mrs. O'Connor, the subject of In re O'Connor, had several times expressed her desire not to be placed on life-support if she were not going to be able to care for herself. However, both of her daughters testified that they did not know whether their mother would want to decline artificial nutrition and hydration under her present circumstances. Cf. n. 13, *supra*. Moreover, despite damage from several strokes, Mrs. O'Connor was conscious and capable of responding to simple questions and requests, and the medical testimony suggested she might improve to some extent. Cf. *supra*, at 301. The New York Court of Appeals also denied permission to terminate blood transfusions for a severely retarded man with terminal cancer because there was no evidence of a treatment choice made by the man when competent, as he had never been competent. See *In re Storar*, 52 N.Y.2d 363, 438 N.Y.S.2d 266, 420 N.E.2d 64, cert. denied, 454 U.S. 858 (1981). Again, the court relied on evidence that the man was conscious, functioning in the way he always had, and that the transfusions did not cause him substantial pain (although it was clear he did not like them).

C

I do not suggest that States must sit by helplessly if the choices of incompetent patients are in danger of being ignored. See *ante* at 281. Even if the Court had ruled that Missouri's rule of decision is unconstitutional, as I believe it should have, States would nevertheless remain free to fashion procedural protections to safeguard the interests of incompetents under these circumstances. The Constitution provides merely a framework here: protections must be genuinely aimed at ensuring decisions commensurate with the will of the patient, and must be reliable as instruments to that end. Of the many States which have instituted such protections, Missouri is virtually the only one to have fashioned a rule that lessens the likelihood of accurate determinations. In contrast, nothing in the Constitution prevents States from reviewing the advisability of a family decision by requiring a court proceeding or by appointing an impartial guardian ad litem.

There are various approaches to determining an incompetent patient's treatment choice in use by the several States today, and there may be advantages and disadvantages to each, and other approaches not yet envisioned. The choice, in largest part, is and should be left to the States, so long as each State is seeking, in a reliable manner, to discover what the patient would want. But with such momentous interests in the balance, States must avoid procedures that will prejudice the decision. "To err either way—to keep a person alive under circumstances under which he would rather have been allowed to die, or to allow that person to die when he would have chosen to cling to life—would be deeply unfortunate." *In re Conroy*, 98 N.J. at 343, 486 A.2d at 1 220.

D

Finally, I cannot agree with the majority that where it is not possible to determine what choice an incompetent patient would make, a State's role as *parens patriae* permits the State automatically to make that choice itself. See *ante* at 286 (explaining that the Due Process Clause does not require a State to confide the decision to "anyone but the patient herself"). Under fair rules of evidence, it is improbable that a court could not determine what the patient's choice would be. Under the rule of decision adopted by Missouri and upheld today by this Court, such occasions might be numerous. But in neither case does it follow that it is constitutionally acceptable for the State invariably to assume the role of deciding for the patient. A State's legitimate interest in safeguarding a patient's choice cannot be furthered by simply appropriating it.

The majority justifies its position by arguing that, while close family members may have a strong feeling about the ques-

tion, "there is no automatic assurance that the view of close family members will necessarily be the same as the patient's would have been had she been confronted with the prospect of her situation while competent." *Ibid.* I cannot quarrel with this observation. But it leads only to another question: Is there any reason to suppose that a State is more likely to make the choice that the patient would have made than someone who knew the patient intimately? To ask this is to answer it. As the New Jersey Supreme Court observed: "Family members are best qualified to make substituted judgments for incompetent patients not only because of their peculiar grasp of the patient's approach to life, but also because of their special bonds with him or her. . . . It is . . . they who treat the patient as a person, rather than a symbol of a cause." *In re Jobes*, 108 N.J. 394, 416, 529 A.2d 434, 445 (1987). The State, in contrast, is a stranger to the patient.

A State's inability to discern an incompetent patient's choice still need not mean that a State is rendered powerless to protect that choice. But I would find that the Due Process Clause prohibits a State from doing more than that. A State may ensure that the person who makes the decision on the patient's behalf is the one whom the patient himself would have selected to make that choice for him. And a State may exclude from consideration anyone having improper motives. But a State generally must either repose the choice with the person whom the patient himself would most likely have chosen as proxy or leave the decision to the patient's family.[23]

IV

As many as 10,000 patients are being maintained in persistent vegetative states in the United States, and the number is expected to increase significantly in the near future. See Cranford, *supra*, n. 2, at 27, 31. Medical technology, developed over the past 20 or so years, is often capable of resuscitating people after they have stopped breathing or their hearts have stopped beating. Some of those people are brought fully back to life. Two decades ago, those who were not and could not swallow and digest food died. Intravenous solutions could not provide sufficient calories to maintain people for more than a short time. Today, various forms of artificial feeding have been developed that are able to keep people metabolically alive for years, even decades. See Spencer & Palmisano, Specialized Nutritional Support of Patients—A Hospital's Legal Duty?, 11 Quality Rev.Bull. 160, 160–161 (1985). In addition, in this century, chronic or degenerative ailments have replaced communicable diseases as the

---

[23]Only in the exceedingly rare case where the State cannot find any family member or friend who can be trusted to endeavor genuinely to make the treatment choice the patient would have made does the State become the legitimate surrogate decision maker.

primary causes of death. See R. Weir, Abating Treatment with Critically Ill Patients 12–13 (1989); President's Commission 15–16. The 80% of Americans who die in hospitals are

> "likely to meet their end . . . 'in a sedated or comatose state; betubed nasally, abdominally and intravenously; and far more like manipulated objects than like moral subjects.'" [24] A fifth of all adults surviving to age 80 will suffer a progressive dementing disorder prior to death. See Cohen & Eisdorfer, Dementing Disorders, in The Practice of Geriatrics 194 (E. Calkins, P. Davis, & A. Ford eds. 1986).

> "[L]aw, equity and justice must not themselves quail and be helpless in the face of modern technological marvels presenting questions hitherto unthought of." *In re Quinlan*, 70 N.J. 10, 44, 355 A.2d 647, 665, cert. denied, 429 U.S. 922 (1976).

The new medical technology can reclaim those who would have been irretrievably lost a few decades ago and restore them to active lives. For Nancy Cruzan, it failed, and for others with wasting incurable disease it may be doomed to failure. In these unfortunate situations, the bodies and preferences and memories of the victims do not escheat to the State; nor does our Constitution permit the State or any other government to commandeer them. No singularity of feeling exists upon which such a government might confidently rely as *parens patriae*. The President's Commission, after years of research, concluded:

"In few areas of health care are people's evaluations of their experiences so varied and uniquely personal as in their assessments of the nature and value of the processes associated with dying. For some, every moment of life is of inestimable value; for others, life without some desired level of mental or physical ability is worthless or burdensome. A moderate degree of suffering may be an important means of personal growth and religious experience to one person, but only frightening or despicable to another." President's Commission 276.

Yet Missouri and this Court have displaced Nancy's own assessment of the processes associated with dying. They have discarded evidence of her will, ignored her values, and deprived her of the right to a decision as closely approximating her own choice as humanly possible. They have done so disingenuously in her name, and openly in Missouri's own. That Missouri and this Court may truly be motivated only by concern for incompetent patients makes no matter. As one of our most prominent jurists warned us decades ago: "Experience should teach us to be most on our guard to protect liberty when the government's purposes are beneficent. . . . The greatest dangers to liberty lurk in insidious encroachment by men of zeal, well meaning but without understanding." *Olmstead v. United States*, 277 U.S. 438, 479 (1928) (Brandeis, J., dissenting).

I respectfully dissent.

[Other dissenting opinions omitted]

---

[24]Fadiman, The Liberation of Lolly and Gronky, Life Magazine, Dec. 1986, p. 72 (quoting medical ethicist Joseph Fletcher).

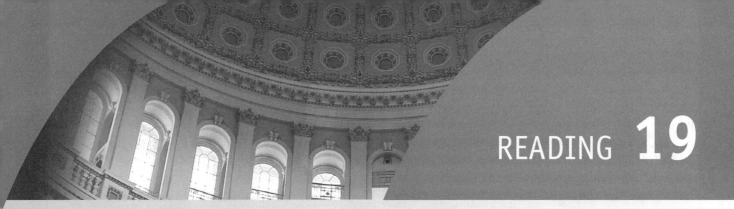

Case Law: *Washington v. Glucksberg* (Physician-Assisted Suicide)

WASHINGTON ET AL. *v.* GLUCKSBERG ET AL.

CERTIORARI TO THE UNITED STATES COURT OF APPEALS FOR THE NINTH CIRCUIT

No. 96-110. Argued January 8, 1997–Decided June 26, 1997

REHNQUIST, C. J., delivered the opinion of the Court, in which O'CONNOR, SCALIA, KENNEDY, and THOMAS, JJ., joined. O'CONNOR, J., filed a concurring opinion, in which GINSBURG and BREYER, JJ., joined in part, *post*, p. 736. STEVENS, J., *post*, p. 738, SOUTER, J., *post*, p. 752, GINSBURG, J., *post*, p. 789, and BREYER, J., *post*, p. 789, filed opinions concurring in the judgment.

CHIEF JUSTICE REHNQUIST delivered the opinion of the Court.

The question presented in this case is whether Washington's prohibition against "caus[ing]" or "aid[ing]" a suicide offends the Fourteenth Amendment to the United States Constitution. We hold that it does not.

It has always been a crime to assist a suicide in the State of Washington. In 1854, Washington's first Territorial Legislature outlawed "assisting another in the commission of self-murder."[1] Today, Washington law provides: "A person is guilty of promoting a suicide attempt when he knowingly causes or aids another person to attempt suicide." Wash. Rev. Code § 9A.36.060(1)

(1994). "Promoting a suicide attempt" is a felony, punishable by up to five years' imprisonment and up to a $10,000 fine. §§ 9A.36.060(2) and 9A.20.021(1)(c). At the same time, Washington's Natural Death Act, enacted in 1979, states that the "withholding or withdrawal of life-sustaining treatment" at a patient's direction "shall not, for any purpose, constitute a suicide." Wash. Rev. Code § 70.122.070(1).[2]

Petitioners in this case are the State of Washington and its Attorney General. Respondents Harold Glucksberg, M. D., Abigail Halperin, M. D., Thomas A. Preston, M. D., and Peter Shalit, M. D., are physicians who practice in Washington. These doctors occasionally treat terminally ill, suffering patients, and declare that they would assist these patients in ending their lives if not for Washington's assisted-suicide ban.[3] In January 1994, respondents, along with three gravely ill, pseudonymous plaintiffs who have since died and Compassion in Dying, a nonprofit organization that counsels people considering physician-assisted suicide, sued in the United States District Court, seeking a declaration that Wash. Rev. Code § 9A.36.060(1)

---

[1]Act of Apr. 28, 1854, § 17, 1854 Wash. Laws 78 ("Every person deliberately assisting another in the commission of self-murder, shall be deemed guilty of manslaughter"); see also Act of Dec. 2, 1869, § 17, 1869 Wash. Laws 201; Act of Nov. 10, 1873, § 19, 1873 Wash. Laws 184; Criminal Code, ch. 249, §§ 135–136, 1909 Wash. Laws, 11th Sess., 929.

[2]Under Washington's Natural Death Act, "adult persons have the fundamental right to control the decisions relating to the rendering of their own health care, including the decision to have life-sustaining treatment withheld or withdrawn in instances of a terminal condition or permanent unconscious condition." Wash. Rev. Code § 70.122.010 (1994). In Washington, "[a]ny adult person may execute a directive directing the withholding or withdrawal of life-sustaining treatment in a terminal condition or permanent unconscious condition," § 70.122.030, and a physician who, in accordance with such a directive, participates in the withholding or withdrawal of life-sustaining treatment is immune from civil, criminal, or professional liability, § 70.122.051.

[3]Glucksberg Declaration, App. 35; Halperin Declaration, id., at 49–50; Preston Declaration, id., at 55–56; Shalit Declaration, id., at 73–74.

(1994) is, on its face, unconstitutional. *Compassion in Dying* v. *Washington*, 850 F. Supp. 1454, 1459 (WD Wash. 1994).[4]

The plaintiffs asserted "the existence of a liberty interest protected by the Fourteenth Amendment which extends to a personal choice by a mentally competent, terminally ill adult to commit physician-assisted suicide." *Ibid.* Relying primarily on *Planned Parenthood of Southeastern Pa.* v. *Casey*, 505 U.S. 833 (1992), and *Cruzan* v. *Director, Mo. Dept. of Health*, 497 U.S. 261 (1990), the District Court agreed, 850 F. Supp., at 1459–1462, and concluded that Washington's assisted-suicide ban is unconstitutional because it "places an undue burden on the exercise of [that] constitutionally protected liberty interest." *Id.,* at 1465.[5] The District Court also decided that the Washington statute violated the Equal Protection Clause's requirement that "'all persons similarly situated . . . be treated alike.'" *Id.,* at 1466 (quoting *Cleburne* v. *Cleburne Living Center, Inc.,* 473 U.S. 432, 439 (1985)).

A panel of the Court of Appeals for the Ninth Circuit reversed, emphasizing that "[i]n the two hundred and five years of our existence no constitutional right to aid in killing oneself has ever been asserted and upheld by a court of final jurisdiction." *Compassion in Dying* v. *Washington*, 49 F. 3d 586, 591 (1995). The Ninth Circuit reheard the case en banc, reversed the panel's decision, and affirmed the District Court. *Compassion in Dying* v. *Washington*, 79 F. 3d 790, 798 (1996). Like the District Court, the en banc Court of Appeals emphasized our *Casey* and *Cruzan* decisions. 79 F. 3d, at 813–816. The court also discussed what it described as "historical" and "current societal attitudes" toward suicide and assisted suicide, id., at 806–812, and concluded that "the Constitution encompasses a due process liberty interest in controlling the time and manner of one's death—that there is, in short, a constitutionally-recognized 'right to die.'" *Id.,* at 816. After "[w]eighing and then balancing" this interest against Washington's various interests, the court held that the State's assisted-suicide ban was unconstitutional "as applied to terminally ill competent adults who wish to hasten their deaths with medication prescribed by their physicians." *Id.,* at 836, 837.[6] The court did not reach the

District Court's equal protection holding. *Id.,* at 838.[7] We granted certiorari, 518 U.S. 1057 (1996), and now reverse.

I

We begin, as we do in all due process cases, by examining our Nation's history, legal traditions, and practices. See, *e.g., Casey, supra,* at 849–850; *Cruzan, supra,* at 269–279; *Moore* v. *East Cleveland*, 431 U.S. 494, 503 (1977) (plurality opinion) (noting importance of "careful 'respect for the teachings of history'"). In almost every State—indeed, in almost every western democracy—it is a crime to assist a suicide.[8] The States' assisted-suicide bans are not innovations. Rather, they are longstanding expressions of the States' commitment to the protection and preservation of all human life. *Cruzan, supra,* at 280 ("[T]he States—indeed, all civilized nations—demonstrate their commitment to life by treating homicide as a serious crime. Moreover, the majority of States in this country have laws imposing criminal penalties on one who assists another to commit suicide"); see *Stanford* v. *Kentucky*, 492 U.S. 361, 373 (1989) ("[T]he primary and most reliable indication of [a national] consensus is . . . the pattern of enacted laws"). Indeed, opposition to and condemnation of suicide—and, therefore,

---

[4]John Doe, Jane Roe, and James Poe, plaintiffs in the District Court, were then in the terminal phases of serious and painful illnesses. They declared that they were mentally competent and desired assistance in ending their lives. Declaration of Jane Roe, *id.,* at 23–25; Declaration of John Doe, *id.,* at 27–28; Declaration of James Poe, *id.,* at 30–31; *Compassion in Dying*, 850 F. Supp., at 1456–1457.

[5]The District Court determined that *Casey's* "undue burden" standard, 505 U.S., at 874 (joint opinion), not the standard from *United States* v. *Salerno*, 481 U.S. 739, 745 (1987) (requiring a showing that "no set of circumstances exists under which the [law] would be valid"), governed the plaintiffs' facial challenge to the assisted-suicide ban. 850 F. Supp., at 1462–1464.

[6]Although, as JUSTICE STEVENS observes, *post,* at 739 (opinion concurring in judgments), "[the court's] analysis and eventual holding that the statute

was unconstitutional was not limited to a particular set of plaintiffs before it," the court did note that "[d]eclaring a statute unconstitutional as applied to members of a group is atypical but not uncommon." 79 F. 3d, at 798, n. 9, and emphasized that it was "not deciding the facial validity of [the Washington statute]," *id.,* at 797–798, and nn. 8–9. It is therefore the court's holding that Washington's physician-assisted suicide statute is unconstitutional as applied to the "class of terminally ill, mentally competent patients," *post,* at 750 (STEVENS, J., concurring in judgments), that is before us today.

[7]The Court of Appeals did note, however, that "the equal protection argument relied on by [the District Court] is not insubstantial," 79 F. 3d, at 838, n. 139, and sharply criticized the opinion in a separate case then pending before the Ninth Circuit, *Lee* v. *Oregon*, 891 F. Supp. 1429 (Ore. 1995) (Oregon's Death With Dignity Act, which permits physician-assisted suicide, violates the Equal Protection Clause because it does not provide adequate safeguards against abuse), vacated, *Lee* v. *Oregon*, 107 F. 3d 1382 (CA9 1997) (concluding that plaintiffs lacked Article III standing). *Lee*, of course, is not before us, any more than it was before the Court of Appeals below, and we offer no opinion as to the validity of the *Lee* courts' reasoning. In *Vacco* v. *Quill, post*, p. 793, however, decided today, we hold that New York's assisted-suicide ban does not violate the Equal Protection Clause.

[8]See *Compassion in Dying* v. *Washington*, 79 F. 3d 790, 847, and nn. 10–13 (CA9 1996) (Beezer, J., dissenting) ("In total, forty-four states, the District of Columbia and two territories prohibit or condemn assisted suicide") (citing statutes and cases); *Rodriguez* v. *British Columbia (Attorney General)*, 107 D. L. R. (4th) 342, 404 (Can. 1993) ("[A] blanket prohibition on assisted suicide . . . is the norm among western democracies") (discussing assisted-suicide provisions in Austria, Spain, Italy, the United Kingdom, the Netherlands, Denmark, Switzerland, and France). Since the Ninth Circuit's decision, Louisiana, Rhode Island, and Iowa have enacted statutory assisted-suicide bans. La. Rev. Stat. Ann. § 14:32.12 (West Supp. 1997); R. 1. Gen. Laws §§ 11-60-1,11-60-3 (Supp. 1996); Iowa Code Ann. §§ 707 A.2, 707 A.3 (Supp. 1997). For a detailed history of the States' statutes, see Marzen, O'Dowd, Crone, & Balch, Suicide: A Constitutional Right?, 24 Duquesne L. Rev. 1, 148–242 (1985) (App.) (hereinafter Marzen).

of assisting suicide—are consistent and enduring themes of our philosophical, legal, and cultural heritages. See generally Marzen 17–56; New York State Task Force on Life and the Law, When Death is Sought: Assisted Suicide and Euthanasia in the Medical Context 77–82 (May 1994) (hereinafter New York Task Force).

More specifically, for over 700 years, the Anglo-American common-law tradition has punished or otherwise disapproved of both suicide and assisting suicide.[9] *Cruzan,* 497 U.S., at 294–295 (SCALIA, J., concurring). In the 13th century, Henry de Bracton, one of the first legal-treatise writers, observed that "[j]ust as a man may commit felony by slaying another so may he do so by slaying himself." 2 Bracton on Laws and Customs of England 423 (f. 150) (G. Woodbine ed., S. Thorne transl., 1968). The real and personal property of one who killed himself to avoid conviction and punishment for a crime were forfeit to the King; however, thought Bracton, "if a man slays himself in weariness of life or because he is unwilling to endure further bodily pain . . . [only] his movable goods [were] confiscated." *Id.,* at 423–424 (f. 150). Thus, "[t]he principle that suicide of a sane person, for whatever reason, was a punishable felony was . . . introduced into English common law."[10] Centuries later, Sir William Blackstone, whose Commentaries on the Laws of England not only provided a definitive summary of the common law but was also a primary legal authority for 18th- and 19th-century American lawyers, referred to suicide as "self-murder" and "the pretended heroism, but real cowardice, of the Stoic philosophers, who destroyed themselves to avoid those ills which they had not the fortitude to endure. . . ." 4 W. Blackstone, Commentaries *189. Blackstone emphasized that "the law has . . . ranked [suicide] among the highest crimes," ibid.,

although, anticipating later developments, he conceded that the harsh and shameful punishments imposed for suicide "borde[r] a little upon severity." *Id.,* at *190.

For the most part, the early American Colonies adopted the common-law approach. For example, the legislators of the Providence Plantations, which would later become Rhode Island, declared, in 1647, that "[s]elf-murder is by all agreed to be the most unnatural, and it is by this present Assembly declared, to be that, wherein he that doth it, kills himself out of a premeditated hatred against his own life or other humor: . . . his goods and chattels are the king's custom, but not his debts nor lands; but in case he be an infant, a lunatic, mad or distracted man, he forfeits nothing." The Earliest Acts and Laws of the Colony of Rhode Island and Providence Plantations 1647–1719, p. 19 (J. Cushing ed. 1977). Virginia also required ignominious burial for suicides, and their estates were forfeit to the Crown. A. Scott, Criminal Law in Colonial Virginia 108, and n. 93, 198, and n. 15 (1930).

Over time, however, the American Colonies abolished these harsh common-law penalties. William Penn abandoned the criminal-forfeiture sanction in Pennsylvania in 1701, and the other Colonies (and later, the other States) eventually followed this example. *Cruzan, supra,* at 294 (SCALIA, J., concurring). Zephaniah Swift, who would later become Chief Justice of Connecticut, wrote in 1796:

"There can be no act more contemptible, than to attempt to punish an offender for a crime, by exercising a mean act of revenge upon lifeless clay, that is insensible of the punishment. There can be no greater cruelty, than the inflicting [of] a punishment, as the forfeiture of goods, which must fall solely on the innocent offspring of the offender. . . . [Suicide] is so abhorrent to the feelings of mankind, and that strong love of life which is implanted in the human heart, that it cannot be so frequently committed, as to become dangerous to society. There can of course be no necessity of any punishment." 2 Z. Swift, A System of the Laws of the State of Connecticut 304 (1796).

This statement makes it clear, however, that the movement away from the common law's harsh sanctions did not represent an acceptance of suicide; rather, as Chief Justice Swift observed, this change reflected the growing consensus that it was unfair to punish the suicide's family for his wrongdoing. *Cruzan, supra,* at 294 (SCALIA, J., concurring). Nonetheless, although States moved away from Blackstone's treatment of suicide, courts continued to condemn it as a grave public wrong. See, *e.g., Bigelow* v. *Berkshire Life Ins. Co.,* 93 U.S. 284, 286 (1876) (suicide is "an act of criminal self destruction"); *Von Holden* v. *Chapman,* 87 App. Div. 2d 66, 70–71, 450 N. Y. S. 2d 623, 626–627 (1982); *Blackwood* v. *Jones,* 111 Fla. 528, 532, 149 So. 600, 601 (1933) ("No sophistry is tolerated . . . which seek[s]

---

[9]The common law is thought to have emerged through the expansion of pre-Norman institutions sometime in the 12th century. J. Baker, An Introduction to English Legal History 11 (2d ed. 1979). England adopted the ecclesiastical prohibition on suicide five centuries earlier, in the year 673 at the Council of Hereford, and this prohibition was reaffirmed by King Edgar in 967. See G. Williams, The Sanctity of Life and the Criminal Law 257 (1957).

[10]Marzen 59. Other late-medieval treatise writers followed and restated Bracton; one observed that "man-slaughter" may be "[o]f [one]self; as in case, when people hang themselves or hurt themselves, or otherwise kill themselves of their own felony" or "[o]f others; as by beating, famine, or other punishment; in like cases, all are man-slayers." A. Horne, The Mirrour of Justices, ch. 1, § 9, pp. 41–42 (w. Robinson ed. 1903). By the mid-16th century, the Court at Common Bench could observe that "[suicide] is an Offence against Nature, against God, and against the King .... [T]o destroy one's self is contrary to Nature, and a Thing most horrible." *Hales* v. *Petit,* 1 Plowd. Com. 253,261,75 Eng. Rep. 387, 400 (1561–1562). In 1644, Sir Edward Coke published his Third Institute, a lodestar for later common lawyers. See T. Plucknett, A Concise History of the Common Law 281–284 (5th ed. 1956). Coke regarded suicide as a category of murder, and agreed with Bracton that the goods and chattels—but not, for Coke, the lands—of a sane suicide were forfeit. 3 E. Coke, Institutes *54. William Hawkins, in his 1716 Treatise of the Pleas of the Crown, followed Coke, observing that "our laws have always had ... an abhorrence of this crime." 1 W. Hawkins, Pleas of the Crown, ch. 27, §4, p. 164 (T. Leach ed. 1795).

to justify self-destruction as commendable or even a matter of personal right").

That suicide remained a grievous, though nonfelonious, wrong is confirmed by the fact that colonial and early state legislatures and courts did not retreat from prohibiting assisting suicide. Swift, in his early 19th-century treatise on the laws of Connecticut, stated that "[i]f one counsels another to commit suicide, and the other by reason of the advice kills himself, the advisor is guilty of murder as principal." 2 Z. Swift, A Digest of the Laws of the State of Connecticut 270 (1823). This was the well-established common-law view, see *In re Joseph G.,* 34 Cal. 3d 429, 434–435, 667 P. 2d 1176, 1179 *(1983); Commonwealth* v. *Mink,* 123 Mass. 422, 428 (1877) ("Now if the murder of one's self is felony, the accessory is equally guilty as if he had aided and abetted in the murder") (quoting Chief Justice Parker's charge to the jury in *Commonwealth* v. *Bowen,* 13 Mass. 356 (1816)), as was the similar principle that the consent of a homicide victim is "wholly immaterial to the guilt of the person who cause[d] [his death]," 3 J. Stephen, A History of the Criminal Law of England 16 (1883); see 1 F. Wharton, Criminal Law §§ 451–452 (9th ed. 1885); *Martin* v. *Commonwealth,* 184 Va. 1009, 10181019, 37 S. E. 2d 43, 47 (1946) ("The right to life and to personal security is not only sacred in the estimation of the common law, but it is inalienable"). And the prohibitions against assisting suicide never contained exceptions for those who were near death. Rather, "[t]he life of those to whom life ha[d] become a burden—of those who [were] hopelessly diseased or fatally wounded—nay, even the lives of criminals condemned to death, [were] under the protection of the law, equally as the lives of those who [were] in the full tide of life's enjoyment, and anxious to continue to live." *Blackburn* v. *State,* 23 Ohio St. 146, 163 (1872); see *Bowen, supra,* at 360 (prisoner who persuaded another to commit suicide could be tried for murder, even though victim was scheduled shortly to be executed).

The earliest American statute explicitly to outlaw assisting suicide was enacted in New York in 1828, Act of Dec. 10, 1828, ch. 20, § 4, 1828 N. Y. Laws 19 (codified at 2 N. Y. Rev. Stat. pt. 4, ch. 1, Tit. 2, Art. 1, § 7, p. 661 (1829)), and many of the new States and Territories followed New York's example. Marzen 73–74. Between 1857 and 1865, a New York commission led by Dudley Field drafted a criminal code that prohibited "aiding" a suicide and, specifically, "furnish[ing] another person with any deadly weapon or poisonous drug, knowing that such person intends to use such weapon or drug in taking his own life." *Id.,* at 76–77. By the time the Fourteenth Amendment was ratified, it was a crime in most States to assist a suicide. See *Cruzan,* 497 U.S., at 294–295 (SCALIA, J., concurring). The Field Penal Code was adopted in the Dakota Territory in 1877

and in New York in 1881, and its language served as a model for several other western States' statutes in the late 19th and early 20th centuries. Marzen 76–77, 205–206, 212–213. California, for example, codified its assisted-suicide prohibition in 1874, using language similar to the Field Code's.[11] In this century, the Model Penal Code also prohibited "aiding" suicide, prompting many States to enact or revise their assisted-suicide bans.[12] The code's drafters observed that "the interests in the sanctity of life that are represented by the criminal homicide laws are threatened by one who expresses a willingness to participate in taking the life of another, even though the act may be accomplished with the consent, or at the request, of the suicide victim." American Law Institute, Model Penal Code § 210.5, Comment 5, p. 100 (Official Draft and Revised Comments 1980).

Though deeply rooted, the States' assisted-suicide bans have in recent years been reexamined and, generally, reaffirmed. Because of advances in medicine and technology, Americans today are increasingly likely to die in institutions, from chronic illnesses. President's Comm'n for the Study of Ethical Problems in Medicine and Biomedical and Behavioral Research, Deciding to Forego Life-Sustaining Treatment 16–18 (1983). Public concern and democratic action are therefore sharply focused on how best to protect dignity and independence at the end of life, with the result that there have been many significant changes in state laws and in the attitudes these laws reflect. Many States, for example, now permit "living wills," surrogate health-care decision making, and the withdrawal or refusal of life-sustaining medical treatment. See *Vacco* v. *Quill, post,* at 804–806; 79 F. 3d, at *818–820; People* v. *Kevorkian,* 447 Mich. 436, 478–480, and nn. 53–56, 527 N. W. 2d 714, 731–732, and nn. 53–56 (1994). At the same time, however, voters and legislators continue for the most part to reaffirm their States' prohibitions on assisting suicide.

The Washington statute at issue in this case, Wash. Rev. Code § 9A.36.060 (1994), was enacted in 1975 as part of a revision of that State's criminal code. Four years later, Washington passed its Natural Death Act, which specifically stated that the "withholding or withdrawal of life-sustaining

---

[11]In 1850, the California Legislature adopted the English common law, under which assisting suicide was, of course, a crime. Act of Apr. 13, 1850, ch. 95, 1850 Cal. Stats. 219. The provision adopted in 1874 provided that "[e]very person who deliberately aids or advises, or encourages another to commit suicide, is guilty of a felony." Act of Mar. 30, 1874, ch. 614, § 13,400 (codified at Cal. Penal Code § 400 (T. Hittel ed. 1876)).

[12]"A person who purposely aids or solicits another to commit suicide is guilty of a felony in the second degree if his conduct causes such suicide or an attempted suicide, and otherwise of a misdemeanor." American Law Institute, Model Penal Code § 210.5(2) (Official Draft and Revised Comments 1980).

treatment . . . shall not, for any purpose, constitute a suicide" and that "[n]othing in this chapter shall be construed to condone, authorize, or approve mercy killing. . . ." Natural Death Act, 1979 Wash. Laws, ch. 112, § 8(1), p. 11 (codified at Wash. Rev. Code §§ 70.122.070(1), 70.122.100 (1994)). In 1991, Washington voters rejected a ballot initiative which, had it passed, would have permitted a form of physician-assisted suicide.[13] Washington then added a provision to the Natural Death Act expressly excluding physician-assisted suicide. 1992 Wash. Laws, ch. 98, § 10; Wash. Rev. Code § 70.122.100 (1994).

California voters rejected an assisted-suicide initiative similar to Washington's in 1993. On the other hand, in 1994, voters in Oregon enacted, also through ballot initiative, that State's "Death With Dignity Act," which legalized physician-assisted suicide for competent, terminally ill adults.[14] Since the Oregon vote, many proposals to legalize assisted-suicide have been and continue to be introduced in the States' legislatures, but none has been enacted.[15] And just last year, Iowa and Rhode Island joined the overwhelming majority of States explicitly prohibiting assisted suicide. See Iowa Code Ann. §§ 707 A.2, 707 A.3 (Supp. 1997); R. I. Gen. Laws §§ 11-60-1, 11-60-3 (Supp. 1996). Also, on April 30, 1997, President Clinton signed the Federal Assisted Suicide Funding Restriction Act of 1997, which prohibits the use of federal funds in support of physician-assisted suicide. Pub. L. 105–12, 111 Stat. 23 (codified at 42 U.S.C. § 14401 et seq.).[16]

Thus, the States are currently engaged in serious, thoughtful examinations of physician-assisted suicide and other similar issues. For example, New York State's Task Force on Life and the Law—an ongoing, blue-ribbon commission composed of doctors, ethicists, lawyers, religious leaders, and interested laymen—was convened in 1984 and commissioned with "a broad mandate to recommend public policy on issues raised by medical advances." New York Task Force vii. Over the past decade, the Task Force has recommended laws relating to end-of-life decisions, surrogate pregnancy, and organ donation. *Id.,* at 118–119. After studying physician-assisted suicide, however, the Task Force unanimously concluded that "[l]egalizing assisted suicide and euthanasia would pose profound risks to many individuals who are ill and vulnerable. . . . [T]he potential dangers of this dramatic change in public policy would outweigh any benefit that might be achieved." *Id.,* at 120.

Attitudes toward suicide itself have changed since Bracton, but our laws have consistently condemned, and continue to prohibit, assisting suicide. Despite changes in medical technology and notwithstanding an increased emphasis on the importance of end-of-life decision making, we have not retreated from this prohibition. Against this backdrop of history, tradition, and practice, we now turn to respondents' constitutional claim.

II

The Due Process Clause guarantees more than fair process, and the "liberty" it protects includes more than the absence of physical restraint. *Collins* v. *Harker Heights, 503* U.S. 115, 125 (1992) (Due Process Clause "protects individual liberty against 'certain government actions regardless of the fairness of the procedures used to implement them'") (quoting *Daniels* v. *Williams,* 474 U.S. 327, 331 (1986)). The Clause also provides heightened protection against government interference with

---

[13]Initiative 119 would have amended Washington's Natural Death Act, Wash. Rev. Code § 70.122.010 *et seq.* (1994), to permit "aid-in-dying," defined as "aid in the form of a medical service provided in person by a physician that will end the life of a conscious and mentally competent qualified patient in a dignified, painless and humane manner, when requested voluntarily by the patient through a written directive in accordance with this chapter at the time the medical service is to be provided." App. H to Pet. for Cert. 3–4.

[14]Ore. Rev. Stat. § 127.800 *et seq.* (1996); *Lee* v. *Oregon,* 891 F. Supp. 1429 (Ore. 1995) (Oregon Act does not provide sufficient safeguards for terminally ill persons and therefore violates the Equal Protection Clause), vacated, *Lee* v. *Oregon,* 107 F. 3d 1382 *(CA9 1997).*

[15]See, *e.g.,* Alaska H. B. 371 (1996); Ariz. S. B. 1007 (1996); Cal. A. B. 1080, A. B. 1310 (1995); Colo. H. B. 1185 (1996); Colo. H. B. 1308 (1995); Conn. H. B. 6298 (1995); Ill. H. B. 691, S. B. 948 (1997); Me. H. P. 663 (1997); Me. H. P. 552 (1995); Md. H. B. 474 (1996); Md. H. B. 933 (1995); Mass. H. B. 3173 (1995); Mich. H. B. 6205, S. B. 556 (1996); Mich. H. B. 4134 (1995); Miss. H. B. 1023 (1996); N. H. H. B. 339 (1995); N. M. S. B. 446 (1995); N. Y. S. B. 5024, A. B. 6333 (1995); Neb. L. B. 406 (1997); Neb. L. B. 1259 (1996); R. 1. S. 2985 (1996); Vt. H. B. 109 (1997); Vt. H. B. 335 (1995); Wash. S. B. 5596 (1995); Wis. A. B. 174, S. B. 90 (1995); Senate of Canada, Of Life and Death, Report of the Special Senate Committee on Euthanasia and Assisted Suicide A—156 (June 1995) (describing unsuccessful proposals, between 1991–1994, to legalize assisted suicide).

[16]Other countries are embroiled in similar debates: The Supreme Court of Canada recently rejected a claim that the Canadian Charter of Rights and Freedoms establishes a fundamental right to assisted suicide, *Rodriguez* v. *British Columbia (Attorney General),* 107 D. L. R. (4th) 342 (1993); the British House of Lords Select Committee on Medical Ethics refused to recommend

any change in Great Britain's assisted-suicide prohibition, House of Lords, Session 1993–94 Report of the Select Committee on Medical Ethics, 12 Issues in Law & Med. 193, 202 (1996) ("We identify no circumstances in which assisted suicide should be permitted"); New Zealand's Parliament rejected a proposed "Death With Dignity Bill" that would have legalized physician-assisted suicide in August 1995, Graeme, MPs Throw out Euthanasia Bill, The Dominion (Wellington), Aug. 17, 1995, p. 1; and the Northern Territory of Australia legalized assisted suicide and voluntary euthanasia in 1995, see Shenon, Australian Doctors Get Right to Assist Suicide, N. Y. Times, July 28, 1995, p. A8. As of February 1997, three persons had ended their lives with physician assistance in the Northern Territory. Mydans, Assisted Suicide: Australia Faces a Grim Reality, N. Y. Times, Feb. 2, 1997, p. A3. On March 24,1997, however, the Australian Senate voted to overturn the Northern Territory's law. Thornhill, Australia Repeals Euthanasia Law, Washington Post, Mar. 25, 1997, p. A14; see Euthanasia Laws Act 1997, No. 17, 1997 (Austl.). On the other hand, on May 20, 1997, Colombia's Constitutional Court legalized voluntary euthanasia for terminally ill people. C-239/97 de Mayo 20, 1997, Corte Constitucional, M. P. Carlos Gaviria Diaz; see Colombia's Top Court Legalizes Euthanasia, Orlando Sentinel, May 22, 1997, p. A1S.

certain fundamental rights and liberty interests. *Reno v. Flores*, 507 U.S. 292, 301–302 (1993); *Casey*, 505 U.S., at 851. In a long line of cases, we have held that, in addition to the specific freedoms protected by the Bill of Rights, the "liberty" specially protected by the Due Process Clause includes the rights to marry, *Loving v. Virginia*, 388 U.S. 1 (1967); to have children, *Skinner v. Oklahoma ex rel. Williamson*, 316 U.S. 535 (1942); to direct the education and upbringing of one's children, *Meyer v. Nebraska*, 262 U.S. 390 (1923); *Pierce v. Society of Sisters*, 268 U.S. 510 (1925); to marital privacy, *Griswold v. Connecticut*, 381 U.S. 479 (1965); to use contraception, *ibid.*; *Eisenstadt v. Baird*, 405 U.S. 438 (1972); to bodily integrity, *Rochin v. California*, 342 U.S. 165 (1952), and to abortion, *Casey, supra.* We have also assumed, and strongly suggested, that the Due Process Clause protects the traditional right to refuse unwanted lifesaving medical treatment. *Cruzan*, 497 U.S., at 278–279.

But we "ha[ve] always been reluctant to expand the concept of substantive due process because guideposts for responsible decision making in this unchartered area are scarce and open-ended." *Collins*, 503 U.S., at 125. By extending constitutional protection to an asserted right or liberty interest, we, to a great extent, place the matter outside the arena of public debate and legislative action. We must therefore "exercise the utmost care whenever we are asked to break new ground in this field," *ibid.*, lest the liberty protected by the Due Process Clause be subtly transformed into the policy preferences of the Members of this Court, *Moore*, 431 U.S., at 502 (plurality opinion).

Our established method of substantive-due-process analysis has two primary features: First, we have regularly observed that the Due Process Clause specially protects those fundamental rights and liberties which are, objectively, "deeply rooted in this Nation's history and tradition," *id.*, at 503 (plurality opinion); *Snyder v. Massachusetts*, 291 U.S. 97, 105 (1934) ("so rooted in the traditions and conscience of our people as to be ranked as fundamental"), and "implicit in the concept of ordered liberty," such that "neither liberty nor justice would exist if they were sacrificed," *Palko v. Connecticut*, 302 U.S. 319, 325, 326 (1937). Second, we have required in substantive-due-process cases a "careful description" of the asserted fundamental liberty interest. *Flores, supra*, at 302; *Collins, supra*, at 125; *Cruzan, supra*, at 277278. Our Nation's history, legal traditions, and practices thus provide the crucial "guideposts for responsible decision making," *Collins, supra*, at 125, that direct and restrain our exposition of the Due Process Clause. As we stated recently in *Flores*, the Fourteenth Amendment "forbids the government to infringe . . . 'fundamental' liberty interests at *all*, no matter what process is provided, unless the infringement is narrowly tailored to serve a compelling state interest." 507 U.S., at 302.

JUSTICE SOUTER, relying on Justice Harlan's dissenting opinion in *Poe v. Ullman*, 367 U.S. 497 (1961), would largely abandon this restrained methodology, and instead ask "whether [Washington's] statute sets up one of those 'arbitrary impositions' or 'purposeless restraints' at odds with the Due Process Clause of the Fourteenth Amendment," *post*, at 752 (quoting *Poe, supra*, at 543 (Harlan, J., dissenting)).[17]

In our view, however, the development of this Court's substantive-due-process jurisprudence, described briefly *supra*, at 719–720, has been a process whereby the outlines of the "liberty" specially protected by the Fourteenth Amendment—never fully clarified, to be sure, and perhaps not capable of being fully clarified—have at least been carefully refined by concrete examples involving fundamental rights found to be deeply rooted in our legal tradition. This approach tends to rein in the subjective elements that are necessarily present in due process judicial review. In addition, by establishing a threshold requirement—that a challenged state action implicate a fundamental right—before requiring more than a reasonable relation to a legitimate state interest to justify the action, it avoids the need for complex balancing of competing interests in every case.

Turning to the claim at issue here, the Court of Appeals stated that "[p]roperly analyzed, the first issue to be resolved is whether there is a liberty interest in determining the time and manner of one's death," 79 F. 3d, at 801, or, in other words, "[i]s there a right to die?," *id.*, at 799. Similarly, respondents assert a "liberty to choose how to die" and a right to "control of one's final days," Brief for Respondents 7, and describe the asserted liberty as "the right to choose a humane, dignified death," *id.*, at 15, and "the liberty to shape death," *id.*, at 18. As noted above, we have a tradition of carefully formulating the interest at stake in substantive due-process cases. For example, although *Cruzan* is often described as a "right to die" case, see 79 F. 3d, at 799; *post*, at 745 (STEVENS, J., concurring in judgments) (*Cruzan* recognized "the more specific interest in making decisions about how to confront an imminent death"), we

---

[17]In JUSTICE SOUTER'S opinion, Justice Harlan's *Poe* dissent supplies the "modern justification" for substantive-due-process review. *Post*, at 756, and n. 4 (opinion concurring in judgment). But although Justice Harlan's opinion has often been cited in due process cases, we have never abandoned our fundamental-rights-based analytical method. Just four Terms ago, six of the Justices now sitting joined the Court's opinion in *Reno v. Flores*, 507 U.S. 292, 301–305 (1993); *Poe* was not even cited. And in *Cruzan v. Director, Mo. Dept. of Health*, 497 U.S. 261 (1990), neither the Court's nor the concurring opinions relied on *Poe*; rather, we concluded that the right to refuse unwanted medical treatment was so rooted in our history, tradition, and practice as to require special protection under the Fourteenth Amendment. *Cruzan*, 497 U.S., at 278–279; *id.*, at 287–288 (O'CONNOR, J., concurring). True, the Court relied on Justice Harlan's dissent in *Casey*, 505 U.S., at 848–850, but, as *Flores* demonstrates, we did not in so doing jettison our established approach. Indeed, to read such a radical move into the Court's opinion in *Casey* would seem to fly in the face of that opinion's emphasis on *stare decisis*. 505 U.S., at 854–869.

were, in fact, more precise: We assumed that the Constitution granted competent persons a "constitutionally protected right to refuse lifesaving hydration and nutrition." *Cruzan,* 497 U.S., at 279; *id.,* at 287 (O'CONNOR, J., concurring) ("[A] liberty interest in refusing unwanted medical treatment may be inferred from our prior decisions"). The Washington statute at issue in this case prohibits "aid[ing] another person to attempt suicide," Wash. Rev. Code § 9A.36.060(1) (1994), and, thus, the question before us is whether the "liberty" specially protected by the Due Process Clause includes a right to commit suicide which itself includes a right to assistance in doing So.[18]

We now inquire whether this asserted right has any place in our Nation's traditions. Here, as discussed *supra,* at 710719, we are confronted with a consistent and almost universal tradition that has long rejected the asserted right, and continues explicitly to reject it today, even for terminally ill, mentally competent adults. To hold for respondents, we would have to reverse centuries of legal doctrine and practice, and strike down the considered policy choice of almost every State. See *Jackman v. Rosenbaum Co.,* 260 U.S. 22, 31 (1922) ("If a thing has been practised for two hundred years by common consent, it will need a strong case for the Fourteenth Amendment to affect it"); *Flores,* 507 U.S., at 303 ("The mere novelty of such a claim is reason enough to doubt that 'substantive due process' sustains it").

Respondents contend, however, that the liberty interest they assert *is* consistent with this Court's substantive-due-process line of cases, if not with this Nation's history and practice. Pointing to *Casey* and *Cruzan,* respondents read our jurisprudence in this area as reflecting a general tradition of "self-sovereignty," Brief for Respondents 12, and as teaching that the "liberty" protected by the Due Process Clause includes "basic and intimate exercises of personal autonomy," *id.,* at 10; see *Casey,* 505 U.S., at 847 ("It is a promise of the Constitution that there is a realm of personal liberty which the government may not enter"). According to respondents, our liberty jurisprudence, and the broad, individualistic principles it reflects, protects the "liberty of competent, terminally ill adults to make end-of-life decisions free of undue government interference." Brief for Respondents 10. The question presented in this case, however, is whether the protections of the Due Process Clause include a right to commit suicide with another's assistance. With this "careful description" of respondents' claim in mind, we turn to *Casey* and *Cruzan.*

In *Cruzan,* we considered whether Nancy Beth Cruzan, who had been severely injured in an automobile accident and was in a persistive vegetative state, "ha[d] a right under the United States Constitution which would require the hospital to withdraw life-sustaining treatment" at her parents' request. 497 U.S., at 269. We began with the observation that "[a]t common law, even the touching of one person by another without consent and without legal justification was a battery." *Ibid.* We then discussed the related rule that "informed consent is generally required for medical treatment." *Ibid.* After reviewing a long line of relevant state cases, we concluded that "the common-law doctrine of informed consent is viewed as generally encompassing the right of a competent individual to refuse medical treatment." *Id.,* at 277. Next, we reviewed our own cases on the subject, and stated that "[t]he principle that a competent person has a constitutionally protected liberty interest in refusing unwanted medical treatment may be inferred from our prior decisions." *Id.,* at 278. Therefore, "for purposes of [that] case, we assume[d] that the United States Constitution would grant a competent person a constitutionally protected right to refuse lifesaving hydration and nutrition." *Id.,* at 279; see *id.,* at 287 (O'CONNOR, J., concurring). We concluded that, notwithstanding this right, the Constitution permitted Missouri to require clear and convincing evidence of an incompetent patient's wishes concerning the withdrawal of life-sustaining treatment. *Id.,* at 280–281.

Respondents contend that in *Cruzan* we "acknowledged that competent, dying persons have the right to direct the removal of life-sustaining medical treatment and thus hasten death," Brief for Respondents 23, and that "the constitutional principle behind recognizing the patient's liberty to direct the withdrawal of artificial life support applies at least as strongly to the choice to hasten impending death by consuming lethal medication," *id.,* at 26. Similarly, the Court of Appeals concluded that "*Cruzan,* by recognizing a liberty interest that includes the refusal of artificial provision of life-sustaining food and water, necessarily recognize[d] a liberty interest in hastening one's own death." 79 F. 3d, at 816.

The right assumed in *Cruzan,* however, was not simply deduced from abstract concepts of personal autonomy. Given the common-law rule that forced medication was a battery, and the long legal tradition protecting the decision to refuse unwanted medical treatment, our assumption was entirely consistent with this Nation's history and constitutional traditions. The decision to commit suicide with the assistance of another may be just as personal and profound as the decision to refuse

---

[18]See, *e.g., Quill* v. *Vacco,* 80 F. 3d 716, 724 *(CA2* 1996) ("right to assisted suicide finds no cognizable basis in the Constitution's language or design"); *Compassion in Dying* v. *Washington,* 49 F. 3d 586, 591 *(CA9* 1995) (referring to alleged "right to suicide," "right to assistance in suicide," and "right to aid in killing oneself"); *People* v. *Kevorkian,* 447 Mich. 436,476, n. 47, 527 N. W. 2d 714, 730, n. 47 (1994) ("[T]he question that we must decide is whether the [C]onstitution encompasses a right to commit suicide and, if so, whether it includes a right to assistance").

unwanted medical treatment, but it has never enjoyed similar legal protection. Indeed, the two acts are widely and reasonably regarded as quite distinct. See *Quill* v. *Vacco, post,* at 800–808. In *Cruzan* itself, we recognized that most States outlawed assisted suicide—and even more do today—and we certainly gave no intimation that the right to refuse unwanted medical treatment could be somehow transmuted into a right to assistance in committing suicide. 497 U.S., at 280.

Respondents also rely on *Casey.* There, the Court's opinion concluded that "the essential holding of *Roe* v. *Wade* [410 U.S. 113 (1973)] should be retained and once again reaffirmed." 505 U.S., at 846. We held, first, that a woman has a right, before her fetus is viable, to an abortion "without undue interference from the State"; second, that States may restrict postviability abortions, so long as exceptions are made to protect a woman's life and health; and third, that the State has legitimate interests throughout a pregnancy in protecting the health of the woman and the life of the unborn child. *Ibid.* In reaching this conclusion, the opinion discussed in some detail this Court's substantive-due-process tradition of interpreting the Due Process Clause to protect certain fundamental rights and "personal decisions relating to marriage, procreation, contraception, family relationships, child rearing, and education," and noted that many of those rights and liberties "involv[e] the most intimate and personal choices a person may make in a lifetime." *Id.,* at 851.

The Court of Appeals, like the District Court, found *Casey* "highly instructive" and "almost prescriptive" for determining "what liberty interest may inhere in a terminally ill person's choice to commit suicide":

"Like the decision of whether or not to have an abortion, the decision how and when to die is one of 'the most intimate and personal choices a person may make in a lifetime,' a choice 'central to personal dignity and autonomy.'" 79 F. 3d, at 813–814.

Similarly, respondents emphasize the statement in *Casey* that:

"At the heart of liberty is the right to define one's own concept of existence, of meaning, of the universe, and of the mystery of human life. Beliefs about these matters could not define the attributes of personhood were they formed under compulsion of the State." 505 U.S., at 851.

Brief for Respondents 12. By choosing this language, the Court's opinion in *Casey* described, in a general way and in light of our prior cases, those personal activities and decisions that this Court has identified as so deeply rooted in our history and traditions, or so fundamental to our concept of constitutionally ordered liberty, that they are protected by the Fourteenth Amendment.[19] The opinion moved from the recognition that liberty necessarily includes freedom of conscience and belief about ultimate considerations to the observation that "though the abortion decision may originate within the zone of conscience and belief, it is *more than a philosophic exercise.*" *Casey,* 505 U.S., at 852 (emphasis added). That many of the rights and liberties protected by the Due Process Clause sound in personal autonomy does not warrant the sweeping conclusion that any and all important, intimate, and personal decisions are so protected, *San Antonio Independent School Dist.* v. *Rodriguez,* 411 U.S. 1, 33–35 (1973), and *Casey* did not suggest otherwise.

The history of the law's treatment of assisted suicide in this country has been and continues to be one of the rejection of nearly all efforts to permit it. That being the case, our decisions lead us to conclude that the asserted "right" to assistance in committing suicide is not a fundamental liberty interest protected by the Due Process Clause. The Constitution also requires, however, that Washington's assisted suicide ban be rationally related to legitimate government interests. See *Heller* v. *Doe,* 509 U.S. 312, 319–320 (1993); *Flores,* 507 U.S., at 305. This requirement is unquestionably met here. As the court below recognized, 79 F. 3d, at 816–817,[20] Washington's assisted-suicide ban implicates a number of state interests.[21] See 49 F. 3d, at 592–593; Brief for State of California et al. as *Amici Curiae* 26–29; Brief for United States as *Amicus Curiae* 16–27.

First, Washington has an "unqualified interest in the preservation of human life." *Cruzan,* 497 U.S., at 282. The

---

[19]See *Moore* v. *East Cleveland,* 431 U.S. 494, 503 (1977) ("[T]he Constitution protects the sanctity of the family *precisely because* the institution of the family is deeply rooted in this Nation's history and tradition" (emphasis added)); *Griswold* v. *Connecticut,* 381 U.S. 479, 485–486 (1965) (intrusions into the "sacred precincts of marital bedrooms" offend rights "older than the Bill of Rights"); id., at 495–496 (Goldberg, J., concurring) (the law in question "disrupt[ed] the traditional relation of the family—a relation as old and as fundamental as our entire civilization"); *Loving* v. *Virginia,* 388 U.S. 1, 12 (1967) ("The freedom to marry has long been recognized as one of the vital personal rights essential to the orderly pursuit of happiness"); *Turner* v. *Safley,* 482 U.S. 78, 95 (1987) ("[T]he decision to marry is a fundamental right"); *Roe* v. *Wade,* 410 U.S. 113, 140 (1973) (stating that at the founding and throughout the 19th century, "a woman enjoyed a substantially broader right to terminate a pregnancy"); *Skinner* v. *Oklahoma ex rel. Williamson,* 316 U.S. 535, 541 (1942) ("Marriage and procreation are fundamental"); *Pierce* v. *Society of Sisters,* 268 U.S. 510, 535 (1925); *Meyer* v. *Nebraska,* 262 U.S. 390, 399 (1923) (liberty includes "those privileges long recognized at common law as essential to the orderly pursuit of happiness by free men").

[20]The court identified and discussed six state interests: (1) preserving life; (2) preventing suicide; (3) avoiding the involvement of third parties and use of arbitrary, unfair, or undue influence; (4) protecting family members and loved ones; (5) protecting the integrity of the medical profession; and (6) avoiding future movement toward euthanasia and other abuses. 79 F. 3d, at 816–832.

[21]Respondents also admit the existence of these interests, Brief for Respondents 28–39, but contend that Washington could better promote and protect them through regulation, rather than prohibition, of physician assisted suicide. Our inquiry, however, is limited to the question whether the State's prohibition is rationally related to legitimate state interests.

State's prohibition on assisted suicide, like all homicide laws, both reflects and advances its commitment to this interest. See *id.*, at 280; Model Penal Code § 210.5, Comment 5, at 100 ("[T]he interests in the sanctity of life that are represented by the criminal homicide laws are threatened by one who expresses a willingness to participate in taking the life of another").[22] This interest is symbolic and aspirational as well as practical:

"While suicide is no longer prohibited or penalized, the ban against assisted suicide and euthanasia shores up the notion of limits in human relationships. It reflects the gravity with which we view the decision to take one's own life or the life of another, and our reluctance to encourage or promote these decisions." New York Task Force 131–132.

Respondents admit that "[t]he State has a real interest in preserving the lives of those who can still contribute to society and have the potential to enjoy life." Brief for Respondents 35, n. 23. The Court of Appeals also recognized Washington's interest in protecting life, but held that the "weight" of this interest depends on the "medical condition and the wishes of the person whose life is at stake." 79 F. 3d, at 817. Washington, however, has rejected this sliding-scale approach and, through its assisted-suicide ban, insists that all persons' lives, from beginning to end, regardless of physical or mental condition, are under the full protection of the law. See *United States* v. *Rutherford*, 442 U.S. 544, 558 (1979) (". . . Congress could reasonably have determined to protect the terminally ill, no less than other patients, from the vast range of self-styled panaceas that inventive minds can devise"). As we have previously affirmed, the States "may properly decline to make judgments about the 'quality' of life that a particular individual may enjoy," *Cruzan, supra*, at 282. This remains true, as *Cruzan* makes clear, even for those who are near death.

Relatedly, all admit that suicide is a serious public-health problem, especially among persons in otherwise vulnerable groups. See Washington State Dept. of Health, Annual Summary of Vital Statistics 1991, pp. 29–30 (Oct. 1992) (suicide is a leading cause of death in Washington of those between the ages of 14 and 54); New York Task Force 10,23–33 (suicide rate in the general population is about one percent, and suicide is especially prevalent among the young and the

elderly). The State has an interest in preventing suicide, and in studying, identifying, and treating its causes. See 79 F. 3d, at 820; *id.*, at 854 (Beezer, J., dissenting) ("The state recognizes suicide as a manifestation of medical and psychological anguish"); Marzen 107–146.

Those who attempt suicide—terminally ill or not—often suffer from depression or other mental disorders. See New York Task Force 13–22, 126–128 (more than 95% of those who commit suicide had a major psychiatric illness at the time of death; among the terminally ill, uncontrolled pain is a "risk factor" because it contributes to depression); Physician Assisted Suicide and Euthanasia in the Netherlands: A Report of Chairman Charles T. Canady to the Subcommittee on the Constitution of the House Committee on the Judiciary, 104th Cong., 2d Sess., 10–11 (Comm. Print 1996); cf. Back, Wallace, Starks, & Pearlman, Physician-Assisted Suicide and Euthanasia in Washington State, 275 JAMA 919, 924 (1996) ("[I]ntolerable physical symptoms are not the reason most patients request physician-assisted suicide or euthanasia"). Research indicates, however, that many people who request physician-assisted suicide withdraw that request if their depression and pain are treated. H. Hendin, Seduced by Death: Doctors, Patients and the Dutch Cure 24–25 (1997) (suicidal, terminally ill patients "usually respond well to treatment for depressive illness and pain medication and are then grateful to be alive"); New York Task Force 177–178.

The New York Task Force, however, expressed its concern that, because depression is difficult to diagnose, physicians and medical professionals often fail to respond adequately to seriously ill patients' needs. *Id.*, at 175. Thus, legal physician-assisted suicide could make it more difficult for the State to protect depressed or mentally ill persons, or those who are suffering from untreated pain, from suicidal impulses.

The State also has an interest in protecting the integrity and ethics of the medical profession. In contrast to the Court of Appeals' conclusion that "the integrity of the medical profession would [not] be threatened in any way by [physician-assisted suicide]," 79 F. 3d, at 827, the American Medical Association, like many other medical and physicians' groups, has concluded that "[p]hysician-assisted suicide is fundamentally incompatible with the physician's role as healer." American Medical Association, Code of Ethics § 2.211 (1994); see Council on Ethical and Judicial Affairs, Decisions Near the End of Life, 267 JAMA 2229,2233 (1992) ("[T]he societal risks of involving physicians in medical interventions to cause patients' deaths is too great"); New York Task Force 103–109 (discussing physicians' views). And physician-assisted suicide could, it is argued, undermine the trust that is essential to the doctor-patient relationship by blurring the time-honored line

---

[22]The States express this commitment by other means as well: "[N]early all states expressly disapprove of suicide and assisted suicide either in statutes dealing with durable powers of attorney in health-care situations, or in 'living will' statutes. In addition, all states provide for the involuntary commitment of persons who may harm themselves as the result of mental illness, and a number of states allow the use of nondeadly force to thwart suicide attempts." *People* v. *Kevorkian,* 447 Mich., at 478–479, and nn. 53–56, 527 N. W. 2d, at 731–732, and nn. 53–56.

between healing and harming. Assisted Suicide in the United States, Hearing before the Subcommittee on the Constitution of the House Committee on the Judiciary, 104th Cong., 2d Sess., 355–356 (1996) (testimony of Dr. Leon R. Kass) ("The patient's trust in the doctor's whole-hearted devotion to his best interests will be hard to sustain").

Next, the State has an interest in protecting vulnerable groups—including the poor, the elderly, and disabled persons—from abuse, neglect, and mistakes. The Court of Appeals dismissed the State's concern that disadvantaged persons might be pressured into physician-assisted suicide as "ludicrous on its face." 79 F. 3d, at 825. We have recognized, however, the real risk of subtle coercion and undue influence in end-of-life situations. *Cruzan*, 497 U.S., at 281. Similarly, the New York Task Force warned that "[l]egalizing physician-assisted suicide would pose profound risks to many individuals who are ill and vulnerable. . . . The risk of harm is greatest for the many individuals in our society whose autonomy and well-being are already compromised by poverty, lack of access to good medical care, advanced age, or membership in a stigmatized social group." New York Task Force 120; see *Compassion in Dying*, 49 F. 3d, at 593 ("An insidious bias against the handicapped—again coupled with a cost-saving mentality—makes them especially in need of Washington's statutory protection"). If physician-assisted suicide were permitted, many might resort to it to spare their families the substantial financial burden of end-of-life health-care costs.

The State's interest here goes beyond protecting the vulnerable from coercion; it extends to protecting disabled and terminally ill people from prejudice, negative and inaccurate stereotypes, and "societal indifference." 49 F. 3d, at 592. The State's assisted-suicide ban reflects and reinforces its policy that the lives of terminally ill, disabled, and elderly people must be no less valued than the lives of the young and healthy, and that a seriously disabled person's suicidal impulses should be interpreted and treated the same way as anyone else's. See New York Task Force 101–102; Physician-Assisted Suicide and Euthanasia in the Netherlands: A Report of Chairman Charles T. Canady, *supra*, at 9, 20 (discussing prejudice toward the disabled and the negative messages euthanasia and assisted suicide send to handicapped patients).

Finally, the State may fear that permitting assisted suicide will start it down the path to voluntary and perhaps even involuntary euthanasia. The Court of Appeals struck down Washington's assisted-suicide ban only "as applied to competent, terminally ill adults who wish to hasten their deaths by obtaining medication prescribed by their doctors." 79 F. 3d, at 838. Washington insists, however, that the impact of the court's decision will not and cannot be so limited. Brief for Petitioners

44–47. If suicide is protected as a matter of constitutional right, it is argued, "every man and woman in the United States must enjoy it." *Compassion in Dying*, 49 F. 3d, at 591; see *Kevorkian*, 447 Mich., at 470, n. 41, 527 N. W. 2d, at 727–728, n. 41. The Court of Appeals' decision, and its expansive reasoning, provide ample support for the State's concerns. The court noted, for example, that the "decision of a duly appointed surrogate decision maker is for all legal purposes the decision of the patient himself," 79 F. 3d, at 832, n. 120; that "in some instances, the patient may be unable to self-administer the drugs and . . . administration by the physician . . . may be the only way the patient may be able to receive them," *id.*, at 831; and that not only physicians, but also family members and loved ones, will inevitably participate in assisting suicide, *id.*, at 838, n. 140. Thus, it turns out that what is couched as a limited right to "physician-assisted suicide" is likely, in effect, a much broader license, which could prove extremely difficult to police and contain.[23] Washington's ban on assisting suicide prevents such erosion.

This concern is further supported by evidence about the practice of euthanasia in the Netherlands. The Dutch government's own study revealed that in 1990, there were 2,300 cases of voluntary euthanasia (defined as "the deliberate termination of another's life at his request"), 400 cases of assisted suicide, and more than 1,000 cases of euthanasia without an explicit request. In addition to these latter 1,000 cases, the study found an additional 4,941 cases where physicians administered lethal morphine overdoses without the patients' explicit consent. Physician-Assisted Suicide and Euthanasia in the Netherlands: A Report of Chairman Charles T. Canady, *supra*, 12–13 (citing Dutch study). This study suggests that, despite the existence of various reporting procedures, euthanasia in the Netherlands

---

[23]JUSTICE SOUTER concludes that "[t]he case for the slippery slope is fairly made out here, not because recognizing one due process right would leave a court with no principled basis to avoid recognizing another, but because there is a plausible case that the right claimed would not be readily containable by reference to facts about the mind that are matters of difficult judgment, or by gatekeepers who are subject to temptation, noble or not." *Post*, at 785 (opinion concurring in judgment). We agree that the case for a slippery slope has been made out, but—bearing in mind Justice Cardozo's observation of "[t]he tendency of a principle to expand itself to the limit of its logic," The Nature of the Judicial Process 51 (1932)—we also recognize the reasonableness of the widely expressed skepticism about the lack of a principled basis for confining the right. See Brief for United States as *Amicus Curiae* 26 ("Once a legislature abandons a categorical prohibition against physician assisted suicide, there is no obvious stopping point"); Brief for Not Dead Yet et al. as *Amici Curiae* 21–29; Brief for Bioethics Professors as *Amici Curiae* 23–26; Report of the Council on Ethical and Judicial Affairs, App. 133, 140 ("[I]f assisted suicide is permitted, then there is a strong argument for allowing euthanasia"); New York Task Force 132; Kamisar, The "Right to Die"; On Drawing (and Erasing) Lines, 35 Duquesne L. Rev. 481 (1996); Kamisar, Against Assisted Suicide—Even in a Very Limited Form, 72 U. Det. Mercy L. Rev. 735 (1995).

has not been limited to competent, terminally ill adults who are enduring physical suffering, and that regulation of the practice may not have prevented abuses in cases involving vulnerable persons, including severely disabled neonates and elderly persons suffering from dementia. *Id.,* at 16–21; see generally C. Gomez, Regulating Death: Euthanasia and the Case of the Netherlands (1991); H. Hendin, Seduced By Death: Doctors, Patients, and the Dutch Cure (1997). The New York Task Force, citing the Dutch experience, observed that "assisted suicide and euthanasia are closely linked," New York Task Force 145, and concluded that the "risk of ... abuse is neither speculative nor distant," *id.,* at 134. Washington, like most other States, reasonably ensures against this risk by banning, rather than regulating, assisted suicide. See *United States* v. 12 *200ft. Reels* of Super 8MM. Film, 413 U.S. 123, 127 (1973) ("Each step, when taken, appear[s] a reasonable step in relation to that which preceded it, although the aggregate or end result is one that would never have been seriously considered in the first instance").

We need not weigh exactly the relative strengths of these various interests. They are unquestionably important and legitimate, and Washington's ban on assisted suicide is at least reasonably related to their promotion and protection. We therefore hold that Wash. Rev. Code § 9A.36.060(1) (1994) does not violate the Fourteenth Amendment, either on its face or "as applied to competent, terminally ill adults who wish to hasten their deaths by obtaining medication prescribed by their doctors." 79 F. 3d, at 838.[24]

Throughout the Nation, Americans are engaged in an earnest and profound debate about the morality, legality, and practicality of physician-assisted suicide. Our holding permits this debate to continue, as it should in a democratic society. The decision of the en banc Court of Appeals is reversed, and the case is remanded for further proceedings consistent with this opinion.

It is so ordered.

---

[24]JUSTICE STEVENS states that "the Court does conceive of respondents' claim as a facial challenge—addressing not the application of the statute to a particular set of plaintiffs before it, but the constitutionality of the statute's categorical prohibition. . . ." *Post,* at 740 (opinion concurring in judgments). We emphasize that we today reject the Court of Appeals' specific holding that the statute is unconstitutional "as applied" to a particular class. See n. 6, supra. JUSTICE STEVENS agrees with this holding, see *post,* at 750, but would not "foreclose the possibility that an individual plaintiff seeking to hasten her death, or a doctor whose assistance was sought, could prevail in a more particularized challenge," ibid. Our opinion does not absolutely foreclose such a claim. However, given our holding that the Due Process Clause of the Fourteenth Amendment does not provide heightened protection to the asserted liberty interest in ending one's life with a physician's assistance, such a claim would have to be quite different from the ones advanced by respondents here.

Case Law: *Vacco v. Quill* (Physician-Assisted Suicide)

VACCO, ATTORNEY GENERAL OF NEW YORK, ET AL. *v.* QUILL ET AL.

CERTIORARI TO THE UNITED STATES COURT OF APPEALS FOR THE SECOND CIRCUIT

No. 95-1858. Argued January 8, 1997-Decided June 26,1997

REHNQUIST, C. J., delivered the opinion of the Court, in which O'CONNOR, SCALIA, KENNEDY, and THOMAS, JJ., joined. O'CONNOR, J., filed a concurring opinion, in which GINSBURG and BREYER, JJ., joined in part, *ante*, p. 736. STEVENS, J., *ante*, p. 738, SOUTER, J., *post*, p. 809, GINSBURG, J., *ante*, p. 789, and BREYER, J., *ante*, p. 789, filed opinions concurring in the judgment.

CHIEF JUSTICE REHNQUIST delivered the opinion of the Court.

In New York, as in most States, it is a crime to aid another to commit or attempt suicide,[1] but patients may refuse even lifesaving medical treatment.[2] The question presented by this case is whether New York's prohibition on assisting suicide

therefore violates the Equal Protection Clause of the Fourteenth Amendment. We hold that it does not.

Petitioners are various New York public officials. Respondents Timothy E. Quill, Samuel C. Klagsbrun, and Howard A. Grossman are physicians who practice in New York. They assert that although it would be "consistent with the standards of [their] medical practice[s]" to prescribe lethal medication for "mentally competent, terminally ill patients" who are suffering great pain and desire a doctor's help in taking their own lives, they are deterred from doing so by New York's ban on assisting suicide. App. 25–26.[3] Respondents, and three gravely ill patients who have since died,[4] sued the State's Attorney General in the United States District Court. They urged that because New York permits a competent person to refuse life-sustaining medical treatment, and because the refusal of such treatment is "essentially the same thing" as physician-assisted suicide, New York's assisted-suicide ban violates the Equal Protection Clause. *Quill v. Koppell,* 870 F. Supp. 78, 84–85 (SDNY 1994).

The District Court disagreed: "[I]t is hardly unreasonable or irrational for the State to recognize a difference between allowing nature to take its course, even in the most severe situations, and intentionally using an artificial death producing

---

[1]New York Penal Law § 125.15 (McKinney 1987) ("Manslaughter in the second degree") provides: "A person is guilty of manslaughter in the second degree when . . . (3) He intentionally causes or aids another person to commit suicide. Manslaughter in the second degree is a class C felony." Section 120.30 ("Promoting a suicide attempt") states: "A person is guilty of promoting a suicide attempt when he intentionally causes or aids another person to attempt suicide. Promoting a suicide attempt is a class E felony." See generally *Washington* v. *Glucksberg, ante*, at 710–719.

[2]"It is established under New York law that a competent person may refuse medical treatment, even if the withdrawal of such treatment will result in death." *Quill* v. *Koppell,* 870 F. Supp. 78, 84 (SDNY 1994); see N. Y. Pub. Health Law, §§ 2960–2979 (McKinney 1993 and Supp. 1997) ("Orders Not to Resuscitate") (regulating right of "adult with capacity" to direct issuance of orders not to resuscitate); *id.*, §§ 2980–2994 ("Health Care Agents and Proxies") (allowing appointment of agents "to make . . . health care decisions on the principal's behalf," including decisions to refuse lifesaving treatment).

[3]Declaration of Timothy E. Quill, M. D., App. 42–49; Declaration of Samuel C. Klagsbrun, M. D., id., at 68–74; Declaration of Howard A. Grossman, M. D., id., at 84–89; 80 F. 3d 716, 719 (CA2 1996).

[4]These three patients stated that they had no chance of recovery, faced the "prospect of progressive loss of bodily function and integrity and increasing pain and suffering," and desired medical assistance in ending their lives. App. 25–26; Declaration of William A. Barth, *id.*, at 96–98; Declaration of George A. Kingsley, *id.*, at 99–102; Declaration of Jane Doe, *id.*, at 105–109.

device." *Id.*, at 84. The court noted New York's "obvious legitimate interests in preserving life, and in protecting vulnerable persons," and concluded that "[u]nder the United States Constitution and the federal system it establishes, the resolution of this issue is left to the normal democratic processes within the State." *Id.*, at 84–85.

The Court of Appeals for the Second Circuit reversed. 80 F. 3d 716 (1996). The court determined that, despite the assisted-suicide ban's apparent general applicability, "New York law does not treat equally all competent persons who are in the final stages of fatal illness and wish to hasten their deaths," because "those in the final stages of terminal illness who are on life-support systems are allowed to hasten their deaths by directing the removal of such systems; but those who are similarly situated, except for the previous attachment of life-sustaining equipment, are not allowed to hasten death by self-administering prescribed drugs." *Id.*, at 727, 729. In the court's view, "[t]he ending of life by [the withdrawal of life-support systems] is *nothing more nor less than assisted suicide.*" *Id.*, at 729 (emphasis added). The Court of Appeals then examined whether this supposed unequal treatment was rationally related to any legitimate state interests,[5] and concluded that "to the extent that [New York's statutes] prohibit a physician from prescribing medications to be self-administered by a mentally competent, terminally-ill person in the final stages of his terminal illness, they are not rationally related to any legitimate state interest." *Id.*, at 731. We granted certiorari, 518 U.S. 1055 (1996), and now reverse.

The Equal Protection Clause commands that no State shall "deny to any person within its jurisdiction the equal protection of the laws." This provision creates no substantive rights. *San Antonio Independent School Dist.* v. *Rodriguez*, 411 U.S. 1, 33 (1973); *id.*, at 59 (Stewart, J., concurring). Instead, it embodies a general rule that States must treat like cases alike but may treat unlike cases accordingly. *Plyler* v. *Doe*, 457 U.S. 202, 216 (1982) ("'[T]he Constitution does not require things which are different in fact or opinion to be treated in law as though they were the same'") (quoting *Tigner* v. *Texas*, 310 U.S. 141, 147 (1940)). If a legislative classification or distinction "neither burdens a fundamental right nor targets a suspect class, we will uphold [it] so long as it bears a rational relation to some legitimate end." *Romer* v. *Evans*, 517 U.S. 620, 631 (1996).

New York's statutes outlawing assisting suicide affect and address matters of profound significance to all New Yorkers alike. They neither infringe fundamental rights nor involve suspect classifications. *Washington* v. *Glucksberg, ante,* at 719–728; see 80 F. 3d, at 726; *San Antonio School Dist.*, 411 U.S., at 28 ("The system of alleged discrimination and the class it defines have none of the traditional indicia of suspectness"); *id.*, at 33–35 (courts must look to the Constitution, not the "importance" of the asserted right, when deciding whether an asserted right is "fundamental"). These laws are therefore entitled to a "strong presumption of validity." *Heller* v. *Doe,* 509 U.S. 312, 319 (1993).

On their faces, neither New York's ban on assisting suicide nor its statutes permitting patients to refuse medical treatment treat anyone differently from anyone else or draw any distinctions between persons. *Everyone,* regardless of physical condition, is entitled, if competent, to refuse unwanted lifesaving medical treatment; *no one* is permitted to assist a suicide. Generally speaking, laws that apply evenhandedly to all "unquestionably comply" with the Equal Protection Clause. *New York City Transit Authority* v. *Beazer,* 440 U.S. 568, 587 (1979); see *Personnel Administrator of Mass.* v. *Feeney,* 442 U.S. 256, 271–273 (1979) ("[M]any [laws] affect certain groups unevenly, even though the law itself treats them no differently from all other members of the class described by the law").

The Court of Appeals, however, concluded that some terminally ill people—those who are on life-support systems—are treated differently from those who are not, in that the former may "hasten death" by ending treatment, but the latter may not "hasten death" through physician-assisted suicide. 80 F. 3d, at 729. This conclusion depends on the submission that ending or refusing lifesaving medical treatment "is nothing more nor less than assisted suicide." *Ibid.* Unlike the Court of Appeals, we think the distinction between assisting suicide and withdrawing life-sustaining treatment, a distinction widely recognized and endorsed in the medical profession[6] and in our legal

---

[5]The court acknowledged that because New York's assisted-suicide statutes "do not impinge on any fundamental rights [or] involve suspect classifications," they were subject only to rational-basis judicial scrutiny. 80 F. 3d, at 726–727.

[6]The American Medical Association emphasizes the "fundamental difference between refusing life-sustaining treatment and demanding a life-ending treatment." American Medical Association, Council on Ethical and Judicial Affairs, Physician-Assisted Suicide, 10 Issues in Law & Medicine 91, 93 (1994); see also American Medical Association, Council on Ethical and Judicial Affairs, Decisions Near the End of Life, 267 JAMA 2229, 2230–2231, 2233 (1992) ("The withdrawing or withholding of life-sustaining treatment is not inherently contrary to the principles of beneficence and nonmaleficence," but assisted suicide "is contrary to the prohibition against using the tools of medicine to cause a patient's death"); New York State Task Force on Life and the Law, When Death is Sought: Assisted Suicide and Euthanasia in the Medical Context 108 (1994) ("[Professional organizations] consistently distinguish assisted suicide and euthanasia from the withdrawing or withholding of treatment, and from the provision of palliative treatments or other medical care that risk fatal side effects"); Brief for American Medical Association et al. as *Amici Curiae* 18–25. Of course, as respondents' lawsuit demonstrates, there are differences of opinion within the medical profession on this question. See New York Task Force, *supra*, at 104–109.

traditions, is both important and logical; it is certainly rational. See *Feeney, supra,* at 272 ("When the basic classification is rationally based, uneven effects upon particular groups within a class are ordinarily of no constitutional concern").

The distinction comports with fundamental legal principles of causation and intent. First, when a patient refuses life-sustaining medical treatment, he dies from an underlying fatal disease or pathology; but if a patient ingests lethal medication prescribed by a physician, he is killed by that medication. See, *e.g., People* v. *Kevorkian,* 447 Mich. 436, 470–472, 527 N. W. 2d 714, 728 (1994), cert. denied, 514 U.S. 1083 (1995); *Matter of Conroy,* 98 N. J. 321, 355, 486 A. 2d 1209, 1226 (1985) (when feeding tube is removed, death "result[s] . . . from [the patient's] underlying medical condition"); *In re Colyer,* 99 Wash. 2d 114, 123, 660 P. 2d 738, 743 (1983) ("[D]eath which occurs after the removal of life sustaining systems is from natural causes"); American Medical Association, Council on Ethical and Judicial Affairs, Physician-Assisted Suicide, 10 Issues in Law & Medicine 91, 93 (1994) ("When a life-sustaining treatment is declined, the patient dies primarily because of an underlying disease").

Furthermore, a physician who withdraws, or honors a patient's refusal to begin, life-sustaining medical treatment purposefully intends, or may so intend, only to respect his patient's wishes and "to cease doing useless and futile or degrading things to the patient when [the patient] no longer stands to benefit from them." Assisted Suicide in the United States, Hearing before the Subcommittee on the Constitution of the House Committee on the Judiciary, 104th Cong., 2d Sess., 368 (1996) (testimony of Dr. Leon R. Kass). The same is true when a doctor provides aggressive palliative care; in some cases, painkilling drugs may hasten a patient's death, but the physician's purpose and intent is, or may be, only to ease his patient's pain. A doctor who assists a suicide, however, "must, necessarily and indubitably, intend primarily that the patient be made dead." *Id.,* at 367. Similarly, a patient who commits suicide with a doctor's aid necessarily has the specific intent to end his or her own life, while a patient who refuses or discontinues treatment might not. See, *e.g., Matter of Conroy, supra,* at 351, 486 A. 2d, at 1224 (patients who refuse life-sustaining treatment "may not harbor a specific intent to die" and may instead "fervently wish to live, but to do so free of unwanted medical technology, surgery, or drugs"); *Superintendent of Belchertown State School* v. *Saikewicz,* 373 Mass. 728, 743, n. 11, 370 N. E. 2d 417, 426, n. 11 (1977) ("[I]n refusing treatment the patient may not have the specific intent to die").

The law has long used actors' intent or purpose to distinguish between two acts that may have the same result. See, *e.g., United States* v. *Bailey,* 444 U.S. 394, 403–406 (1980) ("[T]he . . .

common law of homicide often distinguishes . . . between a person who knows that another person will be killed as the result of his conduct and a person who acts with the specific purpose of taking another's life"); *Morissette* v. *United States,* 342 U.S. 246, 250 (1952) (distinctions based on intent are "universal and persistent in mature systems of law"); M. Hale, 1 Pleas of the Crown 412 (1847) ("If A. with an intent to prevent a gangrene beginning in his hand doth without any advice cut off his hand, by which he dies, he is not thereby *felo de se* for tho it was a voluntary act, yet it was not with an intent to kill himself"). Put differently, the law distinguishes actions taken "because of" a given end from actions taken "in spite of" their unintended but foreseen consequences. *Feeney,* 442 U.S., at 279; *Compassion in Dying* v. *Washington,* 79 F. 3d 790, 858 (CA9 1996) (Kleinfeld, J., dissenting) ("When General Eisenhower ordered American soldiers onto the beaches of Normandy, he knew that he was sending many American soldiers to certain death. His purpose, though, was to . . . liberate Europe from the Nazis").

Given these general principles, it is not surprising that many courts, including New York courts, have carefully distinguished refusing life-sustaining treatment from suicide. See, *e.g., Fosmire* v. *Nicoleau,* 75 N. Y. 2d 218, 227, and n. 2, 551 N. E. 2d 77, 82, and n. 2 (1990) ("[M]erely declining medical care . . . is not considered a suicidal act").[7] In fact, the first state-court decision explicitly to authorize withdrawing lifesaving treatment noted the "real distinction between the self-infliction of deadly harm and a self-determination against artificial life support." *In re Quinlan,* 70 N. J. 10, 43, 52, and n. 9, 355 A. 2d 647, 665, 670, and n. 9, cert. denied *sub nom. Garger* v. *New Jersey,* 429 U.S. 922 (1976). And recently, the Michigan Supreme Court also rejected the argument that the distinction "between acts that artificially sustain life and acts that artificially curtail life" is merely a "distinction without constitutional significance—a meaningless exercise in semantic gymnastics," insisting that "the *Cruzan* majority disagreed and so do we." *Kevorkian,* 447 Mich., at 471, 527 N. W. 2d, at 728.[8]

---

[7]Thus, the Second Circuit erred in reading New York law as creating a "right to hasten death"; instead, the authorities cited by the court recognize a right to refuse treatment, and nowhere equate the exercise of this right with suicide. *Schloendorff* v. *Society of New York Hospital,* 211 N. Y. 125, 129–130, 105 N. E. 92, 93 (1914), which contains Justice Cardozo's famous statement that "[e]very human being of adult years and sound mind has a right to determine what shall be done with his own body," was simply an informed-consent case. See also *Rivers* v. *Katz,* 67 N. Y. 2d 485, 495, 495 N. E. 2d 337, 343 (1986) (right to refuse antipsychotic medication is not absolute, and may be limited when "the patient presents a danger to himself"); *Matter of Storar,* 52 N. Y. 2d 363, 377, n. 6, 420 N. E. 2d 64, 71, n. 6, cert. denied, 454 U.S. 858 (1981).

[8]Many courts have recognized this distinction. See, *e. g., Kevorkian* v. *Thompson,* 947 F. Supp. 1152, 1178, and nn. 20–21 (ED Mich. 1997); *In re Fiori,* 543 Pa. 592, 602, 673 A. 2d 905, 910 (1996); *Singletary* v. *Costello,* 665 So.

Similarly, the overwhelming majority of state legislatures have drawn a clear line between assisting suicide and withdrawing or permitting the refusal of unwanted lifesaving medical treatment by prohibiting the former and permitting the latter. *Glucksberg, ante,* at 710–711, 716–719. And "nearly all states expressly disapprove of suicide and assisted suicide either in statutes dealing with durable powers of attorney in healthcare situations, or in 'living will' statutes." *Kevorkian, supra,* at 478–479, and nn. 53–54, 527 N. W. 2d, at 731–732, and nn. 53–54.[9] Thus, even as the States move to protect and promote patients' dignity at the end of life, they remain opposed to physician-assisted suicide.

New York is a case in point. The State enacted its current assisted-suicide statutes in 1965.[10] Since then, New York has acted several times to protect patients' common law right to refuse treatment. Act of Aug. 7, 1987, ch. 818, § 1, 1987 N. Y. Laws 3140 ("Do Not Resuscitate Orders") (codified as amended at N. Y. Pub. Health Law §§ 2960–2979 (McKinney 1993 and Supp. 1997)); Act of July 22, 1990, ch. 752, § 2, 1990 N. Y. Laws 3547 ("Health Care Agents and Proxies") (codified as amended at N. Y. Pub. Health Law §§ 2980–2994 (McKinney 1993 and Supp. 1997)). In so doing, however, the State has neither endorsed a general right to "hasten death" nor approved physician-assisted suicide. Quite the opposite: The State has reaffirmed the line between "killing" and "letting die." See N. Y. Pub. Health Law § 2989(3) (McKinney 1993) ("This article is not intended to permit or promote suicide, assisted suicide, or euthanasia"); New York State Task Force on Life and the Law, Life Sustaining Treatment: Making Decisions and Appointing a Health Care Agent 36–42 (July 1987); Do Not Resuscitate Orders: The Proposed Legislation and Report of the New York State Task Force on Life and the Law 15 (Apr. 1986). More recently, the New York State Task Force on Life and the Law studied assisted suicide and euthanasia and, in 1994, unanimously recommended against legalization. When Death is Sought: Assisted Suicide and Euthanasia in the Medical Context vii (1994). In the Task Force's view, "allowing decisions to forgo life-sustaining treatment and allowing assisted suicide or euthanasia have radically different consequences and meanings for public policy." *Id.,* at 146.

This Court has also recognized, at least implicitly, the distinction between letting a patient die and making that patient

2d 1099, 1106 (Fla. App. 1996); *Laurie v. Senecal,* 666 A. 2d 806, 808–809 (R. I. 1995); *State ex rel. Schuetzle* v. *Vogel,* 537 N. W. 2d 358, 360 (N. D. 1995); *Thor* v. *Superior Court,* 5 Cal. 4th 725, 741–742, 855 P. 2d 375, 385–386 (1993); *DeGrella* v. *Elston,* 858 S. W. 2d 698, 707 (Ky. 1993); *People* v. *Adams,* 216 Cal. App. 3d 1431, 1440, 265 Cal. Rptr. 568, 573–574 *(1990); Guardianship of Jane Doe,* 411 Mass. 512, 522–523, 583 N. E. 2d 1263, 1270, cert. denied *sub nom. Doe* v. *Gross,* 503 U.S. 950 (1992); *In re L. W,* 167 Wis. 2d 53, 83, 482 N. W. 2d 60, 71 (1992); *In re Rosebush,* 195 Mich. App. 675, 681, n. 2, 491 N. W. 2d 633, 636, n. 2 (1992); *Donaldson* v. *Van de Kamp,* 2 Cal. App. 4th 1614, 1619–1625, 4 Cal. Rptr. 2d 59, 61–64 *(1992); In re Lawrance,* 579 N. E. 2d 32, 40, n. 4 (Ind. 1991); *McKay* v. *Bergstedt,* 106 Nev. 808, 822–823, 801 P. 2d 617, 626–627 (1990); *In re Browning,* 568 So. 2d 4, 14 (Fla. 1990); *McConnell* v. *Beverly Enterprises Connecticut, Inc.,* 209 Conn. 692, 710, 553 A. 2d 596, 605 (1989); *State* v. *McAfee,* 259 Ga. 579, 581, 385 S. E. 2d 651, 652 (1989); *In re Grant, 109* Wash. 2d 545, 563, 747 P. 2d 445, 454–455 (1987); *In re Gardner,* 534 A. 2d 947, 955–956 (Me. 1987); *Matter of Farrell,* 108 N. J. 335, 349–350, 529 A. 2d 404, 411 (1987); *Rasmussen* v. *Fleming,* 154 Ariz. 207, 218, 741 P. 2d 674, 685 (1987); *Bouvia* v. *Superior Court,* 179 Cal. App. 3d 1127, 1144–1145, 225 Cal. Rptr. 297, 306 (1986); *Von Holden* v. *Chapman,* 87 App. Div. 2d 66, 70, 450 N. Y. S. 2d 623, 627 (1982); *Bartling* v. *Superior Court, 163* Cal. App. 3d 186, 196–197, 209 Cal. Rptr. 220, 225–226 (1984); *Foody* v. *Manchester Memorial Hospital,* 40 Conn. Supp. 127, 137, 482 A. 2d 713, 720 (1984); *In re P. V. W,* 424 So. 2d 1015, 1022 (La. 1982); *Leach* v. *Akron General Medical Center,* 68 Ohio Misc. 1, 10, 426 N. E. 2d 809, 815 (Ohio Comm. Pleas 1980); *In re Severns,* 425 A. 2d 156, 161 (Del. Ch. 1980); *Satz* v. *Perlmutter,* 362 So. 2d 160, 162–163 (Fla. App. 1978); *Application of the President and Directors of Georgetown College,* 331 F. 2d 1000, 1009 (CADC), cert. denied, 377 U.S. 978 (1964); *Brophy* v. *New England Sinai Hospital,* 398 Mass. 417, 439, 497 N. E. 2d 626, 638 (1986). The British House of Lords has also recognized the distinction. *Airedale N. H. S. Trust* v. *Bland,* 2 W. L. R. 316, 368 (1993).

[9]See Ala. Code §22-8A-1O (1990); Alaska Stat. Ann. §§ 18. 12.080(a), (f) (1996); Ariz. Rev. Stat. Ann. § 36-3210 (Supp. 1996); Ark. Code Ann. §§ 2013-905(a), (f), 20-17-210(a), (g) (1991 and Supp. 1995); Cal. Health & Safety Code Ann. §§ 7191.5(a), (g) (West Supp. 1997); Cal. Prob. Code Ann. § 4723 (West Supp. 1997); Colo. Rev. Stat. §§ 15-14-504(4),15-18-112(1),15-18.5101(3), 15-18.6-108 (1987 and Supp. 1996); Conn. Gen. Stat. § 19a-575 (Supp. 1996); Del. Code Ann., Tit. 16, § 2512 (Supp. 1996); D. C. Code Ann. §§ 6-2430,21-2212 (1995 and Supp. 1996); Fla. Stat. §§ 765.309(1), (2) (Supp. 1997); Ga. Code Ann. §§31-32-11(b), 31-36-2(b) (1996); Haw. Rev. Stat. §327D-13 (1996); Idaho Code §39-152 (Supp. 1996); Ill. Compo Stat., ch. 755, §§35/9(f), 40/5, 40/50, 45/2–1 (1992); Ind. Code §§ 16-36-1-13, 16-364-19,30-5-5-17 (1994 and Supp. 1996); Iowa Code §§ 144A.11.1-144A.11.6, 144B.12.2 (1989 and Supp. 1997); Kan. Stat. Ann. § 65-28,109 (1985); Ky. Rev. Stat. Ann. §311.638 (Baldwin Supp. 1992); La. Rev. Stat. Ann. § 40: 1299.58.10(A), (B) (West 1992); Me. Rev. Stat. Ann., Tit. 18-A, §§ 5813(b), (c) (Supp. 1996); Md. Health Code Ann. § 5-611(c) (1994); Mass. Gen. Laws 20m, § 12 (Supp. 1997); Mich. Compo Laws Ann. § 700.496(20) (West 1995); Minn. Stat. §§ 145B.14, 145C.14 (Supp. 1997); Miss. Code Ann. §§4141-117(2), 41-41-119(1) (Supp. 1992); Mo. Rev. Stat. §§459.015.3, 459.055(5) (1992); Mont. Code Ann.

§§ 50-9-205(1), (7), 50-10-104(1), (6) (1995); Neb. Rev. Stat. §§ 20-412(1), (7), 30-3401(3) (1995); Nev. Rev. Stat. § 449.670(2) (1996); N. H. Rev. Stat. Ann. §§ 137-H:10, 137-H:13, 137-J:1 (1996); N. J. Stat. Ann. §§26:2H-54(d), (e), 26:2H-77 (West 1996); N. M. Stat. Ann. §§24-7A-13(B)(1), (C) (Supp. 1995); N. Y. Pub. Health Law §2989(3) (McKinney 1993); N. C. Gen. Stat. §§ 90-320(b), 90-321(f) (1993); N. D. Cent. Code §§ 23-06.4-01, 23-06.5-01 (1991); Ohio Rev. Code Ann. §§ 2133.12(A), (D) (Supp. 1996); Okla. Stat., Tit. 63, §§ 3101.2(C), 3101.12(A), (G) (1997); 20 Pa. Cons. Stat. § 5402(b) (Supp. 1996); R. I. Gen. Laws §§ 23-4.10-9(a), (f), 23-4. 11-1O(a), (f) (1996); S. C. Code Ann. §§44-77-130, 44-78-50(A), (C), 62-5-504(0) (Supp. 1996); S. D. Codified Laws §§34-12D-14, 34-12D-20 (1994); Tenn. Code Ann. §§32-11-110(a), 39-13-216 (Supp. 1996); Tex. Health & Safety Code Ann. §§ 672.017, 672.020, 672.021 (1992); Utah Code Ann. §§ 75-2-1116,75-2-1118 (1993); Vt. Stat. Ann., Tit. 18, § 5260 (1987); Va. Code Ann. § 54.1-2990 (1994); V. I. Code Ann., Tit. 19, §§ 198(a), (g) (1995); Wash. Rev. Code §§ 70.122.070(1), 70.122.100 (Supp. 1997); W. Va. Code §§ 16-30-10, 16-30A-16(a), 16-30B-2(b), 16-30B-13, *16-30C-14* (1995); Wis. Stat. §§ 154.11(1), (6), 154.25(7), 155.70(7) (Supp. 1996); Wyo. Stat. §§3-5-211, 35-22-109, 35-22-208 (1994 and Supp. 1996). See also 42 U.S.C. §§ 14402(b)(1), (2), (4) (1994 ed., Supp. III) ("Assisted Suicide Funding Restriction Act of 1997").

[10]It has always been a crime, either by statute or under the common law, to assist a suicide in New York. See Marzen, O'Dowd, Crone, & Balch, Suicide: A Constitutional Right?, 24 Duquesne L. Rev. 1, 205–210 (1985) (App.).

die. In *Cruzan v. Director, Mo. Dept. of Health*, 497 U.S. 261, 278 (1990), we concluded that "[t]he principle that a competent person has a constitutionally protected liberty interest in refusing unwanted medical treatment may be inferred from our prior decisions," and we assumed the existence of such a right for purposes of that case, *id.*, at 279. But our assumption of a right to refuse treatment was grounded not, as the Court of Appeals supposed, on the proposition that patients have a general and abstract "right to hasten death," 80 F. 3d, at 727–728, but on well-established, traditional rights to bodily integrity and freedom from unwanted touching, *Cruzan*, 497 U.S., at 278–279; *id.*, at 287-288 (O'CONNOR, J., concurring). In fact, we observed that "the majority of States in this country have laws imposing criminal penalties on one who assists another to commit suicide." *Id.*, at 280. *Cruzan* therefore provides no support for the notion that refusing life-sustaining medical treatment is "nothing more nor less than suicide."

For all these reasons, we disagree with respondents' claim that the distinction between refusing lifesaving medical treatment and assisted suicide is "arbitrary" and "irrational." Brief for Respondents 44.[11] Granted, in some cases, the line between the two may not be clear, but certainty is not required, even were it possible.[12] Logic and contemporary practice support New York's judgment that the two acts are different, and New York may therefore, consistent with the Constitution, treat them differently. By permitting everyone to refuse unwanted medical treatment while prohibiting anyone from assisting a suicide, New York law follows a longstanding and rational distinction.

New York's reasons for recognizing and acting on this distinction—including prohibiting intentional killing and preserving life; preventing suicide; maintaining physicians' role as their patients' healers; protecting vulnerable people from indifference, prejudice, and psychological and financial pressure to end their lives; and avoiding a possible slide towards euthanasia—are discussed in greater detail in our opinion in *Glucksberg, ante.* These valid and important public interests easily satisfy the constitutional requirement that a legislative classification bear a rational relation to some legitimate end.[13]

The judgment of the Court of Appeals is reversed.

It is so ordered.

---

[11]Respondents also argue that the State irrationally distinguishes between physician-assisted suicide and "terminal sedation," a process respondents characterize as "induc[ing] barbiturate coma and then starv[ing] the person to death." Brief for Respondents 48–50; see 80 F. 3d, at 729. Petitioners insist, however, that "'[a]lthough proponents of physician-assisted suicide and euthanasia contend that terminal sedation is covert physician-assisted suicide or euthanasia, the concept of sedating pharmacotherapy is based on informed consent and the principle of double effect.'" Reply Brief for Petitioners 12 (quoting P. Rousseau, Terminal Sedation in the Care of Dying Patients, 156 Archives Internal Med. 1785, 1785–1786 (1996)). Just as a State may prohibit assisting suicide while permitting patients to refuse unwanted lifesaving treatment, it may permit palliative care related to that refusal, which may have the foreseen but unintended "double effect" of hastening the patient's death. See New York Task Force, When Death is Sought, *supra* n. 6, at 163 ("It is widely recognized that the provision of pain medication is ethically and professionally acceptable even when the treatment may hasten the patient's death, if the medication is intended to alleviate pain and severe discomfort, not to cause death").

[12]We do not insist, as JUSTICE STEVENS suggests, *ante,* at 750 (opinion concurring in judgments), that "in all cases there will in fact be a significant difference between the intent of the physicians, the patients, or the families [in withdrawal-of-treatment and physician-assisted-suicide cases]." See *supra,* at 801–802 ("[A] physician who withdraws, or honors a patient's refusal to begin, life-sustaining medical treatment purposefully intends, *or may so intend,* only to respect his patient's wishes. . . . The same is true when a doctor provides aggressive palliative care; . . . the physician's purpose and intent is, *or may be,* only to ease his patient's pain" (emphasis added)). In the absence of omniscience, however, the State is entitled to act on the reasonableness of the distinction.

[13]Justice Stevens observes that our holding today "does not foreclose the possibility that some applications of the New York statute may impose an intolerable intrusion on the patien'ts freedom." *Ante,* at 16 (concurring opinion). This is true, but as we observe in *Glucksberg, ante,* at 31–32, n. 24, a particular case would need to present different and considerably stronger arguments than those advanced by respondents here.

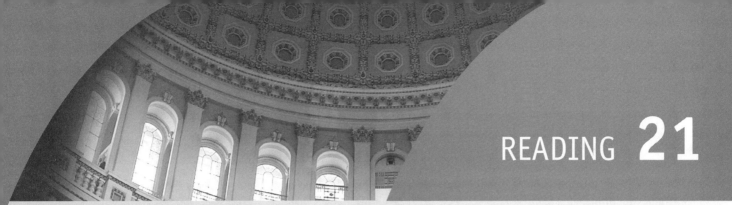

The Oregon Death with Dignity Act Statute, Regulations, and State's Report on Its Use

THE OREGON DEATH WITH DIGNITY ACT

OREGON REVISED STATUTES

(GENERAL PROVISIONS)

(Section 1)

Note: The division headings, subdivision headings and leadlines for 127.800 to 127.890, 127.895 and 127.897 were enacted as part of Ballot Measure 16 (1994) and were not provided by Legislative Counsel.

127.800 §1.01. Definitions. The following words and phrases, whenever used in ORS 127.800 to 127.897, have the following meanings:

(1) "Adult" means an individual who is 18 years of age or older.

(2) "Attending physician" means the physician who has primary responsibility for the care of the patient and treatment of the patient's terminal disease.

(3) "Capable" means that in the opinion of a court or in the opinion of the patient's attending physician or consulting physician, psychiatrist or psychologist, a patient has the ability to make and communicate health care decisions to health care providers, including communication through persons familiar with the patient's manner of communicating if those persons are available.

(4) "Consulting physician" means a physician who is qualified by specialty or experience to make a professional diagnosis and prognosis regarding the patient's disease.

(5) "Counseling" means one or more consultations as necessary between a state licensed psychiatrist or psychologist and a patient for the purpose of determining that the patient is capable and not suffering from a psychiatric or psychological disorder or depression causing impaired judgment.

(6) "Health care provider" means a person licensed, certified or otherwise authorized or permitted by the law of this state to administer health care or dispense medication in the ordinary course of business or practice of a profession, and includes a health care facility.

(7) "Informed decision" means a decision by a qualified patient, to request and obtain a prescription to end his or her life in a humane and dignified manner, that is based on an appreciation of the relevant facts and after being fully informed by the attending physician of:
   (a) His or her medical diagnosis;
   (b) His or her prognosis;
   (c) The potential risks associated with taking the medication to be prescribed;
   (d) The probable result of taking the medication to be prescribed; and
   (e) The feasible alternatives, including, but not limited to, comfort care, hospice care and pain control.

(8) "Medically confirmed" means the medical opinion of the attending physician has been confirmed by a consulting physician who has examined the patient and the patient's relevant medical records.

(9) "Patient" means a person who is under the care of a physician.

(10) "Physician" means a doctor of medicine or osteopathy licensed to practice medicine by the Board of Medical Examiners for the State of Oregon.

(11) "Qualified patient" means a capable adult who is a resident of Oregon and has satisfied the requirements of ORS 127.800 to 127.897 in order to obtain a prescription for medication to end his or her life in a humane and dignified manner.

(12) "Terminal disease" means an incurable and irreversible disease that has been medically confirmed and will, within reasonable medical judgment, produce death within six months. [1995 c.3 §1.01; 1999 c.423 §1]

(Written Request for Medication to End One's Life in a Humane and Dignified Manner)

(Section 2)

127.805 §2.01. Who may initiate a written request for medication.

(1) An adult who is capable, is a resident of Oregon, and has been determined by the attending physician and consulting physician to be suffering from a terminal disease, and who has voluntarily expressed his or her wish to die, may make a written request for medication for the purpose of ending his or her life in a humane and dignified manner in accordance with ORS 127.800 to 127.897.

(2) No person shall qualify under the provisions of ORS 127.800 to 127.897 solely because of age or disability. [1995 c.3 §2.01; 1999 c.423 §2]

127.810 §2.02. Form of the written request.

(1) A valid request for medication under ORS 127.800 to 127.897 shall be in substantially the form described in ORS 127.897, signed and dated by the patient and witnessed by at least two individuals who, in the presence of the patient, attest that to the best of their knowledge and belief the patient is capable, acting voluntarily, and is not being coerced to sign the request.

(2) One of the witnesses shall be a person who is not:
   (a) A relative of the patient by blood, marriage or adoption;
   (b) A person who at the time the request is signed would be entitled to any portion of the estate of the qualified patient upon death under any will or by operation of law; or

   (c) An owner, operator or employee of a health care facility where the qualified patient is receiving medical treatment or is a resident.

(3) The patient's attending physician at the time the request is signed shall not be a witness.

(4) If the patient is a patient in a long term care facility at the time the written request is made, one of the witnesses shall be an individual designated by the facility and having the qualifications specified by the Department of Human Services by rule. [1995 c.3 §2.02]

(Safeguards)

(Section 3)

127.815 §3.01. Attending physician responsibilities.

(1) The attending physician shall:
   (a) Make the initial determination of whether a patient has a terminal disease, is capable, and has made the request voluntarily;
   (b) Request that the patient demonstrate Oregon residency pursuant to ORS 127.860;
   (c) To ensure that the patient is making an informed decision, inform the patient of:
      (A) His or her medical diagnosis;
      (B) His or her prognosis;
      (C) The potential risks associated with taking the medication to be prescribed;
      (D) The probable result of taking the medication to be prescribed; and
      (E) The feasible alternatives, including, but not limited to, comfort care, hospice care and pain control;
   (d) Refer the patient to a consulting physician for medical confirmation of the diagnosis, and for a determination that the patient is capable and acting voluntarily;
   (e) Refer the patient for counseling if appropriate pursuant to ORS 127.825;
   (f) Recommend that the patient notify next of kin;
   (g) Counsel the patient about the importance of having another person present when the patient takes the medication prescribed pursuant to ORS 127.800 to 127.897 and of not taking the medication in a public place;
   (h) Inform the patient that he or she has an opportunity to rescind the request at any time and in any manner, and offer the patient an opportunity to rescind at

the end of the 15 day waiting period pursuant to ORS 127.840;

(i) Verify, immediately prior to writing the prescription for medication under ORS 127.800 to 127.897, that the patient is making an informed decision;

(j) Fulfill the medical record documentation requirements of ORS 127.855;

(k) Ensure that all appropriate steps are carried out in accordance with ORS 127.800 to 127.897 prior to writing a prescription for medication to enable a qualified patient to end his or her life in a humane and dignified manner; and

(l)

(A) Dispense medications directly, including ancillary medications intended to facilitate the desired effect to minimize the patient's discomfort, provided the attending physician is registered as a dispensing physician with the Board of Medical Examiners, has a current Drug Enforcement Administration certificate and complies with any applicable administrative rule; or

(B) With the patient's written consent:

(i) Contact a pharmacist and inform the pharmacist of the prescription; and

(ii) Deliver the written prescription personally or by mail to the pharmacist, who will dispense the medications to either the patient, the attending physician or an expressly identified agent of the patient.

(2) Notwithstanding any other provision of law, the attending physician may sign the patient's death certificate. [1995 c.3 §3.01; 1999 c.423 §3]

127.820 §3.02. Consulting physician confirmation. Before a patient is qualified under ORS 127.800 to 127.897, a consulting physician shall examine the patient and his or her relevant medical records and confirm, in writing, the attending physician's diagnosis that the patient is suffering from a terminal disease, and verify that the patient is capable, is acting voluntarily and has made an informed decision. [1995 c.3 §3.02]

127.825 §3.03. Counseling referral. If in the opinion of the attending physician or the consulting physician a patient may be suffering from a psychiatric or psychological disorder or depression causing impaired judgment, either physician shall refer the patient for counseling. No medication to end a patient's life in a humane and dignified manner shall be prescribed until the person performing the counseling determines that the patient is not suffering from a psychiatric or psycho-

logical disorder or depression causing impaired judgment. [1995 c.3 §3.03; 1999 c.423 §4]

127.830 §3.04. Informed decision. No person shall receive a prescription for medication to end his or her life in a humane and dignified manner unless he or she has made an informed decision as defined in ORS 127.800 (7). Immediately prior to writing a prescription for medication under ORS 127.800 to 127.897, the attending physician shall verify that the patient is making an informed decision. [1995 c.3 §3.04]

127.835 §3.05. Family notification. The attending physician shall recommend that the patient notify the next of kin of his or her request for medication pursuant to ORS 127.800 to 127.897. A patient who declines or is unable to notify next of kin shall not have his or her request denied for that reason. [1995 c.3 §3.05; 1999 c.423 §6]

127.840 §3.06. Written and oral requests. In order to receive a prescription for medication to end his or her life in a humane and dignified manner, a qualified patient shall have made an oral request and a written request, and reiterate the oral request to his or her attending physician no less than fifteen (15) days after making the initial oral request. At the time the qualified patient makes his or her second oral request, the attending physician shall offer the patient an opportunity to rescind the request. [1995 c.3 §3.06]

127.845 §3.07. Right to rescind request. A patient may rescind his or her request at any time and in any manner without regard to his or her mental state. No prescription for medication under ORS 127.800 to 127.897 may be written without the attending physician offering the qualified patient an opportunity to rescind the request. [1995 c.3 §3.07]

127.850 §3.08. Waiting periods. No less than fifteen (15) days shall elapse between the patient's initial oral request and the writing of a prescription under ORS 127.800 to 127.897. No less than 48 hours shall elapse between the patient's written request and the writing of a prescription under ORS 127.800 to 127.897. [1995 c.3 §3.08]

127.855 §3.09. Medical record documentation requirements. The following shall be documented or filed in the patient's medical record:

(1) All oral requests by a patient for medication to end his or her life in a humane and dignified manner;

(2) All written requests by a patient for medication to end his or her life in a humane and dignified manner;

(3) The attending physician's diagnosis and prognosis, determination that the patient is capable, acting voluntarily and has made an informed decision;

(4) The consulting physician's diagnosis and prognosis, and verification that the patient is capable, acting voluntarily and has made an informed decision;

(5) A report of the outcome and determinations made during counseling, if performed;

(6) The attending physician's offer to the patient to rescind his or her request at the time of the patient's second oral request pursuant to ORS 127.840; and

(7) A note by the attending physician indicating that all requirements under ORS 127.800 to 127.897 have been met and indicating the steps taken to carry out the request, including a notation of the medication prescribed. [1995 c.3 §3.09]

127.860 §3.10. Residency requirement. Only requests made by Oregon residents under ORS 127.800 to 127.897 shall be granted. Factors demonstrating Oregon residency include but are not limited to:

(1) Possession of an Oregon driver license;

(2) Registration to vote in Oregon;

(3) Evidence that the person owns or leases property in Oregon; or

(4) Filing of an Oregon tax return for the most recent tax year. [1995 c.3 §3.10; 1999 c.423 §8]

127.865 §3.11. Reporting requirements.

(1)
　(a) The Department of Human Services shall annually review a sample of records maintained pursuant to ORS 127.800 to 127.897.
　(b) The department shall require any health care provider upon dispensing medication pursuant to ORS 127.800 to 127.897 to file a copy of the dispensing record with the department.

(2) The department shall make rules to facilitate the collection of information regarding compliance with ORS 127.800 to 127.897. Except as otherwise required by law, the information collected shall not be a public record and may not be made available for inspection by the public.

(3) The department shall generate and make available to the public an annual statistical report of information collected under subsection (2) of this section. [1995 c.3 §3.11; 1999 c.423 §9; 2001 c.104 §40]

127.870 §3.12. Effect on construction of wills, contracts and statutes.

(1) No provision in a contract, will or other agreement, whether written or oral, to the extent the provision would affect whether a person may make or rescind a request for medication to end his or her life in a humane and dignified manner, shall be valid.

(2) No obligation owing under any currently existing contract shall be conditioned or affected by the making or rescinding of a request, by a person, for medication to end his or her life in a humane and dignified manner. [1995 c.3 §3.12]

127.875 §3.13. Insurance or annuity policies. The sale, procurement, or issuance of any life, health, or accident insurance or annuity policy or the rate charged for any policy shall not be conditioned upon or affected by the making or rescinding of a request, by a person, for medication to end his or her life in a humane and dignified manner. Neither shall a qualified patient's act of ingesting medication to end his or her life in a humane and dignified manner have an effect upon a life, health, or accident insurance or annuity policy. [1995 c.3 §3.13]

127.880 §3.14. Construction of Act. Nothing in ORS 127.800 to 127.897 shall be construed to authorize a physician or any other person to end a patient's life by lethal injection, mercy killing or active euthanasia. Actions taken in accordance with ORS 127.800 to 127.897 shall not, for any purpose, constitute suicide, assisted suicide, mercy killing or homicide, under the law. [1995 c.3 §3.14]

(Immunities and Liabilities)

(Section 4)

127.885 §4.01. Immunities; basis for prohibiting health care provider from participation; notification; permissible sanctions. Except as provided in ORS 127.890:

(1) No person shall be subject to civil or criminal liability or professional disciplinary action for participating in good faith compliance with ORS 127.800 to 127.897. This includes being present when a qualified patient takes the prescribed medication to end his or her life in a humane and dignified manner.

(2) No professional organization or association, or health care provider, may subject a person to censure, discipline, suspension, loss of license, loss of privileges, loss of membership or other penalty for participating or refusing to

participate in good faith compliance with ORS 127.800 to 127.897.

(3) No request by a patient for or provision by an attending physician of medication in good faith compliance with the provisions of ORS 127.800 to 127.897 shall constitute neglect for any purpose of law or provide the sole basis for the appointment of a guardian or conservator.

(4) No health care provider shall be under any duty, whether by contract, by statute or by any other legal requirement to participate in the provision to a qualified patient of medication to end his or her life in a humane and dignified manner. If a health care provider is unable or unwilling to carry out a patient's request under ORS 127.800 to 127.897, and the patient transfers his or her care to a new health care provider, the prior health care provider shall transfer, upon request, a copy of the patient's relevant medical records to the new health care provider.

(5)

(a) Notwithstanding any other provision of law, a health care provider may prohibit another health care provider from participating in ORS 127.800 to 127.897 on the premises of the prohibiting provider if the prohibiting provider has notified the health care provider of the prohibiting provider's policy regarding participating in ORS 127.800 to 127.897. Nothing in this paragraph prevents a health care provider from providing health care services to a patient that do not constitute participation in ORS 127.800 to 127.897:

(b) Notwithstanding the provisions of subsections (1) to (4) of this section, a health care provider may subject another health care provider to the sanctions stated in this paragraph if the sanctioning health care provider has notified the sanctioned provider prior to participation in ORS 127.800 to 127.897 that it prohibits participation in ORS 127.800 to 127.897:

(A) Loss of privileges, loss of membership or other sanction provided pursuant to the medical staff bylaws, policies and procedures of the sanctioning health care provider if the sanctioned provider is a member of the sanctioning provider's medical staff and participates in ORS 127.800 to 127.897 while on the health care facility premises, as defined in ORS 442.015, of the sanctioning health care provider, but not including the private medical office of a physician or other provider;

(B) Termination of lease or other property contract or other nonmonetary remedies provided by lease contract, not including loss or restriction of medical staff privileges or exclusion from a provider panel, if the sanctioned provider participates in ORS 127.800 to 127.897 while on the premises of the sanctioning health care provider or on property that is owned by or under the direct control of the sanctioning health care provider; or

(C) Termination of contract or other nonmonetary remedies provided by contract if the sanctioned provider participates in ORS 127.800 to 127.897 while acting in the course and scope of the sanctioned provider's capacity as an employee or independent contractor of the sanctioning health care provider. Nothing in this subparagraph shall be construed to prevent:

(i) A health care provider from participating in ORS 127.800 to 127.897 while acting outside the course and scope of the provider's capacity as an employee or independent contractor; or

(ii) A patient from contracting with his or her attending physician and consulting physician to act outside the course and scope of the provider's capacity as an employee or independent contractor of the sanctioning health care provider.

(c) A health care provider that imposes sanctions pursuant to paragraph (b) of this subsection must follow all due process and other procedures the sanctioning health care provider may have that are related to the imposition of sanctions on another health care provider.

(d) For purposes of this subsection:

(A) "Notify" means a separate statement in writing to the health care provider specifically informing the health care provider prior to the provider's participation in ORS 127.800 to 127.897 of the sanctioning health care provider's policy about participation in activities covered by ORS 127.800 to 127.897.

(B) "Participate in ORS 127.800 to 127.897" means to perform the duties of an attending physician pursuant to ORS 127.815, the consulting physician function pursuant to ORS 127.820 or the counseling function pursuant to ORS 127.825.

"Participate in ORS 127.800 to 127.897" does not include:

(i) Making an initial determination that a patient has a terminal disease and informing the patient of the medical prognosis;

(ii) Providing information about the Oregon Death with Dignity Act to a patient upon the request of the patient;

(iii) Providing a patient, upon the request of the patient, with a referral to another physician; or

(iv) A patient contracting with his or her attending physician and consulting physician to act outside of the course and scope of the provider's capacity as an employee or independent contractor of the sanctioning health care provider.

(6) Suspension or termination of staff membership or privileges under subsection (5) of this section is not reportable under ORS 441.820. Action taken pursuant to ORS 127.810, 127.815, 127.820 or 127.825 shall not be the sole basis for a report of unprofessional or dishonorable conduct under ORS 677.415 (2) or (3).

(7) No provision of ORS 127.800 to 127.897 shall be construed to allow a lower standard of care for patients in the community where the patient is treated or a similar community. [1995 c.3 §4.01; 1999 c.423 §10]

Note: As originally enacted by the people, the leadline to section 4.01 read "Immunities." The remainder of the leadline was added by editorial action.

127.890 §4.02. Liabilities.

(1) A person who without authorization of the patient willfully alters or forges a request for medication or conceals or destroys a rescission of that request with the intent or effect of causing the patient's death shall be guilty of a Class A felony.

(2) A person who coerces or exerts undue influence on a patient to request medication for the purpose of ending the patient's life, or to destroy a rescission of such a request, shall be guilty of a Class A felony.

(3) Nothing in ORS 127.800 to 127.897 limits further liability for civil damages resulting from other negligent conduct or intentional misconduct by any person.

(4) The penalties in ORS 127.800 to 127.897 do not preclude criminal penalties applicable under other law for conduct which is inconsistent with the provisions of ORS 127.800 to 127.897. [1995 c.3 §4.02]

127.892 Claims by governmental entity for costs incurred. Any governmental entity that incurs costs resulting from a person terminating his or her life pursuant to the provisions of ORS 127.800 to 127.897 in a public place shall have a claim against the estate of the person to recover such costs and reasonable attorney fees related to enforcing the claim. [1999 c.423 §5a]

(Severability)

(Section 5)

127.895 §5.01. Severability. Any section of ORS 127.800 to 127.897 being held invalid as to any person or circumstance shall not affect the application of any other section of ORS 127.800 to 127.897 which can be given full effect without the invalid section or application. [1995 c.3 §5.01]

(Form of the Request)

(Section 6)

127.897 §6.01. Form of the request. A request for a medication as authorized by ORS 127.800 to 127.897 shall be in substantially the following form: [Exhibit 1]

PENALTIES

127.990: [Formerly part of 97.990; repealed by 1993 c.767 §29]

127.995 Penalties.

(1) It shall be a Class A felony for a person without authorization of the principal to willfully alter, forge, conceal or destroy an instrument, the reinstatement or revocation of an instrument or any other evidence or document reflecting the principal's desires and interests, with the intent and effect of causing a withholding or withdrawal of life-sustaining procedures or of artificially administered nutrition and hydration which hastens the death of the principal.

(2) Except as provided in subsection (1) of this section, it shall be a Class A misdemeanor for a person without authorization of the principal to willfully alter, forge, conceal or destroy an instrument, the reinstatement or revocation of an instrument, or any other evidence or document reflecting the principal's desires and interests with the intent or effect of affecting a health care decision. [Formerly 127.585]

Department of Human Services, Public Health

Exhibit 1-1

Request for Medication to End My Life in a Humane and Dignified Manner

I, _____, am an adult of sound mind.

I am suffering from _____, which my attending physician has determined is a terminal disease and which has been medically confirmed by a consulting physician.

I have been fully informed of my diagnosis, prognosis, the nature of medication to be prescribed and potential associated risks, the expected result, and the feasible alternatives, including comfort care, hospice care and pain control.

I request that my attending physician prescribe medication that will end my life in a humane and dignified manner.

INITIAL ONE:

_____ I have informed my family of my decision and taken their opinions into consideration.

_____ I have decided not to inform my family of my decision.

_____ I have no family to inform of my decision.

I understand that I have the right to rescind this request at any time.

I understand the full import of this request and I expect to die when I take the medication to be prescribed. I further understand that although most deaths occur within three hours, my death may take longer and my physician has counseled me about this possibility.

I make this request voluntarily and without reservation, and I accept full moral responsibility for my actions.

Signed: _____

Dated: _____

DECLARATION OF WITNESSES

We declare that the person signing this request:

(a) Is personally known to us or has provided proof of identity;

(b) Signed this request in our presence;

(c) Appears to be of sound mind and not under duress, fraud or undue influence;

(d) Is not a patient for whom either of us is attending physician.

_____ Witness 1/Date

_____ Witness 2/Date

Note: One witness shall not be a relative (by blood, marriage or adoption) of the person signing this request, shall not be entitled to any portion of the person's estate upon death and shall not own, operate or be employed at a health care facility where the person is a patient or resident. If the patient is an inpatient at a health care facility, one of the witnesses shall be an individual designated by the facility.

[1995 c.3 §6.01; 1999 c.423 §11]

TABLE 21-1 Reporting Requirements of the Oregon Death with Dignity Act

333-009-0000

Definitions

For the purpose of OAR 333-009-0000 through 333-009-0030, the following definitions apply.

(1) "Act" means the "Oregon Death with Dignity Act" or Measure 16 as adopted by the voters on November 8, 1994.

(2) "Adult" means an individual who is 18 years of age or older.

(3) "Attending Physician" means the physician who has primary responsibility for the care of the patient and treatment of the patient's terminal disease.

(4) "Capable" means that in the opinion of a court or in the opinion of the patient's attending physician or consulting physician, psychiatrist or psychologist, a patient has the ability to make and communicate health care decisions to health care providers, including communication through persons familiar with the patient's manner of communicating, if those persons are available.

(5) "Consulting physician" means a physician who is qualified by specialty or experience to make a professional diagnosis and prognosis regarding the patient's disease.

(6) "Counseling" means one or more consultations as necessary between a state licensed psychiatrist or psychologist and a patient for the purpose of determining that the patient is capable and not suffering from a psychiatric or psychological disorder or depression causing impaired judgment.

(7) "Dispensing Record" means a copy of the pharmacy dispensing record form.

(8) "Department" means the Department of Human Services.

(9) "Health Care Facility" shall have the meaning given in ORS 442.015.

(10) "Health Care Provider" means a person licensed, certified or otherwise authorized or permitted by the law of this state to administer health care or dispense medication in the ordinary course of business or practice of a profession and includes a health care facility.

(11) "Patient" means a person who is under the care of a physician.

(12) "Physician" means a doctor of medicine or osteopathy licensed to practice medicine by the Board of Medical Examiners for the State of Oregon.

(13) "Qualified patient" means a capable adult who is a resident of Oregon and has satisfied the requirements of this Act in order to obtain a prescription for medication to end his or her life in a humane and dignified manner.

Stat. Auth.: ORS 127.865

Stats. Implemented: ORS 127.800-127.995 Hist.: HD 15-1997(Temp), f. & cert. ef. 11-6-97; OHD 4-1998, f. & cert. ef. 5-4-98; OHD 12-1999, f. & cert. ef. 12-28-99

333-009-0010

Reporting

(1) To comply with ORS 127.865(2), within seven calendar days of writing a prescription for medication to end the life of a qualified patient the attending physician shall send the following completed, signed and dated documentation by mail to the State Registrar, Center for Health Statistics, 800 NE Oregon Street, Suite 205, Portland OR 97232, or by facsimile to (971) 673-1201:

(a) The patient's completed written request for medication to end life, either using the "Written Request for Medication to End My Life in a Humane and Dignified Manner" form prescribed by the Department or in substantially the form described in ORS 127.897;

(b) One of the following reports prescribed by the Department:

(A) "Attending Physician's Compliance Form"; or

(B) "Attending Physician's Compliance Short Form" accompanied by a copy of the relevant portions of the patient's medical record documenting all actions required by the Act;

(c) "Consulting Physician's Compliance Form" prescribed by the Department; and

(d) "Psychiatric/Psychological Consultant's Compliance Form" prescribed by the Department, if an evaluation was performed.

(2) Within 10 calendar days of a patient's ingestion of lethal medication obtained pursuant to the Act, or death from any other cause, whichever comes first, the attending physician shall complete the "Oregon Death with Dignity Act Attending Physician Interview" form prescribed by the Department.

continues

TABLE 21-1 Reporting Requirements of the Oregon Death with Dignity Act (continued)

(3) To comply with ORS 127.865(1)(b), within 10 calendar days of dispensing medication pursuant to the Death with Dignity Act, the dispensing health care provider shall file a copy of the "Pharmacy Dispensing Record Form" prescribed by the Department with the State Registrar, Center for Health Statistics, 800 NE Oregon St., Suite 205, Portland, OR 97232 or by facsimile to (971) 673-1201. Information to be reported to the Department shall include:

(a) Patient's name and date of birth;

(b) Prescribing physician's name and phone number;

(c) Dispensing health care provider's name, address and phone number;

(d) Medication dispensed and quantity;

(e) Date the prescription was written; and

(f) Date the medication was dispensed.

Stat. Auth.: ORS 127.865

Stats. Implemented: ORS 127.800 - ORS 127.995 Hist.: HD 15-1997(Temp), f. & cert. ef. 11-6-97; OHD 4-1998, f. & cert. ef. 5-4-98; OHD 12-1999, f. & cert. ef. 12-28-99 Forms referenced are available from the agency at http://egov.oregon.gov/DRS/ph/pas/pasforms.shtml.

333-009-0020

Record Review/Annual Report

(1) The Department shall annually review records maintained pursuant to this Act.

(2) The Department shall generate and make available to the public an annual statistical report of information collected under this Act.

Stat. Auth.: ORS 127.865 Stats. Implemented: ORS 127.800 - ORS 127.995 and 432.060 Hist.: HD 15-1997(Temp), f. & cert. ef. 11-6-97; OHD 4-1998, f. & cert. ef. 5-4-98

333-009-0030

Confidentiality /Liability

(1) All information collected pursuant to ORS 127.800 to 127.897 including, but not limited to, the identity of patients, physicians and other health care providers, and health care facilities shall not be a public record and may not be made available for inspection by the public.

(2) All information collected pursuant to ORS 127.800 to 127.897 and the annual statistical report referred to in 333-009-0020(2) shall be considered a special morbidity and mortality study under ORS 432.060. Summary information released in statistical reports shall be aggregated to prevent identification of individuals, physicians, or health care facilities.

(3) Pursuant to ORS 432.060, providing morbidity and mortality information to the Department does not subject any physician, hospital, health care facility or other organization or person furnishing such information to an action for damages.

(4) Access to death certificate information shall be in accordance with OAR 333-011-0096 pursuant to ORS 432.121.

Stat. Auth.: ORS 127.865 Stats. Implemented: ORS 127.800–ORS 127.995,432.060, and 432.121. Hist.: HD 15-1997(Temp), f. & cert. ef. 11-6-97; OHD 4-1998, f. & cert. ef. 5-4-98

Eighth Annual Report on Oregon's Death with Dignity Act

For more information contact:

Darcy Niemeyer
Department of Human Services, Oregon State Public Health
Office of Disease Prevention and Epidemiology
800 N.E. Oregon Street, Suite 730
Portland, OR 97232

E-mail: darcy.niemeyer@state.or.us
Phone: 971-673-0982
Fax: 971-673-0994
http://www.oregon.gov/DHS/ph/pas/index.shtml

Contributing Editor: Richard Leman, MD
Data Analysis: David Hopkins, MS
State Epidemiologist: Melvin A. Kohn, MD, MPH

ACKNOWLEDGMENTS

This assessment was conducted as part of the required surveillance and public health practice activities of the Department of Human Services and was supported by Department funds.

TABLE OF CONTENTS

SUMMARY

Physician-assisted suicide (PAS) has been legal in Oregon since November 1997, when Oregon voters approved the Death with Dignity Act (DWDA) for the second time (see *History*, page 6). The Department of Human Services (DHS) is legally required to collect information regarding compliance with the Act and make the information available on a yearly basis. In this eighth annual report, we characterize the 38 Oregonians who died in 2005 following ingestion of medications prescribed under provisions of the Act, and look at whether the numbers and characteristics of these patients differ from those who used PAS in prior years. Patients choosing PAS were identified through mandated physician and pharmacy reporting. Our information comes from these reports, physician interviews and death certificates. We also compare the demographic characteristics of patients participating during 1998–2005 with other Oregonians who died of the same underlying causes.

In 2005, 39 physicians wrote a total of 64 prescriptions for lethal doses of medication. In 1998, 24 prescriptions were written, followed by 33 in 1999, 39 in 2000, 44 in 2001, 58 in 2002, 68 in 2003, and 60 in 2004. Thirty-two of the 2005 pre-scription recipients died after ingesting the medication. Of the 32 recipients who did not ingest the prescribed medication in 2005, 15 died from their illnesses, and 17 were alive on December 31, 2005. In addition, six patients who received prescriptions during 2004 died in 2005 as a result of ingesting the prescribed medication, giving a total of 38 PAS deaths during 2005. One 2004 prescription recipient, who ingested the prescribed medication in 2005, became unconscious 25 minutes after ingestion, then regained consciousness 65 hours later. This person did not obtain a subsequent prescription and died 14 days later of the underlying illness (17 days after ingesting the medication).

After an initial increase in PAS use during the first five years the Act was in effect, the number of Oregonians who use PAS remained relatively stable since 2002. In 1998, 16 Oregonians used PAS, followed by 27 in 1999, 27 in 2000, 21 in 2001, 38 in 2002, 42 in 2003, and 37 in 2004. The ratio of PAS deaths to total deaths trended upward during 1998–2003, peaking at 13.6 in 2003 and has since remained stable. In 1998 there were 5.5 PAS deaths per every 10,000 total deaths, followed by 9.2 in 1999, 9.1 in 2000, 7.1 in 2001, 12.2 in 2002, 13.6 in 2003, 12.3 in 2004, and an estimated 12/10,000 in 2005.[1–7]

Compared to all Oregon decedents in 2005, PAS participants were more likely to have malignant neoplasms (84% vs. 24%), to be younger (median age 70 vs. 78 years), and to have more formal education (37% vs. 15% had at least a baccalaureate degree).

During the past eight years, the 246 patients who took lethal medications differed in several ways from the 74,967 Oregonians dying from the same underlying diseases. Rates of participation in PAS decreased with age, although over 65% of PAS users were age 65 or older. Rates of participation were higher among those who were divorced or never married, those with more years of formal education, and those with amyotrophic lateral sclerosis, HIV/AIDS, or malignant neoplasms (see *Patient Characteristics*, page 12).

Physicians indicated that patient requests for lethal medications stemmed from multiple concerns, with eight in 10 patients having at least three concerns. The most frequently mentioned end-of-life concerns during 2005 were: a decreasing ability to participate in activities that made life enjoyable, loss of dignity, and loss of autonomy (see *End-of-Life Concerns*, page 14).

Complications were reported for three patients during 2005; two involved regurgitation, and, as noted above, one patient regained consciousness after ingesting the prescribed medication. None involved seizures (see *Complications*, page 13). Fifty percent of patients became unconscious within five minutes of ingestion of the lethal medication and the same percentage died within 26 minutes of ingestion. The range of time from ingestion to death was from five minutes to 9.5 hours. Emergency Medical Services were called for one patient in order to pronounce death.

The number of terminally ill patients using PAS has remained small, with about 1 in 800 deaths among Oregonians in 2005 resulting from physician-assisted suicide.

INTRODUCTION

This eighth annual report presents data on participation in Oregon's Death with Dignity Act (DWDA), which legalizes physician-assisted suicide (PAS) for terminally ill Oregon residents. This report summarizes the information collected from physician reports, interviews, and death certificates.

History

The Oregon Death with Dignity Act was a citizen's initiative first passed by Oregon voters in November 1994 with 51% in favor. Implementation was delayed by a legal injunction, but after proceedings that included a petition denied by the United States Supreme Court, the Ninth Circuit Court of Appeals lifted the injunction on October 27, 1997. In November 1997, a measure asking Oregon voters to repeal the Death with Dignity Act was placed on the general election ballot (Measure 51, authorized by Oregon House Bill 2954). Voters rejected this measure by a margin of 60% to 40%, retaining the Death with Dignity Act. After voters reaffirmed the DWDA in 1997, Oregon became the only state allowing legal physician-assisted suicide.[8]

Although physician-assisted suicide has been legal in Oregon for eight years, it remains highly controversial. On November 6, 2001, U.S. Attorney General John Ashcroft issued a new interpretation of the Controlled Substances Act, which would prohibit doctors from prescribing controlled substances for use in physician-assisted suicide. To date, all the medications prescribed under the Act have been barbiturates, which are controlled substances and, therefore, would be prohibited by this ruling for use in PAS. In response to a lawsuit filed by the State of Oregon on November 20, 2001, a U.S. district court issued a temporary restraining order against Ashcroft's ruling pending a new hearing. On April 17, 2002, U.S. District Court Judge Robert Jones upheld the Death with Dignity Act. On September 23, 2002, Attorney General Ashcroft filed an appeal, asking the Ninth U.S. Circuit Court of Appeals to overturn the District Court's ruling. The appeal was denied on May 26, 2004 by a three-judge panel. On July 13, 2004, Ashcroft filed an appeal requesting that the Court rehear his previous motion with an 11-judge panel; on August 13, 2004, the Court declined to rehear the case. On November 9, 2004, Ashcroft asked the U.S. Supreme Court to re-

view the Ninth Circuit's decision. On October 5, 2005, the Supreme Court heard arguments in the case, and on January 17, 2006 it affirmed the lower court's decision. At this time, Oregon's Death with Dignity Act remains in effect.

Requirements

The Death with Dignity Act allows terminally ill Oregon residents to obtain and use prescriptions from their physicians for self-administered, lethal medications. Under the Act, ending one's life in accordance with the law does not constitute suicide. However, we use "physician-assisted suicide" because that terminology is used in medical literature to describe ending life through the voluntary self-administration of lethal medications prescribed by a physician for that purpose. The Death with Dignity Act legalizes PAS, but specifically prohibits euthanasia, where a physician or other person directly administers a medication to end another's life.[8]

To request a prescription for lethal medications, the Death with Dignity Act requires that a patient must be:

- An adult (18 years of age or older),
- A resident of Oregon,
- Capable (defined as able to make and communicate health care decisions), and
- Diagnosed with a terminal illness that will lead to death within six months.

Patients meeting these requirements are eligible to request a prescription for lethal medication from a licensed Oregon physician. To receive a prescription for lethal medication, the following steps must be fulfilled:

- The patient must make two oral requests to his or her physician, separated by at least 15 days.
- The patient must provide a written request to his or her physician, signed in the presence of two witnesses.
- The prescribing physician and a consulting physician must confirm the diagnosis and prognosis.
- The prescribing physician and a consulting physician must determine whether the patient is capable.
- If either physician believes the patient's judgment is impaired by a psychiatric or psychological disorder, the patient must be referred for a psychological examination.
- The prescribing physician must inform the patient of feasible alternatives to assisted suicide, including comfort care, hospice care, and pain control.
- The prescribing physician must request, but may not require, the patient to notify his or her next-of-kin of the prescription request.

To comply with the law, physicians must report to the Department of Human Services (DHS) all prescriptions for lethal medications.[9] Reporting is not required if patients begin the request process but never receive a prescription. In 1999, the Oregon legislature added a requirement that pharmacists must be informed of the prescribed medication's intended use. Physicians and patients who adhere to the requirements of the Act are protected from criminal prosecution, and the choice of legal physician-assisted suicide cannot affect the status of a patient's health or life insurance policies. Physicians, pharmacists, and health care systems are under no obligation to participate in the Death with Dignity Act.[8]

The Oregon Revised Statutes specify that action taken in accordance with the Death with Dignity Act does not constitute suicide, mercy killing or homicide under the law.[8]

METHODS

The Reporting System

DHS is required by the Act to develop and maintain a reporting system for monitoring and collecting information on PAS.[8] To fulfill this mandate, DHS uses a system involving physician and pharmacist compliance reports, death certificate reviews, and follow-up interviews.[9]

When a prescription for lethal medication is written, the physician must submit to DHS information that documents compliance with the law. We review all physician reports and contact physicians regarding missing or discrepant data. DHS Vital Records files are searched periodically for death certificates that correspond to physician reports. These death certificates allow us to confirm patients' deaths, and provide patient demographic data (e.g., age, place of residence, educational attainment).

In addition, using our authority to conduct special studies of morbidity and mortality, DHS conducts telephone interviews with prescribing physicians after receipt of the patients' death certificates.[10] Each physician is asked to confirm whether the patient took the lethal medications. If the patient took the medications, we ask for information that was not available from previous physician reports or death certificates—including insurance status and enrollment in hospice. We ask why the patient requested a prescription, specifically exploring concerns about the financial impact of the illness, loss of autonomy, decreasing ability to participate in activities that make life enjoyable, being a burden, loss of control of bodily functions, uncontrollable pain, and loss of dignity. We collect information on the time from ingestion to unconsciousness and death, and ask about any adverse reactions. Because physicians are not legally required to be present when a patient ingests the med-

ication, not all have information about what happened when the patient ingested the medication. If the prescribing physician was not present, we accept information they have based on discussions with family members, friends or other health professionals who attended the patients' deaths. We also accept information directly from these individuals. We do not interview or collect any information from patients prior to their death. In lieu of the telephone interview, physicians have the option of printing the questionnaire from our website, completing it at their convenience, and mailing the document to us. Reporting forms and the physician questionnaire are available at: http://www.oregon.gov/DHS/ph/pas/pasforms.shtml

Data Analysis

We classified patients by year of participation based on when they ingested the legally-prescribed lethal medication. Using demographic information from 1997–2004 Oregon death certificates (the most recent years for which complete data are available), we compared patients who used legal PAS with other Oregonians who died from the same diseases. Demographic- and disease-specific PAS rates were computed using the number of deaths from the same causes as the denominator. The overall PAS rates by year were computed using the total number of resident deaths. Annual rates were calculated using numerator and denominator data from the same year, except for 2005 where the number of resident deaths from 2004 was used as the denominator. SPSS, release 12 and PEPI, version 4.0 were used in data analysis. Statistical significance was determined using Fisher's exact test, the chi-square test, the chi-square for trend test, and the Mann-Whitney test.

RESULTS

Both the number of prescriptions written and the number of Oregonians using PAS vary annually but have been relatively stable since 2002. In 2005, 39 physicians wrote 64 prescriptions for lethal doses of medication. In 1998, 24 prescriptions were written, followed by 33 in 1999, 39 in 2000, 44 in 2001, 58 in 2002, 68 in 2003, and 60 in 2004. (Figure 1.)

Thirty-two of the 2005 prescription recipients died after ingesting the medication. Of the 32 recipients who did not ingest the prescribed medication in 2005, 15 died from their illnesses, and 17 were alive on December 31, 2005. In addition, six patients who received prescriptions during 2004 died in 2005 as a result of ingesting their medication, giving a total of 38 PAS deaths during 2005.

In 1998, 16 Oregonians used PAS, followed by 27 in 1999, 27 in 2000, 21 in 2001, 38 in 2002, 42 in 2003, and 37 in 2004. Ratios of PAS deaths to total deaths have shown a similar trend: in 1998 there were 5.5 PAS deaths for every 10,000 total deaths,

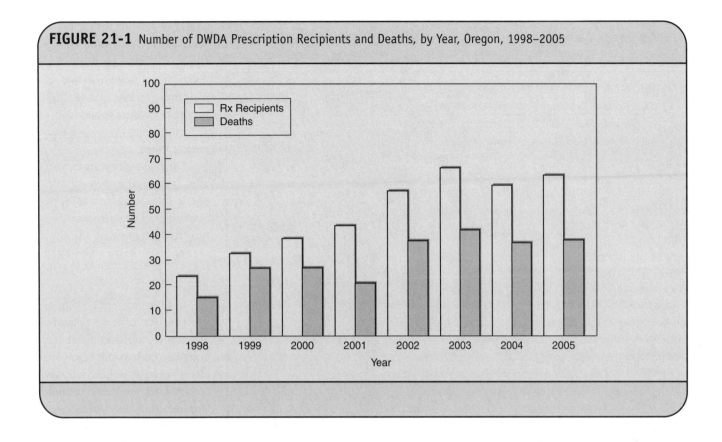

FIGURE 21-1 Number of DWDA Prescription Recipients and Deaths, by Year, Oregon, 1998–2005

followed by 9.2 in 1999, 9.1 in 2000, 7.0 in 2001, 12.2 in 2002, 13.6 in 2003, 12.3, in 2004, and an estimated 12/10,000 in 2005.

The percentage of patients referred to a specialist for psychological evaluation beyond that done by a hospice team has declined, falling from 31% in 1998 to 5% in 2005.

Patient Characteristics

There were no statistically significant differences between Oregonians who used PAS in 2005 and those from prior years. For a comparison, see Table 1.

Although year-to-year variations occur, certain demographic patterns have become evident over the past eight years. Males and females have been equally likely to take advantage of the DWDA. Divorced and never-married persons were more likely to use PAS than married and widowed residents. A higher level of education has been strongly associated with the use of PAS; Oregonians with a baccalaureate degree or higher were 7.9 times more likely to use PAS than those without a high school diploma. Conversely, several groups have emerged as being less likely to use PAS. These include people age 85 or older, people who did not graduate from high school, people who are married or widowed, and Oregon residents living east of the Cascade Range.

Patients with certain terminal illnesses were more likely to use PAS (Table 3). The ratio of DWDA deaths to all deaths resulting from the same underlying illness was highest for three conditions: amyotrophic lateral sclerosis (ALS) (269.5 per 10,000), HIV/AIDS (218.3), and malignant neoplasms (39.9). Among the causes associated with at least five deaths, the lowest rate (8.7) was for patients with chronic lower respiratory diseases (CLRD), such as emphysema.

During 2005, 36 patients died at home, and two died at assisted living facilities. All individuals had some form of health insurance (Table 4). As in previous years, most (92%) of the patients who used PAS in 2005 were enrolled in hospice care. The median length of the patient-physician relationship was 8 weeks.

Physician Characteristics

The prescribing physicians of patients who used PAS during 2005 had been in practice a median of 26 years (range 3–55). Their medical specialties included: family medicine (62%), oncology (23%), internal medicine (10%), and other (5%). Family medicine physicians represent 15% of all physicians in Oregon, oncologists 0.9%, and internists 16%.

Seventy-four percent of the physicians who wrote prescriptions for lethal medication during 2005 wrote a

TABLE 21-1 Demographic characteristics of 246 DWDA patients who died after ingesting a lethal dose of medication, by year, Oregon, 1998–2005

Characteristics	2005 (N = 38)*	1998–2004 (N = 208)*	Total (N = 246)*
Sex			
Male (%)	23 (61)	108 (52)	131 (53)
Female (%)	15 (39)	100 (48)	115 (47)
Age			
18–44 (%)	1 (3)	9 (4)	10 (4)
45–64 (%)	11 (29)	60 (29)	71 (29)
65–84 (%)	21 (55)	123 (59)	144 (59)
85+ (%)	5 (13)	16 (8)	21 (9)
Median years (Range)	70 (42–90)	69 (25–94)	69 (25–94)
Race			
White (%)	36 (95)	203 (98)	239 (97)
Asian (%)	1 (3)	5 (2)	6 (2)
Native American (%)	1 (3)	0	1 (<1)
Marital status			
Married (%)	20 (53)	90 (43)	110 (45)
Widowed (%)	8 (21)	47 (23)	55 (22)
Divorced (%)	8 (21)	56 (27)	64 (26)
Never married (%)	2 (5)	15 (7)	17 (7)
Education			
Less than high school (%)	3 (8)	18 (9)	21 (9)
High school graduate (%)	9 (24)	62 (30)	71 (29)
Some college (%)	12 (32)	40 (19)	52 (21)
Baccalaureate or higher (%)	14 (37)	88 (42)	102 (41)
Residence			
Metro counties (%)**	12 (32)	83 (40)	95 (39)
Coastal counties (%)***	2 (5)	17 (8)	19 (8)
Other W. counties (%)	21 (55)	96 (46)	117 (48)
E. of the Cascades (%)	3 (8)	12 (6)	15 (6)
Underlying illness			
Malignant neoplasms (%)	32 (84)	164 (79)	196 (80)
Lung and bronchus (%)	8 (21)	40 (19)	48 (20)
Breast (%)	4 (11)	19 (9)	23 (9)
Pancreas (%)	2 (5)	18 (9)	20 (8)
Colon (%)	4 (11)	12 (6)	16 (7)
Other (%)	14 (37)	75 (36)	89 (36)
Amyotrophic lateral sclerosis (%)	4 (11)	16 (8)	20 (8)
Chronic lower respiratory disease (%)	1 (3)	10 (5)	11 (4)
HIV/AIDS (%)	0	5 (2)	5 (2)
Illnesses listed below (%)	1 (3)	13 (6)	14 (6)

* Unknowns are excluded when calculating percentages.
** Clackamas, Multnomah, and Washington counties.
*** Excluding Douglas and Lane counties.
# Includes amyloidosis of the kidney, aortic stenosis, congestive heart failure, diabetes mellitus with renal complications, digestive organ neoplasm of unknown behavior, emphysema, hepatitis C, myelodysplastic syndrome, pulmonary disease with fibrosis, scleroderma, and Shy-Drager syndrome.

single prescription. Of the 39 physicians who wrote prescriptions in 2005, 29 wrote one prescription, three wrote two prescriptions, three wrote three prescriptions, three wrote four prescriptions, and one wrote eight prescriptions.

During the first three years after the legalization of PAS, physicians were present at the patient's ingestion of lethal medication half or more of the time. During 2005, the prescribing physician was present 23% of the time.

It is the policy of DHS to report cases to the Oregon Board of Medical Examiners when required forms have not been completed correctly or have not been received in a timely fashion. During 2005, four cases were referred to the Oregon Board of Medical Examiners, one involving witnessing of signatures and three others for failure to file required documentation in a timely manner.

One case, in which a patient awakened after ingesting the prescribed medication, was referred to the Board of Pharmacy.

Lethal Medication

During 1998–2004, secobarbital was the lethal medication prescribed for 101 of the 208 patients (49%). During 2005, as during previous years, all lethal medications prescribed under the provisions of the DWDA were barbiturates. In 2005, 34 patients (89%) used pentobarbital and 4 patients (11%) used secobarbital. Since the DWDA was implemented, 56% of the PAS patients used pentobarbital, 43% used secobarbital, and 2% used

TABLE 21-2 Demographic characteristics of 246 patients who died during 1998–2005 after ingesting a lethal dose of medication, compared with 74,967 Oregonians dying from the same underlying diseases

Characteristics	PAS patients 1998–2005 (N = 246)*	Oregon deaths, same diseases (N = 74,967)*	DWDA deaths per 10,000	Rate ratio (95% CI**)
Sex				
Male (%)	131 (53)	37,847 (50)	34.6	1.1 (0.9–1.4)
Female (%)	115 (47)	37,120 (500)	31.0	1.0
Age				
18–44 (%)	10 (4)	1,815 (2)	55.1	4.1 (1.9–8.7)#
45–64 (%)	71 (29)	14,445 (19)	49.2	3.6 (2.2–5.9)
65–84 (%)	144 (59)	42,956 (57)	33.5	2.5 (1.6–3.9)
85+ (%)	21 (9)	15,751 (21)	13.3	1.0
Median years	69 (25–94)	76		
Race				
White (%)	239 (97)	72,799 (97)	32.8	1.0
Asian (%)	6 (2)	802 (1)	74.8	2.3 (0.8–5.1)##
Native American (%)	1 (<1)	507 (1)	19.7	0.6 (0.0–3.4)##
Other (%)	0	849 (1)		
Unknown	0	15		
Marital status				
Married (%)	110 (45)	36,042 (48)	30.5	1.0
Widowed (%)	55 (22)	24,653 (33)	22.3	0.7 (0.5–1.0)
Divorced (%)	64 (26)	10.894 (15)	58.7	1.9 (1.4–2.6)+
Never married (%)	17 (7)	3,202 (4)	53.1	1.7 (1.1–2.9)+
Unknown	*0*	*176*		
Education				
Less than high school (%)	21 (9)	17,403 (24)	12.1	1.0
HS graduate (%)	71 (29)	32,125 (43)	22.1	1.8 (1.1–3.0)
Some college (%)	52 (21)	13,765 (19)	37.8	3.1 (1.9–5.2)
Baccalaureate or higher (%)	102 (41)	10.626 (14)	96.0	7.9 (5.0–12.7)#
Unknown	0	1,048		
Residence				
Metro counties (%)**	95 (39)	26,874 (36)	35.4	1.0
Coastal counties (%)***	19 (8)	6,076 (8)	31.3	0.9 (0.5–1.5)
Other W. counties (%)	117 (48)	31,470 (42)	37.2	1.1 (0.8–1.4)
E. of the Cascades (%)	15 (6)	10.547 (14)	14.2	0.4 (0.2–0.7)+

* Unknowns are excluded when calculating percentages.
** Confidence interval.
# The ratio is statistically significant according to the chi-square test for trend.
Confidence intervals calculated with Fisher's exact test.
+ The ratio is statistically significant according to the chi-square test.

other medications. (Three used secobarbital/amobarbital, and one used secobarbital and morphine).

Complications

During 2005, physicians reported that three patients experienced complications: two patients vomited some of the medication, one of whom died 15 minutes after ingestion and the other 90 minutes after ingestion. The former had been vomiting on a daily basis for the week and a half prior to ingestion. One patient became unconscious 25 minutes after ingestion, then regained consciousness 65 hours later. This person did not obtain a subsequent prescription, and died 14 days later of the underlying illness (17 days after ingesting the medication).

None of the patients experienced seizures. Emergency medical services were called to document one death. In no case was EMS called for medical intervention.

End-of-Life Concerns

Providers were asked if, based on discussions with patients, any of seven end-of-life concerns might have contributed to the patients' requests for lethal medication (Table 4). In nearly all cases, physicians reported multiple concerns contributing to the request. The most frequently reported concerns included a decreasing ability to participate in activities that make life enjoyable (89%), loss of dignity (89%), and losing autonomy (79%).

COMMENTS

Since 2002, both the number of prescriptions written for physician-assisted suicide and the number of terminally ill patients taking lethal medication have remained relatively stable with about 1 in 800 deaths among Oregonians in 2005 resulting from physician-assisted suicide. A large population study of dying Oregonians published in 2004 found that 17% considered PAS seriously enough to have discussed the matter with their family and that about 2% of patients formally requested PAS. Of the 1,384 decedents for whom information was gathered, one had received a prescription for lethal medication and did not take it. No unreported cases of PAS were identified.[11]

Overall, smaller numbers of patients appear to use PAS in Oregon compared to the Netherlands.[12] However, as detailed in previous reports, our numbers are based on a reporting system for terminally ill patients who legally receive prescriptions for lethal medications, and do not include patients and physicians who may act outside the provisions of the DWDA.

Over the last eight years, the rate of PAS among patients with ALS in Oregon has been substantially higher than among patients with other illnesses. This finding is consistent with other studies. In the Netherlands, where both PAS and euthanasia are openly practiced, one in five ALS patients died as a result of PAS or euthanasia.[13] A study of Oregon and Washington ALS patients found that one-third of these patients discussed wanting PAS in the last month of life.[14] Though numbers are small, and results must be interpreted with caution, Oregon HIV/AIDS patients are also more likely to use PAS.

Physicians have consistently reported that concerns about loss of autonomy, loss of dignity, and decreased ability to participate in activities that make life enjoyable were important motivating factors in patient requests for lethal medication across all eight years. Interviews with family members during 1999 corroborated physician reports.[2] These findings were supported by a study of hospice nurses and social workers caring for PAS patients in Oregon.[15]

While it may be common for patients with a terminal illness to consider PAS, a request for PAS can be an opportunity for a medical provider to explore with patients their fears and wishes around end-of-life care, and to make patients aware of other options. Often once the provider has addressed a patient's concerns, he or she may choose not to pursue PAS.[16]

TABLE 21-3 Underlying illnesses of 246 patients who died during 1998–2005 after ingesting a lethal dose of medication, compared with 74,967 Oregonians dying from the same underlying diseases

Underlying illnesses	PAS patients 1998–2005 (N = 246)	Oregon deaths, same diseases (N = 74,967)	DWDA deaths per 10,000 Oregon deaths	Rate ratio (95% CI*)
Malignant neoplasms (%)	196 (80)	49,117 (66)	39.9	4.6 (2.5–8.4)[+]
Lung and bronchus (%)	48 (20)	16,160 (22)	29.7	3.4 (1.8–6.6)[+]
Breast (%)	23 (9)	4,102 (5)	56.1	6.4 (3.1–13.2)[+]
Pancreas (%)	20 (8)	2,989 (4)	66.9	7.7 (3.7–16.0)[+]
Colon (%)	16 (7)	4,263 (6)	37.5	4.3 (2.0–9.3)[+]
Prostate (%)	13 (5)	3,491 (5)	37.2	4.3 (1.9–9.5)[++]
Ovary (%)	12 (5)	1,608 (2)	74.6	8.6 (3.5–21.5)[++]
Skin (%)	9 (4)	789 (1)	114.1	13.1 (4.8–35.1)[++]
Other (%)	55 (22)	15,715 (21)	35.0	4.0 (2.1–7.6)[+]
Amyotrophic lateral sclerosis (%)	20 (8)	742 (1)	269.5	31.0 (14.4–73.5)[++]
Chronic lower respiratory dis. (%)	11 (4)	12,596 (17)	8.7	1.0
HIV/AIDS (%)	5 (2)	229 (<1)	218.3	25.1 (6.9–80.4)[++]
Illnesses listed below (%)#	14 (6)	12,283 (16)	11.4	1.3 (0.6–2.9)

* Confidence interval.
# Includes amyloidosis of the kidney, aortic stenosis, cardiomyopathy, congestive heart failure, diabetes mellitus with renal complications, digestive organ neoplasm of unknown behavior, emphysema, hepatitis C, myelodysplastic syndrome, pulmonary disease with fibrosis, scleroderma, and Shy-Drager syndrome.
[+] The ratio is statistically significant according to the chi-square test.
[++] The ratio is statistically significant according to Fisher's exact test.

TABLE 21-4 Death with Dignity end of life care for 246 Oregonians who died after ingesting a lethal dose of medication, by year, 1998–2005

Characteristics	2005 (N = 38)*	1998–2004 (N = 208)*	Total (N = 246)*
End of Life Care			
Hospice			
Enrolled (%)	35 (92)	178 (86)	213 (87)
Not enrolled (%)	3 (8)	28 (14)	31 (13)
Unknown	0	2	2
Insurance			
Private (%)	22 (58)	129 (63)	151 (62)
Medicare or Medicaid (%)	16 (42)	74 (36)	90 (37)
None (%)	0	2 (1)	2 (1)
Unknown	0	3	3
End of Life Concerns*			
Losing autonomy (%)	30 (79)	177 (87)	207 (86)
Less able to engage in activities making life enjoyable (%)	34 (89)	172 (84)	206 (85)
Loss of dignity (%)++	34 (89)	60 (80)	94 (83)
losing control of bodily functions (%)	17 (45)	121 (59)	138 (57)
Burden on family, friends/caregivers (%)	16 (42)	74 (36)	90 (37)
Inadequate pain control or concern about it (%)	9 (24)	45 (22)	54 (22)
Financial implications of treatment (%)	1 (3)	6 (3)	7 (3)
PAS Process			
Referred for psychiatric evaluation (%)	2 (5)	32 (16)	34 (14)
Patient died at Home (patient, family or friend) (%)	36 (95)	196 (94)	232 (94)
Long term care, assisted living or foster care facility (%)	2 (5)	9 (4)	11 (4)
Hospital (%)	0	1 (<1)	1 (<1)
Other (%)	0	2 (1)	2 (1)
Lethal Medication			
Secobarbital (%)	4 (11)	101 (49)	105 (43)
Pentobarbital (%)	34 (89)	103 (50)	137 (56)
Other (%)	0	4 (2)	4 (2)
Health-care provider present when medication ingested†			
Prescribing physician (%)	8 (23)	40 (29)	48 (28)
Other provider, when prescribing physician not present (%)	18 (51)	74 (54)	92 (54)
No provider (%)	9 (26)	22 (16)	31 (18)
Unknown	3	2	5
Complications			
Regurgitated (%)	2 (5)	10 (5)	12 (5)
Seizures (%)	0	0	0
Awakened after taking prescribed medication††	1	0	1
No complications (%)	35 (95)	194 (94)	229 (95)
Unknown	1	4	5

continues

TABLE 21-4 Death with Dignity end of life care for 246 Oregonians who died after ingesting a lethal dose of medication, by year, 1998–2005 (continued)

Characteristics	2005 (N = 38)*	1998–2004 (N = 208)*	Total (N = 246)*
Emergency Medical Services			
Called for intervention after lethal medication ingested (%)	0	0	0
Calls for other reasons (%)**	1 (3)	2 (1)	3 (1)
Not called after lethal medication ingested (%)	36 (97)	203 (99)	239 (99)
Unknown	1	3	4
Timing of PAS Event			
Duration (weeks) of patient-physician relationship			
Median	8	12	12
Range	0–678	0–1065	0–1065
Duration (days) between 1st request and death			
Median	40	38	39
Range	15–1009	15–737	15–1009
Minutes between ingestion and unconsciousness			
Median	5	5	5
Range	2–15	1–38	1–38
Unknown	3	21	24
Time between ingestion and death			
Median (minutes)	26	25	25
Range (minutes–hours)	5m–9.5h	4m–48h	4m–48h
Unknown	2	15	17

* Unknowns are excluded when calculating percentages unless otherwise noted.

** Calls included two to pronounce death and one to help a patient who had fallen.

† The data shown are for 2001–2005. Information about the presence of a health care provider/volunteer, in absence of the prescribing physician, was first collected in 2001. Attendance by the prescribing physician has been recorded since 1998. During 1998–2005 the prescribing physician was present when 35% of the patients ingested the lethal medication.

†† Historically, the Annual Report tables list information on patients who died as a result of ingesting medication prescribed under the provisions of the Death with Dignity Act. Because one patient regained consciousness after ingesting the lethal medication and then died 14 days later from his/her illness rather than from the medication, the complication is recorded here but the patient is not included in the total number of PAS deaths.

+ Affirmative answers only ("Don't know" included in negative answers). Available for 17 patients in 2001.

++ First asked in 2003.

REFERENCES

1. Chin G, Hedberg K, Higginson G, Fleming D. Legalized physician-assisted suicide in Oregon—The first year's experience. N Engl J Med, 1999; 340:577–583.

2. Sullivan AD, Hedberg K, Fleming D. Legalized physician-assisted suicide in Oregon—The second year. N Engl J Med, 2000; 342:598–604.

3. Sullivan AD, Hedberg K, Hopkins D. Legalized physician-assisted suicide in Oregon, 1998–2000. N Engl J Med, 2001; 344:605–607.

4. Hedberg K, Hopkins D, Southwick K. Legalized physician-assisted suicide in Oregon, 2001. N Engl J Med, 2002; 346:450–452.

5. Hedberg K, Hopkins D, Kohn M. Five years of legal physician-assisted suicide in Oregon. N Engl J Med, 2003; 348:961–964.

6. Oregon Department of Human Services. Sixth Annual Report on Oregon's Death with Dignity Act. Office of Disease Prevention and Epidemiology. March 10, 2004. Portland, Oregon. 24 pp. Available at http://www.oregon.gov/DHS/ph/pas/docs/year6.pdf

7. Oregon Department of Human Services. Seventh Annual Report on Oregon's Death with Dignity Act. Office of Disease Prevention and Epidemiology. March 10, 2005. Portland, Oregon. 25 pp. Available at http://www.oregon.gov/DHS/ph/pas/docs/year7.pdf

8. Oregon Revised Statute 127.800–127.995. Available at http://egov.oregon.gov/DHS/ph/pas/ors.shtml

9. Oregon Administrative Rules 333-009-000 to 333-009-0030. Available at http://egov.oregon.gov/DHS/ph/pas/oars.shtml

10. Oregon Revised Statute 432.060. Available at http://www.leg.state.or.us/ors/432.html

11. Tolle SW, Tilden VP, Drach LL, et al. Characteristics and proportion of dying Oregonians who personally consider physician assisted suicide. J Clin Ethics, 2004;15:111–118.

12. Willems DL, Daniels ER, van der Wal G, et al. Attitudes and practices concerning the end of life: A comparison between physicians from the United States and from The Netherlands. Arch Intern Med, 2000;160:63–68.

13. Vledink JH, Wokke JHJ, Van Der Wal G, et al. Euthanasia and physician-assisted suicide among patients with amyotrophic lateral sclerosis in the Netherlands. N Engl J Med, 2002; 346:1638–1644.

14. Ganzini L, Silveira MJ, Johnston WS. Predictors and correlates of interest in assisted suicide in the final month of life among ALS patients in Oregon and Washington. J Pain Symptom Manage, 2002; 3:312–317.

15. Ganzini L, Harvath TA, Jackson A, et al. Experiences of Oregon nurses and social workers with hospice patients who requested assistance with suicide. N Engl J Med, 2002; 347:582–588.

16. Bascom PB, Tolle SW. Responding to requests for physician-assisted suicide: "these are uncharted waters for both of us. . . ." JAMA, 2002; 288:91–98.

Case Law: *Gonzalez v. Oregon* (Physician-Assisted Suicide)

ALBERTO R. GONZALES, ATTORNEY GENERAL, et al., PETITIONERS v. OREGON et al.

ON WRIT OF CERTIORARI TO THE UNITED STATES COURT OF APPEALS FOR THE NINTH CIRCUIT

[January 17, 2006]

Kennedy, J., delivered the opinion of the Court, in which Stevens, O'Connor, Souter, Ginsburg, and Breyer, JJ., joined. Scalia, J., filed a dissenting opinion, in which Roberts, C. J., and Thomas, J., joined. Thomas, J., filed a dissenting opinion.

Justice Kennedy delivered the opinion of the Court.

The question before us is whether the Controlled Substances Act allows the United States Attorney General to prohibit doctors from prescribing regulated drugs for use in physician-assisted suicide, notwithstanding a state law permitting the procedure. As the Court has observed, "Americans are engaged in an earnest and profound debate about the morality, legality, and practicality of physician-assisted suicide." *Washington v. Glucksberg,* 521 U.S. 702, 735 (1997). The dispute before us is in part a product of this political and moral debate, but its resolution requires an inquiry familiar to the courts: interpreting a federal statute to determine whether Executive action is authorized by, or otherwise consistent with, the enactment.

In 1994, Oregon became the first State to legalize assisted suicide when voters approved a ballot measure enacting the Oregon Death With Dignity Act (ODWDA). Ore. Rev. Stat. §127.800 *et seq.* (2003). ODWDA, which survived a 1997 ballot measure seeking its repeal, exempts from civil or criminal liability state-licensed physicians who, in compliance with the specific safeguards in ODWDA, dispense or prescribe a lethal dose of drugs upon the request of a terminally ill patient.

The drugs Oregon physicians prescribe under ODWDA are regulated under a federal statute, the Controlled Substances Act (CSA or Act). 84 Stat. 1242, as amended, 21 U.S.C. § 801 *et seq.* The CSA allows these particular drugs to be available only by a written prescription from a registered physician. In the ordinary course the same drugs are prescribed in smaller doses for pain alleviation.

A November 9, 2001 Interpretive Rule issued by the Attorney General addresses the implementation and enforcement of the CSA with respect to ODWDA. It determines that using controlled substances to assist suicide is not a legitimate medical practice and that dispensing or prescribing them for this purpose is unlawful under the CSA. The Interpretive Rule's validity under the CSA is the issue before us.

I

A

We turn first to the text and structure of the CSA. Enacted in 1970 with the main objectives of combating drug abuse and controlling the legitimate and illegitimate traffic in controlled substances, the CSA creates a comprehensive, closed regulatory regime criminalizing the unauthorized manufacture, distribution, dispensing, and possession of substances classified in any of the Act's five schedules. *Gonzales* v. *Raich,* 545 U.S. ____, ____ (2005) (slip op., at 9–10); 21 U.S.C. § 841 (2000 ed. and Supp. II); 21 U.S.C. § 844. The Act places substances in one of five schedules based on their potential for abuse or dependence, their accepted medical use, and their accepted safety for use under medical supervision. Schedule I contains the most severe restrictions on access and use, and Schedule V the least. *Raich, supra*, at ___ (slip op., at 11); 21 U.S.C. § 812. Congress classified a host of substances when it enacted the CSA, but the statute permits the Attorney General to add, remove, or reschedule substances. He may do so, however, only after making particular findings, and on scientific and medical matters he is required to accept the findings of the Secretary of Health and Human Services (Secretary). These proceedings must be on the record after an opportunity for comment. See 21 U.S.C. A. §811 (main ed. and Supp. 2005).

The present dispute involves controlled substances listed in Schedule II, substances generally available only pursuant to a written, nonrefillable prescription by a physician. 21 U.S.C. § 829(a). A 1971 regulation promulgated by the Attorney General requires that every prescription for a controlled substance "be issued for a legitimate medical purpose by an individual practitioner acting in the usual course of his professional practice." 21 CFR § 1306.04(a) (2005).

To prevent diversion of controlled substances with medical uses, the CSA regulates the activity of physicians. To issue lawful prescriptions of Schedule II drugs, physicians must "obtain from the Attorney General a registration issued in accordance with the rules and regulations promulgated by him." 21 U.S.C. § 822(a)(2). The Attorney General may deny, suspend, or revoke this registration if, as relevant here, the physician's registration would be "inconsistent with the public interest." §824(a)(4); §822(a)(2). When deciding whether a practitioner's registration is in the public interest, the Attorney General "shall" consider:

(1) The recommendation of the appropriate State licensing board or professional disciplinary authority.
(2) The applicant's experience in dispensing, or conducting research with respect to controlled substances.
(3) The applicant's conviction record under Federal or State laws relating to the manufacture, distribution, or dispensing of controlled substances.
(4) Compliance with applicable State, Federal, or local laws relating to controlled substances.
(5) Such other conduct which may threaten the public health and safety. §823(f).

The CSA explicitly contemplates a role for the States in regulating controlled substances, as evidenced by its preemption provision.

"No provision of this subchapter shall be construed as indicating an intent on the part of the Congress to occupy the field in which that provision operates . . . to the exclusion of any State law on the same subject matter which would otherwise be within the authority of the State, unless there is a positive conflict between that provision . . . and that State law so that the two cannot consistently stand together." §903.

B

Oregon voters enacted ODWDA in 1994. For Oregon residents to be eligible to request a prescription under ODWDA, they must receive a diagnosis from their attending physician that they have an incurable and irreversible disease that, within reasonable medical judgment, will cause death within six months. Ore. Rev. Stat. §§127.815, 127.800(12) (2003). Attending physicians must also determine whether a patient has made a voluntary request, ensure a patient's choice is informed, and refer patients to counseling if they might be suffering from a psychological disorder or depression causing impaired judgment. §§127.815, 127.825. A second "consulting" physician must examine the patient and the medical record and confirm the attending physician's conclusions. §127.800(8). Oregon physicians may dispense or issue a prescription for the requested drug, but may not administer it. §§127.815(L), 127.880.

The reviewing physicians must keep detailed medical records of the process leading to the final prescription, §127.855, records that Oregon's Department of Human Services reviews, §127.865. Physicians who dispense medication pursuant to ODWDA must also be registered with both the State's Board of Medical Examiners and the federal Drug Enforcement Administration (DEA). §127.815(1)(L). In 2004, 37 patients ended their lives by ingesting a lethal dose of medication prescribed under ODWDA. Oregon Dept. of Human Servs., Seventh Annual Report on Oregon's Death with Dignity Act 20 (Mar. 10, 2005).

C

In 1997, Members of Congress concerned about ODWDA invited the DEA to prosecute or revoke the CSA registration of Oregon physicians who assist suicide. They contended that hastening a patient's death is not legitimate medical practice, so prescribing controlled substances for that purpose violates the CSA. Letter from Sen. Orrin Hatch and Rep. Henry Hyde to Thomas A. Constantine (July 25, 1997), reprinted in Hearings on S. 2151 before the Senate Committee on the Judiciary, 105th Cong., 2d Sess., 2–3 (1999) (hereinafter Hearings). The letter received an initial, favorable response from the director of the DEA, see Letter from Thomas A. Constantine to Sen. Orrin Hatch (Nov. 5, 1997), Hearings 4–5, but Attorney General Reno considered the matter and concluded that the DEA could not take the proposed action because the CSA did not authorize it to displace the states as the primary regulators of the medical profession, or to override a state's determination as to what constitutes legitimate medical practice, Letter from Attorney General Janet Reno to Sen. Orrin Hatch, on Oregon's Death with Dignity Act (June 5, 1998), Hearings 5–6. Legislation was then introduced to grant the explicit authority Attorney General Reno found lacking; but it failed to pass. See H. R. 4006, 105th Cong., 2d Sess. (1998); H. R. 2260, 106th Cong., 1st Sess. (1999).

In 2001, John Ashcroft was appointed Attorney General. Perhaps because Mr. Ashcroft had supported efforts to curtail assisted suicide while serving as a Senator, see, *e.g.*, 143 Cong. Rec. 5589–5590 (1997) (remarks of Sen. Ashcroft), Oregon Attorney General Hardy Myers wrote him to request a meeting with Department of Justice officials should the Department decide to revisit the application of the CSA to assisted suicide. Letter of Feb. 2, 2001, App. to Brief for Patient-Respondents in Opposition 55a. Attorney General Myers received a reply letter from one of Attorney General Ashcroft's advisers writing on his behalf, which stated

"I am aware of no pending legislation in Congress that would prompt a review of the Department's interpretation of the CSA as it relates to physician-assisted suicide. Should such a review be commenced in the future, we would be happy to include your views in that review." Letter from Lori Sharpe (Apr. 17, 2001), *id.,* at 58a.

On November 9, 2001, without consulting Oregon or apparently anyone outside his Department, the Attorney General issued an Interpretive Rule announcing his intent to restrict the use of controlled substances for physician-assisted suicide. Incorporating the legal analysis of a memorandum he had solicited from his Office of Legal Counsel, the Attorney General ruled "assisting suicide is not a legitimate medical purpose within the meaning of 21 CFR 1306.04 (2001), and that prescribing, dispensing, or administering federally controlled substances to assist suicide violates the Controlled Substances Act. Such conduct by a physician registered to dispense controlled substances may render his registration . . . inconsistent with the public interest and therefore subject to possible suspension or revocation under 21 U.S.C. 824(a)(4). The Attorney General's conclusion applies regardless of whether state law authorizes or permits such conduct by practitioners or others and regardless of the condition of the person whose suicide is assisted." 66 Fed. Reg. 56608 (2001).

There is little dispute that the Interpretive Rule would substantially disrupt the ODWDA regime. Respondents contend, and petitioners do not dispute, that every prescription filled under ODWDA has specified drugs classified under Schedule II. A physician cannot prescribe the substances without DEA registration, and revocation or suspension of the registration would be a severe restriction on medical practice. Dispensing

controlled substances without a valid prescription, furthermore, is a federal crime. See, *e.g.,* 21 U.S.C. § 841(a)(1) (2000 ed., Supp. II); *United States* v. *Moore,* 423 U.S. 122 (1975).

In response the State of Oregon, joined by a physician, a pharmacist, and some terminally ill patients, all from Oregon, challenged the Interpretive Rule in federal court. The United States District Court for the District of Oregon entered a permanent injunction against the Interpretive Rule's enforcement.

A divided panel of the Court of Appeals for the Ninth Circuit granted the petitions for review and held the Interpretive Rule invalid. *Oregon* v. *Ashcroft,* 368 F.3d 1118 (2004). It reasoned that, by making a medical procedure authorized under Oregon law a federal offense, the Interpretive Rule altered the "usual constitutional balance between the States and the Federal Government" without the requisite clear statement that the CSA authorized such action. *Id.,* at 1124–1125 (quoting *Gregory* v. *Ashcroft,* 501 U.S. 452, 460 (1991) (in turn quoting *Atascadero State Hospital* v. *Scanlon,* 473 U.S. 234, 242 (1985))). The Court of Appeals held in the alternative that the Interpretive Rule could not be squared with the plain language of the CSA, which targets only conventional drug abuse and excludes the Attorney General from decisions on medical policy. 368 F.3d, at 1125–1129.

We granted the Government's petition for certiorari. 543 U.S. 1145 (2005).

II

Executive actors often must interpret the enactments Congress has charged them with enforcing and implementing. The parties before us are in sharp disagreement both as to the degree of deference we must accord the Interpretive Rule's substantive conclusions and whether the Rule is authorized by the statutory text at all. Although balancing the necessary respect for an agency's knowledge, expertise, and constitutional office with the courts' role as interpreter of laws can be a delicate matter, familiar principles guide us. An administrative rule may receive substantial deference if it interprets the issuing agency's own ambiguous regulation. *Auer* v. *Robbins,* 519 U.S. 452, 461–463 (1997). An interpretation of an ambiguous statute may also receive substantial deference. *Chevron U.S. A. Inc.* v. *Natural Resources Defense Council, Inc.,* 4, 842–845 (1984). Deference in accordance with *Chevron,* however, is warranted only "when it appears that Congress delegated authority to the agency generally to make rules carrying the force of law, and that the agency interpretation claiming deference was promulgated in the exercise of that authority." *United States* v. *Mead Corp.,* 533 U.S. 218, 226–227 (2001). Otherwise, the interpretation is "entitled to respect" only to the extent it has the power to persuade. *Skidmore* v. *Swift & Co.,* 323 U.S. 134, 140 (1944).

A

The Government first argues that the Interpretive Rule is an elaboration of one of the Attorney General's own regulations, 21 CFR § 1306.04 (2005), which requires all prescriptions be issued "for a legitimate medical purpose by an individual practitioner acting in the usual course of his professional practice." As such, the Government says, the Interpretive Rule is entitled to considerable deference in accordance with *Auer*.

In our view *Auer* and the standard of deference it accords to an agency are inapplicable here. *Auer* involved a disputed interpretation of the Fair Labor Standards Act of 1938 as applied to a class of law enforcement officers. Under regulations promulgated by the Secretary of Labor, an exemption from overtime pay depended, in part, on whether the employees met the "salary basis" test. 519 U.S., at 454–455. In this Court the Secretary of Labor filed an *amicus* brief explaining why, in his view, the regulations gave exempt status to the officers. *Id.*, at 461. We gave weight to that interpretation, holding that because the applicable test was "a creature of the Secretary's own regulations, his interpretation of it is, under our jurisprudence, controlling unless plainly erroneous or inconsistent with the regulation." *Ibid.* (internal quotation marks omitted).

In *Auer*, the underlying regulations gave specificity to a statutory scheme the Secretary was charged with enforcing and reflected the considerable experience and expertise the Department of Labor had acquired over time with respect to the complexities of the Fair Labor Standards Act. Here, on the other hand, the underlying regulation does little more than restate the terms of the statute itself. The language the Interpretive Rule addresses comes from Congress, not the Attorney General, and the near-equivalence of the statute and regulation belies the Government's argument for *Auer* deference.

The Government does not suggest that its interpretation turns on any difference between the statutory and regulatory language. The CSA allows prescription of drugs only if they have a "currently accepted medical use," 21 U.S.C. § 812(b); requires a "medical purpose" for dispensing the least controlled substances of those on the schedules, §829(c); and, in its reporting provision, defines a "valid prescription" as one "issued for a legitimate medical purpose," §830(b)(3)(A)(ii). Similarly, physicians are considered to be acting as practitioners under the statute if they dispense controlled substances "in the course of professional practice." §802(21). The regulation uses the terms "legitimate medical purpose" and "the course of professional practice," *ibid.*, but this just repeats two statutory phrases and attempts to summarize the others. It gives little or no instruction on a central issue in this case: Who decides whether a particular activity is in "the course of professional practice" or done for a "legitimate medical purpose?" Since the regula-

tion gives no indication how to decide this issue, the Attorney General's effort to decide it now cannot be considered an interpretation of the regulation. Simply put, the existence of a parroting regulation does not change the fact that the question here is not the meaning of the regulation but the meaning of the statute. An agency does not acquire special authority to interpret its own words when, instead of using its expertise and experience to formulate a regulation, it has elected merely to paraphrase the statutory language.

Furthermore, as explained below, if there is statutory authority to issue the Interpretive Rule it comes from the 1984 amendments to the CSA that gave the Attorney General authority to register and deregister physicians based on the public interest. The regulation was enacted before those amendments, so the Interpretive Rule cannot be justified as indicative of some intent the Attorney General had in 1971. That the current interpretation runs counter to the "intent at the time of the regulation's promulgation," is an additional reason why *Auer* deference is unwarranted. *Thomas Jefferson Univ.* v. *Shalala,* 512 U.S. 504, 512 (1994) (internal quotation marks omitted). Deference under *Auer* being inappropriate, we turn to the question whether the Interpretive Rule, on its own terms, is a permissible interpretation of the CSA.

B

Just as the Interpretive Rule receives no deference under *Auer*, neither does it receive deference under *Chevron*. If a statute is ambiguous, judicial review of administrative rule making often demands *Chevron* deference; and the rule is judged accordingly. All would agree, we should think, that the statutory phrase "legitimate medical purpose" is a generality, susceptible to more precise definition and open to varying constructions, and thus ambiguous in the relevant sense. *Chevron* deference, however, is not accorded merely because the statute is ambiguous and an administrative official is involved. To begin with, the rule must be promulgated pursuant to authority Congress has delegated to the official. *Mead*, 533 U.S., at 226–227.

The Attorney General has rulemaking power to fulfill his duties under the CSA. The specific respects in which he is authorized to make rules, however, instruct us that he is not authorized to make a rule declaring illegitimate a medical standard for care and treatment of patients that is specifically authorized under state law.

The starting point for this inquiry is, of course, the language of the delegation provision itself. In many cases authority is clear because the statute gives an agency broad power to enforce all provisions of the statute. See, *e.g., National Cable & Telecommunications Assn.* v. *Brand X Internet Services,* 545 U.S. ___, ___ (2005) (slip op., at 8) (explaining that a Federal

Communications Commission regulation received *Chevron* deference "because Congress has delegated to the Commission the authority to . . . 'prescribe such rules and regulations as may be necessary in the public interest to carry out the provisions' of the Act" (quoting 47 U.S.C. § 201(b))); *Household Credit Services, Inc.* v. *Pfennig*, 541 U.S. 232, 238 (2004) (giving *Chevron* deference to a Federal Reserve Board regulation where "Congress has expressly delegated to the Board the authority to prescribe regulations . . . as, in the judgment of the Board, 'are necessary or proper to effectuate the purposes of'" the statute (quoting 15 U.S.C. § 1604(a))). The CSA does not grant the Attorney General this broad authority to promulgate rules.

The CSA gives the Attorney General limited powers, to be exercised in specific ways. His rulemaking authority under the CSA is described in two provisions: (1) "The Attorney General is authorized to promulgate rules and regulations and to charge reasonable fees relating to the registration and control of the manufacture, distribution, and dispensing of controlled substances and to listed chemicals," 21 U.S.C. A. §821 (Supp. 2005); and (2) "The Attorney General may promulgate and enforce any rules, regulations, and procedures which he may deem necessary and appropriate for the efficient execution of his functions under this subchapter," 21 U.S.C. § 871(b). As is evident from these sections, Congress did not delegate to the Attorney General authority to carry out or effect all provisions of the CSA. Rather, he can promulgate rules relating only to "registration" and "control," and "for the efficient execution of his functions" under the statute.

Turning first to the Attorney General's authority to make regulations for the control of drugs, this delegation cannot sustain the Interpretive Rule's attempt to define standards of medical practice. Control is a term of art in the CSA. "As used in this subchapter," §802—the subchapter that includes §821— "The term 'control' means to add a drug or other substance, or immediate precursor, to a schedule under part B of this subchapter, whether by transfer from another schedule or otherwise." §802(5).

To exercise his scheduling power, the Attorney General must follow a detailed set of procedures, including requesting a scientific and medical evaluation from the Secretary. See 21 U.S.C. A. §§811, 812 (main ed. and Supp. 2005). The statute is also specific as to the manner in which the Attorney General must exercise this authority: "Rules of the Attorney General under this subsection [regarding scheduling] shall be made on the record after opportunity for a hearing pursuant to the rule making procedures prescribed by [the Administrative Procedure Act, 5 U.S.C. § 553]." 21 U.S.C. § 811(a). The Interpretive Rule now under consideration does not concern the scheduling of substances and was not issued after the re-

quired procedures for rules regarding scheduling, so it cannot fall under the Attorney General's "control" authority.

Even if "control" in §821 were understood to signify something other than its statutory definition, it would not support the Interpretive Rule. The statutory references to control outside the scheduling context make clear that the Attorney General can establish controls "against diversion," *e.g.*, §823(a)(1), but do not give him authority to define diversion based on his view of legitimate medical practice. As explained below, the CSA's express limitations on the Attorney General's authority, and other indications from the statutory scheme, belie any notion that the Attorney General has been granted this implicit authority. Indeed, if "control" were given the expansive meaning required to sustain the Interpretive Rule, it would transform the carefully described limits on the Attorney General's authority over registration and scheduling into mere suggestions.

We turn, next, to the registration provisions of the CSA. Before 1984, the Attorney General was required to register any physician who was authorized by his State. The Attorney General could only deregister a physician who falsified his application, was convicted of a felony relating to controlled substances, or had his state license or registration revoked. See 84 Stat. 1255. The CSA was amended in 1984 to allow the Attorney General to deny registration to an applicant "if he determines that the issuance of such registration would be inconsistent with the public interest." 21 U.S.C. § 823(f). Registration may also be revoked or suspended by the Attorney General on the same grounds. §824(a)(4). In determining consistency with the public interest, the Attorney General must, as discussed above, consider five factors, including: the State's recommendation; compliance with state, federal, and local laws regarding controlled substances; and public health and safety. §823(f).

The Interpretive Rule cannot be justified under this part of the statute. It does not undertake the five-factor analysis and concerns much more than registration. Nor does the Interpretive Rule on its face purport to be an application of the registration provision in §823(f). It is, instead, an interpretation of the substantive federal law requirements (under 21 CFR § 1306.04 (2005)) for a valid prescription. It begins by announcing that assisting suicide is not a "legitimate medical purpose" under §1306.04, and that dispensing controlled substances to assist a suicide violates the CSA. 66 Fed. Reg. 56608 (2001). Violation is a criminal offense, and often a felony, under 21 U.S.C. § 841 (2000 ed. and Supp. II). The Interpretive Rule thus purports to declare that using controlled substances for physician-assisted suicide is a crime, an authority that goes well beyond the Attorney General's statutory power to register or deregister.

The Attorney General's deregistration power, of course, may carry implications for criminal enforcement because if a physician dispenses a controlled substance after he is deregistered, he violates §841. The Interpretive Rule works in the opposite direction, however: it declares certain conduct criminal, placing in jeopardy the registration of any physician who engages in that conduct. To the extent the Interpretive Rule concerns registration, it simply states the obvious because one of the five factors the Attorney General must consider in deciding the "public interest" is "[c]ompliance with applicable State, Federal, or local laws relating to controlled substances." 21 U.S.C. § 823(f)(4). The problem with the design of the Interpretive Rule is that it cannot, and does not, explain why the Attorney General has the authority to decide what constitutes an underlying violation of the CSA in the first place. The explanation the Government seems to advance is that the Attorney General's authority to decide whether a physician's actions are inconsistent with the "public interest" provides the basis for the Interpretive Rule.

By this logic, however, the Attorney General claims extraordinary authority. If the Attorney General's argument were correct, his power to deregister necessarily would include the greater power to criminalize even the actions of registered physicians, whenever they engage in conduct he deems illegitimate. This power to criminalize—unlike his power over registration, which must be exercised only after considering five express statutory factors—would be unrestrained. It would be anomalous for Congress to have so painstakingly described the Attorney General's limited authority to deregister a single physician or schedule a single drug, but to have given him, just by implication, authority to declare an entire class of activity outside the course of professional practice, and therefore a criminal violation of the CSA. See *Federal Maritime Comm'n* v. *Seatrain Lines, Inc.,* 411 U.S. 726, 744 (1973) ("In light of these specific grants of . . . authority, we are unwilling to construe the ambiguous provisions . . . to serve this purpose [of creating further authority]—a purpose for which it obviously was not intended").

Sutton v. *United Air Lines, Inc.,* 527 U.S. 471 (1999), is instructive. The statute at issue was the Americans with Disabilities Act of 1990 (ADA), which, like the CSA, divides interpretive authority among various Executive actors. The Court relied on the "terms and structure of the ADA" to decide that neither the Equal Employment Opportunity Commission, nor any other agency had authority to define "disability" in the ADA. *Id.,* at 479. Specifically, the delegating provision stated that the EEOC "shall issue regulations . . . to carry out this subchapter," 42 U.S.C. § 12116 and the section of the statute defining "disability" was in a different subchapter. The Court did not accept the idea that because "the employment subchapter, *i.e.,*

'*this* subchapter,' includes other provisions that use the defined terms, . . . [t]he EEOC might elaborate, through regulations, on the meaning of 'disability' . . . if elaboration is needed in order to 'carry out' the substantive provisions of 'this subchapter.' " 527 U.S., at 514 (Breyer, J., dissenting). See also *Adams Fruit Co.* v. *Barrett,* 494 U.S. 638, 649–650 (1990) (holding that a delegation of authority to promulgate motor vehicle safety "*standards*" did not include the authority to decide the pre-emptive scope of the federal statute because "[n]o such delegation regarding [the statute's] enforcement provisions is evident in the statute").

The same principle controls here. It is not enough that the terms "public interest," "public health and safety," and "Federal law" are used in the part of the statute over which the Attorney General has authority. The statutory terms "public interest" and "public health" do not call on the Attorney General, or any other Executive official, to make an independent assessment of the meaning of federal law. The Attorney General did not base the Interpretive Rule on an application of the five-factor test generally, or the "public health and safety factor" specifically. Even if he had, it is doubtful the Attorney General could cite the "public interest" or "public health" to deregister a physician simply because he deemed a controversial practice permitted by state law to have an illegitimate medical purpose.

As for the federal law factor, though it does require the Attorney General to decide "[c]ompliance" with the law, it does not suggest that he may decide what the law says. Were it otherwise, the Attorney General could authoritatively interpret "State" and "local laws," which are also included in 21 U.S.C. § 823(f), despite the obvious constitutional problems in his doing so. Just as he must evaluate compliance with federal law in deciding about registration, the Attorney General must as surely evaluate compliance with federal law in deciding whether to prosecute; but this does not entitle him to *Chevron* deference. See *Crandon* v. *United States,* 494 U.S. 152, 177 (1990) (Scalia, J., concurring in judgment) ("The Justice Department, of course, has a very specific responsibility to determine for itself what this statute means, in order to decide when to prosecute; but we have never thought that the interpretation of those charged with prosecuting criminal statutes is entitled to deference").

The limits on the Attorney General's authority to define medical standards for the care and treatment of patients bear also on the proper interpretation of §871(b). This section allows the Attorney General to best determine how to execute "his functions." It is quite a different matter, however, to say that the Attorney General can define the substantive standards of medical practice as part of his authority. To find a delegation of this extent in §871 would put that part of the statute in considerable tension with the narrowly defined delegation concerning control and registration. It would go, moreover, against the plain language of the text to treat a delegation for the "execution" of his functions as a further delegation to define other functions well beyond the statute's specific grants of authority. When Congress chooses to delegate a power of this extent, it does so not by referring back to the administrator's functions but by giving authority over the provisions of the statute he is to interpret. See, *e.g., National Cable & Telecommunications Assn.,* 545 U.S. ___; *Household Credit Services,* 541 U.S. 232.

The authority desired by the Government is inconsistent with the design of the statute in other fundamental respects. The Attorney General does not have the sole delegated authority under the CSA. He must instead share it with, and in some respects defer to, the Secretary, whose functions are likewise delineated and confined by the statute. The CSA allocates decisionmaking powers among statutory actors so that medical judgments, if they are to be decided at the federal level and for the limited objects of the statute, are placed in the hands of the Secretary. In the scheduling context, for example, the Secretary's recommendations on scientific and medical matters bind the Attorney General. The Attorney General cannot control a substance if the Secretary disagrees. 21 U.S.C. § 811(b). See H. R. Rep. No. 91–1444, pt. 1, p. 33 (1970) (the section "is not intended to authorize the Attorney General to undertake or support medical and scientific research [for the purpose of scheduling], which is within the competence of the Department of Health, Education, and Welfare").

In a similar vein the 1970 Act's regulation of medical practice with respect to drug rehabilitation gives the Attorney General a limited role; for it is the Secretary who, after consultation with the Attorney General and national medical groups, "determine[s] the appropriate methods of professional practice in the medical treatment of . . . narcotic addiction." 42 U.S.C. § 290bb–2a; see 2(g) (2000 ed. and Supp. II) (stating that the Attorney General shall register practitioners who dispense drugs for narcotics treatment when the Secretary has determined the applicant is qualified to treat addicts and the Attorney General has concluded the applicant will comply with record keeping and security regulations); *Moore,* 423 U.S., at 144 (noting that in enacting the addiction-treatment provisions, Congress sought to change the fact "that 'criminal prosecutions' in the past had turned on the opinions of federal prosecutors"); H. R. Rep. No. 93–884, p. 6 (1974) ("This section preserves the distinctions found in the [CSA] between the functions of the Attorney General and the Secretary . . . . All decisions of a medical nature are to be made by the Secretary. . . . Law enforcement decisions respecting the security of stocks of narcotics drugs and the maintenance of records on such drugs are to be made by the Attorney General").

Postenactment congressional commentary on the CSA's regulation of medical practice is also at odds with the Attorney General's claimed authority to determine appropriate medical standards. In 1978, in preparation for ratification of the Convention on Psychotropic Substances, Feb. 21, 1971, [1979–1980] 32 U. S. T. 543, T. I. A. S. No. 9725, Congress decided it would implement the United States' compliance through "the framework of the procedures and criteria for classification of substances provided in the CSA." 21 U.S.C. § 801a(3). It did so to ensure that "nothing in the Convention will interfere with ethical medical practice in this country as determined by [the Secretary] on the basis of a consensus of the views of the American medical and scientific community." *Ibid.*

The structure of the CSA, then, conveys unwillingness to cede medical judgments to an Executive official who lacks medical expertise. In interpreting statutes that divide authority, the Court has recognized: "Because historical familiarity and policy making expertise account in the first instance for the presumption that Congress delegates interpretive lawmaking power to the agency rather than to the reviewing court, we presume here that Congress intended to invest interpretive power in the administrative actor in the best position to develop these attributes." *Martin* v. *Occupational Safety and Health Review Comm'n,* 499 U.S. 144, 153 (1991) (citations omitted). This presumption works against a conclusion that the Attorney General has authority to make quintessentially medical judgments.

The Government contends the Attorney General's decision here is a legal, not a medical, one. This generality, however, does not suffice. The Attorney General's Interpretive Rule, and the Office of Legal Counsel memo it incorporates, place extensive reliance on medical judgments and the views of the medical community in concluding that assisted suicide is not a "legitimate medical purpose" See 66 Fed. Reg. 56608 (noting the medical distinctions between assisting suicide and giving sufficient medication to alleviate pain); Memorandum from Office of Legal Counsel to Attorney General (June 27, 2001), App. to Pet. for Cert. 121a–122a, and n. 17 (discussing the "Federal medical policy" against physician-assisted suicide), *id.,* at 124a–130a (examining views of the medical community). This confirms that the authority claimed by the Attorney General is both beyond his expertise and incongruous with the statutory purposes and design.

The idea that Congress gave the Attorney General such broad and unusual authority through an implicit delegation in the CSA's registration provision is not sustainable. "Congress, we have held, does not alter the fundamental details of a regulatory scheme in vague terms or ancillary provisions—it does not, one might say, hide elephants in mouseholes." *Whitman* v.

American Trucking Assns., Inc., 531 U.S. 457, 468 (2001); see *FDA* v. *Brown & Williamson Tobacco Corp.*, 529 U.S. 120, 160 (2000) (["W]e are confident that Congress could not have intended to delegate a decision of such economic and political significance to an agency in so cryptic a fashion").

The importance of the issue of physician-assisted suicide, which has been the subject of an "earnest and profound debate" across the country, *Glucksberg*, 521 U.S., at 735, makes the oblique form of the claimed delegation all the more suspect. Under the Government's theory, moreover, the medical judgments the Attorney General could make are not limited to physician-assisted suicide. Were this argument accepted, he could decide whether any particular drug may be used for any particular purpose, or indeed whether a physician who administers any controversial treatment could be deregistered. This would occur, under the Government's view, despite the statute's express limitation of the Attorney General's authority to registration and control, with attendant restrictions on each of those functions, and despite the statutory purposes to combat drug abuse and prevent illicit drug trafficking.

We need not decide whether *Chevron* deference would be warranted for an interpretation issued by the Attorney General concerning matters closer to his role under the CSA, namely preventing doctors from engaging in illicit drug trafficking. In light of the foregoing, however, the CSA does not give the Attorney General authority to issue the Interpretive Rule as a statement with the force of law.

If, in the course of exercising his authority, the Attorney General uses his analysis in the Interpretive Rule only for guidance in deciding when to prosecute or deregister, then the question remains whether his substantive interpretation is correct. Since the Interpretive Rule was not promulgated pursuant to the Attorney General's authority, its interpretation of "legitimate medical purpose" does not receive *Chevron* deference. Instead, it receives deference only in accordance with *Skidmore*. "The weight of such a judgment in a particular case will depend upon the thoroughness evident in its consideration, the validity of its reasoning, its consistency with earlier and later pronouncements, and all those factors which give it power to persuade, if lacking power to control." 323 U.S., at 140; see also *Mead*, 533 U.S., at 235 (noting that an opinion receiving *Skidmore* deference may "claim the merit of its writer's thoroughness, logic, and expertness, its fit with prior interpretations, and any other sources of weight"). The deference here is tempered by the Attorney General's lack of expertise in this area and the apparent absence of any consultation with anyone outside the Department of Justice who might aid in a reasoned judgment. In any event, under *Skidmore*, we follow an agency's rule only to the extent it is persuasive, see *Christensen* v. *Harris*

County, 529 U.S. 576, 587 (2000); and for the reasons given and for further reasons set out below, we do not find the Attorney General's opinion persuasive.

III

As we have noted before, the CSA "repealed most of the earlier antidrug laws in favor of a comprehensive regime to combat the international and interstate traffic in illicit drugs." *Raich*, 545 U.S., at ___ (slip op., at 9). In doing so, Congress sought to "conquer drug abuse and to control the legitimate and illegitimate traffic in controlled substances." *Ibid*. It comes as little surprise, then, that we have not considered the extent to which the CSA regulates medical practice beyond prohibiting a doctor from acting as a drug "pusher" instead of a physician. *Moore*, 423 U.S., at 143. In *Moore*, we addressed a situation in which a doctor "sold drugs, not for legitimate purposes, but primarily for the profits to be derived therefrom." *Id.*, at 135 (quoting H. R. Rep. No. 91–1444, pt. 1, at 10; internal quotation marks omitted). There the defendant, who had engaged in large-scale overprescribing of methadone, "concede[d] in his brief that he did not observe generally accepted medical practices." 423 U.S., at 126. And in *United States* v. *Oakland Cannabis Buyers Cooperative*, 532 U.S. 483 (2001), Congress' express determination that marijuana had no accepted medical use foreclosed any argument about statutory coverage of drugs available by a doctor's prescription.

In deciding whether the CSA can be read as prohibiting physician-assisted suicide, we look to the statute's text and design. The statute and our case law amply support the conclusion that Congress regulates medical practice insofar as it bars doctors from using their prescription-writing powers as a means to engage in illicit drug dealing and trafficking as conventionally understood. Beyond this, however, the statute manifests no intent to regulate the practice of medicine generally. The silence is understandable given the structure and limitations of federalism, which allow the States "great latitude under their police powers to legislate as to the protection of the lives, limbs, health, comfort, and quiet of all persons." *Medtronic, Inc.* v. *Lohr*, 518 U.S. 470, 475 (1996) (quoting *Metropolitan Life Ins. Co.* v. *Massachusetts*, 471 U.S. 724, 756 (1985)).

The structure and operation of the CSA presume and rely upon a functioning medical profession regulated under the States police powers. The Attorney General can register a physician to dispense controlled substances "if the applicant is authorized to dispense . . . controlled substances under the laws of the State in which he practices." 21 U.S.C. § 823(f). When considering whether to revoke a physician's registration, the Attorney General looks not just to violations of federal drug laws; but he "shall" also consider "[t]he recommendation of the appropriate state licensing board or professional disciplinary authority" and the registrant's compliance with state and local drug laws. *Ibid.* The very definition of a "practitioner" eligible to prescribe includes physicians "licensed, registered, or otherwise permitted, by the United States or the jurisdiction in which he practices" to dispense controlled substances. §802(21). Further cautioning against the conclusion that the CSA effectively displaces the States' general regulation of medical practice is the Act's pre-emption provision, which indicates that, absent a positive conflict, none of the Act's provisions should be "construed as indicating an intent on the part of the Congress to occupy the field in which that provision operates . . . to the exclusion of any State law on the same subject matter which would otherwise be within the authority of the State." §903.

Oregon's regime is an example of the state regulation of medical practice that the CSA presupposes. Rather than simply decriminalizing assisted suicide, ODWDA limits its exercise to the attending physicians of terminally ill patients, physicians who must be licensed by Oregon's Board of Medical Examiners. Ore. Rev. Stat. §§127.815, 127.800(10) (2003). The statute gives attending physicians a central role, requiring them to provide prognoses and prescriptions, give information about palliative alternatives and counseling, and ensure patients are competent and acting voluntarily. §127.815. Any eligible patient must also get a second opinion from another registered physician, §127.820, and the statute's safeguards require physicians to keep and submit to inspection detailed records of their actions, §§127.855, 127.865.

Even though regulation of health and safety is "primarily, and historically, a matter of local concern," *Hillsborough County v. Automated Medical Laboratories, Inc.,* 471 U.S. 707, 719 (1985), there is no question that the Federal Government can set uniform national standards in these areas. See *Raich, supra,* at ___ (slip op., at 6). In connection to the CSA, however, we find only one area in which Congress set general, uniform standards of medical practice. Title I of the Comprehensive Drug Abuse Prevention and Control Act of 1970, of which the CSA was Title II, provides that

"[The Secretary], after consultation with the Attorney General and with national organizations representative of persons with knowledge and experience in the treatment of narcotic addicts, shall determine the appropriate methods of professional practice in the medical treatment of the narcotic addiction of various classes of narcotic addicts, and shall report thereon from time to time to the Congress." §4, 84 Stat. 1241, codified at 42 U.S.C. § 290bb–2a.

This provision strengthens the understanding of the CSA as a statute combating recreational drug abuse, and also indi-

cates that when Congress wants to regulate medical practice in the given scheme, it does so by explicit language in the statute.

In the face of the CSA's silence on the practice of medicine generally and its recognition of state regulation of the medical profession it is difficult to defend the Attorney General's declaration that the statute impliedly criminalizes physician-assisted suicide. This difficulty is compounded by the CSA's consistent delegation of medical judgments to the Secretary and its otherwise careful allocation of powers for enforcing the limited objects of the CSA. See Part II–B, *supra.* The Government's attempt to meet this challenge rests, for the most part, on the CSA's requirement that every Schedule II drug be dispensed pursuant to a "written prescription of a practitioner." 21 U.S.C. § 829(a). A prescription, the Government argues, necessarily implies that the substance is being made available to a patient for a legitimate medical purpose. The statute, in this view, requires an anterior judgment about the term "medical" or "medicine." The Government contends ordinary usage of these words ineluctably refers to a healing or curative art, which by these terms cannot embrace the intentional hastening of a patient's death. It also points to the teachings of Hippocrates, the positions of prominent medical organizations, the Federal Government, and the judgment of the 49 States that have not legalized physician-assisted suicide as further support for the proposition that the practice is not legitimate medicine. See Brief for Petitioners 22–24; Memorandum from Office of Legal Counsel to Attorney General, App. to Pet. for Cert. 124a–130a.

On its own, this understanding of medicine's boundaries is at least reasonable. The primary problem with the Government's argument, however, is its assumption that the CSA impliedly authorizes an Executive officer to bar a use simply because it may be inconsistent with one reasonable understanding of medical practice. Viewed alone, the prescription requirement may support such an understanding, but statutes "should not be read as a series of unrelated and isolated provisions." *Gustafson* v. *Alloyd Co.,* 513 U.S. 561, 570 (1995). The CSA's substantive provisions and their arrangement undermine this assertion of an expansive federal authority to regulate medicine.

The statutory criteria for deciding what substances are controlled, determinations which are central to the Act, consistently connect the undefined term "drug abuse" with addiction or abnormal effects on the nervous system. When the Attorney General schedules drugs, he must consider a substance's psychic or physiological dependence liability. 21 U.S.C. § 811(c)(7). To classify a substance in Schedules II through V, the Attorney General must find abuse of the drug leads to psychological or physical dependence. §812(b). Indeed, the differentiation of Schedules II through V turns in large part on a substance's habit-forming potential: The more addictive a substance, the stricter the controls. *Ibid.* When Congress wanted to extend the CSA's regulation to substances not obviously habit forming or psychotropic, moreover, it relied not on Executive ingenuity, but rather on specific legislation. See §1902(a) of the Anabolic Steroids Control Act of 1990, 104 Stat. 4851 (placing anabolic steroids in Schedule III).

The statutory scheme with which the CSA is intertwined further confirms a more limited understanding of the prescription requirement. When the Secretary considers FDA approval of a substance with "stimulant, depressant, or hallucinogenic effect," he must forward the information to the Attorney General for possible scheduling. Shedding light on Congress' understanding of drug abuse, this requirement appears under the heading "Abuse potential." 21 U.S.C. § 811(f). Similarly, when Congress prepared to implement the Convention on Psychotropic Substances, it did so through the CSA. §801a.

The Interpretive Rule rests on a reading of the prescription requirement that is persuasive only to the extent one scrutinizes the provision without the illumination of the rest of the statute. See *Massachusetts* v. *Morash,* 490 U.S. 107, 114–115 (1989). Viewed in its context, the prescription requirement is better understood as a provision that ensures patients use controlled substances under the supervision of a doctor so as to prevent addiction and recreational abuse. As a corollary, the provision also bars doctors from peddling to patients who crave the drugs for those prohibited uses. See *Moore,* 423 U.S., at 135, 143. To read prescriptions for assisted suicide as constituting "drug abuse" under the CSA is discordant with the phrase's consistent use throughout the statute, not to mention its ordinary meaning.

The Government's interpretation of the prescription requirement also fails under the objection that the Attorney General is an unlikely recipient of such broad authority, given the Secretary's primacy in shaping medical policy under the CSA, and the statute's otherwise careful allocation of decision-making powers. Just as the conventions of expression indicate that Congress is unlikely to alter a statute's obvious scope and division of authority through muffled hints, the background principles of our federal system also belie the notion that Congress would use such an obscure grant of authority to regulate areas traditionally supervised by the States' police power. It is unnecessary even to consider the application of clear statement requirements, see, *e.g., United States* v. *Bass,* 404 U.S. 336, 349 (1971); cf. *BFP* v. *Resolution Trust Corporation,* 511 U.S. 531, 544–546 (1994), or presumptions against pre-emption, see, *e.g., Rush Prudential HMO, Inc.* v. *Moran,* 536 U.S. 355, 387 (2002), to reach this commonsense conclusion. For all these reasons, we conclude the CSA's prescription requirement does not authorize the Attorney General to bar dispensing controlled substances for assisted suicide in the face of a state medical regime permitting such conduct.

IV

The Government, in the end, maintains that the prescription requirement delegates to a single Executive officer the power to effect a radical shift of authority from the States to the Federal Government to define general standards of medical practice in every locality. The text and structure of the CSA show that Congress did not have this far-reaching intent to alter the federal-state balance and the congressional role in maintaining it.

The judgment of the Court of Appeals is
Affirmed.
[Dissenting opinions omitted.]

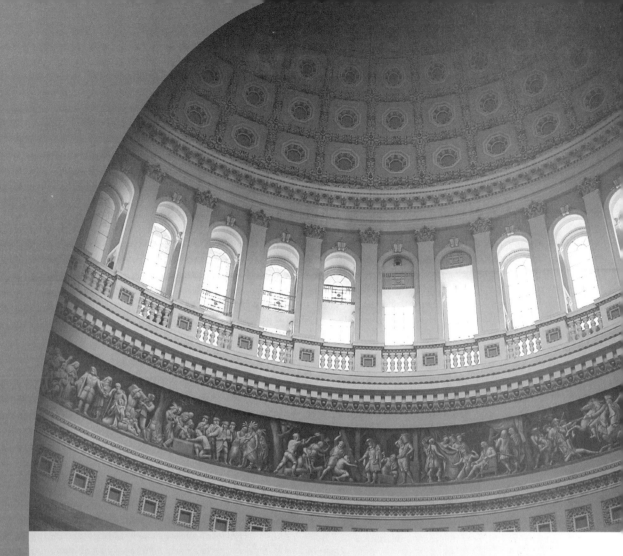

PART **IV**

Rethinking the Public Health and Health Care Systems

If there is one thing many people can agree on, it is that there is room for significant improvement in the public health and health care systems. Unfortunately, there is little agreement about how to reform them. For example, a recent tracking poll by the Kaiser Family Foundation found that Democrats prefer to focus on expanding coverage for the uninsured, whereas Republicans are more concerned about containing health care costs, and Independents are split between the two issues.[1] Even within the topic of covering the uninsured, a separate study revealed a wide range of views among respondents about their willingness to subsidize coverage of the uninsured and about the proper role of government to provide health insurance.[2] This lack of consensus suggests that health reform will remain on the political agenda for years to come. This Part includes a series of articles designed to improve readers' understanding of key health reform issues and to provoke discussion about whether and how to reform the public health and health care systems.

The section opens with "Morality, Politics, and Health Policy," in which James Morone considers the place of community and morality in American politics. This article examines what community—a central aspect of public health—means to this country and how it has impacted the development of health policy. As preparation for considering reform proposals, it will be useful to try to answer the question posed by Thomas Rice in "Can Markets Give Us the Health System We Want?" In an excerpt from this article, Rice reviews basic economic theory of market competition and discusses how the assumptions underlying this theory apply to the health care field.

The section then turns to a discussion of the health care *safety net*, the term used to describe health care providers who care for the uninsured and other vulnerable populations. Given the lack of universal insurance coverage in this country and the existence of racial and ethnic health disparities, the safety net has become an increasingly important component of the health care system. "Health Centers and Health Insurance: Complements, Not Alternatives," by Sara Wilensky and Dylan Roby, maintains that successful health reform will include both a strong health center safety net system and universal health insurance coverage. This article is followed by "Health Reform and the Safety Net: Big Opportunities; Major Risks." In it, Bruce Siegel, Marsha Regenstein, and Peter Shin discuss the importance of the safety net as well as current threats to its survival.

These thematic articles are followed by a discussion of specific health reform proposals and enacted legislation. "An Analysis of

Leading Congressional Health Care Bills, 2005–2007: Part 1, Insurance Coverage," by the Commonwealth Foundation, outlines the types of national health reform proposals that have recently been under consideration.

Next, this Part steps away from health reform proposals on the federal level and considers options developed by individual states and lessons to be learned from the approaches adopted by other countries. In the absence of comprehensive health reform at the federal level, states have acted in a variety of innovative ways to address the problems of uninsurance and rising health care costs. "State of the States 2007: Building Hope, Raising Expectations" reviews state-level solutions to health care problems and identifies lessons for policy-makers to consider before adopting these strategies. "Comparing Health Systems in Four Countries: Lessons for the United States" discusses how Canada, France, Germany, and Great Britain address coverage, funding, costs, and other health care issues. In "Learning From High Performance Health Systems Around the Globe," Karen Davis provides useful data and graphics about lessons other countries can teach the United States as it tries to repair its own damaged health systems.

IN THIS SECTION

James Morone, "Morality, Politics, and Health Policy" from *Policy Challenges in Modern Health Care*

Thomas Rice, "Can Markets Give Us the Health System We Want?"

Sara Wilensky and Dylan Roby, "Health Centers and Health Insurance: Complements, Not Alternatives"

Bruce Siegel, Marsha Regenstein, and Peter Shin, "Health Reform and the Safety Net: Big Opportunities; Major Risks"

Sara Collins, Karen Davis, and Jennifer Kriss, "An Analysis of Leading Congressional Health Care Bills, 2005-2007: Part 1, Insurance Coverage"

State Coverage Initiative, "State of the States: Building Hope, Raising Expectations"

Lawrence Brown, "Comparing Health Systems in Four Countries: Lessons for the United States"

Karen Davis, invited testimony to the U.S. Senate Health, Education, Labor and Pension Committee, "Learning from high performance health systems around the globe"

---

[1]Kaiser Family Foundation. Kaiser Health Tracking Poll: Election 2008. Available at http://www.kff.org/kaiserpolls/upload/7655.pdf. Accessed on August 14, 2007.

[2]Kaiser Family Foundation. Kaiser Public Opinion Spotlight: Public Opinion on the Uninsured. Available at http://www.kff.org/spotlight/uninsured/index.cfm. Accessed on August 14, 2007.

Morality, Politics, and Health Policy from *Policy Challenges in Modern Health Care*

James A. Morone

Source: By permission of Rutgers University Press. Reprinted from Morone, JA. Morality, Politics and Health Policy. In: Mechanic, D, Rogut, LB, Colby, DC, Knickman, JR, eds. *Policy Challenges in Modern Health Care.* Piscataway, NJ: Rutgers University Press, 2005. Copyright © 2005 by Rutgers, the State University.

American health care policy is different from health policy in other industrial nations. The United States has no national health insurance, of course. However, that difference simply reflects a deeper contrast in the ways we Americans think about politics and health care. European health policy analysts regularly invoke a "solidarity culture"—a staunch belief in sharing resources and concern for what might be called "the people's health" (Morone 2000). European political cultures and institutions often reflect this collective ideal.

What most observers first notice about the American process is the unabashed pursuit of self-interest. In our dynamic (some would say raucous) system, stakeholders and interest groups jockey for advantage on every issue. One wily nineteenth-century politician put it famously after double-crossing a rival: "Politics is not a branch of the Sunday school business" (Morone 1998). This process poses a challenge for health specialists: groups pushing their own interests will stand up and oppose even the most unambiguous scientific findings.

Both scholars and laypeople usually view health policy largely through the lens of interest group politics. Stakeholders and politicians pursue their preferences. They negotiate with one another, cajole neutral parties, and mobilize their own supporters. Constitutional rules bound this process, and an elaborate network of rights protects each individual. The entire political system lurches along, operating its celebrated checks, balancing public programs with private, markets, blunting radical changes, and producing incremental adjustments to the status quo. From this perspective, health science constantly wrestles with self-interested politics. Even robust findings are only as good as the policy coalition that assembles around them.

However, interest group politics is only the most obvious story. Two other traditions run through policymaking in the United States. First, Americans also share an intermittent legacy of cooperation—one that grows especially vivid during a crisis. National service programs (such as VISTA and AmeriCorps), town hall meetings (often employed by political campaigns), and attempts to stimulate citizen participation are all familiar efforts to tap the American communal legacy. Public health advocates, in particular, often try to move beyond competition and appeal to shared interests and values.

Morality offers Americans still another powerful political framework. As foreign observers often point out, the United States remains the industrial world's foremost Puritan nation (Morone 2003a). The Puritan colonists bequeathed America a tendency to turn political differences into moral disputes. The debates that gust up around our social programs often directly concern the moral worth of the beneficiaries: Are they deserving? Such questions put vivid and contested moral images—of virtue and vice, good and evil, us and them—at the heart of American health care politics and policies.

TRADITIONAL MODELS OF AMERICAN POLITICS

Individualism

Why are Americans so committed to individualism (or what political theorists call classical liberalism)? One of our great national myths offers a popular answer: the first colonists sailed away from old world tyranny and settled a vast "unpopulated" land—the place almost thrust freedom on them. American settlers did not have to push aside kings or nobles to get ahead. Instead, as Tocqueville famously put it, "Americans were born equal instead of becoming so" (Tocqueville 1969, 509; Hartz 1955; Greenstone 1986). Men (and maybe women; the myth gets a bit shaky here) faced extraordinary opportunities. The land and its riches awaited; success simply required a little capital and a lot of work. The irresistible result would be the nation's celebrated individualism, a deep faith in free economic markets (some foreign observers see almost a cult), and a corresponding belief in limited government.

The U.S. Constitution organized this ideology into the nation's political rules. An elaborate system of checks and balances limited national power. But this system also offered political participants many different venues in which to pursue their interests. In the past, political systems had tried to suppress self-interest; the American founders opened the door to it. The answer to the problem of factions, or interests, wrote James Madison in Federalist No. 10 (1787), is injecting an "even greater variety" into the political process. Today political scientists sometimes lament the hyper-pluralism of a system stalemated by competing claims, lobbyists, and lawyers. The practical result is that almost no political arenas stand above the scramble. There are only a very few nonpartisan agencies; there is no prestigious civil service trusted by all sides; and even the judiciary has become another political branch of government (McConnell 1966; Kersh and Morone forthcoming).

The sheer ferocity of this scramble for advantage poses a particular dilemma for health care policy. After all, medical science seeks objective answers to questions about health and health care. It documents, for example, the dangers of smoking, obesity, stress, unsafe sex, and delayed medical care. The surgeon general, the Institute of Medicine, and the Centers for Disease Control and Prevention might issue warnings based on good science. However, any effort to act on those findings simply triggers the politics of self-interest. No cultural mores penalize such a reaction: in politics, economic self-interest is every bit as legitimate as medical science.

The result appears to pose a conflict between medicine and politics. No matter how robust the scientific findings, political interests routinely mobilize and often delay or derail action. The politics of individualism offers health-minded reformers unambiguous advice: use your scientific findings to mobilize your own side. In the political arena, your science is only as strong as your political coalition.

Community

During the 1980s, critics began growing uneasy about unabashed self-interest and untrammeled markets. What happens to the common good when everyone pushes only for number one? Back to early America trooped the social theorists. There they discovered an entirely different American political tradition, one grounded in a robust collective life. In contrast to the legends of rugged individualism, historians documented rich networks of communal assistance. If a barn burned down, townsfolk banded together and helped their neighbor raise another. If iron pots were expensive, families shared them—early American household inventories often list one-half or one-third of a pot or skillet (Morone 2003a, 7).

The communal story sparks enthusiasm across the political spectrum. Here, argue proponents, lies firm ground on which to imagine a renewed civic culture. Americans are not just celebrants of self but partners in a shared public life, not just individualists but communitarians. Conservatives saw an opportunity to restore traditional American values; progressives stressed our obligations to one another, our shared communal fate.

For medical reformers, the legacy of community recalls an often-overlooked public health legacy. After all, American cities have a long history of funding clinics and fighting infectious diseases. A communal heritage—if it can somehow be tapped—opens the prospect of putting self-interest in a larger, civic-minded context (Putnam 2000; Skocpol 2003).

Franklin D. Roosevelt introduced his idea of social security with the classic communal appeal for public health. "The causes of poverty. . . are beyond the control of any individual." So much for the individualistic version of American politics. What was the alternative? Community effort. When a modern civilization faces a disease epidemic, said Roosevelt, "it takes care of the victims after they are stricken." But it also roots out the source of the contagion. Roosevelt proposed an entire social program built on the public health model. He would put aside the "jungle law of economic competition" for "brotherly" cooperation (Roosevelt 1932, 38).

Of course, President Roosevelt introduced his program in response to the Great Depression. The communal alternative has always been the more fragile and intermittent approach, displacing individualism largely during crises and extraordinary circumstances. Moreover, political theorists warn us against romanticizing the American communal tradition. After all, that tradition also animates a painful historical legacy: the urge to reject entire groups based on race, gender, ethnicity, or religion. The Ku Klux Klan, militia groups, and a long, harsh line of nativist organizations that also represent communal thinking (Smith 1997).

Still, the communal vision offers a potential rejoinder to the politics of self-interest. Communitarians were critical of the Clinton administration's health reform effort, for example, because officials tried to sell it by promising one group after another that the plan was in their self-interest. The moral of that story, warned White House advisor Paul Starr, is that with "so many people on board . . . our boat may sink from its own weight." The communitarian perspective would have appealed bluntly to the common good—to the notion that we all share values as residents of the same nation (Hacker 1997, 138).

Could such a collective appeal work? Under what circumstances? What conditions stir America's communal legacy? And what about the ugly urge to reject some Americans? We can find answers to these questions in another tradition: American morality politics.

Morality Politics

Americans take religion and morality more seriously than citizens of most other industrial countries. Some 95 percent of all Americans believe in God—a distinct contrast to Sweden (52 percent), France (62 percent), and Britain (76 percent). While other industrial nations grow secular over time, the United States keeps experiencing religious revivals (Morone 2003a, 22). That social fact has deep consequences for U.S. politics. In a nation marked by moral and religious fervor, partisans often import their faith into politics.[1] Moral fervor drove—drives—an extraordinary range of political movements: civil rights, temperance, tobacco, antiabortion, and many others. Moral judgment seeps into all kinds of political issues in both dramatic and subtle ways.

Moral politics comes with its own founding story. "It seems to me," wrote Alexis de Tocqueville, "that I can see the entire destiny of America contained in the first Puritan who came ashore" (1969, 279). Those first settlers arrived in the New World facing the essential communal question: Who are we? Who were they? The Puritans concocted an extraordinary answer: they were the community of saints. Leadership, in both state and church, went to men who could prove that they were preordained for salvation. The saints could vote, hold office, and enjoy full church membership. (The methodology for proving salvation was complicated, but wealth and health were taken as fairly reliable indicators.) People who were morally uncertain—those who had not demonstrated salvation—were expected to follow the proven saints: they went to church, for example, but did not hold office, vote, or become full church members. And the damned were driven out: witches were hung, Native Americans slaughtered, and heretics sent packing mainly to Rhode Island, the latrina of New England for all its

noxious heresies). In short, moral standing defined leaders, allocated privileges (such as voting), defined communities, and identified the dangerous "other" (Morone 2003a).

The Puritan idea burst out of New England and spread across America thanks to the purest Puritans, the Baptists). The essential Puritan trope still persists and flourishes: moral virtue continues to define the community, still distinguishes "us" from "them." Moral images specify privilege or punishment, inclusion or exclusion, deserving poor or dangerous other. These images of potential beneficiaries—often shifting, constantly contested—lie under every U.S. social policy. "We" get assistance; "they" face social controls.

The traditional individualist model of American politics emphasizes a sharp line between private realm and public sphere. Constitutional rights bar any public authority from meddling in people's private lives. "However strange it may seem," wrote John Locke in 1689, "the lawgiver hath nothing to do with moral virtues and vices." In this view, citizens draw on their private desires and values and then charge into the public, political realm to advance their goals. In the patois of economics, every agent maximizes her own utilities (Locke quoted in Morone 2003a, 6). In contrast, moral politics refuses to honor the private-public distinction. It explicitly enters the private sphere. Individual virtue—character—affects the public good. Citizens' private behavior, ruled right out of politics in traditional models, now becomes crucial. Some group's private behavior (real or imagined) seems to threaten the community.

The Puritans bequeathed the United States two distinct moral visions, two answers to that political bottom line: Whom should we blame for our troubles? I call the two answers the Puritan and the social gospel.

Puritans

The Puritan approach focuses on dangerous sinners lurking in our society. The fears tilt political debates; they sink the communal urge by eroding our sense of common values and shared fate. The policy problem turns instead to protecting us from them.

The personal transgressions—the sins—that ostensibly endanger the nation are most often public health sins. For example, the most sustained moral campaign in U.S. history targeted substance abuse. Temperance crusaders organized in the early nineteenth century, won their first statewide prohibition in 1851, managed national prohibition by 1920, and now inspire a formidable drug war that draws heavily on Prohibition-era jurisprudence (Morone 2003a).

Sexual threats pose another political perennial. The American Medical Association launched its first great political campaign against abortion—a common practice in the mid-nineteenth century, when roughly one abortion occurred for every six live births. Physicians consolidated their own role as social leaders and healers by turning abortion into a crime. Abortions, they argued, were subverting the good community by undermining the white, middle-class birth rate while foreign immigrants multiplied and threatened to swamp American blood (Storer 1867; Morone 2003a).

Similarly, sexually transmitted diseases bred in the urban ghettos and spread into middle-class families. After all, reported the *American Journal of Public Health,* "many . . . white . . . boys are going to sow their wild oats" (Allen 1915, 200). In the South, the black syphilis rate became a standard justification for Jim Crow apartheid. A similar argument reappeared during the first wave of AIDS hysteria; frightened Americans dreamed up all sorts of ways to keep homosexuals from slipping their disease into mainstream culture (Morone 1997).

In each case the same general pattern recurs. Some dangerous personal behavior—drinking, drugs, sexual practices, teen pregnancy, birth control, abortion, the list goes on—threatens the community. The questionable behavior is often associated with some group. Moral politics triggers vibrant stereotypes: Irish drink, Italian immigrants have too many babies, Muslims are terrorists, and black people commit almost every possible sin. Political leaders warn that America faces terrible decline if we don't find a way to rein in the dangerous people and their bad behavior. Standard solutions run to pledges ("just say no" to alcohol, drugs, and sex before marriage), prohibitions, restrictions, regulations, more prisons, and tougher laws.

Of course, all societies impose controls. The political key lies in the emphasis on personal discipline, in the balance between restrictive policies and social welfare benefits. I experienced a vivid illustration of the difference during a debate on the Clinton health reform proposal in 1994.

I was debating a Republican senator who opposed the Clinton plan. We were before a young, liberal audience that was giving the Republican a very chilly hearing. Then, toward the end of the debate, he abruptly turned to face me. The body language said, "Okay, let's quit kidding around." And here's what followed: "Look, professor, you can't expect the hardworking people of suburban Cook County to go into the same health care alliance [a kind of insurance pool] as the crack heads in the city of Chicago." When I turned to face the audience, all set to brush aside this fatuous dichotomy, I saw a room of suddenly sobered liberals. "Yes," they were thinking, "that is a terrible problem." "Hey," I yelped, "those uninsured people in the city of Chicago are college students and hardworking nurses and taxi drivers doing double shifts and single moms holding down two jobs." No dice. In fact, it only got worse. Crack heads and single moms. Our imagined community, struggling together

to fix a troubled health care system, had vanished in an instant. Now it was a hardworking us against a drug-abusing, sexually promiscuous them. Forget about extending health care coverage—what "those people" need is moral discipline. The politics of social policy always turns on the mental images we create of the beneficiaries (Morone 2003a).

The Social Gospel

An alternative moral tradition once offered a sharp alternative to blaming individuals. I call it the social gospel (borrowing from a group of reformers at the end of the nineteenth century). Social gospel thinking shifts the focus from individual sinners to an unjust system. The neo-Puritans blame individual misbehavior for society's troubles; the social gospel approach blames society—or socioeconomic pressures—for individual troubles. The causal arrow runs in precisely the opposite direction: the economic system, race prejudice, underprivilege, and social stress put pressure on people. If those people behave badly (by using illegal drugs, for example), it is largely because social and economic forces have pushed them into a tough corner. The social gospel solution appears in countless variations, but they converge on the same familiar points: fix the system and give every American a fair chance to prosper; don't blame those who fall by the wayside; we all share a common duty to help the disadvantaged.

Thinkers in the late nineteenth and early twentieth century first systematically articulated a version of the social gospel. Reformers like Jane Addams began challenging the dominant Victorian paradigm: poverty caused drunkenness, they said, as much as the other way around. Low salaries and harsh factory conditions—deprivation, not depravity—pushed women into prostitution. This way of thinking came to power with the Roosevelt administration in 1933.[2] Roosevelt constantly articulated the social gospel, and his administration hammered out policies that reflected that approach. The social gospel, like the Puritan perspective, turns on images of health and disease. However, while the neo-Puritans tend to fear contagions, the social gospel seizes on community health as a public policy model.

Roosevelt first introduced the idea of social security while campaigning for president in October 1932. Roosevelt began by declaring that because it was Sunday, he would not be "talking politics" but "preaching a sermon" (Roosevelt 1932, 38). True to his word, the candidate packed his address with religious quotations and allusions. As I noted, he used a public health analogy to draw a picture of the good society, one that protected the weak and the disadvantaged.

Roosevelt brought these generalities down to political earth with sad stories about good people. An 89-year-old neighbor had died while milking a cow, after a blizzard no less;

now it was our collective responsibility to help his "83-year-old kid sister," who was languishing in an insane asylum because she had nowhere else to go. Roosevelt was off and running down a roster of needy innocents who needed help: hungry children in public schools, injured workers, sick men and women, crippled children, the unemployed, and many more (Roosevelt 1932, 38). Each example came with the same political spin: poor people are virtuous neighbors who have fallen on hard times. Roosevelt was consciously displacing the past icons of depravity—undisciplined black men and lazy immigrants lounging about the saloons.

That last example, drinking, carried plenty of baggage, for these were the last days of Prohibition. In the New Dealer's hands, excess drinking turned from sin to illness; dry pledges and national prohibition gave way to treatment and education. The fault line between neo-Puritans and social gospel would run right through the next half-century: vice versus illness, crime versus public health, sin versus social responsibility. The social gospel view reached its high tide during the southern civil rights movement and the Johnson administration's Great Society. "Should we double our wealth and conquer the stars," declared Johnson in his most beautiful speech, "and still be unequal to this issue [of racial inequality] then we will have failed as a people and as a nation. For with a country as with a person; what is a man profited, if he shall gain the whole world, and lose his own soul?" (quoted in Morone 2003a, 426).

The Reagan administration eventually buried the whole approach. Reagan scoffed at the idea of collective responsibility. Instead, he turned personal responsibility—just say no—into a formidable policy mantra. Today the old social gospel idea that drug abuse or crime might stem from underprivilege finds almost no policy traction. Contemporary politics includes plenty of moralizing, but there is scant evidence of the old social gospel idea that we share a collective responsibility to foster social justice for everyone.

MORAL POLITICS IN ACTION

Morality politics are protean and pervasive, springing up in unexpected places and surprising unwary policymakers. Consider two recent cases: school health centers and the politics of obesity.

School-Based Health Clinics

Difficult health problems such as substance abuse, reproductive health, and depression can land teenagers in serious trouble.[3] Given the nature of these problems, perhaps it is not surprising that they are slow to seek care. However, ignoring adolescent health leads to serious problems: one million unintended preg-

nancies a year, three million sexually transmitted diseases, more than four thousand suicides, and terrible incidents of school violence. The United States has a high adolescent and young adult death rate: 1.5 deaths per thousand young males (in contrast to 0.7 in England, 0.6 in Sweden, and 0.9 in Germany).

One policy response that grew increasingly popular in the 1990s sprang from a simple intuition: put the health care where the kids are. Local hospitals, community health centers, and public health departments opened health centers in schools, especially in poor neighborhoods (Morone, Kilbreth, and Langwell 2001).

Across the country school-based health centers immediately set off a political storm, as they inevitably faced issues such as substance abuse and reproductive health. Cultural and religious conservatives feared that providing treatment (possibly without parental notification) would implicitly condone illegal drug use, underage drinking, and premarital sex. Conservatives countered with calls for stronger discipline, personal responsibility (just say no), and abstinence education. By 1997 the Personal Responsibility and Work Opportunity Reconciliation Act (the welfare reform bill) had introduced abstinence education in schools across the United States (Morone 2003b).

Some liberals confronted the moral issues head on, responding that young people needed counseling on sexuality and chemical dependency. If teens were going to have sex, argued these advocates, they ought to be prepared. Dr. Jocelyn Elders set off a firestorm in her first press conference as director of the Arkansas Department of Health: "We are not going to put them on their lunch trays. But yes, we intend to distribute condoms [through] . . . school based clinics" (Elders 1996, 242).

The battle was on. However, liberals soon discovered that cultural (often Christian) conservatives had formed powerful local organizations across the nation. Those groups focused, in particular, on school boards. In the Northeast conservatives found allies in the Catholic bishops, who were chary of birth control. In the South and West conservatives acted with the Christian Coalition. In the Pacific states they allied with anti-tax advocates. When the Christian Coalition helped Mike Foster come from far behind and win the governorship of Louisiana, the organization's first demand was an end to the school health centers.

Parental notification posed another difficult issue. When the California legislature passed a bill guaranteeing privacy in school health centers, critics charged the government with undermining parental control. More than ten thousand people rallied against the bill, which conservative talk-show host Dr. Laura turned into a highly publicized cause. Governor Gray Davis responded by vetoing the legislation.

Yet despite ardent opposition, the clinics survived and flourished. Even the school centers in Louisiana weathered the storm and spread. How? Proponents turned moral politics into a classic interest group issue. Where cultural conservatives opposed reproductive health services and sex education, the centers backed off, usually referring their student patients to other providers. But more important, advocates employed that classic political wisdom: build a constituency. As children started receiving treatment, parents, teachers, and health providers rallied around the centers, countering moral complaints with down-to-earth descriptions of kids getting care.

These respectable locals—parents, teachers, and health care providers—told their legislators heartwarming stories about children and the school clinics. Legislators are always primed to deliver concrete benefits to "responsible" community members, and school clinics have proven a prime constituent service. They combine education and health care. They do not bust the budget. They are simple to understand. They offer fine photo opportunities. And they can be doled out one school at a time (Morone, Kilbreth, and Langwell 2001).

In the end the health centers overcame the opposition and expanded, from some 150 in 1990 to more than 1,300 today. But both sides of the story are important. Although advocates defused the moral attack, the criticism powerfully shaped both the health centers and their politics. The health centers reflect the larger politics of public health. Reviewing the response to AIDS, for example, the *American Journal of Public Health* (*AJPH*) reported that Americans engage in far more premarital sex than their British counterparts while condemning promiscuity at much higher rates (Morone 2003a, 481–482). The colonists still adhere to the old Puritan spirit, chortled the *Economist,* reporting on the *AJPH* survey, and they pay the price (Morone 2003a).

American public health policies must steer carefully between sin and censure. When AIDS hit, the more tolerant and abstemious Europeans quickly launched forceful public health campaigns that included leaflets, television advertisements, and needle exchanges. Across the Atlantic, Americans delayed their efforts while squabbling over the exact moral nuance of their message, particularly the degree of emphasis on abstinence. U.S. incidence of AIDS soon measured ten times higher than Britain's (Morone 2003a, 481). Of course, many factors underlie such differences, and, as with the school health centers, Americans eventually sorted out the tension between education and abstinence. But moral conflict again profoundly shaped the health program and its outcomes.

Obesity

In 2001 Surgeon General David Satcher issued a startling report: over 65 percent of Americans were overweight and 30 percent were clinically obese.[4] Obesity, rising at epidemic rates, threatened to overtake tobacco as the chief cause of preventable death. Americans (in fact, residents of almost every nation) suddenly found themselves bombarded by data on obesity's toll—on our lives, our health, and our budgets (Kersh and Morone 2002a).

The issue first provoked derisive commentaries about "big chocolate" and its "menace." The critics drew on the familiar model of America as a nation of individualists who celebrate free markets and vehemently oppose government meddling in private lives (Kersh and Morone 2002b). What could be more personal than the food one eats? The critics were pointing to a genuine dilemma. How might eager public health advocates make a political issue out of such a private matter?

One classic response lies in the moral realm. Nothing moves the political system like a threat from greedy companies who put profits before the public's welfare. Demonizing providers regularly offers reformers a way to cross into the private sphere and control, limit, or prohibit. In the early twentieth century, temperance advocates gained considerable political mileage by charging breweries and saloons with pouring poison into the American workingman. Tobacco offers a more contemporary example. Public health officials spent years trying to publicize the danger, but for political effect nothing matched revelations that the industry had consciously misled the public about the health effects of smoking.

The same kinds of condemnation rapidly entered the obesity debates. Public health scholars explain the startling rise in obesity by pointing to an "unhealthy food environment." For starters, portion sizes have undergone an extraordinary expansion. In his influential book *Food Fight,* Kelly Brownell describes the growth of the all-American burger. In 1957, he reports, the typical hamburger weighed in at one ounce and 210 calories. Today that burger is up to six ounces and 618 calories—and that's before the bacon, cheese, supersized fries (another 610 calories), and double-gulp (sixty-four-ounce) soft drink (Brownell and Horgen 2003, 183). Highly competitive food service entrepreneurs trumpet ever-larger portions: think Whopper, Xtreme gulp, Big Grab, and the Beast. Each innovation ups the ante in serving sizes. Even ostensibly healthy products come loaded with hidden ingredients: sugar (or high-fructose corn syrup) is the first ingredient in Kellogg's Strawberry Nutri-Grain yogurt bars, and the second in Skippy super-chunk peanut butter (Brownell and Horgen 2003; Nestle 2002; Kersh and Morone forthcoming).

Moving from these analyses to charges of corporate villainy required only a small step. As the most ardent critics put it, a cynical industry targets children and reshapes their eating habits. These companies put soda machines in schools and fast food outlets in lunchrooms. The result, argues Eric Schlosser in *Fast Food Nation,* is "a lifetime of weight problems" and "emotional pain." And that is just the beginning. Fast food, he continues, has trashed the countryside, widened the social gap between rich and poor, and turned the meatpacking industry into a labor nightmare (Schlosser 2001, 240). Schlosser's descriptions of the food business are every bit as horrifying as Upton Sinclair's famous expose *The Jungle.* Schlosser's book became a surprise bestseller, and a steady stream of exposes rapidly followed.

One backlash against fast food muckrakers simply shifts the blame. If some liberals demonize the industry, some conservatives blame overweight individuals. Heavy people lack willpower, they make foolish food choices, they live in unhealthy ways. Like smokers, drug abusers, and heavy drinkers, obese people have made personal choices; they should just say no and push away from the table. The distinct echo from other substance abuse controversies has another unhappy parallel: obesity tends to concentrate in poor and minority communities.

Each picture of blame—the industry versus the individual—carries different policy implications. A focus on the industry suggests requiring better food labels, rethinking school nutrition, restricting advertising, regulating fat content, punishing misleading claims, taxing unhealthy ingredients, and so on. Successfully demonizing big food—directing popular anger at the industry—may cut through the checks and balances of the political system and provoke action.

However, the politics of demonization cuts two ways. Some observers charge that food stamps and school lunches only encourage poor people—who are already fat enough—to overeat (Kaufman 2003). Others have suggested an insurance premium tax on heavy people. Once policymakers begin condemning heavy people, the list of possibilities rapidly grows.

The larger lessons from America's long moral history suggest that demonization is always tempting, since it gets political results, but always dangerous: it fractures communities, limits the range of health policy alternatives, and tends to land hardest on poor and weak populations. In the long run, public health advocates do best when they focus on policies that foster healthy lives and build strong communities.

Past efforts to regulate private behavior, such as alcohol and tobacco use, also take us completely beyond politics and into the cultural realm: Americans dramatically reduced their drinking, their smoking, and even their tolerance for secondhand smoke. When advocates detect a crisis, define a problem, and seek a solution, they are—indirectly, perhaps often unexpectedly—educating the public. The obesity wars are likely to grow, spread, and generate considerable political heat. However, if the history of drinking and smoking serve as a guide, the most important result may lie in the conclusions that citizens draw about their own lifestyles (Kersh and Morone forthcoming).

EPILOGUE

Moral fears and aspirations profoundly affect American politics. Franklin D. Roosevelt and Martin Luther King made moral arguments as they redefined American social policy. President Ronald Reagan asserted a very different moral framework: neo-Puritan rather than social gospel. The force with which he championed his alternative, and the success he met, may be his most enduring domestic legacy.

When it comes to moral politics, every side seizes on health care. The Puritan approach focuses on threats to public health: drinking, drug abuse, out-of-wedlock births, sexually transmitted diseases, and more. Fears often lead to powerful public action: to restrictions, regulations, and prohibitions.

Proponents of the social gospel alternative reframe the problem away from sin and sinners. They see illness rather than crime, addiction rather than moral weakness. They would treat rather than punish; they look past personal behavior and focus on complex social causes. They constantly echo Franklin Roosevelt's Sunday sermon on social security and call for public health solutions. Puritan drug wars elicit social gospel calls for treatment, education, and harm reduction. More broadly, social gospel pushes for social justice; it promotes collective responsibility toward all members of the community. However, today's call for social gospel programs is only a weak echo of the powerful reforming tradition that dominated American politics in the 1930s and 1960s (Morone 2003a, 407).

Still, down through American history and across a wide political spectrum today, every side uses images of health to articulate its hopes and aspirations, to voice its fears and warnings. The problems we face and the solutions we contrive ultimately revolve around our definitions of health and illness and the pictures we construct of one another. In the end, American morality politics simply reminds us of the importance—the cultural power—of health, health care, and health studies in forging a good society.

ACKNOWLEDGMENTS

This chapter is based on my book *Hellfire Nation: The Politics of Sin in American History.* I am grateful to Rogan Kersh and Elizabeth Kilbreth, my collaborators in studying obesity and school health care centers, respectively. Finally, thanks, to John DiIulio, Steve Macedo, Gretchen Ritter, Deborah Stone, Rick Vallely, and Sandra Hackman.

NOTES

1. People often ask me about the constitutional separation of church and state. In fact, that is precisely what fostered the American religious tumult. By keeping government out of the religious sphere (and refusing to privilege any one sect or faith), the Constitution facilitates robust competition—precisely what makes the American religious culture so fluid and vital.

2. Historians would not categorize Roosevelt with the social gospel thinkers. I have redefined the category around its most salient features and applied it more generally. For details, see Morone 2003a, part IV.

3. This discussion of school centers comes from work I have done with Elizabeth Kilbreth. We are grateful to The Robert Wood Johnson Foundation for funding the research.

4. My discussion of obesity is shaped by the insights of my collaborator, Rogan Kersh.

REFERENCES

Allen, L. C. 1915. The Negro Health Problem. *American Journal of Public Health* 5: 194–203.

Brownell, K., and K. B. Horgen. 2003. *Food Fight.* New York: Contemporary Books.

Elders, J. 1996. *Joycelyn Elders, MD.: From Sharecropper's Daughter to Surgeon General of the United States of America.* New York: Avon Books.

Greenstone, D. 1986. Political Culture and American Political Development: Liberty, Union, and the Liberal Bipolarity. *Studies in American Political Development* 1, no. 1: 1–49.

Hacker, J. 1997. *The Road to Nowhere: The Genesis of President Clinton's Plan for Health Security.* Princeton, NJ: Princeton University Press.

Hartz, L. 1955. *The Liberal Tradition in America.* New York: Harcourt, Brace, and World.

Kaufman, Leslie. 2003. Welfare Wars: Are the Poor Suffering from Hunger Anymore? *New York Times,* February 23, WK4.

Kersh, R., and J. A. Morone. 2002a. The Politics of Obesity. *Health Affairs* 20, no. 6 (November/December): 142–153.

——. 2002b. How the Personal Becomes Political: Prohibitions, Public Health, and Obesity. *Studies in American Political Development* 16 (fall): 162–175.

——. Forthcoming. Obesity, Tobacco, and the New Politics of Public Health. *Journal of Health Politics, Policy, and Law.*

Madison, J. 1787. Federalist No. 10. Available at www.constitution.org/fed/federa10.htm.

McConnell, G. 1966. *Private Power and American Democracy.* New York: Knopf.

Morone, J. A. 1997. Enemies of the People: The Moral Dimension to Public Health. *Journal of Health Politics, Policy, and Law* 22, no. 4: 993–1010.

——. 1998. *The Democratic Wish: Popular Participation and the Limits of American Government.* Rev. ed. New Haven, CT: Yale University Press.

——. 2000. Citizens or Shoppers? Solidarity under Siege. *Journal of Health Politics, Policy, and Law* 25 (October): 959–969.

——. 2003a. *Hellfire Nation: The Politics of Sin in American History.* New Haven, CT: Yale University Press.

——. 2003b. American Ways of Welfare. *Perspectives on Politics* 1, no. 1 (March): 137–146.

Morone, J. A., E. Kilbreth, and K. M. Langwell. 2001. Back to School: A Health Care Strategy for Youth. *Health Affairs* 20, no. 1 (January/February): 122–136.

Nestle, M. 2002. *Food Politics: How the Food Industry Influences Nutrition and Health.* Berkeley: University of California Press.

Putnam, R. 2000. *Bowling Alone: The Collapse and Revival of American Community.* New York: Simon and Schuster.

Roosevelt, F. D. 1932. The Philosophy of Social Justice through Social Action. In *The Public Papers and Addresses of Franklin D. Roosevelt.* New York: Random House.

Schlosser, E. 2001. *Fast Food Nation: The Dark Side of the All-American Meal.* New York: Houghton Mifflin.

Skocpol, T. 2003. *Diminished Democracy: From Membership to Management in American Civic Life.* Norman: University of Oklahoma Press.

Smith, R. 1997. *Civic Ideals: Conflicting Ideals of Citizenship in U.S. History.* New Haven, CT: Yale University Press.

Storer, H. R. 1867. *Is It I? A Book for Every Man.* Boston: Lee and Shepherd.

Tocqueville, Alexis de. 1969. *Democracy in America.* New York: Doubleday. (Orig. pub. 1835.)

Can Markets Give Us the Health System We Want?

Thomas Rice

Source: Thomas Rice, "Can Markets Give Us the Health System We Want?", in *Journal of Health Politics, Policy and Law,* UCLA School of Public Health, Vol. 22, No. 2, pp. 383–401. Copyright, 1997, Duke University Press. All rights reserved. Used by permission of the publisher.

The purpose of this article is to reconsider the foundations of health economics as applied to the study of competition. It shows that conclusions concerning the purported desirability of competitive markets are based on a number of assumptions—many of which have heretofore been ignored—that typically are not fulfilled in the health care area. Once this is recognized, market mechanisms no longer necessarily provide the best way to improve social welfare.

The article is divided into two parts: competition and demand. Each of these sections presents and then critiques key assumptions of the conventional economic model, and then provides a number of health applications. It concludes that by not considering the validity of these assumptions in health care applications, researchers and policy analysts will blind themselves to policy options that may be most effective in improving social welfare.

In recent years there has been a surge of interest in reforming health care systems by replacing government regulation with a reliance on market forces. Although much of the impetus has come from the United States, the phenomenon is worldwide. Spurred by ever-increasing health care costs, many analysts and policy makers have embraced the competitive market as the method of choice for reforming health care. This belief stems from economic theory, which purports to show the superiority of markets over government regulation.

This has led advocates to champion a number of policies, including:

- Providing low-income people with subsidies to allow them to purchase health insurance, rather than paying directly for the services they use.
- Having people pay more money out-of-pocket in order to receive health care services, especially for services whose demand is most responsive to price.
- Also requiring that they pay more in premiums to obtain more extensive health insurance coverage.
- Letting the market determine the number and distribution of hospitals and what services they provide, as well as the total number of physicians and their distribution among specialties.
- Removing regulations that control the development and diffusion of medical technologies.
- Eschewing government involvement in determining how much a country spends on health care services.

I would like to thank several friends and colleagues for their helpful comments on a draft of this article: Ronald Andersen, William Comanor, Katherine Desmond, Robert Evans, Rashi Fein, Paul Feldstein, Susan Haber, Diana Hilberman, Donald Light, Harold Luft, David Mechanic, Glenn Melnick, Joseph Newhouse, Mark Peterson, Uwe Reinhardt, John Roemer, Sally Stearns, Greg Stoddart, Pete Welch, and Joseph White. All conclusions are my own and do not reflect those of the reviewers.

This article attempts to show that economic theory does not support the specific belief that such policies will enhance economic efficiency, or the more general one that they will increase social welfare.[1] This is because the theory is based on a large set of assumptions that are not and cannot be met in the health care sector. Although it is well known among economists and noneconomists alike that some set of assumptions needs to be met to ensure that market forces will result in socially desirable outcomes, what is less understood are the specific assumptions that comprise the Iist.[2] This article reviews a number of assumptions that are particularly relevant to health care competition and the theory of demand for care.[3] The above list comprises only a fraction of the total number of assumptions upon which conclusions about the superiority of market forces are based.[4]

This article is aimed at both health economists and noneconomist health policy researchers. It is an attempt to remind economists that it is inappropriate for them to bring into their work any preconceptions that relying on market forces in health care provides the preferred set of social policies. The arguments are also intended to cast doubt on the validity of various tools that health economists often use to analyze the health care sector.

For noneconomists, this article should help clarify what economic theory can and cannot conclude about the desirability of market-based health care reforms. Because economics uses a language of its own, it is often difficult for the other professions to comprehend fully the methods used, and evaluate the conclusions reached, by health economists. (In this regard, Joan Robinson stated, "Study economics to avoid being deceived by economists," quoted in Kuttner 1984: 1.) It is hoped that this article can be used by noneconomists to level the playing field when competing with economists for the ear of policy makers.

The article is divided into two main sections: The first focuses on the economic theory of market competition, and the second on the theory of demand. The competition section discusses three assumptions that affect economic analyses of markets in general, although the applications provided all pertain to health. The section on demand focuses more specifically on applying the assumptions of demand analysis to health care. Each of these two sections is divided into three parts: a short review of the relevant economic theory (which can be skipped by those who are familiar with microeconomics), a discussion of problems with the theory, and implications for health policy.

MARKET COMPETITION
Review of Economic Theory
The field of microeconomics is devoted to the study of competition—mainly its virtues, but also some of its pitfalls.

Although many of the techniques used by economists are fairly new, the emphasis on competition is not, dating back to the writings of Adam Smith over two hundred years ago. Smith believed that people, driven by their own economic interest in the marketplace, are guided by an "invisible hand" to act in a manner that ultimately is most beneficial to society at large.

The notion of competition is intuitively appealing. In a competitive market, people are allowed—but not compelled—to trade their stock of wealth, including their labor, to purchase goods and services. Firms are compelled to produce only those things that people will be willing to purchase, and to do so in the least costly manner. Once everyone stops trading because they see no more advantage, the market is in *equilibrium*. Such an outcome is desirable for several reasons: (a) people are making their own choices; (b) the only goods and services produced are those that people demand, and they are produced without wasting economic resources; and (c) by not engaging in any more trades, people *reveal themselves*[5] to be as satisfied with their economic lot as possible, given the resources with which they began.

There are two facets to competitive theory: consumption and production. In consumer theory, people seek to maximize their *utility*, which is determined by the bundle of goods and services that they possess. To do so, they purchase their ideal bundle based on their desire or *taste* for alternative goods, and based on the prices of these alternatives (subject, of course, to how much income they have available to spend). In production theory, firms seek to maximize profits. To do so, they purchase inputs and transform them into outputs through the application of some sort of technology. How many inputs of each type are purchased depends on how each affects output, as well as their prices.

When both the consumption and production markets are in equilibrium, and when some other conditions are met,[6] the economy will be in a position called *Pareto optimality* (named after Italian economist Vilfredo Pareto). If the economy is in a Pareto optimal state, it is impossible to make someone better off (i.e., increase their welfare) without making someone else worse off. In such a situation, the economy has reached a state of *allocative efficiency*, although as we shall see next, this rests on a number of assumptions.

How does an economy reach Pareto optimality? Economists have shown that if certain conditions are met, a free or competitive market operating on its own will reach such a Pareto optimal state. As a result, allowing competition to occur will result in a situation where it is impossible to make someone better off without making someone else worse off. Taxes and subsidies can then be used to redistribute income so that society's overall welfare can be maximized.

This last point—the need to redistribute income once competition brings about Pareto optimality—is extremely important. A competitive equilibrium can occur when one person has nearly all of the output, and another has almost none. In fact, this can easily occur if the former person begins with the vast majority of initial wealth. This point was made graphically by Amartya Sen (1970: 22), who wrote:

> An economy can be [Pareto] optimal . . . even when some people are rolling in luxury and others are near starvation as long as the starvers cannot be made better off without cutting into the pleasures of the rich. If preventing the burning of Rome would have made Emperor Nero feel worse off, then letting him burn Rome would have been Pareto-optimal. In short, a society or an economy can be Pareto-optimal and still be perfectly disgusting.

Although it might seem desirable to transfer wealth from the rich person to the poor person, this cannot be viewed as improving the economy from a Paretian viewpoint because it will involve making the rich person worse off. If society cares about both efficiency and equity, then it will have to redistribute income—a process that obviously involves value judgments—for it to reach its highest level of welfare.

Problems with the Economic Theory

It would appear that the traditional economic model of competition has a strong grip on health economists. This is supported by a 1989 survey of health economists in the United States and Canada (Feldman and Morrisey 1990). One of the questions asked was whether the competitive model cannot apply to the health care system. Respondents were evenly divided on this question; half thought the model could apply, and half did not. More noteworthy, perhaps, were some of the response patterns to the question. Two-thirds of respondents who received their doctorates from top economics departments thought that the competitive model could apply, versus 53 percent with degrees from other economics departments. Few of those who received their training in noneconomics departments believed that the competitive model could apply to the health care system. Similarly, in his recent survey of health economists, Victor Fuchs (1996) found a great deal of agreement on so-called positive issues, but very little on normative ones, which would presumably include whether health economists believe that the competitive model should be applied to the health care market.

There is thus some evidence that many, if not most, health economists believe that the competitive model is an appropriate means for studying (and perhaps reforming) health care systems. The remainder of this section examines three reasons why such a belief is not warranted; each of these reasons is tied to one of the assumptions around which the purported superiority of the market-based model is based. The following section then applies this to health care.

The Pareto Principle

As noted here, if certain assumptions are met, then allowing competition to occur will result in a state of the world called Pareto optimality, where it is impossible to increase one person's welfare without lowering that of another. Rarely do economists step back and consider whether Pareto optimality is indeed a desirable state of the world. But if the Pareto principle is thought to be problematic, then market competition—which leads to Pareto optimality—would not necessarily be the best way to bring about socially desirable outcomes. Rather, other policies, involving perhaps the regulation of certain industries and even restrictions on what consumers can purchase, could be superior.

It is not hard to see the appeal of the Pareto principle. Why not let people engage in trade until they are satisfied with their lot and no longer wish to engage in further trades? Similarly, why not enact policies that convey benefits to some people and no cost to others? Wouldn't encouraging such trade and enacting such policies be in everyone's best interest?

The answer to this last question is, perhaps surprisingly, "not necessarily." As noted before, under the standard economic theory, consumers derive utility from the quantity of each of the alternative goods that they possess. It is important to think about what is *not* part of this conception of utility. There is no consideration given to how one's bundle of goods and services compares to, and affects or is affected by, those possessed by other people. Stated simply, only one's absolute amount of wealth matters; one's relative standing is irrelevant.

We therefore need to ask, Which conception of utility best represents people's actual behavior—one in which only absolute wealth matters, or one where relative standing is important as well? Intuition would tell us that the Pareto conception, in which only one's own possessions matter, is implausible if not downright wrong. It implies that people are indifferent to their rank or status in society. Rather, all that they care about is what they themselves have, irrespective of whether this is more or less, better or worse, than others with whom they have contact. Suppose that this is not the case, and that people do care about these issues. Then the fact that one person has increased his or her utility by obtaining more goods could in fact lower the utility of another person who does not obtain more goods.

In this regard, A. C. Pigou (1932: 90), one of the founders of modern economics, quoted and affirmed John Stuart Mill's statement that "Men do not desire to be *rich*, but to be richer than other men." In a lighter vein, Robert Frank (1985: 5) noted that "H. L. Mencken once defined wealth as any income that is at least one hundred dollars more a year than the income of one's wife's sister's husband." Lester Thurow (1980: 18) has stated that once incomes exceed the subsistence level, "individual perceptions of the adequacy of their economic performance depend almost solely on relative as opposed to absolute position."

Is there any evidence to *support* the belief that people care about their relative standing in addition to their absolute level of wealth? Richard Easterlin's (1974) study of human happiness in fourteen countries is particularly relevant here. He found that in a given country at a particular time, wealthier people tend to be happier than poorer people. Within a given country over time, however, happiness levels are surprisingly constant, even in the wake of rising real incomes. Furthermore, average levels of happiness are fairly constant across countries; people in poor countries and wealthy countries claim to be about equally happy. The only way such findings can be reconciled is if both relative wealth and absolute wealth matter.[7] Easterlin's findings contradict the notion that people care only about their own level of wealth.

Suppose that one accepts the notion that people are concerned with how they compare with others. It could still be argued that, even so, it is an irrational and/or flawed character trait that should not be respected by the analyst or policy maker. But this argument doesn't hold up for two reasons. First, the traditional economic theory does not evaluate where preferences come from or whether they are good or bad. Instead, it views them as what has to be satisfied in order for an individual, and ultimately, a society to be in a best-off position. Second, concern about one's status, rather than being irrational or even undesirable, is an essential element of human nature allowing not only individuals, but also a society, to prosper. In this regard, Tibor Scitovsky (1976: 115) has written: "The desire to 'live up to the Joneses' is often criticized and its rationality called into question. This is absurd and unfortunate. Status seeking, the wish to belong, the asserting and cementing of one's membership in the group is a deep-seated and very natural drive whose origin and universality go beyond man and are explained by that most basic of drives, the desire to survive." What others have can also be viewed as necessary information for a person in formulating his or her individual desires: It shows what can be had, what is reasonable to expect.

Why is the Pareto principle so important to the belief that markets are superior? It is because markets are able to satisfy individuals only if people care about their absolute bundle of possessions rather than how they stand relative to others. Although health applications will be provided later, an example may help illustrate this. Suppose that an extremely expensive therapy is developed that can substantially reduce the chance of contracting a fatal disease, but only a few people can afford it. Under a market model, this therapy will be available only to those few. This will obviously increase their utility, but it would likely reduce the utility of a far greater group who would know that a life-saving technology was available—but not to them. Relying on markets would therefore tend to reduce overall social welfare. To improve society's overall lot, it might be better if government intervened either to ensure equal access to the technology, or perhaps even to thwart its availability.

Externalities of Consumption

Another assumption necessary for showing the superiority of market competition is that there are no externalities of consumption, or alternatively, that any such externalities are explicitly dealt with through public policy. A consumption externality exists when one person's consumption of a good or service has an effect on the utility of another person. There are positive and negative externalities of consumption. With a positive externality, one person's consumption of a good raises the utility of another person. With a negative externality, it lowers another person's utility.

The existence of important externalities like these means that the operation of a competitive market, by itself, will not result in a socially optimal outcome. One possible way to improve matters is through government intervention. In the case of a positive externality, like immunizations, government can subsidize their provision, even providing them free of charge. By funding such a program through taxes, most taxpayers would help contribute, which would seem desirable because so many people are benefiting. Dealing with a negative consumption externality, like smoking, is somewhat more problematic. Although it is easy to tax smokers by enacting special taxes on the production or consumption of cigarettes, it is much harder to ensure that this revenue is dispersed to those who are most affected by smoking. As a result, governmental bodies in the United States have taken an additional step of prohibiting smoking in many public places.

In this section we will deal with a different type of consumption externality, which has received far less consideration from economists: *concern about the well-being of others*. If we care about other people's needs as well as our own—be they specific ones like food or medical care, or somewhat more vague concerns about how happy they view themselves—then there is a positive externality of consumption.[8] As just mentioned, a competitive market, by itself, will not provide the desirable amount of goods and services for which there is a positive externality. Note that this does not contradict the previous discussion about people feeling envy or having concern about status. It is not unreasonable to believe that people would envy those who have more than they do, and have benevolence toward those who have less.

It is important to understand that this issue is not just about equity: It concerns efficiency as well. Suppose for a moment that I care about poor people and want them to have more food and medical care. In order to increase my own utility, I would want to give some of my resources to the poor.

Why doesn't everyone just donate their optimal amount to charity, which in turn should maximize their personal utility? The problem is that many, if not most, people will attempt to become "free riders," recognizing that the poor will do about as well if everyone except themselves provides donations. This, in turn, will result in less redistribution than is economically efficient; people would feel better if there were a way to redistribute the optimal amount of resources rather than the lesser amount that occurs through the free market.

There is a standard "answer" to this problem in traditional economics. That is to rely on markets to allocate resources efficiently, and then to employ just the right amount of a special kind of tax and subsidy to redistribute income. These are called *lump-sum* taxes and subsidies. It is important to understand the nature of these lump-sum transfers. The idea is to come up with a way to tax, say, the wealthy, to subsidize, perhaps, the poor, without changing in any important way the efficiency-enhancing incentives of a competitive market.

The problem with this lump-sum solution is the virtual impossibility of establishing true lump-sum taxes and subsidies;[9] no such taxes exist that would also be politically acceptable.[10] But if no such methods are feasible, then use of market competition becomes problematic when there are consumption externalities. If we do not redistribute income, the market is inefficient because people want the poor to be better off than they are. But if we do redistribute income—say, by the traditional method, the income tax—we damage the efficiency that the marketplace is designed to create.

Thus, in making policy, it is impossible to separate issues of resource allocation from issues of resource distribution. Rather, they both must be dealt with simultaneously. But this is not in keeping with the traditional method often preached by economists, in which markets are allowed to operate in an unfettered fashion and redistribution is only done afterward, usually through cash transfers rather than through the direct provision of goods and services.

This anomaly—the impossibility of separating allocative and distributional activities of the economy—has been raised, in a variety of contexts, by several economists, but has received little attention from the profession at large.[11] The primary implication for policy makers is a crucially important one: Allocative and distributive decisions by a society should be made in conjunction with each other, not separately.

This concern would be eased if income were redistributed to the degree desired by members of society. But if it is not, then other strategies are necessary to deal with both the inefficiencies and inequities that arise when there are positive externalities of consumption. One of the best ways is to enact policies to ensure that those in need obtain goods and services even if they do not have the economic resources to purchase them in the marketplace. Programs like Medicare and Medicaid, which are not in keeping with some economists' recommendations to rely on competition and then redistribute resources through cash subsidies, offer good examples of how society grapples with problems like these.

Consumer Tastes Are Predetermined

Of all of the assumptions in the traditional economic model, perhaps the one that is most often forgotten is that consumers' tastes are already established when they enter the marketplace. This turns out to be very important; this section will attempt to show that this assumption is not realistic, and that when it is dropped, the competitive model loses many of its advantages.

Economics is almost universally viewed as a social science. The common element among all social sciences is that they seek to understand how individuals and/or groups of people behave, and each has its own way of viewing human behavior. Sociology, for example, focuses on how behavior is affected by society's organization, social stratification, group dynamics, and the like (Mechanic 1979). Political science examines how individuals and groups attempt to obtain what they want through such means as "conflict, influence, and authoritative collective decision making in both public and private settings" (Marmor and Dunham 1983: 3). Social psychology attempts to understand "the influences that people have upon the beliefs or behavior of others" (Aronson 1972: 6).

One facet of these other social sciences is that, in general, they seek to determine how people and groups *actually* behave, not how they *ought to* be behaving. In economics, on the other hand, one commonly sees the word *ought* (e.g., people *ought* to maximize their utility, or otherwise they are being "irrational"; to maximize social welfare, a society *ought* to depend on a competitive marketplace).

In economic theory, individual tastes and preferences "simply exist—fully developed and immutable" (Thurow 1983: 219). This is what Kenneth Boulding (1969: 1) has referred to as the "Immaculate Conception of the Indifference Curve," because "tastes are simply given, and . . . we cannot inquire into the process by which they are formed." Milton Friedman (1962: 13) provided one explanation for this: "Economic theory proceeds largely to take wants as fixed . . . primarily [as] a case of division of labor. The economist has little to say about the formation of wants; this is the province of the psychologist. The economist's task is to trace the consequences of any given set of wants."

Henry Aaron (1994: 7) recently pointed out one of the problems with this viewpoint, when individuals' behavior influences the community and is influenced by it. He noted: "It is then essential to recognize how changes in individual beliefs and values alter the environment in which individual actions occur. The environment is important both because people's preferences are shaped by pressure from peers and neighbors and because community attitudes shape the actual payoffs to various kinds of individual behavior."

The unrealistic nature of the assumption of predetermined tastes is easy to see. Consider the case of advertising. The reader, who is likely well versed in the tactics of the media, probably will admit that most advertising is not aimed at providing objective information so that consumers can obtain the best value. Rather, it is designed to (a) *minimize* the consumer search process, and more generally, (b) change consumer tastes, in part by exerting social pressure. It is hard to claim that the tastes people come to have, as the result of exposure to this sort of advertising, are sacrosanct. In fact, people often make "bad" or nonmaximizing decisions by acting on the message: the hallmark of a successful advertising campaign!

Why, then, does economics consider tastes predetermined rather than subject to the forces of change? Readers who are most familiar with economic theory will understand one possible reason. The primary tenet of modern economics is the sanctity of consumer choice. Most economists believe that the consumer is the best judge of what will maximize his or her utility. Consequently, to maximize overall social welfare, we should set up an economic system that is best at allowing consumer choices to be satisfied. Where these choices come from, as Friedman said, is beside the point.[12]

In contrast, it might be true that your current tastes are determined not on the basis of preferences that are endemic to you, so much as on what you consumed in the past. This implies a strong advantage for whatever is the status quo; familiarity breeds preference (as opposed to contempt), so what exists now will be demanded in the future. But if that is the case, it could be argued that in demanding goods and services in the marketplace, you are *wanting what you got* rather than getting what you want (Pollak 1978).

If what you want depends on what you had in the past, or on the influence of advertisers, then it is not clear that a competitive marketplace is the best way to make people better off. In the following paragraphs, three examples are provided in which people's market behaviors are not predetermined, but rather are a result of their past or present environments. In each case, it is not clear that fulfillment of their personal choices would make them best-off.

The first example, and perhaps the least important of the three given, concerns addiction. Suppose that, while growing up, you are in a peer group that smokes cigarettes, and you become addicted. Once you leave that peer group, you will still have a "taste" for cigarettes and are more likely to demand them than someone who is not addicted. Can we really say, in such an instance, that satisfying this taste through the marketplace is efficient from a societal standpoint—in the same way as satisfying the demand for bread or literature? Might not you be better off if cigarettes are taxed so prohibitively (or even banned) by the government as to make you stop smoking?[13]

A second and much more general application is habit formed by past consumption patterns.[14] Suppose you live in a community that has not discovered the joys of music. A resident of such a place will, therefore, not have developed a taste for music. But, as Alfred Marshall (1920: 94), one of the founders of modern economics, once noted, "the more good music a man hears, the stronger is his taste for it likely to become." The aforementioned resident might likely be better off with music than without, but he or she has not been sufficiently "educated" to know this. Government intervention, in the form, perhaps, of funding for the arts, could make people better off than pure reliance on the marketplace.

The third example concerns occupational choices. In the traditional economic model, it is assumed that people make occupational choices by weighing all alternatives; factors considered would include how much satisfaction they obtain from the work and the wages that it offers. Whatever choice is made in a competitive labor market is assumed to be utility maximizing. But this might not be the case if tastes are a product of one's environment. Suppose, for example, that a person grows up in a factory town and later decides to work in the factory. This might not necessarily be utility-maximizing; it is possibly a poor choice for such a person, which was made because of his or her limited opportunities. As another example, imagine that one person works to perform house cleaning services for another. This may not reflect the personal preferences as much as lack of good alternatives (Buchanan 1977). In this regard, John Roemer (1994: 120) stated that "people learn to live with what they are accustomed to or what is available to them. . . . Thus the slave may have adapted to like slavery; welfare judgments based on individual preferences are clearly impugned in such situations." Again, we see that the status quo would be favored by competitive markets, even though people might be better off if society, in some way, intervened in these choices. A public job training program would be an example of the type of intervention that could be beneficial to society.

If this is true and people's tastes are indeed the product of their environment, why is this an indictment of market forces? It is because people's demand for goods and services might not reflect the things that would make them best-off.[15] In health care, for example, people may not demand certain preventive services that would make them better-off, in part because they grew up in an environment in which more high-tech medical interventions were stressed. In such an instance, having the government provide or subsidize such services would then be superior to relying on the market, where they are not purchased in sufficient quantity. But if consumer tastes are viewed as predetermined, as they are in the market model, people become "stuck" with whatever they demand, because they are assumed to always know best.

Implications for Health Policy

The previous discussion attempted to show that, despite popular belief to the contrary, economic theory does not provide a strong justification for the superiority of market competition in the health care area because the competitive model is based on certain assumptions that do not appear to be met. This section provides some implications of these conclusions for health care policy.

Equalizing Access to Health Care Services

The Pareto principle states that if society can make someone better off without making someone else worse off, it should do so. At first glance, it might appear that most developed countries do believe in the Pareto principle when it comes to health policy. After all, almost all countries, even those with comprehensive universal health insurance programs, allow their citizens to spend their own money on additional health care services if they wish to go outside the government-sanctioned program.

But upon closer examination, it can be demonstrated that health care policy has (and continues to be) conducted on principles quite contrary to the Pareto principle. This is even true in the United States, where, it will be argued, society has not tended to tolerate large differences in access to care.

Evidence supporting this belief dates back many years. Beginning with the post–World War II period, public funding for building and expanding hospitals under the Hill-Burton Act directly reflected a belief that poorer, rural areas of the United States should not be disadvantaged *relative to* wealthier, urban areas of the country. By defining the need for hospitals based on the per capita availability of beds, the philosophy behind Hill-Burton was that no areas of the country should be given greater access than others to hospital care.

Further evidence can be seen by examining the political fallout that arose from the Oregon proposal for Medicaid reform, which was dubbed as requiring "rationing" of services. Early versions of the proposal engendered a great deal of opposition, mainly because program beneficiaries would not be able to receive coverage for the same services as the rest of the insured population. Rather, what services would be paid for would depend on how much money was available. Less cost-effective services would not be covered if program money was exhausted after paying for more cost-effective services. This prompted Bruce Vladeck (1990: 3), who later became director of the federal government's Health Care Financing Administration, to write: "This will be the first system in memory to explicitly plan that poor people with treatable illnesses will die if Medicaid runs out of money or does not budget correctly, and providers will be excused from liability for failing to treat them. The Oregonians argue that it is healthier for society to make such choices explicitly, but it is hardly healthy to establish rules of the game that require such choices." In fact, the proposal was cleared by federal officials only after the methodology was revised to ensure that disabled individuals would not face discrimination in coverage (Fox and Leichter 1993), and after the state made it clear that all essential services would be provided.

A final, and probably the most compelling, example of how health policy operates in conflict with the Pareto principle concerns coverage for new health care technologies. Traditionally, when new and potentially effective technologies become available, they are viewed as experimental until their safety and efficacy are established. But once they are established, insurers almost always cover them; failure to do so first results in strong pressure from policyholders, and eventually lawsuits that the insurer is withholding necessary medical care. Having these technologies covered by public and private insurance ensures their access to the large majority of the population who possess health insurance. In this regard, Uwe Reinhardt (1992: 311) wrote:

> Suppose [that a] new, high-tech medical intervention [is available] and that more of it could be produced without causing reductions in the output of any other commodity. Suppose next, however, that the associated rearrangement of the economy has been such that only well-to-do patients will have access to the new medical procedure. On these assumptions, can we be sure that [this] would enhance overall *social welfare*? Would we not have to assume the absence of *social envy* among the poor and of guilt among the well-to-do? Are these reasonable assumptions? Or should civilized policy analysts refuse to pay heed to base human motives such as envy, prevalent though it may be in any normal society?

If public policy were based on the Pareto principle, then we would see a market-driven gap between the services that are available to the wealthy and those available to the rest of the population. This would likely result in reduced social welfare, as noted by Reinhardt. But we do not see such a gap; once a procedure is found to be safe and effective, everyone with private. health insurance is potentially eligible to receive it. And, if insurers are not sufficiently quick to adopt new procedures, states can and do mandate their provision.[16]

What Comes First: Allocation or Distribution?

In the traditional economic paradigm, a competitive market ensures that resources are allocated efficiently. But if there are positive externalities of consumption, for example, if society wants poorer people to have more resources, then the free-rider effect will prevent a competitive economy from achieving allocative efficiency. The traditional economic solution to this problem is to institute lump-sum taxes and subsidies because they do not distort incentives and reduce efficiency, but in practice, no such mechanisms are available.

Rather than relying on this economic paradigm, what all developed countries do, instead, is confront allocative and distributive issues concurrently. In the United States, public programs like Medicare and Medicaid were established outside the competitive marketplace in order to ensure that their priority—access to medical care services for the elderly and the poor—was met. There is now much discussion about introducing more competition into both programs, and perhaps that will occur. Nevertheless, such proposals have engendered a tremendous amount of opposition because it is contended that the introduction of more competition will jeopardize the principles that formed the basis of these programs in the first place.

The belief that we should start with principles of fairness, and then proceed to considerations of efficiency, is also the foundation upon which most other health care systems have been built. In their comprehensive study of health care financing and equity in nine European countries and the United States, Adam Wagstaff and Eddy van Doorslaer (1992: 363) found that

> There appears to be broad agreement ... among policy-makers in at least eight of the nine European countries ... that payments towards health care should be related to ability to pay rather than to use of medical facilities. Policy makers in all nine European countries also appear to be committed to the notion that all citizens should have access to health care. In many countries this is taken further, it being made clear

that access to and receipt of health care should depend on need, rather than on ability to pay.

No countries have adopted the economic approach of starting with a market system and then engaging in redistribution policies so that the poor can afford to purchase privately provided care. There are many good reasons for this. The key one, however, is that it would provide no assurance that people who find themselves without insurance would purchase it. This, in turn, would lower the welfare of a society where people feel better in knowing that the poor can receive health care services.

Should Cost Control Be a Public Policy?

A larger issue that arises if consumer tastes are pliable concerns cost control. Health economists often point out that we cannot say that a country spends too much of its national income on health care. Who is to say that 14 percent or even 25 percent is "too much"? It is contended that there is nothing necessarily wrong if a society wants to spend more of its money on, say, expensive technologies. But this viewpoint is harder to justify if one views consumer tastes, not as predetermined, but rather as the product of previous experiences.

Take the example of medical technology. People are likely to demand the fruits of new technologies in part because they come to expect them. Dale Rublee (1994) has provided data on the relative availability of six selected medical technologies in Canada, Germany, and the United States. For all six technologies studied, the number of units per million persons is far higher in the United States than in Canada and Germany. With regard to open heart *surgery,* the figures are almost three times as high in the United States as in Canada, and nearly five times as great as in Germany. For magnetic resonance imaging, availability in the United States is ten times as great as in Canada and three times as great as in Germany.

Because of this, the U.S. public—and perhaps more importantly, their physicians—are likely to have developed greater expectations of such technologies. Some analysts argue that it is the growth of these technologies, or, as Joseph Newhouse (1993: 162) termed it, "the enhanced capabilities of medicine," that is primarily responsible for rising health care costs in the United States.

The point—that perhaps people would be equally well-off without so many expensive (not to say duplicative) life-saving interventions—is made only tentatively. One would not want to claim that people want to live longer because they are inculcated into believing that is desirable. Clearly, though, quality-of-life issues become relevant to such a discussion, as does the fact that the United States ranks near the top of the world in only one major vital-statistic category: life expectancy after reaching age 80.[17] One must take pause when considering Easterlin's (1974) results presented earlier—that people in poor countries seem to be equally as happy as those in wealthier ones—or perhaps more relevant to health care, the fact that citizens of other countries, which spend far less money on medical care, tend to be much happier with their health care systems. This latter point is supported by Robert Blendon et al.'s (1990) research on the satisfaction that citizens in ten developed countries have in their health care systems. Only Italians show as low satisfaction levels as do Americans. Ten percent of Americans thought that only minor changes were needed in their health care system, compared to 56 percent of Canadians, 41 percent of Germans, 32 percent of Swedes, and 27 percent of British. Thus, more spending on technologies, in and of itself, does not seem to be increasing utility levels very much.

As was argued previously, if tastes are based on past consumption, then perhaps in demanding things like more medical technology, patients and their physicians are, in part, wanting what they *got* rather than getting what they *want*. It follows that greater medical spending to support more of these technologies might not enhance social welfare so much as it represents the fulfillment of expectations that were built on the availability of such technologies in the past. Having said this, one must be very careful, because in the case of health care, people's utility would appear to depend a great deal on absolutes rather than relatives. (If you feel pain, it is little consolation if your neighbor does too.) Nevertheless, the belief that more and more spending on technologies may not increase utility levels very much—because it raises people's expectations to unrealistic levels—is consistent with a rather sober quotation from E. J. Mishan (1969b: 81):

> As I see it, the main task today of the economist at all concerned with the course of human welfare is that of weaning the public from its postwar fixation on economic growth; of inculcating an awareness of the errors and misconceptions that abound in popular appraisals of the benefits of industrial development; and also, perhaps of voicing an occasional doubt whether the persistent pursuit of material ends, borne onwards today by a tidal wave of unrealisable expectations, can do more eventually than to agitate the current restlessness, and to add to the frustrations and disillusion of ordinary mortals.

[Remainder of article omitted]

NOTES

1. Economic efficiency can be thought of as occurring when the fewest economic resources are used to satisfy consumer demand for alternative goods and services. Social welfare is maximized when the distribution of these goods and services is concordant with society's desires.

2. In this regard, Lester Thurow (1983: 22) has written, "Every economist knows the dozens of restrictive assumptions . . . that are necessary to 'prove' that a free market is the best possible economic game, but they tend to be forgotten in the play of events."

3. I am currently working on a monograph that also evaluates assumptions in two other areas: the theories of supply and redistribution.

4. The assumptions analyzed in this article come from several sources: Graaff 1971; Henderson and Quandt 1980; Mishan 1969a, 1969b; Nath 1969; Ng 1979; and Rowley and Peacock 1975.

5. The section on demand for care will focus on the concept of *revealed preference*.

6. The main one is that consumers' relative desire for different pairs of goods is equal to the economy's ability to transform one good into the other.

7. The idea that relative wealth drives people's behavior was pioneered by James Duesenberry (1952).

8. In this regard, Henry Aaron (1994: 15–16) suggested that people simultaneously possess multiple utility functions: "In one or more of these subfunctions the arguments, as in the standard theory, are particular goods and services. In others the arguments are intangible objectives such as adherence to duty, altruism, or spite."

9. For further discussion of problems in enacting such taxes and subsidies see Graaff 1971: 77–82 and Samuelson [1947] 1976: 247–249.

10. There is, in theory, one sort of tax and subsidy that might work, but it has no practicality; this is a *poll tax*—a tax that is levied on everyone irrespective of income.

11. Some examples of economists who have raised this issue include Arrow (1963), Mishan (l969a; 1969b), Thurow (1983), and Blackorby and Donaldson (1990).

12. For a discussion of alternative models of preference formation, see March 1978.

13. Note that this argument for government intervention does not rely at all on any externalities associated with cigarette smoking.

14. For a good discussion of these issues. see Hahnel and Albert 1990.

15. This line of reasoning is pursued in the second part of the article, which concerns demand for health care.

16. States cannot currently mandate provision of services under employer-sponsored health plans that fall under the jurisdiction of the Employee Retirement Income and Security Act (ERISA). Although this has effectively reduced the strength of state mandates, there is little doubt that such mandates would still exist if ERISA were repealed.

17. Data from twenty-four developed countries show that female life expectancy in the United States at age eighty is rivaled only by Canada, and that male life expectancy at that age is rivaled only by Canada and Iceland. In contrast, fifteen countries exceed the United States in female life expectancy at birth, and seventeen exceed the U.S. in male life expectancy (see Schieber, Poullier, and Greenwald 1992).

REFERENCES

Aaron, H. J. 1994. Public Policy, Values, and Consciousness. *Journal of Economic Perspectives* 8:3–21.

Akerlof, G. A., and W. T. Dickens. 1992. The Economic Consequences of Cognitive Dissonance. *American Economic Review* 72:307–319.

Aronson, E. 1972. *The Social Animal*. San Francisco: W. H. Freeman.

Arrow, K. J. 1963. Uncertainty and the Welfare Economics of Medical Care. *American Economic Review* 53:940–973.

Berk, M. L., and A. C. Monheit. 1992. The Concentration of Health Expenditures: An Update. *Health Affairs* 11(4):145–149.

Blackorby, C., and D. Donaldson. 1990. A Review Article: The Case against the Use of the Sum of Compensating Variations in Cost-Benefit Analysis. *Canadian Journal of Economics* 23:471–494.

Blendon, R. J., R. Leitman, R. Morrison, and K. Donelan. 1990. Satisfaction with Health Systems in Ten Nations. *Health Affairs* 9(2):185–192.

Boulding, Kenneth E. 1969. Economics as a Moral Science. *American Economic Review* 59(1):1–12.

Buchanan, J. M. 1977. Political Equality and Private Property: The Distributional Paradox. In *Markets and Morals*, ed. G. Dworkin, G. Bermant, and P. G. Brow. Washington, DC: Hemisphere.

Dranove, D. 1995. A Problem with Consumer Surplus Measures of the Cost of Practice Variations. *Journal of Health Economics* 14:243–251.

Duesenberry, J. S. 1952. *Income, Savings, and the Theory of Consumer Behavior*. Cambridge: Harvard University Press.

Easterlin, R. A. 1974. Does Economic Growth Improve the Human Lot? Some Empirical Evidence. In *Nations and Households in Economic Growth: Essays in Honor of Moses Abramovitz*, ed. P. A. David and M. W. Reder. San Diego, CA: Academic Press.

Ellis, R. P., and T. G. McGuire. 1993. Supply-Side and Demand-Side Cost Sharing in Health Care. *Journal of Economic Perspectives* 7:135–151.

Evans, R. G. 1984. *Strained Mercy*. Toronto: Butterworth.

Evans, R. G., M. L. Barer, and G. L. Stoddart. 1993. *It's Not the Money, It's the Principle: Why User Charges for Some Services and Not Others?* University of British Columbia, Vancouver: Centre for Health Services and Policy Research.

Feldman, R., and B. Dowd. 1991. A New Estimate of the Welfare Loss of Excess Health Insurance. *American Economic Review* 81:297–301.

Feldman, R., and M. A. Morrisey. 1990. Health Economics: A Report on the Field. *Journal of Health Politics, Policy and Law* 15:627–646.

Feldstein, P. J. 1988. *Health Care Economics*. New York: Wiley.

Fox, D. M., and H. M. Leichter. 1993. The Ups and Downs of Oregon's Rationing Plan. *Health Affairs* 120(2):66–70.

Frank, R. H. 1985. *Choosing the Right Pond: Human Behavior and the Quest for Status*. New York: Oxford University Press.

Friedman, M. 1962. *Price Theory*. Chicago: Aldine Press.

Fuchs, V. R. 1996. Economics, Values, and Health Care Reform. *American Economic Review* 86:1–24.

Graaff, J. de V. 1971. *Theoretical Welfare Economics*. London: Cambridge University Press.

Hahnel, R., and M. Albert. 1990. *Quiet Revolution in Welfare Economics*. Princeton, NJ: Princeton University Press.

Henderson, J. M., and R. E. Quandt. 1980. *Microeconomic Theory*, 3d. ed. New York: McGraw-Hill.

Hibbard, J. H., and J. J. Jewett. 1996. What Type of Quality Information Do Consumers Want in a Health Care Report Card? *Medical Care Research and Review* 53:28–47.

Hibbard, J. H., and E. C. Weeks. 1989a. The Dissemination of Physician Fee Information: Impact on Consumer Knowledge, Attitudes, and Behaviors. *Journal of Health and Social Policy* 1:75–87.

———. 1989b. Does the Dissemination of Comparative Data on Physician Fees Affect Consumer Use of Services? *Medical Care* 27:1167–1174.

Hoerger, T. J., and L. Z. Howard. 1995. Search Behavior and Choice of Physician in the Market for Prenatal Care. *Medical Care* 33:332–349.

Kuttner, R. 1984. *The Economic Illusion: False Choices between Prosperity and Social Justice*. Boston: Houghton Mifflin.

Leape, L. 1989. Unnecessary Surgery. *Health Services Research* 24:351–407.

Liebenstein, H. 1976. *Beyond Economic Man*. Cambridge: Harvard University Press.

Light, D. W. 1995. *Homo Economicus:* Escaping the Traps of Managed Competition. *European Journal of Public Health* 5:145–154.

Lohr, K. N., R. H. Brook, C. J. Kamberg, G. A. Goldberg, A. Leibowitz, J. Keesey, D. Reboussin, and J. P. Newhouse. 1986. Effect of Cost-Sharing on Use of Medically Effective and Less Effective Care. *Medical Care* 24 (Suppl. S32–S38).

March, J. G. 1978. Bounded Rationality, Ambiguity, and the Engineering of Choice. *Bell Journal of Economics* 9:577–608.

Marmor, T. R., and A. Dunham. 1983. Political Science and the Health Sciences Administration. In *Political Analysis and American Medical Care: Essays*, ed. T. R. Marmor. Cambridge: Cambridge: Cambridge University Press.

Marshall, A. 1920. *Principles of Economics*. London: Macmillan.

Mechanic, D. 1979. *Future Issues in Health Care*. New York: Free Press.

Mishan, E. J. 1969a. *Welfare Economics: Ten Introductory Essays*. New York: Random House.

———. 1969b. *Welfare Economics: An Assessment*. Amsterdam: North-Holland.

———. 1982. *What Is Political Economy All About?* Cambridge: Cambridge University Press.

Nath, S. K. 1969. *A Reappraisal of Welfare Economics*. London: Routledge and Kegan Paul.

Newhouse, J. P. 1993. An Iconoclastic View of Health Cost Containment. *Health Affairs* 10 (Suppl.):152–171.

Newhouse, J. P., and the Insurance Experiment Group. 1993. *Free for All? Lessons from the RAND Health Insurance Experiment*. Cambridge: Harvard University Press.

Ng, Y.-K. 1979. *Welfare Economics*. London: Macmillan.

Pauly, M. V. 1968. The Economics of Moral Hazard. *American Economic Review* 58:231–237.

Phelps, C. E. 1992. *Health Economics*. New York: HarperCollins.

———. 1995. Welfare Loss from Variations: Further Considerations. *Journal of Health Economics* 14:253–260.

Phelps, C. E., and C. Mooney. 1992. Correction and Update on Priority Setting in Medical Technology Assessment in Medical Care. *Medicare Care* 31:744–751.

Phelps, C. E., and S. T. Parente. 1990. Priority Setting in Medical Technology and Medical Practice Assessment. *Medicare Care* 29:703–723.

Pigou, A. C. 1932. *The Economics of Welfare*, 4th ed. New York: Macmillan.

Pollak, R. A. 1978. Endogenous Tastes in Demand and Welfare Analysis. *American Economic Review* 68:374–379.

Reinhardt, U. E. 1992. Reflections on the Meaning of Efficiency: Can Efficiency Be Separated from Equity? *Yale Law and Policy Review* 10:302–315.

Rice, T. 1992. An Alternative Framework for Evaluating Welfare Losses in the Health Care Market. *Journal of Health Economics* 11:85–92.

Rice, T., E. R. Brown, and R. Wyn. 1993. Holes in the Jackson Hole Approach to Health Care Reform. *Journal of the American Medical Association* 270:1357–1362.

Rice, T., and K. R. Morrison. 1994. Patient Cost Sharing for Medical Services: A Review of the Literature and Implications for Health Care Reform. *Medical Care Review* 51:235–287.

Robert Wood Johnson Foundation. 1994. *Annual Report: Cost Containment*. Princeton, NJ: Robert Wood Johnson Foundation.

Roemer, J. E. 1994. *Egalitarian Perspectives*. Cambridge: Cambridge University Press.

Rowley, C. K., and A. T. Peacock. 1975. *Welfare Economics: A Liberal Restatement*. New York: Wiley.

Rublee, D. A. 1994. Medical Technology in Canada, Germany, and the United States: An Update. *Health Affairs* 13(4):113–117.

Samuelson, P. A. 1938. A Note on the Pure Theory of Consumers' Behavior. *Economica* 5:61–71.

———. [1947] 1976. *Foundations of Economic Analysis*. New York: Atheneum.

Schieber, G. J., J.-P. Poullier, and L. M. Greenwald. 1992. U.S. Health Expenditure Performance: An International Comparison. *Health Care Financing Review* 13:1–87.

Scitovsky, T. 1976. *The Joyless Economy*. New York: Oxford University Press.

Sen, A. K. 1970. *Collective Choice and Social Welfare*. San Francisco: Holden-Day.

———. 1982. *Choice, Welfare and Measurement*. Cambridge: MIT Press.

———. 1987. *On Ethics and Economics*. Oxford, England: Basil Blackwell.

———. 1992. *Inequality Revisited*. Cambridge: Harvard University Press.

Siu, A. L., F. A. Sonnenberg, W. G. Manning, G. A. Goldberg, E. S. Bloomfield, J. P. Newhouse, and R. H. Brook. 1986. Inappropriate Use of Hospitals in a Randomized Trial of Health Insurance Plans. *New England Journal of Medicine* 315:1259–1266.

Sugden, R. 1993. Welfare, Resources, and Capabilities: A Review of Inequality Reexamined by Amartya Sen. *Journal of Economic Literature* 31:1947–1962.

Thurow, L. C. 1980. *The Zero-Sum Society*. New York: Penguin Books.

———. 1983. *Dangerous Currents: The State of Economics*. New York: Random House.

Vladeck, B. C. 1990. *Simple, Elegant, and Wrong*. New York: United Hospital Fund.

Voltaire, F. [1759] 1981. *Candide*. Trans. L. Bair. New York: Bantam Books.

Wagstaff, A., and E. van Doorslaer. 1992. Equity in the Finance of Health Care: Some International Comparisons. *Journal of Health Economics* 11:361–387.

Weisbrod, B. A. 1978. *Competition in the Health Care Sector: Past, Present, and Future*, ed. W. Greenberg. Washington, DC: Bureau of Economics, Federal Trade Commission.

Health Centers and Health Insurance: Complements, Not Alternatives

Sara Wilensky and Dylan H. Roby

Source: Health Centers and Health Insurance: Complements, Not Alternatives. Sara Wilensky, JD, MPP; Dylan H. Roby, MPhil. *Journal of Ambulatory Care Management,* Vol. 28, No. 4: 348-356 (October–December 2005)

Abstract: While some consider health centers and universal health insurance to be opposing concepts, we consider them to be complementary. Health centers play a vital role regardless of the type of insurance system in place because they reduce barriers to care and provide quality culturally competent care to vulnerable populations. The current private employer-based US healthcare system does not create incentives for providers to care for low-income and vulnerable populations. Even in countries with universal health coverage, health centers increase access to care and improve health outcomes. Instead of arguing whether health centers or health insurance should be expanded, the debate should focus on how best to use safety net providers as health insurance coverage expands. **Key words:** *community health centers, insurance, Medicaid, Medicare, reimbursement, underserved populations, uninsured, universal coverage*

Over the 40 years since health centers were created, nationally elected officials have had varied views of how the US healthcare system should be shaped and advocates have had to continually make the case to retain health centers. The Johnson Administration supported the first significant federal foray into the healthcare system with the passage of Medicaid and Medicare in 1965. Attempts at creating a national health insurance system rose to the forefront of the Nixon and Clinton Administrations. The Reagan era was marked by significant re-

ductions in spending on domestic programs. The current Bush Administration prefers a private market model that moves away from the employer-based system through which most Americans receive their health insurance. Despite these wide-ranging views of how the healthcare system should evolve, health centers have survived because of strong bipartisan support for their mission. President G. W. Bush has proposed and Congress has been funding a health center expansion program designed to double the number of sites and serve 6.1 million new patients by 2006. Health centers garner support across the political spectrum because their value does not depend on design of the health system. Whether they are part of a fully public universal health insurance system, a completely private one, or somewhere in between, the health center mission of providing quality, culturally competent care to the medically underserved and vulnerable populations remains vital.

This article provides a brief overview of the history of the health center program as it relates to insurance and demonstrates why health centers are not designed to replace insurance, in the same way that insurance coverage could never replace health centers. Some may not agree that both are needed. They would argue that a neat, silver-bullet approach exists and finding that approach would eliminate the complicated financing and administrative healthcare system that exists in the United States. Others may be concerned that increasing the use of health centers means supporting a 2-tiered system where the poor receive lesser care. We argue that both of those positions are faulty. Although insurance is an important component of the US healthcare system, insuring all Americans would not solve all of our healthcare problems.

Creating a system of universal insurance coverage would not address important issues affecting healthcare and health status, such as access, specialized services, discrimination, and poverty that are dealt with by health centers on a regular basis. Furthermore, numerous studies have shown that health centers provide high-quality care, on par with other, often more expensive, providers. The 2 systems—health centers and health insurance—play a complementary role in each other's existence, and to eliminate one or the other would be detrimental to the health of our nation.

HEALTH CENTERS AND HEALTH INSURANCE— A BRIEF HISTORY

After starting as the Neighborhood Health Center Program (NHCP) demonstration project in 1965, Community Health Centers were authorized as a separate program under Section 330 of the Public Health Service Act in 1975. This legislation was designed to expand care to low-income and minority populations who had difficulty accessing traditional sources of care by requiring the health centers to be located in urban and rural areas designated as either medically underserved areas or health professional shortage areas (Sardell, 1988). Other key features of health centers include the following:

- The provision of comprehensive primary care services to all;
- The provision of enabling services such as translation, transportation, and community outreach, designed to increase access to care;
- The provision of services targeted to the specific needs of their community, including providing care in a manner consistent with the cultures in the community;
- The use of a sliding fee scale that bases charges on the patient's income level; and
- A mandate that health center patients make up the majority of the center's governing board.

While open to all patients, NHCP was created to work in concert with the newly enacted Medicaid program to provide healthcare to both the newly insured low-income population as well as the uninsured (Hawkins & Rosenbaum, 1998). NHCP proponents assumed Medicaid and Medicare would provide the bulk of the funding needed to run the centers. However, for numerous reasons that was not the case. It took some time for Medicaid and Medicare to become established; even when it was fully operational, Medicaid reimbursement was lower for health centers than some other providers, covered health center services were part of the optional category of services that did not have to be included in state plans, Medicaid did not provide reimbursement for some important health center ser-

vices, not all health center patients were eligible for Medicaid, health centers were not adept at collecting fees from their low-income patients, and Medicare did not recognize health centers as qualified providers until 1973 and even then, Medicare only reimbursed centers with sophisticated accounting capability (Sardell, 1988). In short, health centers were heavily reliant on federal grant support during the early years.

Despite these circumstances, the Nixon administration sought to reduce federal funding for social programs such as community health centers. A 1973 Department of Health, Education, and Welfare regulation required health centers to recover as much funding as possible from other sources (Sardell, 1988). Two significant events increased Medicaid's role in health center funding. The 1977 Rural Health Clinic Services Act created all-inclusive Medicare and Medicaid rates for nurse practitioner, nurse midwife, and physician assistant services in rural health clinics. While this act did not focus on health centers, rural health centers could take advantage of the act's provisions to gain better reimbursement. In 1990, all health centers received their own cost-related Medicaid rate through the Federally Qualified Health Center Program. Finally, 25 years after the demonstration project began, Medicaid became the significant revenue source for health centers as envisioned by its first supporters.

As a result, the proportion of health center revenue from federal grants fell from 41% to 26% between 1990 and 1998 while the proportion from Medicaid grew from 21% to 34%. In 2003, Medicaid accounted for 36% of total health center revenue and 64% of third-party collections (National Association of Community Health Centers [NACHC], 2004a). Since the health center patient population is primarily children and women of childbearing age, Medicare has remained a relatively small percentage of health center revenue. In 2003, only 7% of health center patients were on Medicare, bringing in 10% of health center's third-party collections (NACHC, 2004a). However, these figures may shift in the near future as increasingly larger proportions of health center patients are near-elderly (ages 45–65).

As health centers celebrate their 40th anniversary, a new era of reimbursement has begun. Since 2001, the new Prospective Payment System (PPS) created a baseline prospective per patient rate on the basis of each health center's historical costs and adjusted by an inflationary factor each year (Medicare, Medicaid, SCHIP Benefits Improvement and Protection Act, 2000). While the PPS system has brought some security to health centers, given their heavy reliance on public financing, health centers remain in a precarious position as states look to reduce program benefits and eligibility during difficult economic times.

HEALTH INSURANCE

It would be difficult to design a health insurance system more complex than the one in the United States. The variation in patient characteristics, the numerous funding sources for healthcare, and the gaps in the healthcare system serve to separate patient groups in terms of their access to care and health outcomes. Although numerous reimbursement policies are in place to assist safety net providers, more needs to be done to ensure that health centers and other safety net providers are able to provide care for vulnerable populations.

Health Insurance and Health Status

Health insurance became a more common benefit in the 1930s and by the 1960s approximately two thirds of the general population had private insurance (Institute of Medicine [IOM], 2004). Yet, lack of health insurance has remained a persistent problem for a significant portion of the nonelderly population in the United States. The proportion of the nonelderly without health insurance grew from 13.7% in 1987 to 16.9% in 1997 to 17.7% in 2003 (IOM, 2004). Some contend that there would be no need for health centers, or other safety net providers, if everyone had insurance coverage. Or, conversely, that the role of safety net providers is simply to care for the uninsured in the United States (Perry et al., 2000). This view of health centers does not capture either the full scope of health center activities or the effects of how health insurance is provided and utilized in the United States.

Health insurance, for those who have it, is provided through a combination of government-run insurance programs, large privately run employment-based insurance, private individual insurance plans, and a variety of government, private, and philanthropic funding sources (Hadley & Holohan, 2004). While most nonelderly Americans still obtain health insurance through their employers, the proportion of the nonelderly with employer-based health insurance decreased from 65% in 2001 to 61% in 2004, reflecting a downward trend over the last few years in the proportion of employers offering health insurance benefits (Kaiser Family Foundation and Health Research and Education Trust, 2004).

Individuals may cycle between types of insurance or between being insured and uninsured because of the increasing cost of insurance, losing eligibility for public programs, changing or losing jobs, and other life events. Changing insurance plans or falling off of insurance completely makes it difficult to maintain continuity of care and receive appropriate care. Individuals often lose access to their private providers, resulting in lower health outcomes in individuals without continuous coverage (IOM, 2004).

Privately insured, government-insured, and uninsured individuals all have very different characteristics—not only in terms of demographics, but also in their access to healthcare, health status, ability to pay for services, and healthcare behaviors. Generally, privately insured patients have the best outcomes, uninsured patients have the highest proportion of late-stage diagnosis, and Medicaid beneficiaries fall in between. Children on Medicaid have higher utilization rates than poor children without insurance, but less than nonpoor privately insured children (Newacheck et al., 1998). While the proportion of children with a usual source of care is much higher for Medicaid (95.6%) than uninsured poor children (73.8%), the gap is quite small between Medicaid children and nonpoor privately insured children (97.4%) (Newacheck et al., 1998). However, some studies have found health outcomes of Medicaid beneficiaries are comparable to that of the uninsured, possibly due to cycling on and off the program (IOM, 2004). Overall, Medicaid and uninsured patients generally have lower incomes, worse health status, and need more medical care than their privately insured counterparts.

These differences exist for various reasons. The Medicaid population is extremely poor and has health needs associated with or accompanying their poverty (Kotranski et al., 2004). Studies have found that uninsured individuals are more likely to report being in fair or poor health, lack a regular source of care, and are less likely to receive preventive screening and appropriate routine care for chronic conditions (IOM, 2004). When compared to the insured, the uninsured are more likely to spend a higher proportion of their healthcare costs out of their own pocket, and to forgo care because of cost (IOM, 2004). In addition, Medicaid and uninsured patients are more likely to be minorities and have English language limitations (Kaiser Family Foundation, 2004).

Public and Private Reimbursement Policies

The significant and varied healthcare needs of the uninsured and publicly insured patients are often not dealt with by conventional providers, as noted by our colleagues Fiscella and Shin elsewhere in this journal. Private providers have discretion to accept or refuse patients for almost any reason, including ability to pay, demographics, or specific health conditions. One important reason private providers shy away from low-income, uninsured, and publicly insured patients is concern about reimbursement, both in terms of variation in benefits covered by public and private insurance and the level of reimbursement by public programs.

In terms of benefits covered, private insurance generally does not provide reimbursement for the enabling services, such as translation or transportation services that are so important to reducing barriers to care for vulnerable populations. Therefore, providers with mostly low-income or special need patients are left with the choices of providing uncompensated enabling services to patients, trying to shift the cost of enabling services onto privately insured patients, or trying to treat publicly and privately insured patients without these important services.

Public programs generally reimburse providers at a much lower rate than private insurance when care is delivered in a private setting. This leads to private providers limiting access to patients on public programs, such as Medicaid and Medicare. Various studies have shown that significant numbers of providers are refusing to accept Medicaid and Medicare patients. For example, one study found that only half of the physicians surveyed would accept all new Medicaid patients and one fifth refused to accept any (Cunningham, 2002). Another recent study found that 40% have restricted access to new Medicaid patients because of billing and reimbursement issues. While most physicians continue to accept all new Medicare patients, the number willing to accept all new fee-for-service Medicare patients has declined since 1999 (Schoenman & Feldman, 2002). Simply having public insurance coverage is not sufficient to ensure access to a provider.

Safety net providers—such as public hospitals, community health centers, and other local and state clinics—are best equipped to deal with the needs of poor and uninsured patients. They are able to offer quality care for the uninsured and publicly insured patients because they focus on providing culturally competent care and provide additional services such as transportation, translation, extended hours, mobile clinics, case management, and other services that are built into the design of these safety net programs through their mandates.

In recognition of the extra services provided and high-need populations served by community health centers, public insurance programs give additional per patient funding to these providers. For example, Medicaid currently pays and Medicare will pay starting in 2006 a health center-managed care wraparound payment to make up the difference between the cost of providing care to health center patients and the reimbursement amount given by managed care organizations. In addition, under cost-related reimbursement health centers are paid on a per-visit rate that usually exceeds what private providers will be reimbursed, due to the additional costs health centers incur when providing enabling services. The health center PPS that took effect in 2001 requires reimbursement to be on a prospective basis unless both the state and individual health center agree to use a cost-based formula or other alternative payment methodology. PPS protects health centers from cuts in Medicaid reimbursement in ways that other providers

are not because the prospective formula provides a federally guaranteed minimum for reimbursement (regardless of what kind of payment methodology is used). This minimum includes an annual increase based on the Medicare Economic Index. However, the extent of this protection is not clear since as least one state has used a federal waiver to avoid paying the PPS rate for a new optional population.

As a result of these reimbursement policies, Medicaid and Medicare managed care patients end up bringing in more revenue to health centers than privately insured patients—the opposite result experienced by private providers. Medicaid reimburses health centers at a higher rate than private plans, most likely because of a combination of wraparound payments and the extensive services offered by health centers (Rosenbaum et al., 2001). Another explanation could be that private managed care patients seen at health centers may be underinsured (i.e., have high deductibles and fewer benefits than Medicaid), thus rendering the patient essentially uninsured and the health center unpaid for delivering these services until the deductible is met or until the insurance will cover a limited amount of care. For these reasons, health centers are highly reliant on Medicaid patients who account for over a third of their total revenue.

As noted elsewhere in this journal, these public policies reflect the understanding that poor and uninsured patients often have multiple health issues, low health status, and numerous nonhealth barriers to accessing needed healthcare services. More than just providing insurance coverage, health centers are designed to be a continuous source of high-quality, culturally competent care to these vulnerable populations.

HEALTH CENTERS AND HEALTH INSURANCE— COMPLEMENTS, NOT ALTERNATIVES

The health center design recognizes that just having insurance is not enough to ensure adequate care. Even though some may think that universal insurance is a panacea for our healthcare woes, several studies suggest otherwise. Having insurance does not guarantee access to care, providers willing to accept all insurance, ability to pay cost-sharing requirements, coverage for all medically necessary services, ability to obtain culturally competent care, or satisfaction with the care received. Anecdotal evidence shows that many previously uninsured health center patients continue to seek care at health centers after they have gained insurance coverage because of the continuity of care, range of services offered, longer hours, and flexibility of the provider to meet patient needs (Nolan et al., 2002). The need for both health centers and health insurance is illustrated by understanding the interaction between having a usual source of care and insurance, and by exploring why countries with universal coverage find it necessary and useful to have health centers provide care to their residents.

Usual Source of Care

Whether or not one is insured, it is crucial to have a usual source of care. Having a usual source of care is positively associated with better and more timely access to care, better chronic disease management, fewer emergency department visits, fewer lawsuits against emergency departments, increased utilization rates, and increased cancer screenings for women (Starfield & Shi, 2004). In fact, lack of a usual source of care is an even greater predictor than insurance status in delay in seeking care (Sox et al., 1998).

Does that mean that providing a usual source of care for everyone is an adequate replacement for universal insurance? No. Having health insurance and a usual source of care are complementary, not substitute factors in providing better, more accessible healthcare to patients. Numerous studies have shown that having both health insurance and a usual source of care result in improved health of the population (NACHC, 2004b).

One recent study reviewing 1996 Medical Expenditure Panel Survey data found that more patients with both insurance and a usual source of care received preventive services than individuals with only insurance or only a usual source of care (DeVoe et al., 2003). When comparing *insured* patients with a usual source of care to *uninsured* patients with a usual source of care, a higher percentage of the insured patients received care in each of 7 preventive care categories studied— blood pressure (85% vs 70%), cholesterol check (59% vs 45%), physical exam (54% vs 38%), dental checkup (41% vs 19%), papanicolaou tests (67% vs 49%), breast exams (71% vs 47%), and mammogram (57% vs 36%). Having a usual source of care and insurance had "independent, additive effects" on the receipt of care (DeVoe et al., 2003). In other words, patients in the best position were those with both insurance and a usual source of care.

Another study considered the impact of having a usual source of care in a country with universal healthcare (Menec et al., 2005). The authors evaluated the benefits of continuity of care on the population of Winnipeg, Canada, by looking at the number of visits to family physicians. Even though the Canadian healthcare system provides free access to healthcare services, their study found that having an ongoing relationship with a single family physician makes a difference in health outcomes. Patients with high continuity of care had better preventive care and a reduced likelihood of emergency department visits as compared to those with low continuity of care (Menec et al., 2005). The authors conclude that because it is up to the patients whether they use the healthcare system, family physicians play a key role in educating, promoting, and monitoring use of health services.

Furthermore, they found that socioeconomic status was a key factor to accessing care even in a universal healthcare system. Those living in more affluent neighborhoods were twice as likely to have a mammogram and half as likely to visit the emergency department as those living in the poorest neighborhoods (Menec et al., 2005). Even though everyone has an equal right to healthcare in Canada, additional safeguards are needed to make sure that their poorer citizens have equal access.

Where patients usually receive their care is also important. Health centers are designed to catch the patients who might otherwise fall through the cracks of the healthcare system. As compared to uninsured American patients nationwide, uninsured patients at health centers are less likely to delay seeking care because of cost, go without needed care, or fail to fill prescriptions for needed medicine (Politzer et al., 2001). Uninsured health center patients are also more likely to receive health education and health promotion services than uninsured adults nationwide (Politzer et al.).

Health centers also effectively serve insured patients. Approximately 60% of health center patients are insured (NACHC, 2004a). Compared to other providers such as office-based physicians, outpatient departments, and emergency departments, health centers scored highest in the proportion of Medicaid pediatric patients who received preventive services in one study (Stuart et al., 1995). Among women with Medicaid, 96% of those seen by health centers received mammograms as compared to 75% nationally (NACHC, 2004b). Overall, health center women are more likely to receive mammograms, clinical breast exams, and papanicolaou tests than women not using health centers (Politzer et al., 2001). The health center model, focused on community needs and providing quality culturally competent care, is important to insured as well as uninsured patients (Kominski et al., 2005). As discussed in more detail elsewhere in this journal by Michelle Proser, health centers have been very successful in reaching their target population, providing high-quality healthcare, and improving health outcomes. Fears that promoting health centers means a 2-tiered system of care are unfounded.

For these reasons, another study concluded that policymakers should pursue the dual strategy of expanding both health insurance and health centers (Cunningham & Hadley, 2004). They found access to care was highest in communities with both strong insurance and strong health center presence. In particular, low-income individuals had best access and faced the fewest perceived barriers to care in these communities. Even though insurance expansion can be a primary tool for eliminating *financial* concerns, health centers "play an important role in filling" the gaps for vulnerable populations and in underserved areas by their location and by providing additional services and culturally competent care necessary to increase access to care. (Cunningham & Hadley, 2004).

Health Centers in Countries with National Health Systems

Perhaps, most telling of the ways health centers and health insurance are complementary is illustrated by the use of community-based providers designed with features that are similar to health centers in countries with universal or near universal health insurance coverage. A literature review of countries with national health insurance systems and economies similar to that of the United States, found that 9 of 11 countries* evaluated employ a health center-style program (Hawkins et al., 2001). These countries use health centers in a variety of ways. For example, Scandinavian countries rely on health centers to provide primary care because of their geographic accessibility and holistic approach to healthcare. In Australia, health centers are more likely than private physicians to engage in group health promotion activities and community development initiatives. In Canada, health centers have the lead responsibility for home care, postoperative care, hospital follow-up, and vaccination campaigns.

As in the United States, other countries—even those with national health insurance systems—use health centers to serve the hard-to-reach and vulnerable populations. Several studies indicate that health centers abroad focus on serving special populations such as the homeless, disabled, elderly, mentally ill, and persons with substance abuse related health problems. Also, health centers in Canada and Australia are used to provide care to culturally distinct subpopulations, such as aboriginal populations, who have different healthcare traditions and preferences than the rest of the country (Hawkins et al., 2001). Thus, even under national insurance, certain populations would still remain underserved because of complex barriers to care. Regardless of the size of the country, the health system used, or the specific needs of the community, the health center model has proven to be effective in providing quality care and culturally competent care to vulnerable populations.

* These countries with health centers are as follows: United Kingdom, Canada, Spain, Australia, New Zealand, Sweden, Finland, Switzerland (limited used), and Japan. The countries without health centers are France and Germany.

CONCLUSION

Given the current political and economic climate, it is unlikely that universal health insurance coverage is on the horizon in the United States. As we debate the best means for improving access to care for the underserved, it is essential to understand that funding safety net providers and supporting expanded health insurance coverage are not opposing choices. As we have seen, private providers are not as well equipped to deal with the type of patients that make their medical home at community health centers. A health center is better able to handle the primary care needs for any patient that walks through the door, due to their mission to be located in medically underserved areas and provide culturally competent, comprehensive primary care services, regardless of insurance status or ability to pay. Of course, insurance is also important in ensuring access to care. Health center growth does not undercut the need for insurance. Rather, both are vital to ensure improved access to care for the largest number of people.

Instead, the debate should be about how best to use safety net providers in the event that health insurance coverage expands. It is essential that health centers remain adequately funded through direct operational subsidies from the federal government and sufficient Medicaid reimbursement, as well as reimbursement from any universal coverage system that may be implemented. In the future, assuming that an expanded or universal health insurance program would be an adequate payer, there are several ways to use health center funds. As more people gain health insurance, funding pools that had been used to cover the uninsured could be targeted to cover even more enabling services that have proved so crucial for minority, poor, and underserved populations. Additional efforts could focus on improving how health centers and local hospitals and private, office-based physicians work together to treat at-risk populations who tend to have lower health status in their communities, with the goal of reducing the use of emergency departments for ambulatory care-sensitive conditions. Health center grants could be used to provide higher reimbursement rates to health centers, open more health center access points, and offer increased services that were previously limited or had not been available, such as dental services or behavioral healthcare. Whatever choices are made, options must be considered with the awareness that health centers will continue to be necessary to reach vulnerable populations regardless of the type of healthcare system in place.

REFERENCES

Cunningham, P., & Hadley, J. (2004). Expanding care versus expanding coverage: How to improve access to care. *Health Affairs. 23*(4), 234–244.

Cunningham, P. J. (2002). *Mounting pressures: Physicians serving Medicaid patients and the uninsured. 1997–2001* (Trucking Report No. 6). Washington, DC: Center for Studying Health Systems Change.

DeVoe, D., Fryer, G., Phillips, R., & Green, L. (2003). Receipt of preventive care among adults: Insurance status and usual source of care. *American Journal of Public Health, 93*(5), 786–791.

Hadley, J., & Holohan, J. (2004). The *cost of care for the uninsured. What do we spend, who pays, and what would full coverage add to Medicaid spending?* Menlo Park, CA: Kaiser Commission on Medicaid and the Uninsured.

Hawkins, D.. Gevorgyan, M., Lopes, A., & Rosenbaum, S. (2001). *The use of community health centers in countries with national health insurance: A synthesis of the literature.* Washington, DC: National Association of Community Health Centers.

Hawkins, D. R., Jr., & Rosenbaum, S. (1998). The challenges facing health centers in a changing healthcare system. In S. Altman, U. Reinhardt, & A. Shields (Eds.), *The future U.S. healthcare system: Who will care for the poor and uninsured* (pp. 99–122). Chicago: Health Administration Press.

Institute of Medicine. (2004). *Insuring America's health: Principles and recommendations.* Washington, DC: National Academy Press.

Kaiser Family Foundation. (2004, June 12). *Key facts: Race, ethnicity, and medical care.* Analysis of 2003 California Health Interview Survey. Retrieved March 10, 2005, from www.askchis.com.

Kaiser Family Foundation and Health Research and Education Trust. (2004). *Employer health benefits 2004 annual survey.* Retrieved August 11, 2005, from http://www.kff.org/insurance/7148/upload/2004-Employer-Health-Benefits-Survey-Full-Report.pdf.

Kominski, G., Roby, D., & Kincheloe, J. (2005). *Cost of insuring California's uninsured.* Los Angeles: UCLA Center for Health Policy Research.

Kotranski, L., Axler, F., & Beraima, A. (2004). *Health status of women Medicaid recipients before and after welfare reform.* Paper presented at annual meeting of the American Public Health Association, Washington, DC.

Medicare, Medicaid, SCHIP Benefits Improvement and Protection Act, 42 USC 1396a(bb) (2002).

Menec, V., Sirski, M., & Attawar, D. (2005). Does continuity of care matter in a universally insured population? *Health Services Research, 40*(2), 389–400.

National Association of Community Health Centers. (2004a) *Health center fact sheet 2004.* Retrieved March 10, 2005, from http://www.nachc.com/research/ Files/IntrotoHealthCenters8.04.pdf.

National Association of Community Health Centers. (2004b). *A nation's health at risk II: A front row seat in a changing health care system.* Retrieved March 10, 2005, from http://www.nachc.com/press/files/Nations HealthIISTIB7.pdf.

Newacheck, P. W., Pearl, M., Hughes, D. C., & Halfon, N. (1998). The role of Medicaid in ensuring children's access to care. *JAMA, 280*(20), 1789–1793.

Nolan, L., Harvey, J., Jones, K., Vaquerano, L., & Zuvekas, A. (2002). *The impact of the state children's health insurance program (SCHIP) on community health centers.* Washington, DC: The George Washington University Center for Health Services Research and Policy.

Perry, M., Kannel, S., & Castillo, E. (2000). *Barriers to health coverage for Hispanic workers: Focus group findings.* New York, NY: The Commonwealth Fund Task Force on the Future of Health Insurance.

Politzer, R. M., Yoon, J., Shi, L., Hughes, R. G., Regan, J., & Gaston, M. H. (2001). Inequality in America: The contribution of health centers in reducing and eliminating disparities in access to care. *Medicine Care Research and Review, 58*(2), 234–248.

Rosenbaum, S., Wilensky, S., Shin, P., & Roby, D. (2001). *Managed care and health centers: An overview and analysis.* Bethesda, MD: The Bureau of Primary Health Care, Health Services and Resources Administration.

Sardell, S. (1988). *The U.S. experiment in social medicine: The community health center program, 1965–1986.* Pittsburgh: University of Pittsburgh Press.

Schoenman, J., & Feldman, J. (2002). *Results of the Medicare payment advisory commission's 2002 survey of physicians.* Bethesda, MD: The Project HOPE Center for Health Affairs.

Sox, C., Swartz, K., Burstin, H., & Brennan, T. (1998). Insurance or regular physician: Which is the most powerful predictor of health care? *American Journal of Public Health, 88*(3), 364–370.

Starfield, B., & Shi, L. (2004). The medical home, access to care, and insurance: A review of evidence. *Pediatrics, 113*(5), 1493–1498.

Stuart, M., Steinwachs, D., Starfield, B., Orr, S., & Kerns, A. (1995). Improving Medicaid pediatric care. *Journal of Public Health Management Practice, 1*(2), 31–38.

Health Reform and the Safety Net: Big Opportunities; Major Risks

Bruce Siegel, Marsha Regenstein, and Peter Shin

Source: Health Reform and the Safety Net: Big Opportunities; Major Risks. Bruce Siegel, Marsha Regenstein, Peter Shin. *The Journal of Law, Medicine & Ethics,* Symposium: National Health Reform and America's Uninsured, pp. 426–432 (Fall 2004).

Millions of Americans are dependent on what is often called the "safety net." These loosely-organized networks of health and social service providers serve the many Americans who are uninsured, dependent on public coverage, or for a variety of reasons unable to access other private systems of care. The Institute of Medicine (IOM) report, *America's Health Care Safety Net: Intact but Endangered,* called attention to both the fragility and the resilience of this health care safety net.[1] The IOM report underscored the critical importance of the safety net to the health and well-being of millions of individuals and called for efforts to strengthen it and improve the nation's ability to monitor its viability.[2] Given this central role, any health care reform efforts need to be fully informed by an understanding of what the safety net includes, how it is financed, and how it is responding to a series of challenges it now faces. They also must consider the nature of the role of the health care safety net in radical health care reform, like universal coverage. As this article discusses, universal coverage would change, not eliminate, the need for the safety net. It may offer opportunities for these providers to better meet their core missions, but such reform potentially poses major risks as well.

STRUCTURE AND FUNCTION OF THE SAFETY NET

Populations that rely on the safety net include many of our nation's most vulnerable individuals, including the uninsured, low-income and homeless families who are at higher risk for serious illnesses than the general population, migrant farm workers, undocumented immigrants, persons with chronic illnesses, and substance abusers.[3] Safety net users may also reside in medically underserved areas where residents present a variety of health challenges related to high rates of unemployment, poverty, inadequate health care infrastructure, lack of access to needed services, and poor working and living conditions.[4] High infant mortality rates, poor perinatal outcomes, domestic violence, tobacco and alcohol related morbidity and mortality, poor dental hygiene and care, substantial mental health problems, and diet and nutritionally-related illness and disease all commonly contribute to the health problems seen in communities that rely heavily on the safety net.[5]

There is no true concensus on what constitutes the safety net. One representative definition refers to the set of providers who organize and deliver a significant level of health care and other health-related services to uninsured, Medicaid, and other vulnerable patients.[6] Some of these providers are mandated by law to provide services regardless of a patient's coverage or ability to pay. Others are considered safety net providers by virtue of their organizational mission to serve uninsured, publicly insured or otherwise vulnerable patients. The composition of local safety nets is highly variable but generally includes some combination of providers such as public or non-profit hospitals, community health centers, public health department clinics, rural health clinics, free clinics and sometimes individual physician practices. For our purposes we will focus on two of the largest and most visible elements: community health centers and public hospitals.

The Role of Community Health Centers in the Safety Net

Community health centers (CHCs) are the backbone of the primary care safety net in the U.S. CHCs grew out of the Civil Rights movement in the 1960s and the desire to provide accessible and affordable health care to low-income and otherwise disenfranchised community residents who were often unable to access care through private physicians' offices. CHCs are congressionally-mandated to provide care for low-income and minority persons who cannot afford access to health care.[7] Virtually all CHCs are non-profit entities. At least 51 percent of the members of the CHC's governing body must be patients who use the center's services. This requirement serves as a safeguard to ensure that the CHC remains responsive to the medical and social needs of the community.[8]

As of 2002, there were nearly 850 CHCs that provided care to over 11.3 million patients, the majority of whom were low-income.[9] A single CHC often provides services through multiple delivery sites, and they are currently located in over 3500 urban and rural communities.[10]

About 39 percent of CHC patients are uninsured and another 36 percent are covered by the Medicaid program.[11] According to 2002 data, more than 621,000 CHC patients are homeless and over 708,000 are migrant workers. Two-thirds of CHC patients nationwide are members of racial or ethnic minority groups.[12]

Because they care for such a vulnerable group of patients, CHCs provide a variety of services beyond preventive and primary health care. These include interpreter services to enable patients who speak languages other than English to communicate effectively with health center staff and providers; outreach efforts to screen for illnesses and high-risk individuals; case management for individuals with complex health and social service needs; and child care, housing assistance, and other enabling services that make health care more accessible and effective.[13] In 2002, medical services accounted for 77 percent of total CHC encounters, dental services for 8 percent, and enabling services for 8 percent of total services provided. The remaining 7 percent of service encounters went to other professional, mental health, and substance abuse services.[14]

Hospitals in the Safety Net

Public and other safety net hospitals have been serving low-income populations in this country since the eighteenth century.[15] Aside from their governance, they are also characterized by the substantial amount of care they provide to uninsured and publicly-insured individuals. Unlike CHCs, however, they are not organized around, and funded by, a single federal program. Safety net hospitals provide a diverse range of inpatient and outpatient services, including trauma care, psychiatric services, neonatal intensive care, burn care, and state-of-the-art diagnostic services to low-income populations. Unlike CHCs, safety net hospitals see a substantially greater proportion of Medicare patients in greater need of high-cost specialized care. Additionally, the hospital emergency departments (ED) may themselves be safety net providers, given the federal mandate under the Emergency Medical Treatment and Active Labor Act (EMTALA) of 1986.[16] The statute requires appropriate medical screening for all patients and adequate treatment and stabilization for those found to have an emergent condition. In effect, the hospital ED cannot turn away any patients seeking medical care. Between 1996 and 2000, the number of ED visits increased nearly 20 percent from 91 million to 108 million.[17] Although privately-insured patients account for a majority of the growth in ED visits, the uninsured are four times more likely than privately-insured patients to use the ED as a source of primary care.[18]

How Do We Pay for the Safety Net?

Safety net providers have long been dependent on governmental sources of financing to support care for low-income populations. That support is most likely a blend of Medicaid, federal and state grants, Disproportionate Share Hospital (DSH) funding, and local taxpayer support. Public financing will become even more important in light of the growing uninsured population in this country, which reached 43.6 million in 2002.[19]

The need for special finance systems is demonstrated by the stark difference in uncompensated care costs between the safety net and the rest of the health care system. Uncompensated costs average about six percent of total hospital costs in the U.S.[20] But this figure is very different for hospitals in the safety net. Uncompensated care costs account for 17.6 percent of major public teaching hospital costs, 14.2 percent for urban government hospitals, and 26 percent for public hospitals.[21] High uncompensated care in hospitals accompanies high numbers of publicly insured individuals: Hospitals that serve a larger share of Medicaid patients also provided the greatest share of uncompensated care.[22]

Medicaid is the major source of funding for the safety net. Indeed, Medicaid accounted for approximately 35 percent of CHCs' operating revenues in 2002[23] and 38 percent of safety net hospital revenues in 2001.[24] For hospitals, Medicaid DSH payments also represent major sources of support for uncompensated care: The federal payments totaled approximately $8.6 billion in 2003.[25] While this may seem like a substantial amount, there is evidence that these DSH payments are inadequate to match the increasing burden of uncompensated care or to support institutions with the greatest uncompensated care burden.[26] Even with these payments, average margins at safety net hospitals were under one percent in 2001, compared to 4.5 percent among hospitals nationally.[27]

For CHCs, federal grants are the second largest source of revenue. In 2004, the federal Bureau of Primary Health Care provided CHCs over $1.62 billion to cover costs of care for the uninsured.[28] Although grants and subsidies on which these publicly-funded entities depend remained stagnant in real terms in the 1990s, the Bush administration spearheaded efforts to significantly increase funding for new CHCs and expansions of existing centers.[29] Under this expansion program, the federal government aims to double the number of CHC sites to serve 6.1 million new patients by 2006. The CHCs are on pace to meet this target. Since 2001, over 2.6 million additional persons were served.[30]

State and local subsidies are also critical in financing care for the uninsured and low-income population.[31] According to the National Association of Public Hospitals and Health Systems, state and local funds financed 38 percent of public hospitals' uncompensated care costs in 2001.[32] In 2002, CHCs received over $531 million from state and local sources.[33]

In the end, safety net providers must piece together a myriad of funding sources to provide services to low-income residents because there is no stable and adequate source of financing for the nation's uninsured population.

THE SAFETY NET UNDER REFORM: OPPORTUNITIES AND CHALLENGES

Safety nets face a complex set of challenges. Given their reliance on public funding, they are exquisitely sensitive to policy and political decisions at all levels of government, especially when those decisions affect the funding of care for uninsured and publicly insured individuals. They also face the challenge of meeting their historic missions in an increasingly market-driven health care economy, which falls to recognize the costs of care for the poor, the great capital investments and expenses required to adopt and provide new technologies, and the expenses of training future health professionals. With the effects of a downturn in the U.S. economy, increasingly strapped state budgets, growing numbers of uninsured individuals, and trends in the commercial health insurance market, safety nets and their providers have no shortage of challenges.[34] Any attempts at reform may dispro-

portionately affect the safety net, given the populations it serves and its complex public financing.

Viewed simplistically, any initiatives that increase insurance coverage should have a positive impact on the viability of the safety net, as the uninsured are converted to covered lives. Truly universal health care with meaningful benefits and portability, without onerous cost-sharing, would dramatically reduce the uncompensated care burden of all health care providers. It should most dramatically improve the viability of those with the greatest charity care load, namely those in the safety net. Perhaps more importantly, the benefits to the populations served by the safety net might be impressive. The research on this subject shows a clear and consistent relationship between a lack of health insurance coverage, and reduced access to health services and inferior health outcomes.[35] A recent review of the literature on access to care found insurance status and ability to pay for health care to be the most important predictor of the quality of health care across various groups.[36] The uninsured receive less preventive care, are diagnosed at more advanced disease stages and, once diagnosed, tend to receive less therapeutic care, including pharmaceuticals and surgical interventions.[37] Uninsured children are also at greater risk for poor health outcomes.[38] Major insurance expansions could be expected to ameliorate many of these issues.

Nevertheless, the devil may be in the details for the safety net, given its special circumstances. Health reform that excludes undocumented immigrants, for instance, may be of less benefit to many communities and their safety net providers, where such immigrants make up a large part of the population. It would be hard to imagine that such reform would be particularly effective in large parts of California and Texas, for instance.[39] The vehicle for reform will also be critical. Changes that rely on the use of private insurers may be of less benefit to the safety net, given how private insurers are often less likely to contract with traditional safety net providers. Already, over the past decade, the dramatic shift to managed care for Medicaid has meant that many safety net providers have had to face competition for their Medicaid patients and largest source of revenue, as private plans often contract with many new providers.[40]

Certainly the design of any benefit package will also have differential effects on these populations as well as their systems of care. A "coverage" reform which targets mainly catastrophic benefits will have little ability to increase the use of preventive and primary care services by the poor and uninsured. It will also have much less impact on safety net providers than more comprehensive benefit packages, given the frequent emphasis of those providers on primary care and other outpatient services. Cost-sharing by beneficiaries in the form of high co-payments, deductibles and premium cost-sharing as well as multi-level pharmaceutical pricing schemes[41] all hit low-income individuals the hardest, and create demand for services from insured and uninsured workers alike who turn to the safety net for primary care, specialty care, inpatient services, mental health care, dental services, and a host of other treatments that are beyond their reach in the private market. Even today the increasing demand for emergency department services at many hospitals may reflect the current existence of these trends as greater numbers of Medicaid enrollees and other insured individuals turn to them instead of private providers of primary and specialty care.[42] Any reform which continues these features can be expected to generate the same results.

Other work points to additional reasons why a safety net may still be needed, even under "universal" health care. Recent work demonstrates that health insurance coverage alone does not promise equal access or equal outcomes. There are huge disparities in the health care received by insured individuals and, while some of these disparities are related to the type of insurance involved, others are not explained by factors related to type of insurance or even income. Many are a result of disparate treatment or behavior in some way associated with the patient's race, ethnicity, country of origin, language spoken, or other non-health and non-insurance related variable.[43] The Institute of Medicine's recent report, *Unequal Treatment: Confronting Racial and Ethnic Disparities in Health Care*, has crystallized concern for these issues and recommends moving beyond the process of documenting disparities in favor of comprehensive strategies to eliminate them. Included among these strategies are efforts to increase awareness of disparate care; adhere to clinical guidelines; increase the proportion of underrepresented U.S. racial and ethnic minorities among health professionals; and deconstruct barriers to care by offering transportation assistance, interpreter services, and cross-cultural training.[44] It is doubtful that health care reform will be able to "fix" all these problems in even the long-run.

Thus, expanded health insurance may be viewed as a necessary ingredient in accessing health services, but it appears to be insufficient on its own to guarantee appropriate, or at least equitable, care for millions of individuals, especially members of racial and ethnic minorities. Policymakers who are interested in raising the level of care for all Americans may be surprised by some of the work coming out of community health centers and public hospitals, which indicates that at least some of the safety net is providing high-quality, "disparity-free" service to persons of color and other racial and ethnic minority patients.

Preliminary studies at Denver Health Medical Center found no significant disparities in access to selected preventive and chronic disease management services among patients using the system.[45] Approximately three-quarters of African American, Hispanic and white females (age 52–69) received at least one mammogram in the prior two-year period; half of African American, Hispanic and white patients showed evidence that his or her blood pressure was under control; and for about 70 percent of the same categories of patients, a full lipid profile had been obtained in the prior two-year period. In another example, the New York City Health and Hospitals Corporation (HHC) recently began to measure more than fifty quality of care indicators across its patient populations.[46] Preliminary evidence indicates that African American patients at HHC are much more likely to get certain necessary health services than the average African American patient. For example, while only about 63 percent of African American women are screened for breast cancer nationwide, about 92 percent of HHC patients receive the service. In addition, 92 percent of HHC diabetics receive eye exams, compared to the national average of 44 percent of African American patients with diabetes. And 84 percent of African American patients receive follow-up care after a hospitalization for mental illness; this is 2½ times the national average for African Americans of 33 percent.

Community health center patients also enjoy health care that appears to be less likely to result in access and outcome disparities. Drawing on findings from medical records and patient surveys, Politzer and colleagues found that community health center networks had reduced low-birth weight disparities for African American infants.[47] Overall, the authors contend that health centers have reduced racial, ethnic, income and insurance status disparities in access to primary care and preventive screening services by providing access to a regular and usual source of care. In addition, analyses conducted by the Center for Health Services Research and Policy at George Washington University of the 1999 Uniform Data System[48] and the National Ambulatory Medical Care Survey showed that community health centers provided more mammograms and cervical screenings that their private physician office counterparts.[49]

Given these findings, there may still very much be a role for the safety net even under the most expansive and radical models of health care reform. The safety net may be needed to deliver high-quality services to an array of vulnerable populations, regardless of individuals' insurance status. Reform, depending on how it is structured, may strengthen the safety net's ability to perform these functions; or it may undermine it.

But despite this many key policymakers and coverage proponents continue to separately conceptualize health insurance coverage from access to the safety net, often couching their support for safety net expansions as necessary *in the absence of comprehensive health reform.* Even the Institute of Medicine report, *America's Health Care Safety Net: Intact but Endangered*, prefaced its work by stating that ". . . today's changing healthcare marketplace is placing core safety net providers in many communities at risk of not being able to continue their mission of caring for a growing number of uninsured at a time when other national, federal, state, and local initiatives to expand coverage are still on the drawing board, in a fledging state, or falling short of their promise."[50] For some policymakers, support of the safety net appears to be at odds with their commitment to health coverage for all, a notion that would strike safety net leaders around the country as incomprehensible, at best.

THE SAFETY NET'S RESPONSE

Already faced with reduced resources and rapid changes in the health care marketplace, communities and safety net providers have attempted a number of strategies to try to combat trends that threaten their viability. We could expect many or all of these strategies to be accelerated in the face of significant national health reform, although the nature of that reform will obviously affect which strategies receive the most emphasis. Some of these strategies have involved efforts to increase the viability of a single provider or set of safety net providers in a community through increased public financial support. This might be less critical if new resources actually did flow to these providers through health reform. Adopting a more competitive stance, in an effort to retain existing insured patients (especially those on Medicaid) and attract new ones in order to increase revenues has also been common. These efforts might well need to be redoubled if reform was implemented through a highly competitive, market-driven framework. In some communities, policy makers have tried instead to essentially replace a public "bricks and mortar" safety net (like a public hospital) with a "virtual safety net" in which care for vulnerable populations is financed and spread among a series of remaining institutions, few or none of which may be publicly owned or have a mission of primarily serving these populations. This also might be a very attractive model to some, if large portions of the uninsured were covered. Many of these strategies could be tried in combination, but all are fraught with political, financial and clinical complications, and they may have very different effects on the quality and availability of care for vulnerable populations. We offer these strategies as historical record as well as a guide for what we might expect under reform.

Increasing Community Support

A relatively straightforward but politically difficult strategy is obtaining new or increased funding for the safety net. In some communities, this has already happened as the result of broad-based campaigns to either levy new taxes or access other sources of revenue for the safety net. Often these increases in support are only politically palatable and possible in periods of crisis, during a period of intense media scrutiny with the hospital or clinics in danger of closing. Recent events in Detroit have followed this model. Years of financial losses, hospital closures, massive layoffs, and management reorganizations have finally resulted in a financial lifeline to forestall closure of the principal safety net hospital, Detroit Medical Center. This lifeline took the form of a $50 million emergency aid package from the state that will keep components of the hospital system operating until longer-terms solutions can be identified.[51] Similarly, safety net hospital closures were potentially averted by a voter-approved property tax increase in Los Angeles County in late 2002. In many cases increased support is viewed in the context of the potential loss of services; often the loss of trauma services is the most sensitive topic as they are viewed as a resource for the broad community, not just the poor. Increased support is also often tied to increased public oversight and management changes at the involved provider, as it was in the Detroit example.

All of this might seem irrelevant under potential health reform. Yet reforms that, for instance, lead to the large-scale movement of covered (e.g., Medicaid) patients away from the safety net while leaving those providers with a significant remaining burden of uncompensated care could easily create a scenario in which this specific segment of the health care industry finds itself under increasing distress. Put more bluntly, even if we halve the number of uninsured, the safety net could be endangered if it simultaneously experiences the exodus of its remaining insured patients. Political leaders may find it much more difficult to increase or even continue fiscal support of these systems in the wake of a health reform initiative that was supposed to obviate these issues. Could we really expect the business community, for instance, to continue to support local tax levies for a public hospital after implementation of an employer mandate?

Attempting to Make It in the Competitive Market

Some safety net providers have aggressively tried to meet the competitive market head-on. This direction takes many forms, some of which may be popular and others highly controversial. We could easily envision the continuation and even quickening of these efforts under health care reform that emphasized private market solution like the use of commercial HMOs.

For community health centers and some public hospitals, this strategy has already meant bold (and risky) ventures into the managed care business, in an effort to manage the care and retain the loyalty of the many Medicaid patients they serve, while potentially attracting a broader array of patients. Many safety net providers established major or even exclusive ownership positions in managed care organizations, and by 1998 the majority of community health centers were members of a managed care provider network.[52] This is an attempt to secure an insured population in danger of being attracted to competing private providers, yet it comes with significant financial exposure with fixed premiums. For other safety net providers, the competitive posture has meant a strong focus on improved efficiency and promotion of quality. This drive for efficiency often manifests itself through very unpopular and traumatic workforce downsizing and closures of parts of the system deemed redundant, both of which have recently occurred at Detroit Medical Center in recent years as it cut staff and closed hospitals in its network.[53] Less controversial and more positive competitive strategies include initiatives to strengthen patient satisfaction and quality. The New York City public hospitals have worked to improve ambulatory care access in its extensive outpatient network in concert with the New York Primary Care Development Corporation. This serves as an example of a strategy designed to improve quality while better positioning the provider in the marketplace.[54] Other examples include the community health centers' embrace of quality through the federally-supported Health Disparities Collaboratives designed to improve care for patients with chronic disease.[55] Clearly adapting a more competitive stance can include different strategies which may be perceived very differently within a community.

Reorganizing Corporate Governance

Many institutions have sought to improve their competitive edge by changing their corporate structure or even ownership status. Any health reform that continues or ratchets up competitive market pressures for these providers will continue to provoke this response. Indeed, a simple coverage expansion may lead policymakers and elected officials to the conclusion that there simply isn't a future role for publicly-owned safety net facilities.

Sometimes these changes have taken the form of public hospitals reorganizing themselves as quasi-independent authorities holding greater autonomy from local government, and often exempt from onerous government contracting and personnel policies that are viewed as archaic and inflexible. Two recent examples include the formation of "public benefit corporations" in New York State to govern Westchester Medical Center and Nassau University Medical Center. These reforms have often been viewed as "halfway," with the new entities still beholden to some political entity and often keeping some vestiges of public status, such as public employee unions.[56] More commonly, governance changes involve the actual lease or sale of the public hospital to a private entity, especially in the southeastern part of the country, where literally dozens of formerly county facilities have been transferred.[57] Often these conversions feature some ongoing obligation on the part of the successor entity to provide specialized services (e.g., trauma) or some level of indigent care access. Prominent examples of these conversions include numerous Florida hospitals such as (most recently) Tampa General Health Care. While at least one in-depth study found that these conversions maintained access and improved financial performance,[58] these conversions do not necessarily guarantee viability. Institutions treating large numbers of uninsured, providing high-cost services and training large numbers of health professionals will continue to need high levels of financial support, regardless of their governance structure. Additionally, conversion to a private structure may insulate the provider from negative political pressures, but it may also make it much harder for that provider to call upon public resources in a time of need. Once the provider becomes a "private hospital," it may have a much more difficult time persuading opinion leaders, elected officials and the general public that it is deserving of taxpayer support, even if it has maintained its safety net mission and obligations.

Restricting Access to Staunch the Bleeding

Faced with mounting deficits, some safety net providers have simply moved to restrict access to free or low-cost services. While we might hope that reform would not place these providers in such a predicament, again reforms could very easily actually undermine the safety net by increasing competitive pressures and/or leaving the safety net with the residual uninsured. In June 2003, the Los Angeles County Board of Supervisors voted to require proof of residence from nonemergent patients seeking care in the public health care system. That same year, faced with state budget cuts, the University of Texas Medical Branch in Galveston implemented its "Demand and Access Management Program," or DAMP, requiring strict financial screening of patients, fees before treatment, and restrictions on certain high-cost therapies and drugs.[59] Grady Health System, the flagship safety net network in Atlanta, discontinued the provision of free primary care services to patients residing outside of its Fulton and DeKalb Counties catchment area in early 2004. Maricopa Medical Center in Phoenix instituted "up-front" fees for outpatient visits as well. Note that many of these communities have already moved to competitive models of Medicaid reform, so this history could well be a guide to possible future scenarios.

Critics have been quick to point out the possible effects of such changes in practice, including patients forced to forgo needed care and eventually ending up in already overburdened emergency departments with potentially preventable illnesses. But safety net administrators respond by pointing out that if they do not take these steps, their basic viability will be threatened, resulting essentially in no care for anybody. Political leaders may also find these solutions attractive if they avoid tax increases for local constituents and are couched as making sure that those who can pay, do; or as just not footing the bill for people who cross county lines to get their care for free.

Eliminating the "Bricks and Mortar" Safety Net

Perhaps the most radical response, eliminating the "bricks and mortar" safety net has been tried in a number of U.S. cities including Philadelphia, Washington, DC, Milwaukee and others. In each case, the public hospital was closed with some expectation that other providers would fill the gap. In some cases (though not all), an explicit financing mechanism was put in place to support that care through the remaining providers, recognizing that, without that incentive, the burden might be too much for these institutions to bear.

These responses are particularly relevant to the potential political environment of major health care reform. Many may question why these institutions are still needed and supported if the problems of coverage and access have supposedly been "solved."

In Milwaukee, this strategy has taken the form of the county government providing $30 million annually for indigent and trauma care to a non-profit teaching hospital.[60] In the District of Columbia, the public hospital was essentially replaced with an alliance of contracting private institutions funded with dollars formerly earmarked for that hospital.[61] In all these cases, many observers have raised concerns that the successor system will fail the populations they are intended to serve if funding is insufficient or unstable, and if a cadre of providers with little historic interest in these patients (other than financial) takes the lead in their care. One could easily envision such concerns being raised over health reform schemes. For these observers, this strategy is more akin to abandonment of a historic mission than "reform." Others view it as a prime example of government exiting a competitive business for which it is ill-equipped, and handing this responsibility to a (possibly) more efficient private health care sector. But there is generally little objective data from before and after the reform to allow robust judgments about the real impact on people and communities. Given that, these strategies might well gain widespread acceptance in a post-reform environment.

CONCLUSIONS

The safety net is a complicated web of institutions and services supported by a similarly complex web of payments, subsidies and other supports. Health reform, depending on how it is funded and structured, could have huge impacts on the safety net, some positive, others negative. The belief that simply any coverage expansion will benefit the safety net is ungrounded. Thus responsible health reform needs to be analyzed against its impact on the safety net, and be designed to either bolster it or replace it if need be. That analysis must include an understanding of the differential clinical and fiscal impact of reform on different kinds of providers. It must also include an analysis of the likely political landscape of a post-reform environment: after reform, many local and national health care debates may take on a different tenor, greatly affecting the ability of various actors in the health care system to argue their respective cases. For the safety net, disproportionately dependent on public funding and political leadership, this is especially critical.

The question of whether we need or even want a safety net in the context of significant national health care reform is not trivial. Large-scale coverage expansions might indeed relieve many pressures on the safety net. But even the most aggressive reforms would likely not cover everyone in America, such as undocumented immigrants. Such reforms might also leave many services partially or wholly uncovered, depending on benefit design and the structuring of out-of-pocket expenses. Hence significant uncompensated care might persist, especially for high-cost services and patients with complex medical and social needs. Partial coverage expansions could even have unintended negative consequences for the safety net, if newly insured individuals access health care outside of the safety net, essentially concentrating the remaining uninsured in a set of weakened safety net providers that have lost their paying business. We would find ourselves with a residual set of third-rate safety net providers, unable to provide the most basic services, much less high-quality programs that can address cultural barriers and health disparities for minorities. This would be unfortunate, given that many insured patients (including those on Medicaid) do today choose to use safety net providers. These providers often have expertise in managing chronic disease, rendering culturally-competent care and in serving other needs specific to these populations. We can expect that many would still want and even need these providers, even under a universal health care scenario. Thus, even under some of the most optimistic scenarios, millions of Americans will still turn to a struggling safety net as a matter of choice. Denial of that choice as a result of reform would be a sad result.

REFERENCES

1. M. Lewin and S. Altman, eds., *America's Health Care Safety Net: Intact but Endangered* (Washington, D.C.: National Academy Press, 2000).

2. In response to recommendations in the report concerning safety net monitoring, the Agency for Healthcare Research and Quality issued several data reports on key access and outcome indicators related to the safety net, at http://www.ahrq.gov/data/safetynet (last visited June 21, 2004).

3. M. Lewin and S. Altman, eds., *America's Health Care Safety Net* (Washington, D.C.: National Academy Press, 2000): at 51.

4. Guidelines for Medically Underserved Area and Population Designation, Bureau of Health Professions Website, at http://bhpr.hrsa.gov/shortage/muaguide.htm (last visited June 21, 2004).

5. B.E. Baily et al., *Experts with Experience Community & Migrant Health Centers Highlighting a Decade of Service* (1990–2000) (Washington, D.C.: U.S. Department of Health and Human Services, Health Resources and Services Administration, Bureau of Primary Health Care, 2002): "What kinds of patients go to safety net hospitals?" *Issue Brief* (Washington, D.C.: National Association of Public Hospitals, 2003).

6. M. Lewin and S. Altman, *America's Health Care Safety Net* (Washington, D.C.: National Academy Press, 2000): at 21.

7. Sec. 330 of the Public Health Service Act, 42 USC Sec. 254b.

8. S. Rosenbaum and A. Dievler, *A Literature Review of the Community and Migrant Health Centers Programs* (Washington, D.C.: The George Washington University Center for Health Services Research and Policy, 1992).

9. Uniform Data System (UDS), Department of Health and Human Services, Health Resources and Services Administration (2002); Approximately 97 federally-qualified health center "look-alikes" serve another 1 million patients. Like CHCs, look-alikes are located in medically underserved areas and are eligible for cost-based reimbursement under Medicaid and Medicare. However, look-alikes receive no federal funding. S. Rosenbaum and P. Shin, "Health Centers as Safety Net Providers: An Overview and Assessment of Medicaid's Role," *Issue Brief* (Washington, D.C.: Kaiser Commission on Medicaid and the Uninsured, 2003).

10. D. Hawkins and M. Proser, "A Nation's Health at Risk," *Special Topics Issue Brief* #5 (Washington, D.C.: National Association of Community Health Centers, 2004).

11. See UDS, supra note 9.

12. *Id.*

13. H.H. Schauffler and J. Wolin, "Community Health Clinics under Managed Competition: Navigating Uncharted Waters," *Journal of Health Politics, Policy and Law* 21, no. 3 (1996): 461–488.

14. See UDS, *supra* note 9.

15. P. Starr. *The Social Transformation of American Medicine* (New York, N.Y.: Basic Books, Inc., 1949).

16. Section 1867(a) of the Social Security Act.

17. National Center for Health Statistics, *National Hospital Ambulatory Medical Care Survey*, 1992–2000.

18. P.J. Cunningham and J.H. May, "Insured Americans Drive Surge in Emergency Department Visits," *Issue Brief* no. 70 (Washington, D.C.: Center for Studying Health System Change, 2003).

19. R.J. Mills and S. Bhandari, *Health Insurance Coverage in America: 2002* (Washington, D.C.: US. Census Bureau, 2003).

20. "What is a Safety Net Hospital?" Issue Brief (Washington, D.C.: National Association of Public Hospitals and Health Systems, 2001).

21. *Id.*

22. L.S. Gage, "The Future of Safety Net Hospitals," in S. Altman, U.E. Reinhardt, and A.E. Shields, eds., *The Future U.S. Healthcare System: Who will Care for the Poor and Uninsured* (Chicago, IL: Health Administration Press, 1998).

23. See UDS, *supra* note 9.

24. I. Singer, L. Davison, and L. Fagnani, *America's Safety Net Hospitals and Health Systems, 2001: Results of the 2001 Annual NAPH Member Survey* (Washington, D.C.: National Association of Public Hospitals, 2003).

25. J. Tolbert, ed., *Safety Net Financing: A Source Book for Healthcare Executives* (Washington, D.C.: National Association of Public Hospitals and Health Systems, 2003).

26. The Commonwealth Fund, *A Shared Responsibility: Academic Health Centers and the Provision of Care to the Poor and Uninsured* (New York, N.Y.: The Commonwealth Fund, 2001).

27. Singer, et al., *supra* note 24.

28. Health Resources and Services Administration, "Budget and Appropriations" at http://www.hrsa.gov/budget.htm (last visited June 21, 2004).

29. The Health Care Safety Net Amendments of 2002, P.L. 107-251.

30. See UDS, *supra* note 9.

31. L.E. Felland, J.K. Kinner, and J.F. Hoadley, "The Health Care Safety Net: Money Matters but Savvy Leadership Counts," *Issue Brief* no. 66 (Washington, D.C.: Center for Studying Health System Change, 2003).

32. Singer, et al., *supra* note 24.

33. See UDS, *supra* note 9.

34. "How are Safety Net Hospitals Financed? Who Pays for Free Care?" *Issue Brief* (Washington, D.C.: National Association of Public Hospitals and Health Systems, 2003).

35. See, for example: L. Shi, "The Relation Between Primary Care and Life Chances," *Journal of Health Care for the Poor and Underserved* 2 (1992): 321–35; L. Shi, R. Starfield, B. Kennely, and I. Kavachu, "Income Inequality, Primary Care and Health Indicators," *Journal of Family Practice* 48 (1999): 275–84.

36. B.D. Smedley, A.Y. Stith, and A.R. Nelson, eds., *Unequal Treatment: Confronting Racial and Ethnic Disparities in Health Care* (Washington, D.C.: National Academy Press, 2002).

37. J. Hadley, *Sicker and Poorer: The Consequences of Being Uninsured* (Washington, DC: Kaiser Commission on Medicaid and the Uninsured, May 2002).

38. J. Lave and C. Keane, "The Impact of Lack of Health Insurance on Children," *Journal of Health and Social Policy* 10, no. 2 (1998): 57–73.

39. In 2002, California and Texas reported the largest number of undocumented residents of 2.4 million and 1.1 million, respectively; J.S. Passel, R. Capps, and M. Fix, *Undocumented Immigrants: Facts and Figures* (Washington, D.C.: Urban Institute, 2004).

40. D.J. Gaskin, "Are Urban Safety-Net Hospitals Losing Low-Risk Medicaid Maternity Patients?" *Health Services Research* 36, no. 1, (2001): Part I, 25–51.

41. M.S. Marquis and S.H. Long, "Trends in Managed Care and Managed Competition 1993–1997," *Health Affairs* 18, no. 6 (1999): 75–88: J. Maxwell, P. Temin, and C. Watts, "Corporate Health Care Purchasing among Fortune 500 Firms: The Nation's Largest Employers Have Exacted All of the Savings They Can from Aggressive Purchasing and Switching Employees to Managed Care. What Will Their Next Move Be?" *Health Affairs* 20, no. 3 (2001): 181–188.

42. L.R. Brewster, L.S. Rudell, and C.S. Lesser, "Emergency Room Diversions: A Symptom of Hospitals Under Stress" *Issue Brief* no. 38 (Washington, D.C.: Center for Studying Health System Change, 2001). See also: J.A. Gordon, J. Billings, B.R. Asplin, and K.V. Rhodes, "Safety Net Research in Emergency Medicine: Proceedings of the Academic Emergency Medicine Consensus Conference on The Unraveling Safety Net," *Academic Emergency Medicine* 8, no. 11 (2001): 1024–29.

43. See, for example, K. Fiscella, P. Frank, M.R. Gold, and C.M. Clancy, "Inequality in Quality: Addressing Socioeconomic, Racial and Ethnic Disparities in Health Care," *JAMA* 283 (2000): 2579-84; KS. Collins, D.L. Hughes, M.M. Doty, et al., Diverse Communities, Common Concerns: Assessing Health Care Quality for Minority Americans (New York, N.Y.: The Commonwealth Fund, 2002); S.H. Zuvekas, R.M. Weinick, and J.W. Cohen, "Racial and Ethnic Differences in Access to and Use of Health Care Services, 1977 to 1996," *Medical Care Research and Review* 57, sup. 1 (2000): 36–54.

44. Smedley, et al., *supra* note 36.

45. Presentation by Patricia Gabow, MD, CEO and Medical Director, Denver Health Medical Center, to National Association of Public Hospitals Policy Fellows, March 6, 2002.

46. Presentation by Ben Chu, MD, MPH, President of the New York City Health and Hospitals Corporation, at the National Association of Public Hospitals and Health Systems Annual Meeting, *A Vision for the Safety Net.* June 20, 2002.

47. R.M. Politzer, J.S. Yoon, RG. Hughes, and M.H. Gaston, "Inequality in America: the Contribution of Health Centers in Reducing and Eliminating Disparities in Access to Care," *Medical Care Research and Review* 58, no. 2 (2001): 234–48.

48. The Uniform Data System (UDS) is an annually released dataset on Bureau of Primary Health Care grantee health centers that includes patient demographics, financing, diagnoses, utilization, staffing, and services.

49. S. Rosenbaum, P. Shin, D. Roby, and R. Park, *Health Centers: A National Profile* (Washington, D.C.: The George Washington University Center for Health Services Research and Policy, 2001).

50. M.E. Lewin and S. Altman, eds., *America's Health Care Safety Net: Intact but Endangered* (Washington, D.C.: National Academy Press, 2000): at viii.

51. K. Morris, "Detroit Health Care in Critical Condition" *Detroit Free Press,* October 1, 2003.

52. M. Lewin and S. Altman, eds., *America's Health Care Safety Net* (Washington, D.C.: National Academy Press, 2000): at 138.

53. *Strengthening the Safety Net in Detroit and Wayne County: Report of the Detroit Health Care Stabilization Workgroup* (Detroit, MI: Detroit Health Care Stabilization Workgroup, 2003) available at http://www.michigan.gov/documents/ReportofDetroitHealthCareStabilizationWorkgroup_1_70764_7.pdf.

54. *HHC Ambulatory Care Evolution* 1, no. 1 (New York, N.Y.: Primary Care Development Corporation).

55. T. Bodenheimer, E.H. Wagner, and K. Grumbach, "Improving Primary Care for Patients With Chronic Illness," *Journal of the American Medical Association* 288 (2002): 1775–79.

56. B. Lambert and P. Healy, "At 2 Hospitals, Fiscal Troubles in the Glare of Public View," *New York Times,* January 18, 2004.

57. J. Needleman, D.J. Chollet, and J. Lampere, "Hospital Conversion Trends," *Health Affairs* 16 (1997): 187–195.

58. R.R. Bovbjerg, J.A. Marsteller, and F. C. Ullman, *Health Care for the Poor and Uninsured After a Public Hospital Closure or Conversion* (Washington, D.C.: The Urban Institute, 2000).

59. B. Wysocki, "At One Hospital, A Stark Solution for Allocating Care," *Wall Street Journal* (September 23, 2003).

60. D.P. Andrulis, "The Public Sector in Health Care: Evolution or Dissolution?" *Health Affairs* 16 (1997): 131–140.

61. J. Piotrowski, "How Secure is the Safety Net? Public Hospitals Learn to Survive in an Increasingly Tight Market by Closing, Building, Replacing, and Sometimes Converting," *Modern Healthcare* 32, no. 8 (2002): 34–7.

An Analysis of Leading Congressional Health Care Bills, 2005–2007: Part 1, Insurance Coverage

Sara R. Collins, Karen Davis, and Jennifer L. Kriss

Source: Courtesy of the Commonwealth Fund. An Analysis of Leading Congressional Health Care Bills, 2005–2007: Part I, Insurance Coverage, Sara R. Collins, Karen Davis, and Jennifer L. Kriss, The Commonwealth Fund, March 2007.

Abstract: The first of a two-part series, this report analyzes and compares leading congressional bills and Administration proposals to expand health insurance coverage introduced over 2005–2007. The Commonwealth Fund commissioned The Lewin Group to estimate the effect of the bills on stakeholder and health system costs and the projected number of people who would become newly insured through them. The proposals fall into three categories: those that propose fundamental reform of the health insurance system; those that would expand existing public insurance programs; and those that seek to strengthen employer-based health insurance. The report considers whether the proposals would improve access to care, increase health system efficiency, make the system more equitable, and improve quality of care.

Support for this research was provided by The Commonwealth Fund. The views presented here are those of the authors and not necessarily those of The Commonwealth Fund or its directors, officers, or staff, or of The Commonwealth Fund Commission on a High Performance Health System or its members. This and other Fund publications are available online at www.cmwf.org. To learn more about new publications when they become available, visit the Fund's Web site and register to receive e-mail alerts. Commonwealth Fund pub. no. 1010

The authors gratefully acknowledge the contribution of John Sheils and Randy Haught of The Lewin Group, and Katie Horton, William Scanlon, Steven Stranne, and JoAnne Bailey of Health Policy R&D. The Lewin Group modeled all proposals on which the report is based. Health Policy R&D provided detailed side-by-side comparative analysis of the proposals which informed the model specifications.

EXECUTIVE SUMMARY

The first of a two-part series, this report analyzes and compares leading congressional bills and Administration proposals to expand health insurance coverage introduced over 2005–2007.[1] The Commonwealth Fund commissioned The Lewin Group to estimate the effect of the bills on stakeholder and health system costs and the projected number of people who would become newly insured through them.

All coverage and cost estimates are for 2007 and are based on the assumption of full implementation of the proposals this year. The Lewin Group projects that, under current law, the number of uninsured in the United States will rise to 47.8 million people in 2007 out of a total estimated population of 295.1 million.

The proposals take different approaches to achieve near-universal coverage or more incremental expansions in health insurance. The approaches fall into three broad categories:

- Fundamental reforms of the nation's health insurance system;
- Expansions of existing public insurance programs; and
- Strengthening employer-based health insurance.

FUNDAMENTAL REFORMS OF THE HEALTH INSURANCE SYSTEM

Proposals that would fundamentally reform the U.S. health insurance system include:

- Health insurance tax deduction and tax on employer contribution to health insurance (President Bush);
- Regional insurance exchanges (Senator Wyden);
- Federal-state partnerships to expand health insurance (Senators Bingaman and Voinovich, Representatives Baldwin, Tierney, and Price); and
- Coverage through Medicare (Representative Stark, Senator Kennedy, Representative Dingell).

The proposals vary in design but contain common elements (Table 27-1).

- With the exception of federal–state partnerships, all of the proposals would transform the traditional role of employers by eventually scaling back or eliminating the extent to which they contract directly with health plans for coverage. The president's and Senator Wyden's proposals would achieve this in part by eliminating the tax exemption for employer-provided benefits and replacing it with an income tax deduction. The proposals differ in the extent to which employers would continue to finance coverage.

- With the exception of President Bush's proposal, the plans would require individuals to have health insurance and require employers and individuals to share in the cost.
- All of the proposals except the president's would provide subsidies to people with lower incomes to help defray the costs of premiums.
- All of the proposals except the president's would pool health risks into large groups in order to equalize premium costs across families, regardless of health risk, and increase efficiency in insurance administration.

The proposals vary in the number of people covered, the source of coverage, and in the comprehensiveness and affordability of coverage (Figure 27-1).

- Representative Stark's "AmeriCare" proposal would cover nearly all uninsured, as would Senator Wyden's "Healthy Americans Act."
- Medicare would become the primary source of coverage for all Americans under Representative Stark's bill and private Health Help Agency plans would become the major source under Senator Wyden's bill.
- The state–federal partnerships bills propose state demonstrations to expand health insurance and by definition do not provide sufficient details to permit cost estimates. For purposes of illustration of how such a partnership

---

TABLE 27-1 Major Features of Health Insurance Expansion Bills and Impact on Uninsured, National Expenditures

	President Bush's Tax Reform Plan	Healthy Americans Act[2]	Federal/State Partnership 15 States	AmeriCare
Aims to Cover All People		X		X
Individual Mandate or Auto Enrollment		X	X	X
Employer Shared Responsibility		X	X	X
Public Program Expansion			X	X
Subsidies for Lower Income Families		X	X	X
Risk Pooling		X	X	X
Comprehensive Benefit Package		X	X	X
Quality & Efficiency Measures	X	X	X	X
Uninsured Covered in 2007[1] (in millions)	9.0	45.3	20.3	47.8
Net Health System Cost in 2007 (in billions)	($11.7)	($4.5)	$22.7	($60.7)
Net Federal Budget Cost in 2007 (in billions)	$70.4	$24.3	$22.0	$154.5

[1] Out of an estimated total uninsured in 2007 of 47.8 million.

[2] Estimates reflect a mandatory cash-out of benefit on the part of employers that currently offer coverage.

Source: The Lewin Group for The Commonwealth Fund.

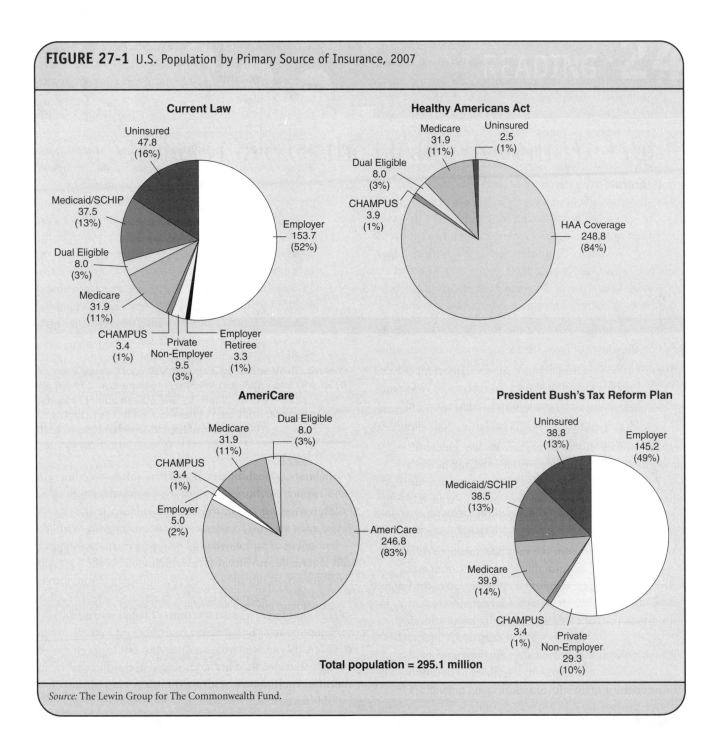

FIGURE 27-1 U.S. Population by Primary Source of Insurance, 2007

Current Law

- Uninsured 47.8 (16%)
- Medicaid/SCHIP 37.5 (13%)
- Dual Eligible 8.0 (3%)
- Medicare 31.9 (11%)
- CHAMPUS 3.4 (1%)
- Private Non-Employer 9.5 (3%)
- Employer Retiree 3.3 (1%)
- Employer 153.7 (52%)

Healthy Americans Act

- Medicare 31.9 (11%)
- Uninsured 2.5 (1%)
- Dual Eligible 8.0 (3%)
- CHAMPUS 3.9 (1%)
- HAA Coverage 248.8 (84%)

AmeriCare

- Medicare 31.9 (11%)
- Dual Eligible 8.0 (3%)
- CHAMPUS 3.4 (1%)
- Employer 5.0 (2%)
- AmeriCare 246.8 (83%)

President Bush's Tax Reform Plan

- Uninsured 38.8 (13%)
- Employer 145.2 (49%)
- Medicaid/SCHIP 38.5 (13%)
- Medicare 39.9 (14%)
- CHAMPUS 3.4 (1%)
- Private Non-Employer 29.3 (10%)

Total population = 295.1 million

Source: The Lewin Group for The Commonwealth Fund.

might work, The Lewin Group assumed a hypothetical model under which 15 states would implement a blended version of Massachusetts's Commonwealth Care and Governor Schwarzenegger's health proposal for California, with federal matching funds provided for Medicaid and State Children's Health Insurance Program (SCHIP) expansions.[2] About 20 million peo-

ple are estimated to gain coverage out of 23.6 million currently uninsured in those states.

- President Bush's proposal to equalize the tax treatment of employer and individual coverage is estimated to cover 9 million previously uninsured people in 2007, mostly through the individual insurance market. The new income tax deduction would be for a fixed amount that would rise annually by the rate of consumer price inflation, which is projected to rise more slowly than premiums. Therefore, the proposal is likely to cover more uninsured people in the first years of the proposal than in future years, when premiums are more likely to exceed the cap and thus be more expensive to taxpayers. Other families may buy increasingly less comprehensive coverage with higher out of pocket costs as the growth in the standard tax deduction lags that of premiums.

- By setting a floor on acceptable levels of health benefits, all of the proposals—with the exception of the president's—would improve coverage for millions of people who are currently underinsured. In addition, Representative Stark's bill, Senator Wyden's bill, and the state–federal partnership model would cap out-of-pocket costs as a share of income and/or subsidize premiums.

The cost of the proposals and how costs are shared depend on the source of coverage, the extent of premium subsidies, how broadly health risk is pooled, and inclusion of other efficiency measures (Table 27-2).[3]

- Representative Stark's AmeriCare bill would increase federal spending by $154.5 billion in 2007. President Bush's proposal would increase the budget deficit by $70.4 billion in 2007, but is expected to generate a surplus within the next ten years. Federal Medicaid and SCHIP matching funds for 15 states would increase federal spending by about $22 billion unless offset by savings measures. Senator Wyden's Healthy Americans Act would increase Federal spending by $165 billion but the

tax revenue effect of the bill's requirement that employers cash-out their health benefits in the first two years of the program would dampen the increase significantly to $24.3 billion in 2007.

- Representative Stark's AmeriCare bill would result in substantial overall health system savings relative to the other approaches: the bill is estimated to reduce national health expenditures by $60.7 billion in 2007, compared with savings of $11.7 billion under the president's proposal and $4.5 billion under Senator Wyden's bill.
- This difference stems primarily from large savings in the cost of administering health insurance under Representative Stark's bill: the total costs of health insurance administration in the United States would decline by $74 billion in 2007. Insuring everyone under Medicare would spread risks across a large risk pool and bring Medicare's lower administrative costs per premium dollar to the full population.
- Senator Wyden's bill also substantially reduces insurance administrative costs by creating large regional groups in which people would buy private coverage. Insurance administration costs are estimated to decline by $57 billion in 2007, though the savings would be offset somewhat by the costs of administering the new program.
- Representative Stark's AmeriCare proposal is also estimated to achieve savings by requiring the federal government to negotiate prescription drug prices with pharmaceutical companies, thus reducing national spending on prescription drugs by $33.9 billion in 2007.

TABLE 27-2 Health Insurance Expansion Bills Change in Health Spending by Stakeholder Group, Billions of Dollars, 2007

	President Bush's Tax Reform Plan	Healthy Americans Act[2]	Federal/State Partnership 15 States	AmeriCare
Total Uninsured Covered, Millions	9.0	45.3	20.3	47.8
Federal Government	$70.4	$24.3	$22.0	$154.5
State and Local Government	($0.3)	($10.2)	$13.4	($57.4)
Private Employers	($50.8)	$60.2	$5.7	($15.2)
Households	($31.0)	($78.8)	($18.4)	($142.6)
Net Health System Cost in 2007 (in billions)	($11.7)	($4.5)	$22.7	($60.7)
Total Uninsured Not Covered,[1] Millions	38.8	2.5	27.5	0

[1] Out of an estimated total uninsured in 2007 of 47.8 million.
[2] Estimates reflect a mandatory cash-out of benefits on the part of employers that currently offer coverage.
Source: The Lewin Group for The Commonwealth Fund.

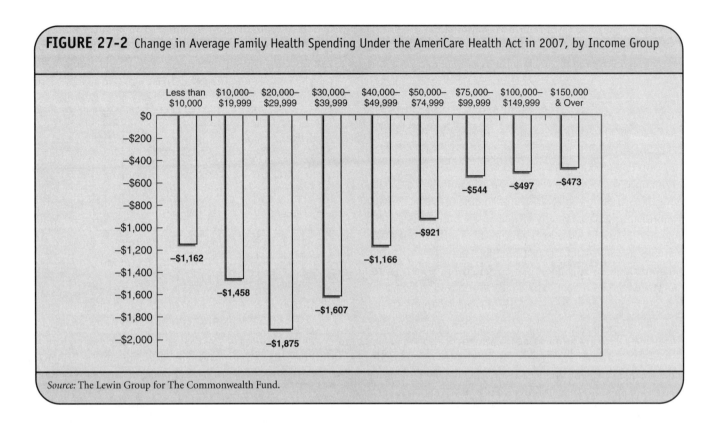

FIGURE 27-2 Change in Average Family Health Spending Under the AmeriCare Health Act in 2007, by Income Group

Source: The Lewin Group for The Commonwealth Fund.

- The president's proposal achieves savings by reducing the comprehensiveness of coverage and inducing lower utilization of services.

Premium subsidies and new tax provisions in the bills greatly affect how family health spending changes.

- Under Representative Stark's bill, households would see a dramatic drop in health care expenditures of $142.6 billion, with the largest savings falling to families with low and moderate incomes (Figure 27-2). However, these savings might be offset if taxes are increased to finance higher federal government spending.
- Under Senator Wyden's bill, household health spending would decline by $78 billion. Spending would decline the most for lower and moderate income households and rise for the highest income earners. Average health spending would fall by $983 per year among families earning less than $10,000 a year and increase by an average $1,562 among families earning $250,000 or more annually (Figure 27-3).
- Under President Bush's proposal, household spending on health care is estimated to fall by a net $31 billion in 2007 due to income tax savings. But tax savings disproportionately accrue to people in higher income brackets: average spending would decline by $23 in 2007

among families with annual incomes of less than $10,000 and by $1,263 a year among those earning $150,000 or more per year. (Figure 27-4). In future years, however, the differential indexing of the deduction and growth in employer premiums would lead to an increase in taxes for households now covered by employer plans.

EXPANSIONS OF EXISTING PUBLIC INSURANCE PROGRAMS

More modest proposals can be important first steps toward universal coverage. Several bills would expand health insurance coverage by building on Medicare, Medicaid, and SCHIP (Table 27-3). These include:

- Medicare buy-in for older adults (Representative Stark);
- Elimination of the Medicare two-year waiting period for people who are disabled (Senator Bingaman and Representative Green);
- Universal coverage for children (Senator Kerry, Representative Waxman, Senator Rockefeller, Representative Stark); and
- Medicaid expansions (Representative Dingell).
- Representative Stark would allow older adults ages 55 to 64 to buy in to Medicare, using tax credits to offset premium costs. This would insure an estimated 3.5 million

FIGURE 27-3 Change in Average Family Health Spending Under the Healthy Americans Act in 2007, by Income Group

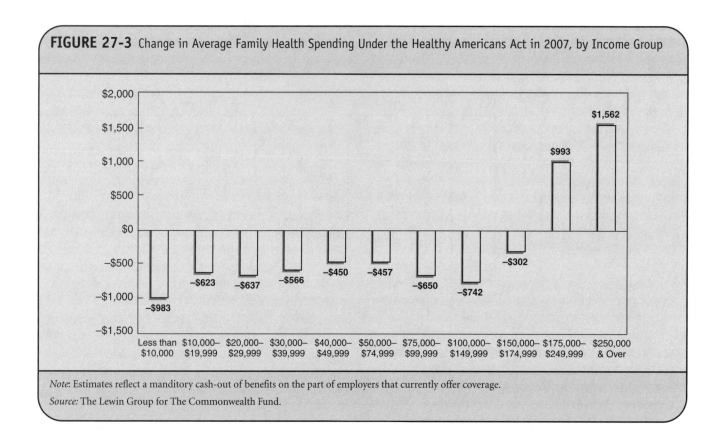

Note: Estimates reflect a mandatory cash-out of benefits on the part of employers that currently offer coverage.

Source: The Lewin Group for The Commonwealth Fund.

FIGURE 27-4 Change in Average Family Health Spending Under President Bush's Health Care Tax Reform Proposal in 2007, by Income Group

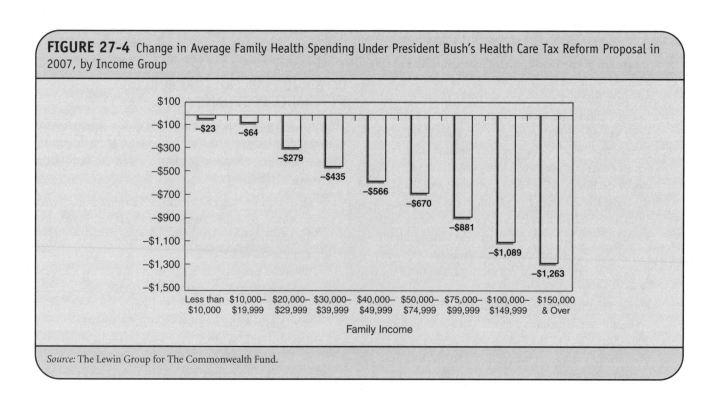

Source: The Lewin Group for The Commonwealth Fund.

TABLE 27-3 Major Features of Health Insurance Expansion Bills and Impact on Uninsured, National Expenditures

	Medicare Buy-in	Eliminate Medicare 2-yr Waiting Period	Universal Coverage for Children	Medicaid/ SCHIP Children & Parents
Aims to Cover All People				
Individual Mandate or Auto Enrollment				
Employer Shared Responsibility	X			
Public Program Expansion	X	X	X	X
Subsidies for Lower Income Families	X		X	
Risk Pooling	X	X	X	X
Comprehensive Benefit Package	X	X	X	X
Quality & Efficiency Measures			X	X
Uninsured Covered in 2007[1] (in millions)	3.5	0.3	5.2	6.2
Net Health System Cost in 2007 (in billions)	$4.9	($0.1)	$3.0	$7.5
Net Federal Budget Cost in 2007 (in billions)	$26.9	$9.1	$19.9	$12.7

[1] Out of an estimated total uninsured in 2007 of 47.8 million.
Source: The Lewin Group for The Commonwealth Fund.

out of 4.8 million uninsured older adults in 2007. The estimated cost to the federal budget is $26.9 billion, with spending on premiums and out-of-pocket costs reduced by $10.6 billion for people who enroll (Table 27-4).

- People who become disabled and cannot work would eventually no longer have to wait 24 months before becoming eligible for Medicare under bills introduced by Senator Bingaman and Representative Green in June 2005. This would help 1.7 million disabled people currently in the waiting period, of whom 15 percent are uninsured. The estimated cost to the federal budget of immediately ending the waiting period in 2007 is $9.1 billion.

TABLE 27-4 Health Insurance Expansion Bills Change in Health Spending by Stakeholder Group, Billions of Dollars, 2007

	Medicare Buy-in	Eliminate 2-yr Medicare Waiting Period	Universal Coverage for Children	Medicaid/ SCHIP Children & Parents
Total Uninsured Covered, Millions	3.5	0.3	5.2	6.2
Federal Government	$26.9	$9.1	$19.9	$12.7
State and Local Government	($2.0)	($3.0)	($8.2)	$3.2
Private Employers	($9.4)	($4.0)	($7.3)	($3.5)
Households	($10.6)	($2.2)	($1.5)	($4.9)
Net Health System Cost in 2007 (in billions)	$4.9	($0.1)	$3.0	$7.5
Total Uninsured Not Covered,[1] Millions	44.3	47.5	42.6	41.6

[1] Out of an estimated total uninsured in 2007 of 47.8 million.
Source: The Lewin Group for The Commonwealth Fund.

- Senator Kerry and Representative Waxman would provide states with incentives to expand coverage through Medicaid and SCHIP for children up to age 21 in families with incomes up to 300 percent of the federal poverty level, and would cap premium costs for children in families with incomes over 300 percent of poverty. The bill is estimated to cover 5.2 million out of 11.1 million uninsured children in 2007. It would increase federal spending by about $20 billion in that year, but reduce state and local government spending by $8.2 billion through increased federal matching funds for poor children.

- Representative Dingell would insure parents of children in Medicaid and SCHIP, thus extending new coverage to an estimated 6.2 million children and adults. The bill would increase federal spending by $12.7 billion in 2007 and state and local government expenditures by $3.2 billion. Family spending on health care would decline by nearly $5 billion as more families gained more comprehensive insurance.

STRENGTHENING EMPLOYER-BASED HEALTH INSURANCE

Several proposals would expand health insurance by building on the employer-based system, which currently covers more than 160 million workers and their dependents, or about 63 percent of the population (Table 27-5). They include:

- Employer mandate for large employers (Representative Pallone); and
- Improving the affordability of health insurance for small employers (President Bush, Representative Johnson, Senator Durbin, Representative Kind, Representative Allen).

  - Representative Pallone would require companies with 50 or more workers to offer and contribute to comprehensive health insurance for their employees and dependents. An estimated 12.3 million workers and their dependents would become newly insured under the proposal. Because workers and their dependents with coverage through public insurance programs are required to enroll in their employers' plans, 9.7 million workers and dependents would move from those programs into employer-based coverage, saving the federal government an estimated $42.6 billion in 2007 (Table 27-6). Employers would face the largest net increase in costs under the bill, of $92.1 billion.

  - The Bush Administration and Representative Johnson would allow trade and other professional associations to create association health plans (AHPs) to provide health insurance to their member employers. The Johnson bill would in effect allow companies to bypass state insurance regulations such as community rating, which are aimed at

TABLE 27-5 Major Features of Health Insurance Expansion Bills and Impact on Uninsured, National Expenditures

	Employer Mandate	Association Health Plans	Small Business Expansion[2]
Aims to Cover All People			
Individual Mandate or Auto Enrollment			
Employer Shared Responsibility	X	X	X
Public Program Expansion			
Subsidies for Lower Income Families			X
Risk Pooling	X		X
Comprehensive Benefit Package	X		X
Quality & Efficiency Measures			X
Uninsured Covered in 2007[1] (in millions)	12.3	(0.3)	0.6
Net Health System Cost in 2007 (in billions)	$28.5	($0.4)	$2.1
Net Federal Budget Cost in 2007 (in billions)	($42.6)	$0.1	$12.0

[1] Out of an estimated total uninsured in 2007 of 47.8 million,

[2] Modeling assumed that firms with under 100 employees are eligible; reinsurance of 90% of costs over $50,000.

Source: The Lewin Group for The Commonwealth Fund.

TABLE 27-6 Health Insurance Expansion Bills Change in Health Spending by Stakeholder Group, Billions of Dollars, 2007

	Employer Mandate	Association Health Plans	Small Business Expansion[2]
Total Uninsured Covered, Millions	12.3	(0.3)	0.6
Federal Government	($42.6)	$0.1	$12.0
State and Local Government	$5.4	$0.6	($0.4)
Private Employers	$92.1	($1.3)	($6.9)
Households	($26.4)	$0.2	($2.6)
Net Health System Cost in 2007 (in billions)	$28.5	($0.4)	$2.1
Total Uninsured Net Covered,[1] Millions	35.5	48.1	47.2

[1] Out of an estimated total uninsured in 2007 of 47.8 million.
[2] Modeling assumed that firms with under 100 employees are eligible; reinsurance of 90% of costs over $50,000.
Source: The Lewin Group for The Commonwealth Fund.

increasing access to the small group market for small businesses with less healthy or older workers. The bill is estimated to make small group coverage more affordable for companies with a young and/or healthy workforce but to significantly increase premiums for companies with older and/or less healthy workforces that must continue to purchase coverage in the small group market. While 2.6 million workers and dependents are estimated to gain employment-based insurance through association health plans, 2.8 million would lose existing employer coverage because of a rise in premiums in the small group market. The number of uninsured is estimated to increase by a net 278,000 under the bill.

- Senator Durbin, Representative Kind, and Representative Allen propose bills that take an entirely different approach than AHPs by establishing pools for small businesses with premium protections and federal reinsurance. But in the absence of state-wide insurance market regulations, the proposals might ultimately have the unintended effect of increasing premiums within the pools, even with the reinsurance and tax credits, as those companies with less healthy and older workforces disproportionately enroll, attracted by the community-rated plans. About 600,000 people become newly insured.

CONCLUSION

To assess these proposals, the public might pose the following criteria: Will the proposals improve access to care, increase

health system efficiency, make the system more equitable, and improve quality of care? Do they promise to set the nation on a path toward longer, healthier, and more productive lives?

Access to Care

- The proposals range in scope from targeted efforts that would cover a defined group of people to those that aim to expand coverage options for everyone. Bills that fundamentally reform the health system vary in their effectiveness (Table 27-7). Representative Stark's AmeriCare proposal and Senator Wyden's Healthy Americans Act would cover nearly all of those currently uninsured. President Bush's proposal would cover less than one of five of those uninsured in 2007, and this number is likely to decline in future years.

- By setting a floor on acceptable levels of health benefits and providing premium assistance for low- and moderate-income families, several of the bills would improve coverage for the estimated 16 million people who are currently underinsured.

Efficiency

- The cost of the proposals and how those costs are distributed across stakeholders is affected by their scope and structure. In general, more targeted proposals are less expensive to the federal government than are more comprehensive coverage plans.

- Yet, the estimated savings to the overall health system from insuring everyone through Medicare or other near-universal mechanisms swamp those from incremental approaches. This results from the administrative savings

TABLE 27-7 Major Features of Health Insurance Expansion Bills

	President Bush's Tax Reform Plan	Healthy Americans Act	Federal/State Partnership 15 States[2]	AmeriCare
Access (% of uninsured covered[1] in 2007)	19%	95%	42%	100%
Efficiency (change in national health system spending in 2007)	($11.7)	($4.5)	$22.7	($60.7)
Equity (change in average family health spending by annual income in 2007)	<$10,000: ($23) >$150,000: ($1,263)	<$10,000: ($983) >$250,000: $1,562	N/A	<$10,000: ($1,162) >$150,000: ($473)
Measures to Improve Quality		Medical home, hospital safety, reward healthy behavior, chronic disease management	State proposals to show improvements in quality, efficiency, and health IT	Uniform electronic claims forms and medical records; electronic national claims data set
Potential to Ensure Long, Healthy, Productive Lives		X	X	X

[1] Out of an estimated total uninsured in 2007 of 47.8 million.
[2] Estimated to cover 86% of the 23.6 million people projected to be uninsured in the 15 states in 2007.
Source: The Lewin Group for The Commonwealth Fund.

from broadly pooling risk as well as other efficiency gains such as negotiating pharmaceutical prices on behalf of the full population.

- The proposals that would enroll people automatically through the tax system or at birth and mandate that people have coverage, such as the Representative Stark's bill and Senator Wyden's bill, are the most likely to ensure that people become enrolled and remain enrolled over their lifespan.

Equity

- The design of new premium subsidies, tax credits, or tax deductions for the purchase of health insurance has dramatic implications for how new costs or savings accrue across households. Representative Stark's AmeriCare proposal and Senator Wyden's Healthy Americans Act would distribute changes in health care expenses equitably, according to family income. Under President Bush's proposal, savings from the new tax deduction accrue disproportionately to those with higher incomes.

- Broad risk pooling; i.e., the sharing of health risks among many participants, also has implications for equity. The proposals that attempt to cover people through existing individual or small group insurance markets ultimately run up against the central dynamic governing those markets—the powerful incentive on the part

of carriers to protect against health risk. To help ensure that everyone, regardless of health risk, has affordable insurance coverage and to prevent escalating premiums, risks should be spread among as large a group as possible, participation should be mandatory, community rating should be imposed for the full state market if one exists outside of the pool, and adequate federal reinsurance should be provided.

Quality

- The ways in which people are insured, the systems that evolve to achieve near-universal coverage, and the role of insurance carriers will be important determinants of whether significant and systematic improvements in quality can be achieved nationally. Proposals that would organize coverage through a central mechanism, such as the Medicare program in Representative Stark's proposal and Health Help Agencies under Senator Wyden's bill, have the potential to improve quality in a number of ways. For example, they could enable development and use of common measures of health care quality, collection of outcome data for the full population, creation of uniform provider payment systems that reward high-quality care, and standardization and broad diffusion of health information technology.

- Most of the bills that would fundamentally reform the health system also include specific quality improvement measures. Senators Bingaman and Voinovich and Representatives Baldwin, Price, and Tierney would require or encourage states proposing coverage expansions to also include plans to improve health care quality and efficiency, and expand the use of health information technology. Senator Wyden would encourage people of all ages to have a "health home," establish an expert panel to ensure quality control in hospitals, reward healthy behavior, and establish a chronic care disease management program. Representative Stark would require uniform electronic claims reporting and electronic medical records and create a national electronic claims data set.

Longer, Healthier, and More Productive Lives

- The ultimate goal of health care reform should be improvements in the length, quality, and productivity of people's lives. The analysis of these proposals demonstrates that universal coverage is feasible and that many proposals and particular elements of the proposals have the potential to yield overall savings in national health expenditures and systematic, long-term improvements in the quality of care nationwide.

- The Institute of Medicine estimates that the millions of people who lack insurance coverage generate between $65 billion and $130 billion annually in costs associated with diminished health and shorter life spans. This provides a stark benchmark against which to compare inaction versus the estimated annual costs and savings in this report of investing in a more rational and equitable system of health care in the United States.

State Coverage Initiative, "State of the States: Building Hope, Raising Expectations"

AcademyHealth, State Coverage Initiatives, State of the States report (January 2007)

PART 1 STATE STRATEGIES: EXPANDING COVERAGE THROUGH INNOVATION, EXPERIENCE, AND COMPROMISE

Early in the year, Massachusetts captured the attention of the nation by enacting groundbreaking reform. Although it is perhaps the best known reform of 2006, Massachusetts is far from alone. In fact, the Commonwealth's efforts are just one example of a larger trend toward bold and comprehensive state health care reform.

Among the current round of state reforms [see Table 28-1] are a variety of new approaches to covering the uninsured, including:

- New mechanisms to subsidize coverage for low-income families;
- New variations of employer and personal responsibility for insurance coverage; and
- New strategies to ease the purchase of health insurance for small employers and individuals without access to employer-sponsored insurance.

Like Massachusetts, several state efforts are characterized as comprehensive because they attempt to reach near universal coverage, accomplishing this task through broad system reforms that include quality initiatives, cost containment efforts, and strategies to control the underlying cost of health care. Other states are moving ahead with incremental approaches such as providing universal coverage for children or public-private partnerships to insure low-income workers or encourage small businesses to offer insurance.

COMPREHENSIVE REFORMS

Northeastern States Break New Ground

The most ambitious reform proposals enacted in 2006 came from the Northeast and demonstrate the capacity for breaking ground in a bi-partisan manner. Massachusetts and Vermont passed comprehensive reforms in 2006 that have ambitious goals for covering the uninsured. Meanwhile Maine, which was one of the few states to take on comprehensive reform in 2003 when most states were dealing with severe deficits, continued to move toward its goal of universal coverage by 2009. When building their current reforms, all three states had relatively low rates of uninsured compared to the nation—due, in part, to a history of previous efforts to reduce the number of uninsured, including establishing relatively generous Medicaid eligibility levels.

The comprehensive reforms in these three states go further toward helping low-income families purchase health insurance than in any other states. One of the key elements shared by all three reforms is that they subsidize coverage for families with annual incomes up to approximately 300 percent of the federal poverty level (FPL). Each has also coupled their subsidized products with other reforms that reflect the distinct priorities in each state.

Massachusetts—Commonwealth Care

Massachusetts' reform legislation is aimed at covering 95 percent of state residents without insurance within three years and represents a culmination of more than a year of

TABLE 28-1 Key Features of State Reforms

State	Initiative	Key Features
Comprehensive Reforms		
Massachusetts	Commonwealth Care	• Individual mandate • Employer Fair Share assessment • Free Rider surcharge • Health Insurance Connector • Insurance market reforms • Commonwealth Care*
Maine (2003)	Dirigo Health	• DirigoChoice* • Cost containment reforms • Maine Quality Forum
Vermont	Catamount Health	• Employer assessment • Premium assistance for low-income workers • Catamount Health Plan* • Chronic care initiatives
Covering All Kids		
Illinois	All Kids	• Universal coverage for children • Sliding scale premiums based on family income
Pennsylvania	Cover All Kids	• Universal coverage for children • Sliding scale premiums based on family income
Tennessee	CoverKids	• Separate stand-alone SCHIP program for children in families with incomes up to 250% FPL • Buy-in for children in families above 250% FPL
Public–Private Partnerships		
Arkansas	ARHealthNet	• Safety Net benefit package • Provided through private insurers • Open to businesses with 2–500 employees that have not offered insurance within last 12 months • Subsidy provided for workers with incomes below 200% FPL
Montana	Insure Montana	• Purchasing pool with a subsidy available to previously uninsured firms (2–9 employees) that have not offered insurance for 24 months • Employer and employee premium subsidies • Tax credit available for currently insured small firms (2–9 employees)
New Mexico	State Coverage Insurance	• New subsidized insurance product delivered by Medicaid managed care organizations • Available to low-income, uninsured, working adults with family income below 200% FPL • An individual may enroll through their employer or as a self-employed individual • Premium paid by employer/employee contributions and state/federal funds
Oklahoma	Oklahoma Employer/ Employee Partnership for Insurance Coverage (O-EPIC)	• Premium assistance voucher available for small firms (2–50 employees) who offer a qualified plan and income eligible employees with incomes below 185% FPL • Individual plan available to uninsured workers whose firm does not offer insurance and self-employed (who earn less than 185% FPL)

continues

TABLE 28-1 Key Features of State Reforms (continued)

State	Initiative	Key Features
Rhode Island	WellCare	• New health plan expected to be 25% below market rates • Assisting Low-Income Small Businesses save an additional 10% through reinsurance pool (legislation passed, but no funding approved) • Making health care cost and quality data more transparent • High Risk Pool • Certificate of Need reform
Tennessee	CoverTN	• New affordable health insurance product for working uninsured and small firms that do not offer coverage • At least two statewide private plans • High Risk Pool • Cost limited to $150/month, split by employer, employee and state
Utah	Utah Premium Partnership for Health Insurance (UPP)	• New premium assistance program under the Primary Care Network • $150 subsidies for low-income workers enrolled in employer-sponsored insurance • Subsidies up to $100 for employee's children

* Includes subsidies for low-income workers

negotiations and compromise between lawmakers and Governor Mitt Romney (R). The need to find compromise and act on comprehensive reform was made more urgent by the potential loss of $385 million in federal matching funds that had been previously used to fund care for the uninsured. In what has been referred to as a demonstration of "unusual political maturity"[20] and a "serendipitous collision of interests,"[21] the state's comprehensive plan includes provisions to increase access to health insurance, contain health care costs, and improve quality. In fact, the very ability of policymakers in Massachusetts to reach bi-partisan consensus on landmark reform fueled new hope for the possibility of health care reform and put state efforts at center stage of the national debate on the uninsured. This notable political feat has many policymakers watching closely as the state finalizes the program design and rolls out the first phases of implementation.

Massachusetts' reform package is built on six key elements:

- **An individual mandate that all who can afford insurance obtain it**
  Massachusetts broke new ground with its requirement that individuals purchase health insurance. Individuals who can afford insurance are required to obtain health insurance by July 1, 2007 or risk the loss of their personal exemption for 2007 income taxes. In subsequent tax years, the penalty will include a fine equaling 50 percent of the monthly cost of health insurance for each month without insurance.

- **An employer requirement for "fair and reasonable" contributions toward employees' health coverage**
  Massachusetts had a high rate of employer-sponsored insurance relative to the rest of the nation prior to the current reforms. Building on this foundation, the state added several provisions to share responsibility with employers. Employers with 11 or more full-time employees (FTE) that do not make a "fair and reasonable" contribution toward their employees' health insurance coverage will be required to make a per-worker contribution, not to exceed approximately $295 per FTE annually. Employers will pass the "fair and reasonable" test if at least 25 percent of full-time employees are enrolled in the company's group health plan and the employer contributes toward the premium. Should employers not meet that criterion, they still can pass if they can demonstrate that they offer to pay at least 33 percent of their full-time employees' health insurance premium.

  In addition, by January 1, 2007, all employers with 11 or more workers must adopt a Section 125 "cafeteria plan" that (as defined in federal law) permits workers to purchase health care with pre-tax dollars, saving approximately 25 percent on the cost of premiums. If these employers do not "offer to contribute toward or arrange for the purchase of health insurance," they may be assessed a "free rider" surcharge if their employees or employees' dependents access free care. The surcharge will exempt the first $50,000 of free care that the employees use but, after that threshold is met, the employer will be charged from 10 to 100 percent of the state's cost of the free care, as determined by the Division of Health Care Finance and Policy.

- **The creation of a Commonwealth Health Insurance Connector Authority to improve availability and affordability of coverage**

  The state coined the term "health care connector," which effectively' communicated how many different elements of a complex reform package must come together. The Commonwealth Health Insurance Connector will be a vehicle to help individuals and small businesses find affordable health coverage. Plans participating in the Connector will be able to develop new benefit packages, designed to make coverage more affordable. The Connector will facilitate the process of small employers offering Section 125 plans. Part-time and seasonal workers can combine employer contributions in the Connector as well. One of the unique features of the Connector is that it allows individuals to keep their policy (and therefore, their health care providers), even if they switch employers.

  The Connector will be the sole entity enrolling uninsured low-income populations in the Commonwealth Care Health Insurance Program.

- **Subsidies to assist low-income populations**

  The Commonwealth Care Health Insurance Program will provide sliding scale subsidies to individuals with incomes below 300 percent FPL beginning January 1, 2007. No premiums will be imposed on those individuals with incomes below $9,800 (100 percent FPL). Additionally, an existing premium assistance program, the Insurance Partnership, will raise eligibility for employee participation from 200 percent to 300 percent FPL. In October 2006, the state announced that the average monthly premiums for products offered through the Connector will range between $276 and $391 before the subsidies are applied.

- **Insurance market reforms designed to reduce premiums and create new options**

  The health care reform bill also includes a number of insurance market reform provisions. Starting in July 2007, the non- and small-group markets will be merged, although a study of this merger must be completed before that date to assist insurers in planning for the tran-

sition. Policymakers estimate that this action will reduce premiums for people currently purchasing in the individual market by at least a quarter of their current cost. The bill also will allow Health Maintenance Organizations (HMOs) to offer coverage plans that are linked to Health Savings Accounts (HSAs) and HMO products with co-insurance. In addition, under the bill, young adults may remain on their parents' policy for two years past the loss of their dependent status, or through age 25, whichever occurs first. Carriers will also be designing new products with fewer benefits, as these products are thought to be more attractive to young adults between the ages of 19 and 26.

- **Financing strategies that rely on state, federal, employer, and individual contributions**

  The reform will be financed via several significant sources. First, $385 million in federal matching funds previously used to fund the safety net and uncompensated care will be redirected to cover the subsidies. Additionally, the state will invest $308 million in general fund revenues over three years and will collect individual and employer contributions as well.

The plan will be implemented in three phases. On October 2, 2006, enrollment began for the nearly 62,000 residents requiring a full subsidy. Starting in January 2007, the state will begin enrolling residents with annual incomes between 100 percent and 300 percent FPL. This group will pay premiums on a sliding-scale basis. Finally, the last phase will occur in July 2007, when the individual mandate becomes effective.

Vermont—Catamount Health

To some degree over-shadowed by Massachusetts' reform, Vermont passed a far reaching health reform plan called Catamount Health in May 2006. Vermont's successful bi-partisan compromise is notable in part because it reflects the determination and the tenacity of state policymakers who pressed forward after the passage, and subsequent gubernatorial veto, of the Green Mountain Health plan in the 2005 legislative session.

The successful Catamount Health plan set a goal of assuring insurance coverage for 96 percent of Vermonters by 2010. The plan includes:

- **Catamount Health Product**

  This new individual market product is designed to be affordable and comprehensive for people who have been uninsured for 12 months (with some exceptions). Coverage is based on the typical non-group market product offered in the state, but with much less cost sharing by the individual or family. The Catamount Health law specifies the specific service and cost benefits that must be included—e.g., for individual coverage, the plan cannot have more than a $250 deductible, 20 percent coinsurance, $10 office visit co-pay, no prescription drug deductible, no out-of-pocket for preventive and chronic care, and an out-of-pocket maximum of $800 per year.[22]

- **Subsidies for low-income, uninsured**
  Catamount Health Plan subsidies will be provided for uninsured individuals and families with incomes up to 300 percent FPL. In addition, the state will provide similar premium assistance to low-income individuals with access to employer-sponsored insurance who have previously been unable to afford insurance.

- **Employer requirements**
  Employers will pay a $365 per FTE annual assessment (with increases allowed as Catamount Health premiums change) based on the following parameters:
  - Employers without a plan that pays some part of the cost of insurance of its workers must pay the health care assessment on all employees.
  - Employers who have coverage must pay the assessment on:
    - Workers who are ineligible to participate in the plan; and
    - Workers who refuse the employer's coverage and do not have coverage from some other source.

The assessment exempts eight FTEs in 2007 and 2008; six FTEs in 2009; and four FTEs thereafter.

- **Vermont's Chronic Care Initiatives**
  This coverage expansion is paired with multiple chronic care initiatives, which are aligned with the state's Blueprint for Health. The Blueprint (see box, Vermont Blueprint for Health), managed by the Vermont Department of Health, is a public-private collaborative approach that seeks to improve the health of Vermonters living with chronic diseases and prevent the increase of chronic disease by utilizing the Chronic Care Model[23] as the framework for system changes. The goal is to take the Blueprint statewide by 2009 by incrementally working

Vermont Blueprint for Health

The Vermont legislature and Governor Jim Douglas (R) recognized the potential to control the growth of health care costs and improve the quality of care delivered in the state by making chronic care management a focus of reform efforts. To provide incentives to residents to focus on monitoring their health, no cost sharing will be imposed for preventive services or use of the management program within Catamount Health. For all Vermonters, the program includes additional benefits that include free immunizations and a Healthy Lifestyles insurance discount.

The Blueprint targets patients, providers, communities, and the health system in the following ways:

- **Patient Self Management**
  Encouragement of the use of decision support tools and other education designed to create informed, active, and prepared patients.
- **Provider Practice**
  Education of providers, office staff, community partners, and other stakeholders to better serve and support patients in self-management of their conditions through the use of evidence-based medicine.
- **Community Activation and Support**
  Support for physical activity and healthy lifestyles by issuing grants to communities to develop evidence-based physical activity programs—and linking these with other community and municipal initiatives to improve the built environment, such as linking walking and biking paths to community centers where people live, work, shop, and go to school.
- **Health Information System**
  Development of a statewide database containing chronic care information and a patient registry for individual and population-based disease management.
- **Health Care System**
  Initiatives to support system change, including payment for quality as a key requirement for Blueprint sustainability. The state Medicaid agency has also been charged with increasing provider reimbursements for primary care and provider participation in care coordination programs.

with hospital service areas and their community partners. In addition, the legislation requires that a chronic care management program, based on Blueprint standards, be implemented for the Medicaid population, and that the new Catamount Health Plan and the state employee health plan have chronic care management programs aligned with Blueprint standards.

- **Funding**

  Funding for the Catamount Health program will come from several sources including an increased tobacco-product tax. Vermont also intends to use federal matching funds that are expected to be available through the Global Commitment to Health waiver approved by CMS in 2005. Under this waiver the state agreed to a cap on Medicaid growth in exchange for the ability to use funds for health care investments such as the Blueprint and expansions of coverage to the uninsured. The state projections assume that the cap negotiated with CMS is sufficient to allow for some of these health care investments.[24] Finally, a portion of the Catamount subsidy will be financed through enrollee premiums and the employer assessment.

Will Comprehensive Reforms Work Here?

The comprehensive health reform plans of 2006 have led to the inevitable question of whether one state's reforms can be replicated elsewhere.

Certainly, states' efforts can test coverage strategies, informing and providing lessons for other states and national leaders. However, the variation among states is far too great for state-by-state reform to result in a comprehensive solution for the 47 million uninsured.

Key Variables:

- **Uninsurance Rate**

  States leading the way with comprehensive solutions all have uninsured rates lower than the national average, largely because of the ongoing strength of employer-based coverage in these states and previous increases in their Medicaid eligibility levels. However, a few states have uninsured populations that are close to a quarter of their population, making it unlikely that they will be able to consider universal coverage goals similar to those states that have pursued comprehensive reform.

- **Funding and Resources**

  There are significant differences in the resources states have at their disposal to address the problem of the uninsured. Substantial variation exists across the states in funding for Medicaid and the safety-net. Maine, Massachusetts, and Vermont all had higher Medicaid eligibility levels for low-income adults than the national average prior to implementing their most recent reforms. Other investments beyond Medicaid, such as charity care funds, can also play a significant role if they can be re-deployed into other programs, as was the case for Massachusetts and the $1 billion it was spending on its safety net fund.

  Conversely, states that have not made significant prior investments in coverage often have to find new funding sources. The search for funding can be the greatest challenge, since there is very different revenue-generating capacity across states, reflecting differences in income distribution as well as historic differences in the states' tax bases. Without federal financial assistance to help low income states, some will be unable to act.

- **Insurance Market Structure**

  States have different insurance markets and regulatory structures that affect how various reforms may work in their state. For example, those familiar with Massachusetts' insurance market have noted that over time, the state implemented various regulatory mechanisms in the small group and non-group insurance markets including guaranteed issue, modified community rating, and medical underwriting prohibitions, creating an environment that makes the individual mandate much more feasible. Other states that use medical underwriting, experience rating, and non-guaranteed issue would find it more challenging to implement a mandate.[28]

  And so, while it is unlikely that comprehensive reforms will be adopted in full by other states, there are elements of these reforms which are more transferable than others.

- **Connector**

  Massachusetts' creation of a health care Connector sparked renewed interest by policymakers in the concept of facilitating the purchase of insurance for small businesses and individuals. While some may consider the Connector to be a purchasing pool, Massachusetts' state officials describe it more as a purchasing mechanism. The Connector does not pool risk. Rather, it streamlines the administrative aspects of purchasing insurance.

  There is a long history of states attempting purchasing pools. Unfortunately, evidence suggests that pools alone are not sufficient to drive down health costs and may actually have a negative impact on the insurance market if they attract a different risk profile than the rest of the market.[29]

  Although new affordable products for small businesses will be accessed inside and outside the Connector, it is the sole mechanism through which individuals can access the subsidized Commonwealth Care insurance product. The state anticipates that the subsidy provided through Commonwealth Care could be as high as 80 percent, providing significant incentive for individuals to seek care through the Connector, if they are eligible. By allowing greater choice and portability for the consumer, the Connector will ease the administrative complexities that come with switching jobs. It also provides a way to reach non-traditional workers such as part-time and seasonal workers.[30] These reasons provide significant incentives for individuals to purchase coverage through the Connector.

  The experience of the Connector will test how purchasing arrangements coupled with subsidies and the other incentives (mainly the individual mandate) will increase enrollment and whether it will build purchasing power. States are likely to continue to look to the Connector as a model, but should recall the limited success of purchasing pools as standalone strategies and consider the Connector as part of a larger strategy to improve insurance coverage.

- **New Benefit Designs and Delivery Mechanisms**

  Many recent state strategies propose new insurance products and programs for currently uninsured individuals and/or small business, experimenting with new ways to encourage coverage. For example, Maine contracts with one insurer to provide their Dirigo product and provides a subsidy for low-income individuals. Vermont will allow at least two private carriers to offer their Catamount subsidized product and rely heavily on chronic care management strategies to encourage healthy behaviors and lower costs. Other states use the Medicaid Managed Care Organizations to deliver a subsidized insurance product to low-wage workers. Arizona is testing a choice of different benefit designs as part of changes they have made to the Healthcare Group, the state's coverage initiative for small businesses. If these benefit designs and delivery mechanisms are able to encourage new businesses to offer coverage or enroll a significant portion of the uninsured, they could serve as examples for other states.

- **Individual mandate**

  Ironically, the individual mandate is the feature of the Massachusetts reform that has generated the most interest nationally, but for several reasons it may be the most difficult element to export to other states. Massachusetts had significantly fewer uninsured (10 percent versus the national average of 16 percent). That, coupled with the state's ability to provide subsidies to address the problem of affordability, made it possible for the state to consider a broad-reaching requirement for individuals to have health insurance.

The efforts in Massachusetts, Maine, and Vermont have demonstrated that compromise is possible. When states consider what elements, if any, they may be able to adapt for their state, they must maintain the appropriate expectations for what any one state can achieve.

Maine—Dirigo Health

Maine is continuing to implement the Dirigo Health Reform Act, which was enacted in 2003. Dirigo, the state motto meaning "I lead" in Latin, includes strategies to control costs, improve quality, and expand coverage. In contrast to the other comprehensive reforms of Massachusetts and Vermont, Maine has relied exclusively on voluntary measures to expand insurance coverage. There is no individual mandate nor are there assessments on employers who do not provide coverage for their employees.

- **The DirigoChoice health insurance product**

  As the centerpiece of the state's efforts to expand coverage to the uninsured, DirigoChoice is available to small businesses, the self-employed, and eligible individuals without access to employer-sponsored insurance. DirigoChoice is available exclusively through Anthem, by far the largest carrier in Maine. The program offers discounts on monthly premiums and reductions in deductibles and out-of-pocket maximums on a sliding scale to enrollees with incomes below 300 percent FPL.

- **Cost-Containment and Quality**

  Maine implemented several cost-containment measures, including rate regulation in the small group market, voluntary caps on cost and operating margin of insurers, hospitals, and practitioners, and a global budget for capital improvements as well as a one-year moratorium on Certificate of Need activity. The Dirigo reforms also created the Maine Quality Forum charged with advocating for high quality health care and helping Maine residents make informed health care choices.

- **Funding**

  Funding for the Dirigo coverage, cost, and quality initiatives combines employer contributions, individual contributions, state general funds, and federal Medicaid matching funds for those individuals who are eligible. The original reform envisioned that future premium subsidies for DirigoChoice would be funded through the "savings offset payment" which is generated through the recovery of bad debt and charity care and other voluntary savings targets set by the state.[25]

Maine was ambitious in its goal of expanding coverage to all uninsured Mainers by 2009. The program drew criticism for enrolling only 12,000 to date, a number much lower than the state had anticipated.[26] However, considering the small population of Maine, the numbers enrolled in the program are impressive. After the first year of operation, most were low-income individuals who were able to benefit from the subsidies available.[27] Still, state officials had hoped for larger enrollment and had not anticipated the continuing resistance from groups that are philosophically opposed to a publicly sponsored insurance initiative and to the program's financing strategy. Improving outreach and marketing strategies for the DirigoChoice program are a main focus of Maine's ongoing efforts to increase enrollment. In addition, state officials are hoping that administrative changes effective in early 2007 will help streamline the subsidy process and make it easier for individuals to participate in the program.

In its second year of operation, Dirigo faced a lawsuit that challenged the savings offset payment. Although the savings offset payments were designed to recapture savings to the health system from the Dirigo reforms, insurance companies and Dirigo officials disagreed about how much savings the program generated and whether offset payments were the best way to finance the program. This disagreement prompted a legal challenge, although the court dismissed it. The case is being appealed. Clearly, Maine's experience underscores how difficult it is to capture and redistribute savings, let alone establish consensus on what constitutes captured savings.

To further the mission of Dirigo Health and ensure that health care continues to be accessible and affordable for the people of Maine, the Governor appointed a new Blue Ribbon Commission in 2006 charged with making "recommendations with respect to long term funding and cost containment methods." The commission will consider various funding alternatives, including the savings offset payment strategy.

INCREMENTAL COVERAGE PROGRAMS

In 2006, several states moved forward on incremental reforms that sought to increase coverage for specific uninsured groups. As in past years, many of these efforts focused on low-wage workers and their lack of access to employer-sponsored insurance. The variety of different approaches states have taken to expand coverage reflects the different regulatory and market environments of each state as well as the compromises that policy leaders were able to craft. The majority of state efforts to expand coverage rely on private insurers to deliver services, including those that use Medicaid funds. Building on the popularity of SCHIP, other incremental strategies focused on making insurance accessible to all uninsured children, regardless of income.

PUBLIC-PRIVATE PARTNERSHIPS: TENNESSEE, RHODE ISLAND, MONTANA, UTAH

Tennessee

In June 2005, as the state began rolling back eligibility under its Medicaid program, TennCare, an estimated 161,000 individuals lost coverage.[31] On the heels of these major changes and reductions, Governor Phil Bredesen (D) proposed the Cover Tennessee initiatives, intended to cover some individuals who lost coverage and also help small businesses to offer coverage.

Aimed at filling in existing coverage gaps for 600,000 uninsured, Cover Tennessee included several strategies to reach different segments of the uninsured population—including high-risk individuals, low-wage workers without access to employer-sponsored insurance, and children. In June 2006, the Governor signed Cover Tennessee into law.

The Cover Tennessee program contains several components.

- **CoverKids**

  The Cover Kids Act creates a separate, stand-alone health care program for all children age 18 and under in Tennessee. This will be a SCHIP Program.

- **CoverTN**

  This program aims to provide new, portable, and affordable coverage for the working uninsured in Tennessee who earn less than $41,000 per year, as well as for small firms that do not currently offer insurance. While CoverTN is a limited benefit plan, covered services will include, at a minimum, physician services, hospital services, outpatient services, mental health services, lab services, and generic pharmaceuticals. Under the CoverTN program, workers would be able to continue participation when they change jobs.

During the first three years of the program, premium amounts charged to employers, employees, and individuals may not increase more than 10 percent per year to maintain affordability. The program is based on the three-share concept whereby participating employers, the State of Tennessee, and the individual each contribute one-third of the premium. The state will contract with statewide carriers to offer two products with an average $150 premium per month. Premiums vary around this average based on age, tobacco use, and weight or body mass index. The benefit package will emphasize primary and preventive services with no deductibles and modest co-pays. At the time this report went to print, the state was in the process of contracting with participating health plans.

- **AccessTN**

The new legislation also creates a high-risk pool called Access Tennessee. Tennessee, prior to TennCare, operated a high-risk pool but it was disbanded when the state chose to cover uninsurable individuals under its TennCare waiver. The new pool will be funded by a combination of premiums, assessments on carriers and third party administrators, state appropriations, and possible federal funds pending grant release from CMS. Premiums charged to pool enrollees will be between 150 percent and 200 percent of a commercial benchmark plan after moderate medical underwriting. The state also authorized a premium assistance program to subsidize individuals who cannot afford the premiums.

The legislation authorizes the administrators of the pool to develop two benefit packages: one modeled after the state employees Preferred Provider Organization (PPO) product, and an alternative option that is a high-deductible health plan coupled with a health savings-account.

- **Other Programs**

The appropriation bill associated with CoverTN also continues funding for Tennessee's safety net program for affordable prescription drugs, with a focus on high priority populations with chronic diseases that require ongoing medication for daily functioning. The drug program will be available for adults who earn less than 250 percent FPL. In addition, the bill includes the Project Diabetes program, which funds endowment grants to high schools and health care entities to combat the epidemic of diabetes and obesity in the state.

Rhode Island

In 2006, Governor Donald Carcieri (R) signed into law a number of new health initiatives including several coverage expansions focused on providing premium relief for small businesses. First, the Health Insurance Commissioner is empowered to work with business, insurance, and other stakeholders to develop a new, affordable health plan, called The Wellness Health Benefit Plan. The legislation sets a target premium of 10 percent of wages, while at the same time providing benefits that meet the following affordability principles outlined in law:

- Promoting primary care, prevention and wellness;
- Actively managing the chronically ill;
- Promoting the use of the least costly, most appropriate setting; and
- Use of evidence-based, quality care.

Meeting this legislatively-defined price point is expected to reduce premiums for all small businesses to approximately 25 percent below market rate through a combination of enhanced negotiating leverage via premium rate controls, administrative cost reductions, and innovative plan design elements. In addition, eligible low-wage small businesses (those with average wages in the bottom quartile) will save an additional 10 percent of premium through a state-sponsored reinsurance program. This reinsurance program passed into law during the 2006 legislative session; however, it is contingent upon the identification of a new funding source during the coming year. Finally, the Health Insurance Commissioner is authorized to seek federal funds for the creation of a high-risk pool in the individual market.

Rhode Island's coverage expansions are part of a larger health care reform package that also includes:

- **Massachusetts Reform Review Task Force:** This panel will explore the potential transferability of the Massachusetts reforms to the State of Rhode Island.
- **Wellness:** The legislation restricts the sale of sweetened beverages in school vending machines, creates an adult flu vaccination program, and encourages insurance coverage of tobacco cessation products.
- **Transparency:** The legislation expands quality and cost data reporting to all licensed health facilities in the state to enable patients with deductibles and co-insurance to make informed decisions.

Montana

Montana also implemented a program in 2006 to reach the growing number of uninsured employees working in the state's small businesses. Insure Montana was a joint initiative of Governor Brian Schweitzer (D) and former State Auditor John Morrison (D). The program, administered by the State Auditor's Office, uses two different mechanisms to assist small businesses of two to nine employees to afford the cost of health insurance.

- **Tax Credits**

  Qualifying small businesses that are currently providing health insurance to their employees are eligible for refundable tax credits. About 600 businesses will be served under the tax credit aspect of the initiative for the first round of funding, totaling approximately 2,200 lives. Approximately 40 percent of the available Insure Montana funding per year is designated for the Employer Tax Credit.

- **Purchasing Pool**

  For qualifying small businesses that previously have been unable to afford health insurance for their employees, Insure Montana provides a monthly assistance payment for both the employer's and the employee's portion of the health insurance premium. This assistance is available to small employers who have not offered insurance in the past 24 months.

Under the purchasing pool program, an employer must pay, before the state Employer Premium Incentive payment, at least 50 percent of an employee-only policy. The Employer Premium Incentive payment pays the employer up to 50 percent of the employer's contribution for each covered employee. Each employee receives a monthly Premium Assistance Payment with amounts ranging from 20 percent to 90 percent, based on a sliding scale tied to the employee's annual family income.

The insurance product wider this program is available through one of the two Blue Cross Blue Shield of Montana plans offered by the State Health Insurance Purchasing Pool or through a qualified Association Plan. The size of each employee's Premium Assistance Payment is determined by Insure Montana staff, based on a formula approved by the Insure Montana Board of Directors.

Utah

In November 2006, Utah announced a revised premium assistance program, the Utah Premium Partnership for Health Insurance (UPP). A prior version of the premium assistance program, called Covered at Work, was initially created in 2002 under the state's Primary Care Network program.[32] The peak monthly enrollment under the initial Covered at Work program was 79 individuals. Many attributed this modest number to the $50 subsidy being too low to attract participants. Now, the new UPP program will provide a significantly larger subsidy of up to $150 per adult for low-income workers enrolled in employer-sponsored insurance whose premiums represent more than 5 percent of their annual income. Subsidies are also available for employees' children at amounts of up to $100. If dental services are covered in their parents' employer-sponsored plan they may be eligible to receive an additional $20 per child. Currently, the state has funding to enroll 1,000 adults and an estimated 250 children.

LEVERAGING MEDICAID TO EXPAND COVERAGE TO WORKING UNINSURED: NEW MEXICO, OKLAHOMA, AND ARKANSAS

New Mexico, Oklahoma, and Arkansas have begun implementation of unique public-private partnerships to cover low-income workers, leveraging individual and employer contributions as well as Medicaid funds.

New Mexico—State Coverage Insurance

New Mexico was the first state to receive a Health Insurance Flexibility and Accountability (HIFA) waiver in 2002 to expand coverage to low-income, uninsured, working adults with Medicaid funds. Because of operational challenges and difficulty securing state matching funds, New Mexico implemented their program, State Coverage Insurance, in July 2005.

The program is now available to low-income, uninsured, working adults with family income below 200 percent FPL. An individual may enroll through their employer or as a self-employed individual. The premium is paid by contributions from the employer and employee in combination with state and federal funds. Self-employed workers must pay the employer as well as the employee portion of the premium. The benefit package is comprehensive, with an annual benefit maximum of $100,000. Services are provided through private managed care organizations and cost sharing is designed to ensure that low-income participants have access to care. The program opened in July 2005 and close to 4,400 workers are currently enrolled in the program.

Oklahoma—Employer/Employee Partnership for Insurance Coverage

On September 30, 2005, Oklahoma received CMS approval of their HIFA waiver, the Oklahoma Employer/Employee Partnership for Insurance Coverage (O-EPIC). O-EPIC is intended to provide health insurance coverage to 50,000 low-wage, working adults in Oklahoma using either a premium assistance program or an individual plan. O-EPIC is funded by state general fund revenues generated by a tobacco tax, along with federal matching funds under Title XIX and employer and employee contributions.

The Premium Assistance program, launched in November 2005, helps qualified employees in small businesses of 50 or fewer employees purchase health insurance coverage through their employer. The employer works with an insurance agent to choose a qualified private health plan to offer its employees. The Premium Assistance program pays 60 percent of the health insurance premium for qualified employees with incomes below 185 percent FPL and 85 percent of the premium for the qualified enrollee's spouse. Employers are expected to contribute 25 percent of the employee's premium and employees are expected to contribute up to 15 percent for themselves and 15 percent for their spouses.

The Individual Plan will be launched shortly and is designed as a safety net health plan for qualified individuals with incomes below 185 percent FPL and who are ineligible to participate in O-EPIC Premium Assistance. The Individual Plan includes self-employed individuals not eligible for small group health coverage; workers at small businesses who are either not eligible to participate in their employer's health plan or whose employer does not offer a qualified health plan; and unemployed individuals who are currently seeking work. The Individual Plan also provides coverage to working individuals with a disability whose income exceeds the Medicaid eligibility level but is below 200 percent FPL, and who meet "ticket to work" requirements.[33] The Individual Plan provides coverage through private managed care plans that also serve the Medicaid program; however, the benefit package is less comprehensive than Medicaid or most products offered in the commercial market.

Arkansas—ARHealthNet

In March 2006, Arkansas received approval from CMS for the establishment of a program that will allow use of state and federal Medicaid funds to provide low-cost health coverage to small businesses. The original application was submitted to CMS in January 2003. During the negotiation phase with CMS, the Arkansas Department of Health and Human Services made some changes to the waiver design; however, the central goal of providing an affordable health coverage option to businesses that are not currently providing insurance remained intact. The new program, ARHealthNet, will be open for employer enrollment in late 2006 with plans to begin offering benefits to enrollees in early 2007. Arkansas is the third state to use a Medicaid HIFA waiver to expand insurance options for businesses and low-wage workers.

ARHealthNet will be open to employers who have not offered group health insurance to their employees during the preceding 12 months. The program requires employers who participate to guarantee coverage for all full-time employees regardless of income. While all employees are eligible to enroll in the new product, a subsidy is only available to those employees with annual incomes below 200 percent FPL.

The ARHealthNet benefit plan, best described as a safety net benefit design, offers limited coverage compared to what would typically be available through commercial plans or through the Medicaid program. It will include six clinician visits, seven hospital days, two outpatient procedures or emergency room visits per year, as well as two prescriptions per month. The state has contracted with a commercial third-party administrator to administer ARHealthNet and to develop and implement a marketing plan using the existing Arkansas private carrier health insurance broker network.

Arkansas originally envisioned that private insurance carriers would accept all medical cost "risk" associated with this plan. However, in acknowledgment that the program represents a new operating model in Arkansas, the state subsequently elected to initially retain the "risk" in order to enhance acceptance by the private marketplace.

The program will be implemented in sequential phases during the five year demonstration period. Phase I will operate for a period of 12 to 24 months with an enrollment cap of 15,000. Phase II will operate for the remainder of the demonstration with enrollment capped based on availability of funding.

COVERING CHILDREN

A growing number of states are interested in covering children above federal SCHIP levels. Since 1997, many have focused on increasing outreach and enrollment for their SCHIP programs. However, states were generally not focused on covering children with family incomes above SCHIP levels. Until recently, Connecticut's Husky B program, the state's SCHIP program, was the only program in the nation that allowed uninsured children in families above 300 percent FPL the opportunity to buy into the program.[34]

In November 2005, Illinois Governor Rod Blagojevich (D) signed the Covering All Kids Health Insurance Act, making insurance coverage available to all uninsured children. The All Kids program was designed to cover an estimated 50 percent of uninsured children in Illinois who reside in families with incomes above 200 percent FPL—the state's SCHIP level. On July 1, 2006, the program officially began covering children. Of the 250,000 eligible uninsured children in Illinois, the state predicts that 50,000 children will enroll in the first year of the program. As of January 2007, All Kids will be available to any

TABLE 28-2 Enrollment Experience of Select State Coverage Programs

Target Population	Program (start date)	Eligibility	Enrollment Fall 2006 (individuals)
Small Business	Maine DirigoChoice (2005)	Small businesses, the self-employed, and eligible individuals without access to employer-sponsored insurance and with incomes below 300 percent FPL	12,000
	Insure Montana (2006)	Previously uninsured firms (2–9 employees) that have not offered insurance for 24 months	6,995
	New Mexico State Coverage Insurance (2005)	Low-income, uninsured, working adults with family income below 200 percent FPL; participating employers must have ≤50 employees and have not voluntarily dropped a commercial health insurance in the past 12 months	4,400
	Oklahoma Employer/ Employee Partnership for Insurance Coverage (2005)	Workers and their spouses, who work in firms with 50 or fewer workers; self-employed; unemployed individuals currently seeking work; and individuals whose employers do not offer health coverage with household incomes at or below 185 percent FPL Small employers must contribute at least 25 percent of eligible employee's premium costs and offer an O-EPIC qualified health plan	1,200
	West Virginia Small Business Plan (2005)	Small businesses (2–50 employees) that have not had health benefit coverage for their employees during the preceding 12 months; employers must pay at least 50 percent of the premium cost	1,200
	Arizona Healthcare Group (1986)	Small business, the self-employed, and political sub-divisions. No income limits apply, but HCG does have employee participation requirements and crowd-out requirements	24,000
	Healthy New York (2001)	Small mployers that have previously not offered insurance and with 30 percent of workers who earn less than $34,000 annually; sole proprietors and working individuals without access to ESI who earn less than 250 percent FPL and have been uninsured 12 months	125,000
Low Income Adults	Washington Basic Health (1988)	Individuals with family incomes below 200 percent FPL	100,000
	Pennsylvania adultBasic (2001)	Adults with incomes up to 200 percent FPL who have been without health insurance for 90 days prior to enrollment	55,000
	Minnesota Care (1992)	Families with children up to 275 percent FPL under Medicaid and childless adults up to 175 percent FPL	117,000
	Maryland Primary Care (2006)	Individuals below 116 percent FPL	23,000
	Utah Primary Care Network (2002)	Adults below 150 percent FPL	Waiver capped at 25,000
	District of Columbia Alliance (2001)	Uninsured individuals with family incomes below 200 percent FPL	35,000
Children Above SCHIP Income Levels	Illinois AllKids (2006)	Any child uninsured for 12 months or more with family income above the SCHIP level (200 percent FPL)	28,600
	Connecticut Husky B Buy-In (1997)	Allows uninsured children in families above 300 percent FPL the opportunity to buy-in to the state's SCHIP program, Husky B	800

child uninsured for 12 months or more, with the cost to the family determined on a sliding scale basis.

The program is funded through enrollee premiums and cost sharing and savings from care management. The state continues to seek federal financial participation for those children that are eligible for KidCare (the state's SCHIP program) and Medicaid. The program is linked with other existing public programs such as FamilyCare (coverage for parents up to 185 percent FPL) and KidCare via their online application. In addition, the state has undertaken a public outreach program called the All Kids Training Tour that will highlight the new and expanded health care programs offered by Illinois.

Illinois' efforts have catalyzed other states to move forward on similar initiatives. Since then, several governors have proposed initiatives targeted at covering all children in their states. The impetus behind such initiatives is fairly simple: covering children is a relatively inexpensive investment, and years of experience with simplifying eligibility and conducting outreach for SCHIP programs are a solid foundation for the successful expansion of children's coverage.

In July 2006, Pennsylvania Governor Edward Rendell (D) announced the development of the Cover All Kids program which will allow families to purchase health insurance on a sliding scale basis relative to their income. The Pennsylvania legislature approved $4.4 million for Cover All Kids for its first year of operation. While CMS has yet to approve the program, the state aims to begin enrollment early in 2007.

Tennessee also passed legislation to cover all children, putting in place a new SCHIP program (SCHIP had previously been a part of the TennCare program). The Cover Kids Act, which became law in Tennessee in 2006, creates a standalone SCHIP program for children in families with incomes up to 250 percent FPL and allows children in higher income families to buy into the program.

Other states are considering similar proposals. In late September, Oregon Governor Ted Kulongoski (D) proposed his plan to cover uninsured children through an expansion of the Oregon Health Plan and a private purchasing arrangement for higher income children. Wisconsin Governor Jim Doyle (D) proposed extending the state's Medicaid program, BadgerCare, to all uninsured children by 2007. Similarly, Washington Governor Christine Gregoire (D) and New Mexico Governor Bill Richardson (D) proposed the goal of insuring all children, but have not yet specified details of how it will be accomplished.

While many of these initiatives still need to be developed in greater detail for enactment or implementation, momentum is clearly building in a number of states to ensure that all children have access to health insurance. The interest in covering all kids is occurring even as many states, including Illinois and Wisconsin, are facing short-term SCHIP federal funding shortfalls. As Congress considers the reauthorization of the SCHIP program, there is rising pressure on federal lawmakers to expand this popular program and address the inadequacy of its current funding.

IMPLEMENTATION OF NEW STATE STRATEGIES: ENROLLMENT AND SUCCESS TAKE TIME AND COMMITMENT

Several states are proposing new strategies to expand coverage to the uninsured and some have bold initiatives that seek to achieve near-universal coverage. Reaching the compromise needed to enact coverage proposals is a significant achievement, but much of the hard work lies ahead for state policymakers as they implement new programs. A long history of state initiatives designed to reduce the number of uninsured suggests that enrollment in these new initiatives may take time and they should be evaluated only after they have had time to mature.

Previous state strategies to expand coverage have resulted in a broad range of enrollment experiences (see Table 28-2). This can largely be explained by the different goals of these programs, the diverse populations these programs intend to cover, the length of time they have been in operation, and the amount of funding the state has provided. However, there are also a number of programmatic design decisions as well as operational practices that impact how many uninsured individuals are ultimately enrolled.

Complex Design

Many of the new state initiatives have fairly complex program design and participation rules. Often the complexity is a result of efforts to target limited resources to specific segments of the uninsured population or to assure that new public programs do not encourage either employers to cease offering coverage or individuals to drop their coverage. However, these participation rules often lead to additional steps in the enrollment process, which can create operational barriers for the target population as well. Income requirements are a fairly standard condition of eligibility. In addition, eligibility is often limited to individuals who have been uninsured for a specific period of time and who work for an employer of a certain size or that does not currently offer coverage. Many also require employers to participate by beginning to offer coverage. With so many factors in play, the underlying complexity of the program design can frustrate success, despite the best efforts to reach out to the eligible population.

The Illinois All Kids program is a notable exception to these complex and targeted efforts. By creating a program that is open to all uninsured children regardless of income, the state can simplify the outreach message to families. The participation rules are very broad, requiring only that the child be uninsured for 12 months, and the state uses the sliding scale premium to target public subsidies to families with incomes below specific thresholds.

Small Businesses Are Hard to Reach

While there has been significant progress by states in improving administrative systems to enroll children in Medicaid or SCHIP, there has been less of a focus on reducing the administrative barriers for initiatives to expand coverage offered by small businesses or to working uninsured individuals. Fewer resources have been available to assist state policymakers in identifying best practices to overcome administrative barriers to enrollment. In the case of initiatives that require employers to begin to offer coverage, it remains unclear what factors inhibit higher enrollment. Two possible explanations are the complex operational barriers to enrollment and the intrinsic challenge of a strategy that focuses only on businesses that have not previously offered coverage and are disinclined to start.

Ramp-Up Time Needed

Regardless of program design, past experience demonstrates that it takes time for new coverage programs to enroll uninsured individuals. Working through a new programs start-up challenges can take time, and states are usually further constrained by both short timeframes for implementation and a lack of funding for administrative functions. The history of the SCHIP program bears this out—initial enrollment in most state SCHIP programs was below expectations and most underspent their federal allotment in the early years. However, current SCHIP enrollment is such that spending exceeds the federal allotment in 40 states.[35]

Small business initiatives may take even more time to build enrollment. For example, Healthy New York, originally established in 2001, is now one of the largest coverage initiatives for small businesses and low-wage workers in the nation. After initial slow enrollment, and following modifications to the design of the program in 2003 that resulted in lower premiums, enrollment grew quickly. In August 2006, enrollment in Healthy New York exceeded 125,000.[36] While the enrollment changes that occurred during this time can be attributed to the more affordable premiums, it also may be due to the amount of time it took for the state to market the program and earn a degree of confidence from businesses and residents. In focus groups, small business leaders have indicated that they are willing to commit to providing health insurance through a state program only after it has demonstrated program stability.[37]

Balancing Vision and Realistic Expectations

It often takes ambitious goals by state policymakers to build support for new coverage strategies. The challenge for policymakers is to balance initial expectations with maintaining support for the initiative in the difficult, early years of implementation. Policymakers' desire to demonstrate early success can make it hard to encourage stakeholders to stay the course over the long term; however, it is only over the long-run that strategies can be fairly evaluated.

STATE COVERAGE STRATEGIES: EVOLVING WITH TIME AND EFFORT

2006

Massachusetts and Vermont demonstrated that bi-partisan compromise and comprehensive reforms are possible at the state level. Several other states approved or began implementing coverage initiatives focused on children and working uninsured adults. Several states also took advantage of the flexibility outlined in the DRA to redesign their Medicaid programs.

Arkansas—CMS approved a waiver to allow Arkansas to receive federal Medicaid funds for a program that will provide low-cost health coverage to small businesses.

Idaho—Taking advantage of the state plan amendment process provided in the DRA, the state split the Medicaid and SCHIP population into three major benefit plans.

Illinois—All Kids program implemented. Many other states propose similar plans to cover all children.

Kansas—Received federal approval for their reform proposal under the DRA.

Kentucky—Moved forward on their Medicaid redesign plans after receiving approval for their state plan amendment under the DRA.

Maryland—Legislature over-rode Governor Ehrlich's veto of the "Fair Share Act." Later in the year, the U.S. District court struck down the bill, declaring the measure was pre-empted by ERISA. The state has appealed the decision.

Maine—Blue Ribbon Commission on Dirigo Health established to evaluate components of the state-subsidized covered program for the uninsured, particularly Dirigo's funding mechanism.

Massachusetts—Passed a landmark comprehensive bill designed to cover 95 percent of the uninsured in the state within the next three years.

Oklahoma—Legislature approved expansion of O-EPIC program to cover businesses with 50 or fewer employees.

Pennsylvania—Legislature approved funding for Cover All Kids, a program allowing families with incomes above the SCHIP eligibility level to purchase health insurance for their children on a sliding scale basis based on income. Implementation to begin January 1, 2007.

Rhode Island—Legislature passed a number of new health initiatives including several coverage expansions focused on providing premium relief for small businesses.

Tennessee—Legislature passed Cover Tennessee program, which includes several expansions to cover children, uninsurable adults, low-income workers, and small businesses.

Utah—Revamped its Covered at Work program and introduced the new Partnership for Health Insurance program, which provides subsidies for low-income workers who are enrolled in coverage provided through their employers.

Vermont—Reached agreement on Catamount Health with goal of reaching universal coverage by 2010. The program includes an employer assessment, a new insurance product with subsidies for individuals below 300 percent FPL, and several chronic disease management initiatives.

West Virginia—Moved forward on Medicaid redesign plans after receiving CMS approval for their state plan amendment under the DRA.

Federal

- Medicare Part D implemented. States are no longer responsible for providing prescription drug coverage to dual eligibles.
- Congress passed the DRA which authorizes states to implement a variety of changes to their Medicaid programs.
- The Medicaid Commission proposed long-term solutions to address Medicaid's escalating costs.

2005

Financial conditions continued to improve for many states and more proposed or implemented coverage initiatives. During this time, the foundation for comprehensive reforms was being laid in Massachusetts and Vermont. Maryland passed "Fair Share" legislation, sparking interest in several states regarding employer responsibility. Spurred by continued budget challenges and the threat of federal changes to the Medicaid program, many states also developed Medicaid reform proposals.

Florida—Received CMS approval for Medicaid redesign plans to be piloted in two counties.

Georgia—Legislature passed minimum benefit legislation.

Illinois—Legislature passed All Kids program, expanding coverage to children above SCHIP levels and continued to phase-in an expansion of coverage for parents up to 185 percent FPL.

Iowa—In exchange for giving up $66 million in Inter-Governmental Transfers, the state received a waiver from CMS to provide a limited set of Medicaid benefits to adults up to 200 percent FPL.

Kansas—Governor Sibelius announced the Kansas Health Care Authority, which streamlined all major health care programs in the state to improve efficiency and allow the state to push for reforms.

Kentucky—Legislature passed minimum benefit legislation.

Maine—Enrollment began in DirigoChoice.

Maryland—Legislature passed the "Fair Share Act," requiring large employers to spend at least 8 percent of their payroll on health care. The bill was vetoed by Governor Ehrlich.

Massachusetts—Several health care reform proposals were introduced and each house in the legislature passed its own version of comprehensive reform. State received approval for Mass Health waiver extension establishing a Safety Net Care Pool.

New Mexico—State Coverage Insurance program, which is available to low-income, uninsured working adults with family incomes below 200 percent FPL, is implemented.

Montana—State implements Insure Montana, an initiative using tax credits and a purchasing pool to help small businesses afford the cost of health insurance.

Oklahoma—The O-EPIC program waiver is approved by CMS.

Pennsylvania—Signed an agreement with Blue Cross Blue Shield insurance plans to spend close to $1 billion in surplus funds over six years on various health programs in the state, including adultBasic.

Tennessee—Granted a waiver amendment to end coverage of uninsured and uninsurable adults in the TennCare program and began disenrolling approximately 320,000 individuals.

Vermont—Governor Douglas vetoed the Green Mountain Health bill, which would have provided primary and preventive services to the uninsured. The state also received approval for their Global Commitment to Health waiver.

West Virginia—The Small Business Plan began enrollment. The state also established the WVAccess high-risk pool.

Federal

- Secretary Leavitt established the Medicaid Commission charged with recommending ways to cut $10 billion from the program over five years.

2004

In 2004, states began to emerge from the severe fiscal crisis of the previous few years and could refocus on coverage strategies. Several states created new funding sources for future expansions, others moved forward on incremental approaches. One state, Maine, continued to work on comprehensive reform plans. Passage of the Medicare Modernization Act (MMA) handed tremendous responsibility to state officials.

California—Voters approved referendum repealing "pay-or-play" law passed in 2003.

Colorado—Voters approved a tobacco tax increase expected to provide $125 million for health programs.

Idaho—Health Insurance Flexibility and Accountability (HIFA) waiver approved, creating the Idaho Access Card and premium assistance programs.

Illinois—Increased family coverage for kids from 185 to 200 percent FPL and for parents from 49 to 133 percent FPL.

Louisiana—Legislature passed minimum benefit legislation.

Maine—Prepared for implementation of the Dirigo reform plan that had been enacted in 2003.

Maryland—Legislature passed minimum benefit legislation.

Michigan—Received CMS approval for Adults Benefit Waiver program covering childless adults at or below 35 percent FPL.

Minnesota—Joined with health purchasers to form the Smart Buy Alliance focusing on health purchasing strategies and rewarding quality and value within the system.

Montana—Voters approved a tobacco tax increase to support a pharmacy program and a coverage program for small businesses.

Oklahoma—Voters approved a tobacco tax increase, which provided funding for a new coverage program.

Texas—Legislature passed minimum benefit legislation.

Washington—Legislature passed minimum benefit legislation.

West Virginia—Legislature passed Small Business Plan, which allowed carriers to access the state's public employees agency reimbursement rates, enabling businesses to find more affordable coverage.

Federal

- The MMA passed in late 2003, providing seniors and people living with disabilities a prescription drug benefit under Medicare and created health savings accounts, part of a growing trend toward broader consumer participation in health care decisions.
- During 2004, state officials sorted out the implications of the new drug benefit and the discount card program.

For more information on state strategies, visit www.state-coverage.net/matrix.

PART II TRENDS IN STATE INITIATIVES AND LESSONS FOR POLICYMAKERS

While the situation and proposed solutions in each state vary widely, a nationwide review of efforts to address the problem of the uninsured reflects current trends and hard learned lessons that can inform future strategies.

Although the reforms of the past year vary in a number of ways, common themes and trends can be seen.

1. **Comprehensive state reforms build off prior efforts and financing mechanisms.**

   States that are attempting to reach near-universal coverage usually build these reforms on prior efforts. The comprehensive reforms in Massachusetts, Vermont, and Maine are all examples of coverage initiatives that built on previous initiatives as a foundation for more comprehensive action. In these states, Medicaid eligibility for adults was expanded over time to income levels well above the national average. Likewise, each had strategies in place to improve access to care or contain costs. In Massachusetts, as much as $1 billion was historically spent annually on the safety net with much of this funding now being shifted to insurance coverage. In Vermont, a prior Medicaid waiver is expected to provide some of the flexibility for funding the new expansion efforts.

2. **Reforms attempt to stem the erosion of employer-sponsored insurance.**

   Many state efforts to expand coverage focus on compelling evidence that the increase in the uninsured is due in large part to the decline in employer-sponsored insurance. During the past several years, many states have collected and analyzed their own data about the uninsured. These state studies, as well as national reports, indicate that more than 80 percent of all nonelderly uninsured are either workers or living in families with working individuals[38]—a finding that has led state leaders to focus most of their efforts to expand coverage to the working uninsured. These strategies either encourage small businesses to offer insurance or target low-income workers or their dependents without access to employer-sponsored insurance.

   States have used a number of voluntary measures to help small businesses to offer insurance. Many allow small employers to offer a more affordable product to their employees either through a group purchasing arrangement, leveraging the buying power of the state, offering subsidies, or allowing insurers to offer limited benefit packages. For example, DirigoChoice in Maine and the Connector in Massachusetts enable small employers to purchase insurance through new purchasing arrangements as well as subsidizing premiums for low-income workers. Massachusetts and Vermont go farther: they are the only states yet to require businesses to pay modest assessments toward state-offered coverage if they fail to provide insurance for their workers. States look to the employer-based system for these coverage strategies for three main reasons. First, employer contributions to premiums can leverage public funds. Second, employers and employees both derive tax advantages from employer-sponsored coverage, offsetting a significant portion of the premium. Finally, where employers are already offering health insurance, the new programs can take advantage of the administrative structures already in place.

What is troubling is that an increasing number of employers are not offering coverage to their workers, and the voluntary strategies states have tried to date have had limited success enticing employers to begin offering coverage. Therefore, many of the new strategies targeted at helping small businesses now also provide a means to assist low-income workers even if their employer is not willing to participate. Oklahoma's O-EPIC Individual Plan, New Mexico's State Coverage Insurance, and all of the comprehensive proposals allow uninsured individuals to enroll if they do not have access to employer-sponsored insurance. Even the states expanding coverage for children are reaching out to working families who no longer have access to employer-sponsored insurance.

3. **Successful efforts to enact reforms often expect shared financial responsibility. Some states are beginning to recognize the need for mandatory participation.**
Even though employer-sponsored insurance has declined, 63 percent of working age adults still get insurance through their employer.[39] Recognizing the essential funding employers provide, none of the efforts to expand coverage in 2006 were exclusively financed with public funds. States have moved forward on initiatives that expect both employers and individuals (based on their income) to contribute. Some also included elements of consumer-driven purchasing to increase consumer involvement.

Many state initiatives include a role for employer contributions to health care coverage on a voluntary basis. However, Massachusetts and Vermont explicitly require employers to contribute to the costs of health care through their employer assessments, albeit only a modest amount compared to the actual cost of health insurance premiums. Maryland's Fair Share Act tried to go further in requiring employer responsibility, but it was struck down by the courts.[40]

The attention given to Massachusetts's requirement that all individuals have health insurance demonstrates a growing recognition that voluntary programs are not likely to reach all of the uninsured. As a result of Massachusetts' groundbreaking reform, policymakers seem more willing to consider mandatory insurance requirements for individuals, sparking a public debate about who is ultimately responsible for assuring coverage.

4. **Expansions in coverage often rely on private insurers to deliver care.**
Whether or not states move forward with incremental or comprehensive reforms, private insurers clearly will continue to play a major role. Commonwealth Care, Catamount Health, and DirigoChoice each contract with private insurers to bear risk. Even states that are largely using Medicaid financing for expansion efforts have carefully crafted the delivery of services through private health insurers, such as New Mexico's State Coverage Insurance and Oklahoma's O-EPIC.

While the aforementioned expansions use private insurers, there continues to be some question whether private plans are the most efficient platform to expand coverage. In the case of Vermont's reform, policymakers questioned the extent to which the expansion of coverage would use private health plans or be administered by the state. A compromise was crafted: the state's commission on health care reform can deem that rates offered by carriers are not a cost-effective method of providing coverage—allowing the state to pursue self-insuring. Maine contracted out DirigoChoice to the largest carrier in the state, Anthem, but has more recently examined whether DirigoChoice should self-insure to achieve greater efficiency.[41] Arkansas made the decision to self-insure but privately administer, at least for the first two years, to avoid uncertainty about the health profile of the population that will enroll.

5. **Medicaid benefits are being redesigned through the DRA, but to date these efforts have not included expansions in coverage.**
A current focus for Medicaid policymakers is the new flexibility that states were given under the DRA to

redesign benefits for current populations. West Virginia, Kentucky, and Idaho were the first states to propose changes to their benefit design for currently covered populations with approved state plan amendments in 2006.

These reforms are likely to have a significant impact on coverage for low-income individuals and may change their access to care. However, to date, none of these reforms change Medicaid beneficiaries' eligibility level for the program. In fact, the flexibility provided to states through the DRA is clearly targeted to currently covered populations versus expansions to wholly new populations.

Medicaid continues to be an important source of funding for strategies to cover the uninsured. Several incremental approaches leverage Medicaid financing to expand coverage. Furthermore, all of the comprehensive reforms include some level of Medicaid financing.

6. **Many state reforms address cost and quality in addition to health insurance coverage.**

As states struggle with reforming their health care systems, the issue of coverage has become more deeply entwined with quality and cost issues than ever before. Access to health care is fundamentally a question of affordability and states are trying to determine the level of efficiency and value they would like the health care system to provide. As such, states are creating programs that go beyond just coverage to include aspects of quality and cost containment.

Early on, Maine concluded that sustainable health care reform required addressing all three issues of access, cost, and quality concurrently. So, while they created DirigoChoice to improve access to insurance through a subsidized insurance product, they also founded the Maine Quality Forum and pursued a number of cost containment initiatives.

A large part of Vermont's reforms addresses the issue of chronic care management both to improve the health of Vermont's population and to help control one of the main underlying cost drivers in the health care system. Other states have created task forces and commissions to focus on cost and quality—including the new Massachusetts Health Care Quality and Cost Council to promote health care quality improvement and cost containment and West Virginia's Interagency Health Council charged with addressing issues related to access, cost control, quality, and equitable financing.

Across the country, many states are collecting data to measure health plan and provider performance and disseminating that information to the public. Medicaid agencies are involved in various activities including performance measurement, financial incentives based on those measures, and encouraging programs to directly improve clinical care for their beneficiaries. In addition, the public health agency in most states is focused on population-based clinical quality improvement. Finally, in some states, the agency that administers the state employee health plan also is working on quality initiatives, many times as part of a larger coalition of other employers in their state.

LESSONS FROM DECADES OF EXPANSION EFFORTS

This is not the first time states have taken the lead in attempting to improve insurance coverage in their states. This recent round of reform builds on at least a decade of state efforts, ranging from comprehensive attempts such as Massachusetts' 1988 pay-or-play requirements to the TennCare expansions and from the Oregon Health Plan to numerous incremental approaches. These efforts have had variable degrees of success and challenges that provide lessons for policymakers considering their own state reforms.

1. **State strategies make a difference because they help people access health care.**

Programs that provide access to coverage for previously uninsured populations make a difference in people's lives. The research demonstrating the link between insurance coverage, access to health care, and improved health outcomes is irrefutable.[42]

State Medicaid and SCHIP growth have prevented what would have otherwise been a larger increase in the uninsured.[43] Many states have used these programs to expand coverage to new populations.

State efforts to expand coverage occur within a broader, more challenging environment. With health insurance premiums growing almost three times faster than workers' wages and a continually declining base of employer-sponsored insurance, it is no surprise that these larger trends in health coverage make it difficult to assess the impact of specific state efforts to improve coverage.[44] Nonetheless, it is clear that more previously uninsured individuals have coverage today as a result of state initiatives (see Table 28-2).

2. **Leadership, opportunity, and readiness to act are all key ingredients to making reform happen.**

No state reform occurred without a champion clearly articulating the need for significant change. Many examples illustrate this imperative—including Massachusetts, where the Governor and legislative leaders were able to come together and make health reform a priority. Making reform happen requires leaders who are committed to a solution, but not so focused on a specific strategy that they are unwilling to look to other options. Ultimately, success requires working through the reality of the political process.

MANDATES: HOW THEY WORK AND WILL THEY WORK?

With continued erosion of employer-sponsored insurance, many states have attempted to encourage employers to offer and contribute to employee health benefits programs through voluntary measures such as tax credits, purchasing pools, and income-based subsidies for low-wage workers. However, because voluntary employer incentives generally have not been able to close the increasing gaps in coverage, some states have begun to consider more mandatory "pay-or-play" strategies, assessing employers that do not provide coverage.[48]

In part, states have reexamined the concept of employer mandates out of concern that the uninsured will end up on public programs or require uncompensated care which results in cost-shifting to those with private coverage. Several states conducted analyses, attempting to determine whether a significant number of uninsured, large-firm employees receive Medicaid, SCHIP, or uncompensated care. Some have discovered that many employees of a few large firms are enrolled in public programs.[49]

The idea of employer mandates to reduce the number of uninsured is not a new concept: many states have enacted legislation calling for an employer mandate but were unable to implement such programs. In 1988, Massachusetts enacted but never implemented an employer mandate, which ultimately was repealed in 1996. Oregon passed an employer mandate in 1989, but it expired before being implemented. Washington followed suit in 1993 with an employer mandate, but it too was repealed in 1995. In 2004, California voters narrowly rejected an employer mandate that would have required businesses with more than 50 employees to pay a fixed fee for workers whom they did not insure.

To date, Hawaii is the only state that has implemented an employer mandate, the Prepaid Health Care Act of 1974, and Hawaii has one of the highest employer offer and coverage rates. The 1974 law required nearly all employers in Hawaii to provide health benefits to employers who work more than 20 hours per week.

MARYLAND'S ATTEMPT AND THE ERISA CHALLENGE

On January 12, 2006, Maryland became the first state to require an employer to spend more on health care for its employees. The Maryland General Assembly over-rode Governor Ehrlich's veto to pass a bill (S.B. 790/H.B. 1284) during the 2005 legislative session requiring private-sector for-profit employers with 10,000 or more employees in the state to spend at least eight percent of their payroll (or six percent in the case of a nonprofit employer) on health care.

It quickly became known as the "Wal-Mart Bill" as Wal-Mart was the only employer in the state on which it would have an effect. According to the bill, those employers that fall below the requirement would be required to pay the difference between their health insurance expenses and the percentage threshold into a new Fair Share Health Care Fund, which would direct the funds into the state's Medicaid program. The Retail Industry Leaders Association (RILA) filed suit against the bill and, in a ruling on July 19, 2006, the Maryland Act was struck down, with the judge declaring that the measure was pre-empted by the Employee Retirement Income Security Act (ERISA) and was therefore invalid.[50]

Nevertheless, Maryland's legislative attempt caught the attention of many other states where bills similar to the Maryland law were introduced in 2006—including a bill in California that was passed by the legislature but was vetoed by the governor in September.[51]

With the court's ruling on the Maryland legislation, few states are likely to pass an employer requirement crafted in the same way. Still, legal experts believe that it is still possible for states to propose ideas that could survive an ERISA challenge.[52] Of note, both Massachusetts and Vermont included requirements on employers in their comprehensive reform plans. Both states have an assessment on employers over a certain size that fail to provide health benefits. Although, in both cases, the employer assessment is well below the cost of actually providing insurance. In Vermont's Catamount Health plan, employers will be required to pay an assessment even for those employees who are eligible for coverage they offer, but are not enrolled and therefore are uninsured. In Massachusetts, such employees will be required to purchase insurance. Vermont will assess the need for an individual mandate in future years.

Massachusetts also requires employers to set up a Section 125 benefit plan (cafeteria plan) or potentially pay a portion of the cost of uncompensated care used by their uninsured employees. Employers are not required to necessarily contribute to the cost of health care, but solely to set up the mechanism for the individual employee to purchase insurance with pre-tax dollars.

The architects of the Massachusetts legislation (see State Strategies section) have commented on the necessity of an individual mandate to effect change.[53] Voluntary measures may not be sufficient to encourage take-up and, despite the presence of a subsidized and affordable insurance product, some people will still go without coverage. Massachusetts survey data indicates that approximately 40 percent of the uninsured earn more than 300 percent FPL and presumably could afford to purchase insurance. The state has engineered a strategy to ensure that every taxpayer contributes to the cost of health care coverage in some fashion and to finance any remaining "free-rider" effect by adding new premium dollars into the health system. In addition, the state is hoping that individuals who are healthy yet currently uninsured will enter the insurance risk pool, stabilizing costs for everyone.

The concept of employer and individual mandates provoke sharp political dialogue about where the balance of responsibility for health insurance coverage lies.

Interest in employer mandates continues as policymakers attempt to reverse the trend in declining employer-sponsored insurance and maintain the largely employer-based insurance system. The interest that has been generated by Massachusetts's passage of an individual mandate portends a readiness by some policymakers to explore focusing responsibility in insurance coverage on individuals.

MORE INFORMATION ON ERISA

More detailed information on ERISA implications for state coverage strategies is available in *ERISA Implications for State Health Care Access Initiatives*. The publication, written by Patricia Butler, JD, DrPH, explores the implications of the recent federal court decision finding that ERISA preempts Maryland's "Fair Share Act." The paper discusses in detail:

- ERISA preemption principles;
- The Maryland law and RILA vs. Fielder court decision;
- Implications for state health care access initiatives involving employers in financing; and
- Arguments that may be raised to challenge and defend such state programs.

ERISA Implications for State Health Care Access Initiatives is part of a continuing series of policy papers on ERISA published by the Robert Wood Johnson Foundation's State Coverage Initiatives program and the National Academy for State Health Policy.

Please visit http://www.statecoverage.net/publicaitons.htm to access a PDF version of the brief.

For better or worse, there is an element of serendipity in the reform process, creating new opportunities to move forward. For both Massachusetts and Vermont there was an alignment of forces in each of the states that pushed forward reforms. Both enacted their reforms after several years of major discussion

with engaged stakeholders driving a reform agenda. In Maine, a new governor came to office with a promise to address health reform and a public mandate for change. However, beyond the opportunity is the ability to act and be prepared to move quickly once the policy window opens. These states had policymakers and analysts who had a profound understanding of the problems they intended to address and an appropriate framework of options to consider.

3. **There are no free solutions.**

States experienced fiscally challenging times during past few years and many states attempted to address the issue of the uninsured and expand coverage using strategies that did not require additional spending— including enacting laws that allowed carriers to sell limited benefit products, creating purchasing pools, and instituting outreach and education initiatives. However, these "no cost" strategies have had little, if any, apparent impact. Significant strides in reducing the number of uninsured require a significant financial investment. As states emerge from their fiscal crisis, some are ready to invest new funds to expand coverage.

4. **There has been little success in addressing underlying costs of health care, but a new focus on chronic care management holds potential.**

Affordability of health insurance is one of the main contributors to a growing uninsured population. The data are compelling. While health insurance premiums are growing more slowly (7.7 percent) than in prior years, they still are growing three times faster than wages.[45] The data for low-income workers are even more striking. The annual premiums for family coverage reached $10,880 in 2005, eclipsing the gross earnings for a full-time minimum-wage worker ($10,712).[46] Providing insurance coverage to all of the uninsured will require more effective strategies to control the growth of underlying health care costs.

Commercial insurers and state programs have responded to rising health care costs with changes in benefit design that shift more financial responsibility to consumers or eliminate benefits altogether.[47] None of those efforts reduce the actual cost of health care.

More recent state reforms have focused on improving services and reducing underlying health care costs. Vermont has led the way by including chronic care management as part of its reform efforts. By targeting patients, payers, communities, and the greater health system, Vermont hopes to control the growth of health care costs and improve the quality of care (see page [17]). Another example is Arkansas which has become a national model for its focus on health and, in particular, for its efforts to halt the obesity epidemic that has been identified as a major contributor to health care cost increases.[54]

While these new strategies hold promise, they still are untested and it will take time to demonstrate outcomes. The question remains whether the current efforts can advance beyond current disease management strategies and contain long term cost growth.

5. **Voluntary purchasing pools, as a standalone strategy, are not likely to be sufficient to expand coverage.**

The creation of a Connector in Massachusetts sparked renewed interest by policymakers in the concept of facilitating the purchase of insurance for small businesses and individuals. While some may consider the Connector to be a purchasing pool, Massachusetts' state officials describe it more as a purchasing mechanism. The Connector does not pool risk. Rather, it streamlines the administrative aspects of purchasing insurance. However, states have a long history of creating pooling arrangements and the evidence suggests that pooling alone is not sufficient to drive down health costs. In fact, voluntary purchasing pools may attract higher risk enrollees than the rest of the market, contributing to a segmentation of risks.[55]

Until recently, California operated one of the largest and longest running purchasing pools— PacAdvantage. Enrollment in PacAdvantage reached more than 100,000 in August 2006, but evaluations of the initiative indicated that it had done little to expand coverage to uninsured individuals.[56] In 2006, PacAdvantage announced that it would cease operations, saying the "withdrawal of participating health plans has left PacAdvantage unable to continue offering competitive healthcare coverage choices for California's small business employees."[57] The withdrawal of plans was caused by numerous factors including an adversely selected risk pool that led to increasing financial losses for those carriers.

Florida's experience with purchasing pools in the 1990s demonstrated the potential harm this strategy can have on the insurance market. Florida created eleven Community Health Purchasing Alliances (CHPA) in 1993 as part of a small-group market reform. Enrollment peaked in 1998 with 92,000 covered lives and an average group size of two. Due to the regulatory environment in Florida, the CHPAs enrolled a disproportionate amount of groups of one as an alternative to the individual market. This raised concerns about adverse selection for the participating health plans. Over time, participating carriers began to withdraw, citing concerns about adverse selection, among other reasons. Subsequently, enrollment fell quickly and premiums increased significantly, leading the CHPAs to disband in July 2000.[58]

It is important to note that Massachusetts' Connector provides several financial incentives to attract enrollees, including providing access to subsidies only available to those covered through the Connector. This may result in a different outcome than prior efforts. The experience of the Connector will test whether purchasing arrangements coupled with financial incentives will affect enrollment and build purchasing power.

FEDERAL PROPOSALS TO SUPPORT STATE INNOVATIONS

The idea of fostering innovation in states is not a new idea for Congress. From 2000–2005, Congress appropriated $76 million dollars for the Health Resources and Services Administration (HRSA) State Planning Grant Program (SPG) which provided funding for state planning efforts related to covering the uninsured. Over the course of the program, the SPG program provided funding for 47 states and four territories to collect new data and study health insurance trends in order to develop coverage options for their uninsured. The program ultimately was defunded, after being evaluated and criticized for not meeting goals that far exceeded what states could have accomplished solely with resources for planning.

However, the seeds of many of today's state innovations have roots in the SPG initiative, which provided state officials from virtually every state with a greater understanding of the uninsured and an increased technical capacity to address the issue. Since the SPG program was dropped from the HHS budget last year, new federal proposals have emerged to foster state innovation.

During the 109th Congress, three bills were introduced that would provide federal grant funds to states to propose and pilot new health reforms. A fourth bill, the Catastrophic Health Protection Act, also allows states to pilot demonstration projects to expand coverage within a federal framework. (See Table 28-3.)

One fundamental issue for fostering state innovation is how new state strategies will be financed— including whether states will be required to find savings to finance expansions in coverage. Some congressional proposals provide federal funding for implementation, but it is not clear whether this is short-term support during the life of the grant or whether federal financing will continue. The potential for on-going federal financial support is an essential consideration for states that would expand coverage under such programs.

Other congressional proposals indicate that state demonstrations will need to be budget neutral, in effect requiring states to fund new initiatives by finding savings elsewhere in their programs. States are already facing difficult choices such as limiting benefits to currently covered individuals or taking funds from an under-funded safety-net system.

The potentially significant costs to the federal government for supporting new coverage initiatives make it difficult to select just a handful of states to pilot strategies. More states will want to follow the lead of successful demonstrations. Therefore, federal policymakers should be prepared to enact and fund strategies that build on successful state demonstrations.

The introduction of these bills clearly bolsters a trend toward developing solutions to the problem of the uninsured at the state level rather than in Washington, D.C. Time will tell whether the new Congress is ready to provide the federal resources necessary to encourage state innovation, whether the status quo will prevail. Regardless of what occurs in the nation's capitol, states are likely to continue to feel public pressure to increase coverage and experiment with new health reforms.

6. **It is difficult to find agreement on what services will be covered.**

As states struggle with declining coverage and growing costs, questions about the level of benefits and services that should be covered are central to the discussion of reform. Benefit design has long been debated within the Medicaid and SCHIP programs, as well as in programs that represent public-private partnerships. In the late-1990s, Oregon had an explicit conversation about which benefits would be covered under

TABLE 28-3 Federal Legislation to Support State Demonstrations

Legislation	Description	Funding
State-Based Health Care Reform Act S. 3776 Sponsor: Sen. Feingold (D-Wis.)	States would apply to a federal health reform task force for state demonstrations to ensure access to high quality health care coverage for uninsured individuals. States would be required to submit a plan to the Task Force designating the specific strategies to achieve their goals and describing the benefits and cost sharing requirements.	Provides $32 billion in federal funds for states to develop 5-year pilot programs. States are required to match 25 percent of costs and meet maintenance of effort requirements.
Health Partnership Through Creative Federalism Act H.R. 5864 Sponsor: Rep. Baldwin (D-Wis.), Co-sponsors: Rep. Price (R-Ga.), et al.	Creates a State Health Coverage Innovation Commission that will review state applications. States could propose a variety of different approaches, but all must have a commitment to cover the uninsured. The commission's recommendations would be "fast-tracked" and receive expedited legislative review.	Funding for federal grants would be determined by congressional appropriation. However, proposals must be budget neutral for the federal government beyond the grant.
Catastrophic Health Coverage Promotion Act S. 3701 Sponsor: Sen. Smith (R-Ore.), Co-sponsor: Sen. Wyden (D-Ore.)	Requires the Secretary of HHS to establish no more than six demonstration projects. The Secretary would design programs to subsidize individuals who earn less than 200 percent FPL, who are not eligible for Medicare or Medicaid, and who have exceeded $10,500 in out-of-pocket health care costs in a year. The programs will subsidize these individuals to purchase catastrophic coverage through a combination of state risk pools, reinsurance, or other public-private partnerships. States would apply to the Secretary to participate in one of these demonstrations.	Up to $50 million in unspent Disproportionate Share Hospital funds may be used for demonstrations.
Health Partnership Act S. 2772 Sponsor: Sen. Voinovich (R-Ohio), Co-sponsors: Sen. Bingaman (D-N.M.), et al.	States would apply to a newly formed State Health Innovation Commission. The commission would evaluate proposals and the commission's recommendations would receive expedited legislative review and procedure. The states have latitude to design coverage expansions.	The legislation does not appropriate a specific amount for grants to states.

Medicaid, developing a "prioritized list" of covered services. However, the limitations envisioned in their process have never been fully tested.

Experimentation with limited benefit designs to reach uninsured individuals and small businesses is not a new phenomenon. Since 2001, at least 13 states have enacted legislation allowing insurance carriers to sell limited-benefit plans to small groups. To date, these products have not sold well; anecdotal evidence suggests that insurers are reluctant to sell these policies, and consumers are uninterested in buying them.[59] Thus, while some states have responded to criticism that too many mandated benefits are increasing costs, savings from eliminating those mandates have not been sufficient to increase take-up rates.

Current reforms continue to struggle with this issue. Massachusetts's individual mandate only applies if there is an "affordable" product and the state is struggling to define in regulation both what affordable means and the benefits such a product should include. Rhode Island must develop a benefit design that is less than 10 percent of workers' average wage level. Tennessee's CoverTN product is envisioned to cost no more than $150 and, while the state is providing broad parameters for that plan, it is leaving the detailed design decisions in the hands of private carriers.

In addition, though the DRA allows states to be more flexible with their Medicaid benefit packages, it remains to be seen what sort of benefit designs may emerge. Some states have already added greater cost sharing and consumer-directed features to the Medicaid benefit packages, provoking a debate about the adequacy of the new benefit designs for low-income populations.

7. **Fully addressing problem of uninsured needs a national solution.**

Recent state efforts to implement comprehensive reforms have fueled optimism that states can lead the way in addressing the problem of the uninsured. Certainly, states' efforts can test coverage strategies both politically and practically, informing and providing lessons for other states and national leaders. However, the variation among states is far too great for state-by-state reform to produce an effective national solution for the uninsured. Without a national solution, it will be virtually impossible for states to bridge the growing gaps in coverage.

[Parts of the article were omitted.]

ENDNOTES

20. McDonough, J. et al. "The Third Wave of Massachusetts Health Care Access Reform," *Health Affairs*, Vol. 25, No. 6, 2006.

21. McGlynn, E. and J. Wasserman. "Massachusetts Health Reform: Beauty Is In the Eye of the Beholder," *Health Affairs*, Vol. 25, No. 6, 2006.

22. Vermont Senate. H. 861 An Act Relating to Health Care Affordability for All Vermonters, May 5, 2006, www.leg.state.vt.us/HealthCare/2006Leg Action.htm.

23. The Chronic Care Model identifies the essential elements of a health care system that encourage high-quality chronic disease care. These elements are the community, the health system, self-management support, delivery system design, decision support, and clinical information systems. Evidence-based change concepts under each element, in combination, foster productive interactions between informed patients who take an active part in their care and providers with resources and expertise. The model can be applied to a variety of chronic illnesses, health care settings, and target populations.

24. Sachs, T. et al. "Uncharted Territory: Current Trends in Section 1115 Demonstrations," State Coverage Initiative Issue Brief, March 2006.

25. The Savings Offset Payment is determined based on all savings that are identified from the Dirigo Health reforms—not just the reduction in uncompensated care. To determine the savings the state measures the savings impact of the moratorium on the Certificate of Need; the implementation of a Capital Investment Fund to limit future Certificate of Needs post-moratorium; the impact of rate regulation in the small-group insurance market; voluntary targets on hospital expenditures; the infusion of new state funds to match Medicaid for increases in physician and hospital payments to reduce cost shifting; and the costs associated with savings in the system resulting from insuring the previously uninsured.

26. Bragdon, T. "Eight Challenges for Dirigo Health in 2006," Dirigo Watch, the Maine Heritage Policy Center, January 30, 2006.

27. Bowe, T. "DirigoChoice Member Survey: A Snapshot of the Program's Early Adopters," Institute of Health Policy, Muskie School of Public Health, USM, August 12, 2005.

28. McDonough, J. et al. "The Third Wave of Massachusetts Health Care Access Reform," *Health Affairs*, Vol. 25, No. 6, 2006.

29. Wicks, E. "Purchasing Pools in a System of Universal Coverage: Facilitating Consumer Choice," New America Foundation Universal Health Insurance Program, May 2004.

30. "The Connector is a breakthrough concept" by Amy Lischko, SCI Summer Meeting, Chicago, IL, August 3, 2006. www.statecoverage.net/0806/lischko. ppt#347,7.

31. According to state officials in Tennessee.

32. The Primary Care Network (PCN) has provided primary and preventive care services to approximately 19,000 low-income adults below 150 percent FPL since 2002.

33. The Ticket to Work and Self-Sufficiency Program is an employment program for individuals with disabilities who are interested in going to work. The Program was authorized under the Ticket to Work and Work Incentives Improvement Act of 1999, which aims to remove barriers for individuals going to work, including the concern about losing health coverage.

34. State Coverage Initiatives Web site, www. statecoverage.net/matrix.

35. "CHIP at 10: A Decade of Covering Children", Senate Finance Subcommittee on Health, July 25, 2006.

36. Swolak, P. "Healthy New York," The Reinsurance Institute.

37. Results from focus groups held by HRSA State Planning Grant states.

38. "The Uninsured: A Primer," Kaiser Commission on Medicaid and the Uninsured, October, 2006.

39. "Changes in Employees' Health Insurance Coverage, 2001–2005," Kaiser Commission on Medicaid and the Uninsured, October 2006.

40. Butler, P. "ERISA Implications for State Health Care Access Initiatives: Impact of the Maryland "Fair Share Act" Court Decision", SCI/NASHP Issue Brief, November 2006. www.statecoverage. net/SCINASHP.pdf.

41. Maine Senate, An Act to Increase Access to Health Insurance Products, L.D. 1845, May 24, 2006.

42. "Coverage Matters: Insurance and Healthcare". Institute of Medicine. October 11, 2001, www.iom. edu/CMS/3809/4660/4662.aspx.

43. The 2005 Current Population Survey, www.census. gov/cps.

44. Palosky, C. and L. Levitt. "Survey Finds Steady Decline in Businesses Offering Health Benefits to Workers Since 2000." Kaiser Family Foundation/ Health Research and Educational Trust. September 2005.

45. Ibid.

46. "Employer Health Benefits 2006 Annual Survey," Kaiser Family Foundation and Health Research and Educational Trust, September 26, 2006.

47. Demchak, C. "Major Changes in Benefit Design: A Plausible Way to Control Costs." AcademyHealth, Vol. IX, No. 6. November 2006.

48. Butler, P. "ERISA Implications for State Health Care Access Initiatives: Impact of the Maryland "Fair Share Act" Court Decision", SCI/NASHP Issue Brief, November 2006, www.statecoverage. net/SCINASHP.pdf.

49. Approximately twenty states have conducted this analysis including Massachusetts and Vermont.

50. Butler, P. "ERISA Implications for State Health Care Access Initiatives: Impact of the Maryland "Fair Share Act" Court Decision, SCI/NASHP Issue Brief, November 2006, www.statecoverage.net/ SCINASHP.pdf.

51. "Special Report: About 30 States Considering 'Fair Share' Health Care Legislation". BNA Pension & Benefits Reporter Vol 22 etc pp. 829–837, March 28, 2006; "California Governor Vetoes Bill Mandating Premium Contribution by Largest Employers," *BNA Pension & Benefits Reporter*, pp. 2232–2233. September 19, 2006.

52. Butler, P. "ERISA Implications for State Health Care Access Initiatives: Impact of the Maryland "Fair Share Act" Court Decision," SCI/NASHP Issue Brief, November 2006. www.statecoverage. net/SCINASHP.pdf.

53. www.roadmaptocoverage.org/pdfs/Roadmap_ Synthesis_Summary.pdf.

54. Thorpe, K. et al. "The Impact of Obesity on Rising Medical Spending," *Health Affairs*, October 2004.

55. Wicks, E. "Purchasing Pools in a System of Universal Coverage: Facilitating Consumer Choice," New America Foundation Universal Health Insurance Program, May 2004.

56. Wicks, et al. March 2000. "Barriers to Small-Group Purchasing Cooperatives" Economic and Social Research Institute: www.esresearch.org/ Documents/HPC.pdf.

57. www.pacadvantage.org/brokers/closure.asp.

58. Wicks, et al. March 2000. "Barriers to Small-Group Purchasing Cooperatives" Economic and Social Research Institute: www.esresearch.org/ Documents/HPC.pdf.

59. Friedenzohn, I. "States' Experience with Benefit Design," State Coverage Initiatives Issue Brief, April 2003.

Comparing Health Systems in Four Countries: Lessons for the United States

Lawrence D. Brown

The Rekindling Reform initiative examined the health systems of 4 countries: Canada, France, Germany, and Great Britain (United Kingdom). From the 4 country reports published in this issue of the *American Journal of Public Health*, 10 crosscutting themes emerge: (1) coverage; (2) funding; (3) costs; (4) providers; (5) integration; (6) markets; (7) analysis; (8) supply; (9) satisfaction; and (10) leadership. Lessons for the United States are presented under each point.

The 4 articles in this issue of the Journal that explore universal-coverage health care systems in (1) Canada, (2) France, (3) Germany, and (4) Great Britain (United Kingdom) are a sophisticated package of generalization, variation, and implication that defies easy synthesis and summation. Nonetheless, this rich cross-national variation yields 10 general themes.

COVERAGE

All 4 nations entitle almost all their citizens to health coverage. Health care is not enough; their images of solidarity, community, and equity insist that how care is obtained, not merely that it be somehow obtainable, matters greatly. Respect for human dignity demands that no one refrain from seeking medical care from fear of the consequences of doing so, and that no one suffer financial adversity as a result of having sought care. The moral foundations of universal coverage are as simple as that.

Although these nations all cover medically necessary and appropriate services, they also debate the limits of publicly defined coverage. In Canada, for example, home health care and drugs lie outside the public system. In France, dental and eye care tend to be covered by supplementary insurance. As medical innovation advances, discussion intensifies about how to define baskets of benefits that distinguish the responsibilities of the national community from those that individuals and families ought to bear personally. Although these deliberations steadily gain prominence and publicity, so far they proceed mainly at the margins of comprehensive systems that show little inclination to cut back covered services. The core values of these systems—solidarity, community, equity, dignity—remain intact and surprisingly little disturbed by rising costs and by gloomy forecasts that aging, technology, and the rest are rendering their systems unaffordable.

The moral and cultural foundations of universal coverage are missing in the United States, as the continuing presence of 40 million uninsured would seem to intimate. Circumstances are not propitious: 85% of the population has medical coverage, much of it funded by private employers; the 15% who lack insurance are not organized, cohesive, or politically active; sizable redistributive shifts by national design are not the political system's strongest suit; and the right-of-center precincts in which that system has lingered for the past 35 years do nothing to ease the struggle. Equally important, Americans "know" that safety net providers care for people who lack coverage—a powerful inhibition to public action in a nation whose welfare state programs aim less at broad-ranging security in health and other policy spheres than at post factum compensation for those who fall through private-sector cracks. Reformist appeals based on human dignity (to which health security is fundamental) resonate very little here. September 11 and rescued miners aside, solidarity finds little place in the national political lexicon. Likewise, in the United States, community is not a spur to national action but rather an alternative to—and an excuse for—declining to pursue it. The brightest and best strategies to build a normative case for universal coverage have failed so far, and no one seems to know how to change these values, which are, by definition, fairly durable.

FUNDING

In all 4 systems the national government sets a statutory framework for financing universal coverage. (In Canada the provinces must meet centrally defined conditions for participation in central/provincial fund-sharing arrangements.) How they raise these monies differs substantially. However: Great Britain's National Health Service draws mainly on general revenues; 70% of Canada's health bill comes from national and provincial general revenues: Germany relies primarily on work-based social insurance contributions; and—the most dramatic evolutionary development in this quartet—France increasingly supports its social insurance regime with general revenues that tap a broad range of wealth. None of these approaches is plainly superior to the others; they all "work," and they all carry their burden of political and economic stress. France and Germany also have various degrees and types of cost sharing by patients.

The good news for the United States is that in essence any major funding approach will serve. The bad news is that no such approach seems close to commanding consensus, and feuding over the merits of funding strategies aggravates the chronic righteous strife among proponents of reform that (given the imposing strength of the opposition) has heavily damaged reform prospects. One contingent contends that a "single payer" (general revenue-based) system is best. Another believes that the success of Social Security and Medicare validates a social insurance strategy. Whereas no other nation believes that universal coverage can be won and sustained without candid debate about taxes, a prominent American reform camp wants to build on the private employer contributions that buy most US health insurance today. (Indeed the Clinton administration's reform plan of 1993 would have mandated such employer "premiums" precisely in order to avoid uttering the dreaded "*t* word.") Meanwhile, the widespread conviction that done right, universal coverage should require no new monies (tax-derived or other) beclouds the US reform debate. The system is said to be replete with waste that can be intelligently squeezed to yield abundant funds to rechannel resources from excessive use and payments to providers and toward coverage for the uninsured. (This too was a premise of the Clinton plan.)

This pastiche of theory and ideology lays down myriad stumbling blocks that reformers must somehow surmount. A workable coalition probably presupposes avoiding fierce redistributive battles over how and where to squeeze and redirect wasteful spending within the status quo, dismissal of employer mandates (and the battles with business they trigger), the political courage to discuss tax increases that (probably) mingle social insurance payments with general revenues, and, not least important, willingness among ardent advocates of diverse financing strategies to rally behind whatever seems to stand some chance of passing. Meanwhile, cost controls can be taken up after the universal deed is done—a prospect that will of course be plain to stakeholders who oppose reform and will take up their political cudgels accordingly.

COSTS

Although the 4 nations spend a smaller share of their national resources on health care than the United States does, cost containment has long been a preoccupation in each and all. (Great Britain is arguably a case apart. There, reorganization and better management of the National Health Service have—until recently—been successfully offered as alternatives to the infusions of cash the Blair government was eventually moved to promise.) The 4 nations pay their physicians less and provide fewer specialized and highly technical services than the United States does, and all expect that structured negotiations between payers and providers will hold the line on costs.

These staples of cost containment seem increasingly insufficient to counter the fundamental challenges all nations face—growing and aging populations, technological progress, inflation, wage pressures, and rising popular expectations[1]—and so in their sundry fashions, the 4 countries try to cap health spending. In Great Britain and Canada, the public health care budget is itself a ceiling. In France, since 1996, Parliament has legislated a national spending target annually. Germany has tried to link health spending increases to the growth of workers' wages. Only in Great Britain have these public constraints generated highly controversial waiting lists, and these, says Light,[2] are mainly limited to elective referrals to specialists. Waiting lists occasionally appear in Canada, but Deber[1] argues that these vary with place and procedure and are a minor, albeit well-publicized, concern. "Rationing" is a nonissue in France and Germany. Containing costs is never easy, but the 4 nations have done it—indeed, in the British case perhaps too well.

Rising health costs are of course a huge headache in the United States, and the likelihood that universal coverage would push them higher and faster is a weighty political burden on reform. Unlike the 4 nations, the United States has rejected all talk of publicly set limits on health spending. Insurers, providers, business interests, and other opponents of reform loudly equate all such aggregate constraints with "rationing," and the equation has dependably terrified public opinion. In 1993, Bill Clinton proposed to harmonize cost control with universal coverage by means of managed competition among health plans, backstopped by caps on health insurance premiums, should market forces fail to hold them down. The Clinton plan was rejected, leaving cost containment to unmanaged competition among health plans, which (to many reformers' surprise) proceeded to "work" in the second half of the 1990s as cost increases slowed dramatically. Health spending moved rapidly upward thereafter, however, leaving purchasers and policymakers wondering what to do for an encore.

This strategic tabula rasa may leave the United States uncommonly receptive to learning from abroad. On the other hand, public budgets and caps, which continue to connote rationing and remain abhorrent to influential stakeholders, do not seem to be gaining a constituency. Adopting them would entail elimination of some politically potent sources of waste that market forces tolerate or aggravate, namely (to borrow from Deber's list): marketing costs, efforts at selective enrollment, stockholders' profits, executives' exorbitant salaries, lobbying expenses, and less widely diffused technology. And if such waste were gone, the fundamental things—growing and aging populations and such—would apply here, as in other nations, as time goes by.

PROVIDERS

Conflict between policymakers (in both health and financial ministries) and providers over terms and levels of payment is a persistent fact of political life in all 4 nations. Within public budgets and fiscal caps, providers negotiate with the state, the sickness funds (health insurance institutions), or both. In Great Britain and Canada, physicians' organizations and individual hospitals bargain directly with government agencies. In Germany, associations of sickness-fund physicians and individual hospitals negotiate with sickness funds within a framework of public rules. In France, unions of physicians bargain separately with the sickness funds as the state moves back and forth between the sidelines and the battlefield. In each of the 4, payers squeeze, providers protest (and sometimes strike), payers relent, costs increase, payers squeeze, and so it goes. Although budget makers invariably spend more than they prefer, providers in all 4 nations earn considerably less than their more specialized US counterparts.

The US medical profession is more lucrative and entrepreneurial than is the case elsewhere. To American providers, collective negotiations with public payers, which imply more than tacit consent to a state-run social enterprise called (or headed toward) national health insurance, have long been anathema.

The United States has coped politically by evolving a bifurcated pattern of payer and provider relations. The main public program, Medicare, shifted from a payment system that mimicked the private sector (retrospective payment of actual hospital costs and usual and customary physician charges) to prospective payment models, steered by commissions in which providers have a voice, and by Congress, which they lobby directly. In the private sector, purchasers have hoped to discipline providers by shopping among and signing on with managed care plans that presumably contract selectively with "efficient" providers and apply organizational reviews and constraints that enforce efficiencies.

The future of these disparate arrangements is a key question for health reform. Would a public system of prospective payment prevail, and could it coexist with the current private managed care model? Must reform mean the end of unmanaged competition among health plans and a belated biting of the bullet on managed competition, and if so, what version of it? As with financing, there appears to be no one right way, but workable reform will have to hold the line on provider payments, and doing so will mean constructing new bargaining machinery with which providers agree to "live," however grudgingly. Today, US providers are more inclined to wish a plague on the payment practices of both Medicare and managed care than they are to think constructively about better ways to negotiate collectively with payers. Most American physicians and hospitals continue to view health insurance as an economic, not a social, enterprise and organize and strategize accordingly.

INTEGRATION

These 4 nations all voice dissatisfaction with the organization of their delivery systems; they all deplore "fragmentation" and aspire to "integration." International literature and their own observations teach that overuse of services is substantial and that, to coin a phrase, care ought to be better managed. Having long allowed physicians and hospitals to practice medicine largely as they pleased—a norm crucial to the quid pro quo in which providers accepted regulation of their payments—these countries now seek efficiencies in production that supposedly accompany organizational innovation. Great Britain's tools of choice, for example, were fundholding among general practitioners and hospital trusts, now giving way to primary care trusts. Indeed, writes Light,[2] the government now plans to "unite specialty care with primary care, unite primary care with community health care, and unite all three with social services," yielding "comprehensive, integrated services that are community based." The French are experimenting with "networks of coordinated care," notes Rodwin.[3] These countries view reorganization (or redisorganization, in health economist Alan Maynard's term) soberly, as "reforms" worth testing as possible sources of better value for money within fundamentally sound systems.

The United States, the esteemed source of much of the theory and practice of the services integration other nations seek to emulate, may be ahead of the international curve but faces integrative challenges of its own. Both here and abroad, proponents of reform sometimes divide over whether the achievement of universal coverage is a necessary *and* sufficient policy objective, over whether to insist that such coverage be encased in a properly designed delivery system. Americans must decide how far to tie reform to managed care, the driver of US-style integration, and increasingly an 800-lb gorilla politically. Will the new system seek to redeem a fee-for-service system, follow Medicare's dubious lead into some variant of choice between a fee-for-service system and managed care, or assume that managed care will be mainstream and fee-for-service payment an exception? Beyond decisions about how far to push managed care lie others on what to do about managed competition, an issue that has vexed US health policy since the 1970s. Is integration—in this case the proliferation of managed care organizations—a natural institutional receipt for better efficiency and quality? Or do these objectives presuppose competition among integrated entities? Can this competition stay loosely managed, as now, or would universal coverage trigger anew the many disputes about managed competition that sunk the Clinton plan a few yew's ago? Ironically, other nations are better equipped to address integration incrementally than the United States is: here it invites a host of radical questions.

MARKETS

American reformers who admire the rest of the West for *its* refusal to treat health care as a commodity to be bought and sold in the marketplace tend to view the growing foreign fascination with market forces in health care as a trip down the garden path. This fascination is unmistakable in all 4 nations, however, as evidenced by Great Britain's internal markets, Germany's regulated competition, France's networks, and Canada's Community Care Access Centres. All the same, foreign attachment to health care markets tends to be clear-eyed and decidedly nonevangelical, is far from taking national health insurance systems by storm, and may already be waning (judging by Light's account[2] of Great Britain, the most market-friendly of the 4). Other nations recognize that competition is difficult, at least in a real world populated by real institutions. Besides breaking important political compacts (for example, that any national health insurance physician may treat any national health insurance patient, a settled norm that pretty much

precludes closed panel plans and selective contracting by payers), competition requires heroic analytic feats, which carry no small price tag: better management information systems, copious consumer information, subtle measures of quality, methods to adjust payments by risk of enrollees, and more. None of these countries views competition as a panacea, and none fantasizes that market forces can supplant the solid regulatory machinery now in place. All 4 worry that even well-designed competition could undercut solidarity, community, and equity, and each wonders candidly whether the market game is worth the social candle.

Although the United States has embraced markets and competition as health care "solutions" with a passion puzzling abroad, it hesitates too. For years, 1 school of market reformers has predicted that competition among managed care plans per se will make the system more efficient, whereas another has contended that such competition must be managed (by and within a sophisticated and extensive framework of public rules) lest it lapse into such market failures as selection of preferred risks, underservice, and geographic segmentation of markets, all of which would damage the public interest. The slow growth of health costs in a strong economy in the latter 1990s cushioned the horns of the dilemma. Today costs rise faster, the economy grows more slowly, and the prospect of incorporating 40 million uninsured into a new reformed system brings competitive disputes to center stage again. Would a new round of reform put managed competition over the political goal line at last? Dare reformers view reform as the great escape from an imprisoning competitive mindset? Must they accept it as part of the strategic furniture they must perforce rearrange? Having gone to market so often, the United States may no longer be capable of a swift, clean U-turn, but if we cannot live without competition, how will reformers live with it?

ANALYSIS

The 4 countries show a strong and growing curiosity about how analytic tools—evidence-based medicine, technology assessment, report cards, and cost-effectiveness analysis, for example—can help policymakers to assess the performance of their health systems and suggest means to improve them. New agencies such as the National Institute for Clinical Excellence in Great Britain and the ANAES (Agence nationale d'accreditation et d'evaluation) in France promote and conduct such evaluative studies. Although foreign policy-makers have suitably modest expectations for these tools, their influence might advance by several different routes—for example, improved performance as measured by analytic criteria could become a condition for increased pay to providers, and continued documentation of overuse of services within these systems might fuel budget makers' determination to manage care—that is, providers—more assertively.

In the United States. the birthplace of many of these tools, expectations are high, but stubborn professional resistance to implementation of practice guidelines and kindred constraints and the befuddlement of most private and some public purchasers over what to do with analytic findings often leave the evaluative enterprise all dressed up with no place to go. In this arena, the United States and the 4 nations may well converge. As cost pressures build, so too will the impulse to find diagnoses and recommendations in neutral expertise and objective evidence. Analytic findings and advice will throw down the gauntlet to providers, who will respond both by seeking to shoot the messenger and by redoubling their efforts to document, define, and perhaps even reconsider their practice patterns. Policymakers will reply that the providers offer too little, too late, and the deployment of analytic weapons in the unending political conflict will escalate.

SUPPLY

The 4 nations all use public authority and planning to control the number and distribution of hospitals and physicians. Contrary to conventional wisdom, such constraints do not necessarily make the system "smaller" or harder to access. Rodwin's Table 2,[3] for example, shows that on most measures of resources and utilization—for instance, active physicians per thousand population: total inpatient hospital beds, physician visits, and hospital days per capita; admission rates to and lengths of stay in hospitals—France surpasses the United States. These limits do make the systems less specialist driven and technology intensive, however, which seems to be how they register savings for the nations in question.

Notwithstanding such programs as certificates of need, the United States relies mainly on a combination of market forces and professional preferences to decide what levels of supply are adequate. The market itself must challenge the hoary conviction that "health is a community affair," meaning in practice a highly entrepreneurial affair in which local providers behave as if more is better, often with the acquiescence of boosterish local business leaders. Hospitals and physicians want bigger and better facilities, the latest and best equipment, deeper market penetration, and more accessible satellite sites, as do the communities they serve. Managed care plans that contract too narrowly risk losing customers. Health "planning," which connotes rationing, waiting lists, and beneficial services foregone, has largely vanished from the American radar screen. Perhaps, however, the cost pressures accompanying universal coverage will so obviously overmatch the disciplinary powers of market forces that US policymakers will rethink their options on this controversial count.

SATISFACTION

In all 4 nations, citizens record high (though not unreserved or uncritical) satisfaction with their health care systems. No one views national health insurance as a big mistake and wants to start over. The vices of the US system—40 million uninsured people, an additional (and sizable) number with inadequate coverage, wide disparities in access and quality—are thought to overwhelm such modest and distinctive virtues as more extensive integration of services and more advanced analytic capacity. The foreign systems' costs are routinely and rhetorically said to be in "crisis." The systems themselves are not.

American public opinion voices no small dissatisfaction with the US system and considerable support for major, even fundamental, changes in it. The rub, however, is that this grousing does not yield a clear mandate for anything very different from the status quo. Despite years of intense opinion polling, policymakers remain unsure precisely what people are upset about (beyond the impossibility of enjoying ready access to fine care at minimal cost) and what they think would work better. Nor is this so odd after all: the same political leaders who quietly pushed arcane payment reforms in public programs have generally declined to launch searching public discussions of the big and touchy redistributive and regulatory issues and tradeoffs on which health reform turns. Bill Clinton's unavailing and politically painful effort to break the pattern reaffirmed it instead. A perplexed public has therefore come to view health care reform as something like shopping for shoes: "We think we are in the mood to buy a health care reform today but not *that* style or fit, so keep showing us others." The technical opacity of the debate, not to mention continuing skepticism of anything "made in Washington," inhibit grassroots mobilization, citizen education, and other key concomitants of vigorous pluralist politics. No one seems to have a clue how to make well-documented dissatisfaction kindle a political fire under health reform.

LEADERSHIP

The 4 countries all recognize that strong, continuing leadership by the central government is the sine qua non of affordable universal coverage. Great Britain is, of course, the home of "socialized medicine." Efforts by France's famously powerful state to reform the health care system have multiplied in the last 2 decades, especially since the Juppe reforms of 1996. Germany's central government is a "supervisor, enabler, facilitator, monitor,"[4] and purveyor of national standards for the health system.

Canada's constitution reserves health duties for the provinces, but the central government uses its financial leverage to enforce on them 5 straightforward principles that protect solidarity and equity for Canadian citizens.

None of the 4 countries, however, supposes that health policy can be run entirely from London, Paris, Berlin, or Ottawa. Germany and Canada are federal systems and, as Altenstetter[4] and Deber[1] explain, a mix of constitutional, political, and informal rules and norms ensure that states and provinces participate extensively in making and running health policies that affect them. With such consultation comes conflict and delay, but federalism and universal coverage are eminently compatible.

Great Britain and France have created new regional and community bodies—the Primary Care Trusts in the former and regional hospital councils and public health conferences in the latter, for instance—that encourage deliberation and coordination closer to the proverbial grass roots. All 4 acknowledge that decentralization and devolution are goals worth pursuing, but they also understand that workable decentralization presupposes effective centralization of political authority.

This latter proposition generally eludes US health polity. Save on rare occasions—for example, the New Deal and the Great Society—when issues of economic and social justice dominate the national agenda, fights over the alleged evils of new central powers quickly upend debate on the ends of reform, health or other. At least in the health sphere, actions may speak louder than words—Medicare, Medicaid, Children's Health Insurance Program, and other public programs control roughly half the dollars in the health care system, after all—but political protocol requires proclaimed allegiance to an official

ideology of market forces and less government even as reformers quietly and incrementally add a new piece of managed care regulation here, expansion of public coverage to another income category there. Much of this (abundant) public action originates in the states or evolves from complex sharing of initiatives, funds, and powers between the national and state governments. Fifty states are a more daunting tableau than 10 provinces, but the United States might infer from the Canadian system that universal coverage in a federal system can be managed by 5 succinct principles, not 50 volumes of the Federal Register. Unfortunately American reformers have been more inclined to admire Canada's "single-payer" financing than its much more instructive central/provincial accommodations.

Where this self-denying activism, this stealthy state leadership, leads is anyone's guess. Perhaps the present pattern—one step forward, one step back, and the nation counting itself lucky if the number of uninsured does not exceed 40 million—will persist. Perhaps incrementalism will proceed and the nation will awake one day to find that enough programmatic pieces are in place to sustain near universal coverage if only the money and leadership can be summoned to add a few more beneficiary categories and raise income thresholds a few more notches. Perhaps another 1932 or 1964 waits right around the corner, and "real" health reform may suddenly arrive on waves of social indignation and political innovation. At this point. however, cross-national learning disappears into the depths of national character.

ABOUT THE AUTHOR

The author is with the Mailman School of Public Health, Columbia University, New York, NY.

REFERENCES

1. Deber, RA. Rekindling Reform: lessons from Canada. *Am J Public Health* 2003;93:20–24.

2. Light, DW. Universal health care: lessons from the British experience. *Am J Public Health* 2003;93:25–30.

3. Rodwin, VG. The health care system under French National Health Insurance: lessons for health reform. *Am J Public Health* 2003;93:31–37.

4. Altenstetter, C. Insights from health care in Germany. *Am J Public Health* 2003;93:38–44.

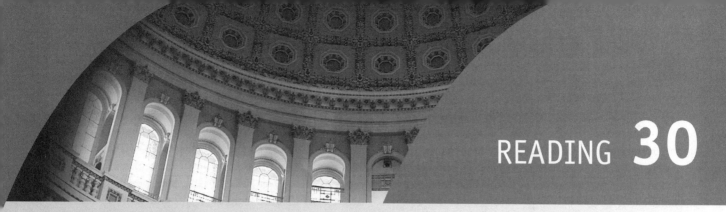

Learning from High Performance Health Systems Around the Globe*

Karen Davis

Source: Courtesy of The Commonwealth Fund. Learning from High Performance Health Systems Around the Globe. Karen Davis, President, The Commonwealth Fund, One East 75th Street, New York, NY 10021. Invited Testimony, Senate Health, Education, Labor, and Pensions Committee, Hearing on "Health Care Coverage and Access: Challenges and Opportunities," January 10, 2007

Acknowledgments: Research assistance from Alyssa L. Holmgren, research associate; comments from Cathy Schoen, senior vice president for research and evaluation, and Robin Osborn, vice president; and editorial assistance from Barry Scholl, vice president for communications and publishing, and Chris Hollander, associate communications director (*all at The Commonwealth Fund*).

This testimony and other Commonwealth Fund publications are online at www.cmwf.org. To learn more about new publications when they become available, visit the Fund's Web site and register to receive e-mail alerts. Commonwealth Fund pub. no. 996.

Thank you, Mr. Chairman and members of the Committee, for this invitation to testify today on a problem of concern to policymakers, employers, health care leaders, and insured and uninsured Americans alike: gaps in health insurance coverage and rising health care costs. The search for effective coverage and cost-containment strategies is of great urgency. One-third of all Americans and two-thirds of low-income Americans are uninsured at some point during the year

or are underinsured.[1] Family health insurance premiums under employer plans have risen 87 percent since 2000 while median family incomes have increased by only 11 percent.[2] As a result, one-third of families now report difficulty paying medical bills or accumulated medical debt, with such problems growing rapidly for middle-class families.[3] We spend 16 percent of our gross domestic product (GDP) on health care, yet we fall short of reaching achievable benchmark levels of quality care.[4]

Broad consensus now exists on the need for action. A recent survey of health care opinion leaders placed expanding coverage for the uninsured and enacting reforms to moderate rising health costs at the top of a list of health care priorities for Congress.[5] Their priorities are the public's priorities as well. Ensuring that all Americans have adequate, reliable health insurance and controlling the rising cost of medical care were cited in a survey of U.S. adults last summer as the top two health care priorities for the president and Congress.[6]

The key question is how to achieve both of these goals while maintaining or improving the quality of care for all. Insight is provided by contrasting the experience of the U.S. with that of other countries. There is now extensive evidence that other countries are achieving universal coverage, much lower spending per capita, and better health outcomes.[7] Given its history, institutions, and preferences, the U.S. is unlikely to adopt another country's health system in all its aspects, but it can learn from examples of practices that contribute to high performance. Today, I would like to share with the Committee what we know about the U.S. health system compared with that of other countries and highlight examples of high

---

*Exhibits not included in article can be found at www.commonwealthfund.org.

performance and innovative practices in countries such as Denmark, the Netherlands, and Germany, among others, that provide potential solutions to the current U.S. challenge of simultaneously achieving better access, higher quality, and greater efficiency.

This assessment of international innovations leading to high performance dovetails with the work of the Commonwealth Fund's Commission on a High Performance Health System, which has identified seven keys to a high performance health system in the U.S.:

- Extending health insurance to all;
- Pursuing excellence in the provision of safe, effective, and efficient care;
- Organizing the care system to ensure coordinated and accessible care to all;
- Increasing transparency and rewarding quality and efficiency;
- Expanding the use of information technology and systems of health information exchange;
- Developing the workforce required to foster patient-centered and primary care; and
- Encouraging leadership and collaboration among public and private stakeholders dedicated to achieving a high performance health system.[8]

NATIONAL HEALTH EXPENDITURES AND VALUE FOR MONEY

Nothing makes it clearer that something is amiss than the contrast between health spending in the U.S. and health spending in other countries. The U.S. spends almost $2 trillion, or $6,700 per person, on health care—more than twice what is spent by other major industrialized countries (Figure 30-1).[9] U.S. health spending is high, even in the context of its substantial economy: the U. S. spends 16 percent of GDP on health care, while other countries spend 8 to 10 percent. Health spending in the U.S. rose faster than in other countries in the last five years, while countries with high spending such as Germany and Canada moderated their growth and countries with low spending such as the U.K. increased outlays as a matter of deliberate public policy.

All countries face rising costs from technological change, higher prices of pharmaceutical products, and aging of the population. In fact, the population in most European countries already has the age distribution that the U.S. will experience in 20 years. Nor is the difference in spending attributable to rationing care. In fact, the U.S. has lower rates of hospitalization and shorter hospital stays than most other countries.[10] One difference is that the U.S. tends to pay higher prices for pre-scription drugs; in other countries governments typically negotiate on behalf of all residents to achieve lower prices.[11]

The U.S. is alone among major industrialized nations in other respects. Over half of health care spending is paid for privately, compared with about one-fourth or less in other countries. Ironically, because the U.S. is so expensive, the government—while it accounts for only 45 percent of all health care spending—spends as much as a percent of GDP on health care as do other countries with publicly financed health systems.[12]

Another striking difference is that the U.S. has fewer physicians per capita than other countries, and many more of our physicians are specialists.[13] Research both within the U.S. and across countries has shown that health care spending is higher and health outcomes worse when there is a lower ratio of primary care to specialist physicians.[14] Compared with patients in other countries, U.S. patients face a more fragmented health care system, are cared for by different physicians for different conditions, have poorer care coordination, and take more medications, all of which contributes to higher rates of medical errors.[15] More things can and do go wrong when care is provided by multiple parties. In fact, in 2006, 42 percent of U.S. adults reported having one of four experiences in the prior two years: their physician ordered a test that had already been done; their physician failed to provide important medical information or test results to other doctors or nurses involved in their care; they incurred a medical, surgical, medication, or lab test error; or their physician recommended care or treatment that in their view was unnecessary.[16]

The bottom line is that the U.S. is not receiving value commensurate to the resources it commits to health care. Many Americans would gladly pay more for health care if it meant longer lives, improved functioning, or better quality of life. Yet, on key health outcome measures, U.S. health performance is average or below average. For example, on mortality from conditions amenable to health care—a measure of death rates before age 75 from diseases and conditions that are preventable or treatable with timely, effective medical care—the U.S. ranked 15th among 19 countries, with a death rate 30 percent higher than in France, Japan, and Spain (Figure 30-2). If U.S. performance were comparable to the best three countries or even the best five states, nearly 90,000 lives a year could be saved.

The Commonwealth Fund supported an international working group on quality indicators, an effort that is now being continued and extended by the Organization for Economic Cooperation and Development. On most measures, the U.S. was neither the best nor the worst on clinical quality outcomes. It had the best outcome among five countries on five-year relative survival rates for breast cancer, but the worst outcome

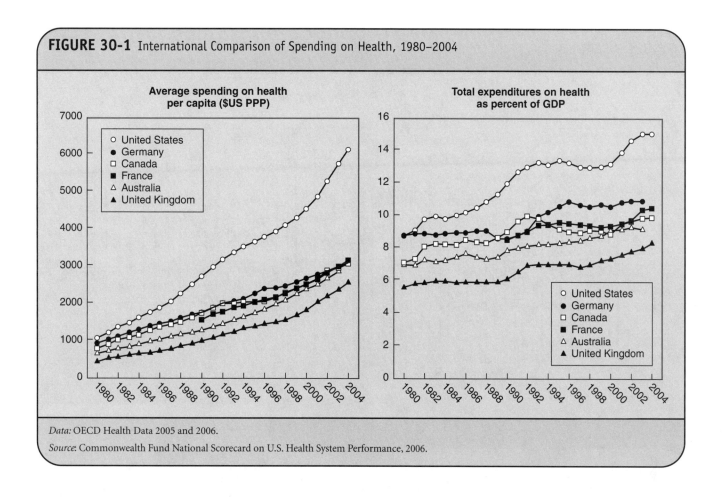

FIGURE 30-1 International Comparison of Spending on Health, 1980–2004

Data: OECD Health Data 2005 and 2006.

Source: Commonwealth Fund National Scorecard on U.S. Health System Performance, 2006.

on five-year relative survival rates for kidney transplants.[17] For the resources it commits to health care, the U.S. should be achieving much better results.

ACCESS TO CARE

The U.S. is also alone among major industrialized nations in failing to provide universal health coverage. This undermines performance of the health system in multiple ways, but the most troubling is the difficulty Americans face in obtaining access to needed care (Figure 30-3). Forty percent of U.S. adults report one of three access problems because of costs: not getting needed care because of the cost of a doctor's visit; skipping medical test, treatment, or follow-up because of costs; or not filling prescription or skipping doses because of cost. Further, Americans pay far more out-of-pocket for health care expenses and are more subject to financial burdens as a result of either no health insurance or inadequate health insurance.

Aside from the evident failure of the U.S. health system to guarantee financial access to care, the organization of care in the U.S. also fails to ensure accessible and coordinated care for all patients. In fact, the U.S. stands out for having patients who report either having no regular doctor or having been with their physician for a short period of time (Table 30-1). Only 42 percent of Americans have been with the same physician for five years or more, compared with over half to three-fourths of patients in other countries. Managed care plans with restricted networks exacerbate poor continuity of care, as patients may need to change physicians when their employers change coverage. By contrast, many other countries encourage or require patients to identify a "medical home," which is their principal source of primary care and is responsible for coordinating specialist care when needed.

Together, these differences in care arrangements and the undersupply of primary care physicians relative to other countries mean that many Americans are unable to get needed care, whether in the doctor's office during the day or on nights and weekends. Among sicker adults—those who rated their health as fair or poor or had a serious illness, surgery, or hospitalization in the past two years—nearly one-fourth of Americans and one-third of Canadians wait six or more days to see a doctor when sick or in need of medical attention, compared with only one of seven or less in New Zealand, Germany, Australia,

FIGURE 30-2 Mortality Amenable to Health Care

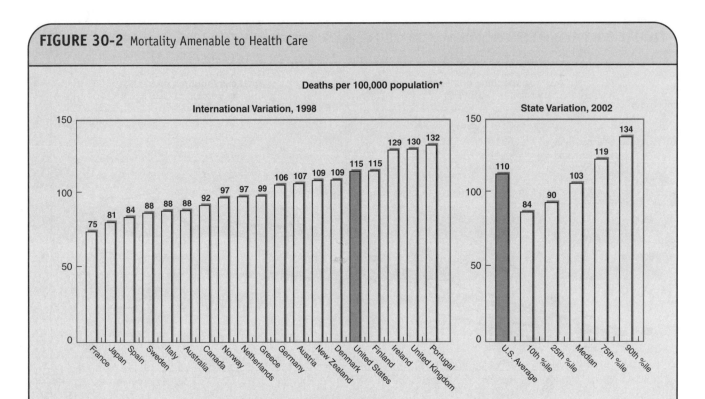

Deaths per 100,000 population*

International Variation, 1998

State Variation, 2002

*Countries' age-standardized death rates, ages 0–74; includes ischemic heart disease.

See Technical Appendix for list of conditions considered amenable to health care in the analysis.

Data: International estimates—World Health Organization, WHO mortality database (Nolte and McKee 2003); State estimates—K. Hempstead, Rutgers University using Nolte and McKee methodology.

Source: Commonwealth Fund National Scorecard on U.S. Health System Performance, 2006.

FIGURE 30-3 Access Problems Because of Costs in Five Countries, Total and by Income, 2004

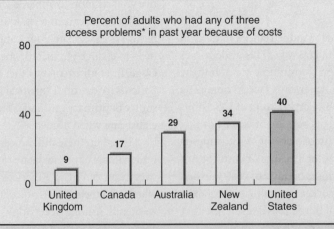

Percent of adults who had any of three
access problems* in past year because of costs

*Did not get medical care because of cost of doctor's visit, skipped medical test, treatment, or follow-up because of cost, or did not fill Rx or skipped doses because of cost.

Data: 2004 Commonwealth Fund International Health Policy Survey of Adults' Experiences with Primary Care (Schoen et al. 2004; Huynh et al. 2006).

Source: Commonwealth Fund National Scorecard on U.S. Health System Performance, 2006.

TABLE 30-1 Length of Time with Regular Doctor

Percent	AUS	CAN	GER	NZ	UK	US
Has regular doctor	92	92	97	94	96	84
Less than 2 years	16	12	6	19	14	17
5 years or more	56	60	76	57	66	42
No regular doctor	8	8	3	6	4	16

Source: 2005 Commonwealth Fund International Health Policy Survey of Sicker Adults.

and the U.K. (Figure 30-4). The U.S. has short waiting times for elective surgery such as hip replacements or cataract operations, but timely access to primary care is rarer in the U.S.

The U.S. also stands out in terms of the level of difficulty in obtaining care on nights and weekends. Three of five Americans report that it is difficult to obtain care off-hours, compared with one of four in Germany and New Zealand (Figure 30-5). In a recent survey, only 40 percent of U.S. primary care physicians say they have an arrangement for after-hours care, compared with virtually all primary care physicians in the Netherlands.

These differences in the accessibility of basic primary care are a reflection of policy decisions made by different countries.[18] Most fundamentally, of course, other countries make primary care financially and physically accessible to their residents. In contrast, the U.S. erects substantial barriers to primary care, including large numbers of uninsured and significant deductibles that pose financial barriers to primary care even for the insured. Other countries provide relatively higher payments to primary care physicians, and support physician practices in organizing after-hours care. These policies increase the attractiveness of primary care practice.

QUALITY OF CARE

The U.S. faces a major increase in chronic conditions as its population ages. Adults with multiple chronic conditions are particularly at risk for experiencing poor-quality or uncoordinated care. Coordination of information across sites of care is essential for safe, effective, and efficient care. Measured by patients saying that test results or medical records were not available at the time of appointments or that physicians duplicated tests, one-third of U.S. patients experience breakdowns in coordination, compared with about one-fifth in other countries (Table 30-2).

Improving the management of patients with chronic disease is key to effective control and prevention of complications.

FIGURE 30-4 Waiting Time to See Doctor When Sick or Need Medical Attention, Sicker Adults in Six Countries, 2005

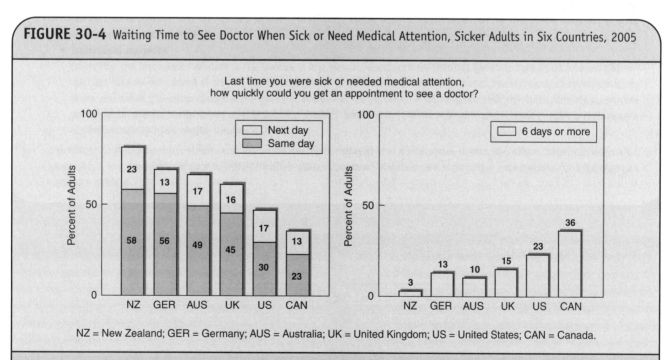

Data: 2005 Commonwealth Fund International Health Policy Survey of Sicker Adults (Schoen et al. 2005a).

Source: Commonwealth Fund National Scorecard on U.S. Health System Performance, 2006.

FIGURE 30-5 Difficulty Getting Care on Nights, Weekends, Holidays Without Going to the ER, Among Sicker Adults in Six Countries, 2005

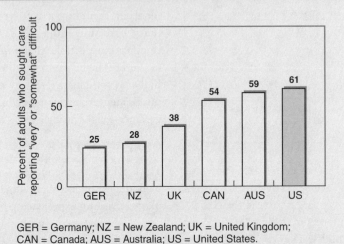

GER = Germany; NZ = New Zealand; UK = United Kingdom;
CAN = Canada; AUS = Australia; US = United States.

Data: 2005 Commonwealth Fund International Health Policy Survey of Sicker Adults (Schoen et al. 2005a).

Source: Commonwealth Fund National Scorecard on U.S. Health System Performance, 2006.

One-third of primary care physicians in the U.S. report routinely giving patients a plan to manage their chronic diseases at home, compared with almost two-thirds in Germany.

Patient safety has received heightened attention in the U.S. in the last five years. Despite this, U.S. patients are more likely to report experiences of medical errors than residents of other countries. These experiences include medical or medication errors, hospital-acquired infections, incorrect lab or diagnostic tests, or delays in communicating abnormal results to patients. Overall one-third of sicker adults in the U.S. reported such errors in 2005, compared with one-fourth in other countries. The frequency of errors was strongly associated with the number of doctors involved in a patient's care: almost half of U.S. sicker adults that were seeing four or more physicians reported such errors.

EFFICIENCY

U.S. physicians are highly trained, and U.S. hospitals are well equipped compared with hospitals in other countries.[19] Some of the waste and missed opportunities to provide high-quality, safe care may be attributable to more limited adoption of information technology in the U.S. About one-fourth of U.S. primary care physician report using electronic medical records compared with more than nine of 10 primary care physicians in the Netherlands, New Zealand, and the U.K. In these countries, physicians are often able to purchase electronic medical record systems through direct financial support from government or reimbursement incentives.

Primary care physicians in other countries not only have basic electronic medical records (EMRs) but an array of health

TABLE 30-2 Patients Report Problems with Care Coordination

Percent saying in the past 2 years	AUS	CAN	GER	NZ	UK	US
Test results or records not available at time of appointment	12	19	11	16	16	23
Duplicate tests: doctor ordered test that had already been done	11	10	20	9	6	18
Percent who experienced either coordination problem	19	24	26	21	19	33

Source: 2005 Commonwealth Fund International Health Policy Survey of Sicker Adults.

information technology, often facilitated by government-arranged systems of information exchange. Less that one-fifth of U.S. primary care physicians routinely send reminder notices to patients about preventive or follow-up care, compared with over nine of 10 in New Zealand. Nine of 10 primary care physicians in the Netherlands, New Zealand, and the U.K. receive electronic alerts about potential problems with prescription drug dosage or interaction, compared with only one-fourth in the U.S. When assessed against 14 different functions of advanced information capacity (EMRs; EMR access to other doctors; access outside office; access by patient; routine use of electronic test ordering; electronic prescriptions; electronic access to test results; electronic access to hospital records; computerized reminders; Rx alerts; prompt tests results; and easy to list diagnoses, medications, and patients due for care), one of five U.S. primary care physicians reported having at least seven of the 14 functions, compared with nine of 10 physicians in New Zealand.

The U.S. relies on market incentives to shape its health care system, yet other countries are more advanced in providing financial incentives to physicians targeted on quality of care. Only 30 percent of U.S. primary care physicians report having the potential to receive financial incentives targeted on quality of care, including the potential to receive payment for: clinical care targets, high patient ratings, managing chronic disease/complex needs, preventive care, or quality improvement activities. By contrast, nearly all primary care physicians in the U.K. and over 70 percent in Australia and New Zealand report such incentives.

The reliance on private insurance and the fragmentation of the U.S. health insurance system—with people moving in and out of coverage and in and out of plans, and changing their usual source of care—all contribute to high administrative costs for insurers and health care providers.[20] In 2005, the U.S. health system spent $143 billion on administrative expenses, not including administrative expenses incurred by health care providers.[21]

The U.S., with its mixed public-private system of financing, devotes a much higher share of health spending to administration than other nations. The U.S. spends 7.3 percent of total health expenditures on insurance administrative expense (Figure 30-6).[22] In 2004, if the U.S. had been able to lower the share of health care spending devoted to insurance overhead to the same level found in the three countries with the lowest rates (France, Finland, and Japan), it would have saved $97 billion a year. If the U.S. had spent what countries with mixed public-private insurance systems, such as Germany and Switzerland, spend on insurance administrative costs, it could have saved $32 billion to $46 billion a year.

INNOVATIONS IN OTHER COUNTRIES THAT PROVIDE EXAMPLES OF HIGH PERFORMANCE

The key question is how the U.S. might achieve improved coverage and greater efficiency while maintaining or improving the quality of care for all. Given its history, institutions, and preferences, the U.S. is unlikely to adopt another country's health system in all its aspects, but it can learn from examples of practices that contribute to high performance. In considering the Commonwealth Fund's nine-year experience conducting comparative surveys of the public as well as health professionals in selected countries and sponsoring annual symposia focused on health care innovations for top government officials and experts, numerous examples of innovative practices and high health system performance stand out. I have also had the opportunity of serving on a team of economists charged with critiquing the Danish health system and preparing a report for the Danish parliament.[23] Drawing on this experience, I'm pleased to share with the Committee innovations for the U.S. to consider, highlighting examples of high performance and innovative practices in Denmark, the Netherlands, Germany, and the U.K.

Let me begin with Denmark, which I visited again last October. Public satisfaction with the health system is higher in Denmark than in any other country in Europe.[24] In my view, this is related to the emphasis Denmark places on patient-centered primary care, which is highly accessible and has an outstanding information system that assists primary care physicians in coordinating care (Table 30-3). Denmark, like most European countries, has a universal health insurance system with no patient cost-sharing for physician or hospital services. Every Dane selects a primary care physician, who receives a monthly payment per patient for serving as the patient's medical home in addition to fees for services provided. Incomes of primary care physicians are slightly higher than those of specialists, who are salaried and employed by hospitals. Primary care physicians own their own practices, which are open from 8 a.m. to 4 p.m., and patients can easily obtain care on the same day if they are sick or need medical attention.

This system of primary care contributes to highly accessible basic and preventive care, as well as lower total health care expenditures. Denmark is rated as one of the best countries on primary care as measured by high levels of first contact accessibility, patient-focused care over time, a comprehensive package of services, and coordination of services when services have to be provided elsewhere.[25]

But what most impresses me about the Danish system is its organized "off-hours service." In every county, clinics see patients at nights and weekends. Physicians sit at phone banks

FIGURE 30-6 Percentage of National Health Expenditures Spent on Health Administration and Insurance, 2003

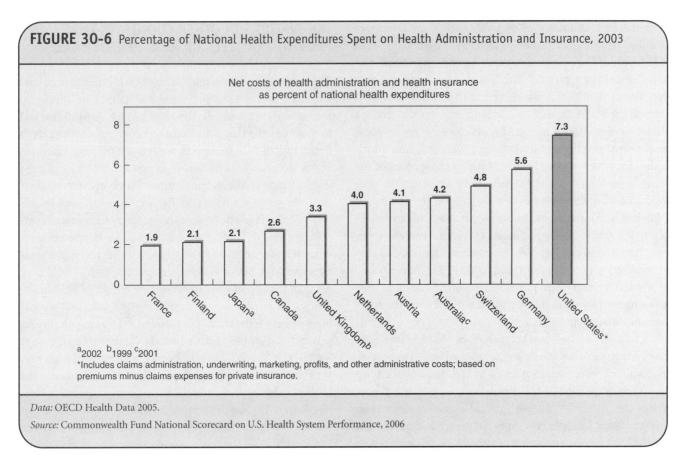

Net costs of health administration and health insurance
as percent of national health expenditures

France	Finland	Japan^a	Canada	United Kingdom^b	Netherlands	Austria	Australia^c	Switzerland	Germany	United States*
1.9	2.1	2.1	2.6	3.3	4.0	4.1	4.2	4.8	5.6	7.3

^a2002 ^b1999 ^c2001
*Includes claims administration, underwriting, marketing, profits, and other administrative costs; based on premiums minus claims expenses for private insurance.

Data: OECD Health Data 2005.

Source: Commonwealth Fund National Scorecard on U.S. Health System Performance, 2006

in the "back office" of the clinic and take direct calls from patients. They sit in front of computer terminals and can access computerized patient records. After listening to a patient's complaint, they can electronically prescribe medications, or ask the patient to come in to see a physician on duty. Physicians are paid for the telephone consultation, and earn a higher fee if the problem can be handled by phone. The patient's own primary care physician receives an e-mail the next day with a record of the consultation.

All primary care physicians (except a few near retirement) are required to have an electronic medical record system, and 98 percent do. Danish physicians are now paid about $8 for

TABLE 30-3 Denmark Leads the Way in Patient-Centered Primary Care

- Blended primary care payment system
  - Fee for service
  - Medical home monthly fee per patient
- Organized off-hours service
  - Physicians staff phone banks nights and weekends with computerized access to patient information; paid for telephone consultations
  - Physicians staff evening and weekend clinics, and
  - Off-hours service physicians do home visits
- Health information technology and information exchange
  - 98% of primary care physicians totally electronic health records and e-prescribing
  - Paid for e-mail with patients
  - All prescriptions, lab and imaging tests, specialist consult reports, hospital discharge letters flow through a single electronic portal (MedCom—a nonprofit organization) accessible to patients, physicians, and home health nurses

e-mail consultations with patients, a service that is growing rapidly. The easy accessibility of physician advice by phone or e-mail, and electronic systems for prescriptions and refills, cuts down markedly on both physician and patient time. Primary care physicians save an estimated 50 minutes a day from information systems that simplify their tasks, a return that easily justifies their investment in an information technology system for their practice.[26]

Physicians, whether seeing patients through the off-hours service or during regular hours, are supported by a nationwide health information exchange, maintained by a nonprofit organization, MedCom. An assessment of health information systems in 10 countries ranks Denmark at the top, and concludes that countries with a single unifying organization to set standards and serve as an information repository have the highest rates of information system functionality.[27] MedCom is a repository of electronic prescriptions, lab and imaging orders and test results, specialist consult reports, and hospital discharge letters that is accessible to patients as well as authorized physicians and home health nurses. It now captures 87 percent of all prescription orders, 88 percent of hospital discharge letters, 98 percent of lab orders, and 60 percent of specialist referrals. Yet, its operating cost is only $2 million a year for a population of 5.3 million Danes, or 40 cents a person a year.

Denmark is not the only country with cutting-edge innovations to improve the quality, accessibility, and efficiency of health care. Germany is a leader in national hospital quality benchmarking, with real-time quality information on all 2,000 German hospitals with over 300 quality indicators for 26 conditions. Peers visit hospitals where quality is substandard and enter into a "dialogue" about why that is the case. Typically, all hospitals come up to high standards within a few years. Germany has instituted disease management programs and clinical guidelines for chronic care, with financial incentives from insurance funds to physicians to enroll patients and be held accountable for care. Initial results show that this system has positive effects on quality.[28] Germany is also experimenting with an all-inclusive global fee for payment of care of cancer patients in Cologne.

The Netherlands stands out for its leadership on transparency in reporting quality data, as well as its own approach to primary care and "after-hours" care arrangements. Although most Dutch primary care practices are solo practices, they support each other through a cooperative, including an after-hours nurse and physician call bank service. The Dutch government funds nurse practitioners based in physician practices to manage chronic disease. Under national reforms implemented in 2006, payments to Dutch doctors now blend capitation, fees for consultations, and payments for performance.

The U.K. General Practitioner contract, which went into effect on April 1, 2004, provides bonuses to primary care physicians for reaching quality targets (Table 30-4). Far more physicians met the targets than anticipated, leading to a controversial cost overrun, but amply demonstrating that financial incentives do change physician behavior.[29] The U.K. National Institute for Health and Clinical Excellence conducts cost-effectiveness review of new drugs and technology. The U.K. also publishes extensive information on hospital quality and surgical results by name of hospital and surgeon.

These are just a few examples of innovative practices that the U.S. might wish to investigate more closely and potentially adapt. Most, however, require leadership on the part of the central government to set standards, ensure the exchange of health information, and reward high performance on quality and efficiency.

CONCLUSION

If we have the world's costliest health system yet still fail to provide everyone with access to care—and fall far short of providing the safe, high-quality care that it is possible to provide—the conclusion that there is room for improvement is inescapable.[30] Only by facing this fact squarely and putting into action the

---

TABLE 30-4 UK: First Year Performance

- Practice by practice results for the Quality and Outcome Framework for England were published on August 31, 2005
- Average score for practices in England in the first year was 959 out of a possible 1050. The maximum score of 1,050 points was achieved by 222 practices (2.6%)
- 8,486 practices in England took part, covering 99.5% of NHS registered patients
- Some of higher performance may have been improved documentation

Source: http://www.ic.nhs.uklservices/qof/data/index_html

best ideas and experiences across the U.S. and around the world can we achieve a vision of American health care that includes: automatic and affordable health insurance for all, accessible care, patient-responsive care, information- and science-based care, and commitment to quality improvement.[31]

Achieving a high performance health care system—high-quality, safe, efficient, and accessible to all—will require a major change in the U.S. system of delivering health services.[32] Steps toward this goal include:

- Extending health insurance to all, in order to improve access, quality, and efficiency;
- Assessing innovations leading to high performance within the U.S. and internationally and adopting best practices;
- Organizing the care system to ensure coordinated and accessible care to all;
- Increasing transparency and rewarding quality and efficiency;
- Expanding the use of information technology and systems of health information exchange;
- Developing the workforce required to foster patient-centered and primary care; and
- Encouraging leadership and collaboration among public and private stakeholders dedicated to achieving a high performance health system.

These steps would take us a long way toward ensuring that the U.S. is a high-performing health system worthy of the 21st century. Thank you very much for the opportunity to join this panel. I look forward to learning from my fellow panelists and answering any questions.

NOTES

1. C. Schoen, K. Davis, S. K. H. How, and S. C. Schoenbaum, "U.S. Health System Performance: A National Scorecard," *Health Affairs* Web Exclusive (Sept. 20, 2006):w457–w475; C. Schoen, M. M. Doty, S. R. Collins, and A. L. Holmgren, "Insured but Not Protected: How Many Adults Are Underinsured?" *Health Affairs* Web Exclusive (June 14, 2005):w289–w302.

2. P. Fronstin and S. R. Collins, *The 2nd Annual EBRI/Commonwealth Fund Consumerism in Health Care Survey, 2006: Early Experience with High-Deductible and Consumer-Driven Health Plans* (New York: The Commonwealth Fund, Dec. 2006).

3. S. R. Collins, K. Davis, M. M. Doty, J. L. Kriss, and A. L. Holmgren, *Gaps in Health Insurance: An All-American Problem* (New York, The Commonwealth Fund, Apr. 2006); S. R. Collins, J. L. Kriss, K. Davis, M. M. Doty, and A. L. Holmgren, *Squeezed: Why Rising Exposure to Health Care Costs Threatens the Health and Financial Well-Being of American Families* (New York: The Commonwealth Fund, Sept. 2006).

4. K. Davis, C. Schoen, S. Guterman, T. Shih, S. C. Schoenbaum, and I. Weinbaum, *Slowing the Growth of U.S. Health Care Expenditures: What Are the Options?* (New York: The Commonwealth Fund, Jan. 2007).

5. A. L. Holmgren, K. Davis, S. Guterman, and B. Scholl, *Health Care Opinion Leaders' Views on Priorities for the New Congress* (New York: The Commonwealth Fund, Jan. 2007).

6. C. Schoen, S. K. H. How, I. Weinbaum, J. E. Craig, Jr., and K. Davis, *Public Views on Shaping the Future of the U.S. Health System* (New York: The Commonwealth Fund, Aug. 2006).

7. C. Schoen, R. Osborn, P. T. Huynh, M. M. Doty, J. Peugh, and K. Zapert, "On the Front Lines of Care: Primary Care Doctors' Office Systems, Experiences, and Views in Seven Countries," *Health Affairs* Web Exclusive (Nov. 2, 2006):w555–w571; C. Schoen, R. Osborn, P. T. Huynh, M. Doty, K. Zapert, J. Peugh, and K. Davis, "Taking the Pulse of Health Care Systems: Experiences of Patients with Health Problems in Six Countries," *Health Affairs* Web Exclusive (Nov. 3, 2005):w509–w525; P. S. Hussey, G .F. Anderson, R. Osborn et al., "How Does the Quality of Care Compare in Five Countries?" *Health Affairs,* May/June 2004 23(3):89–99.

8. The Commonwealth Fund Commission on a High Performance Health System, *Framework for a High Performance Health System for the United States* (New York: The Commonwealth Fund, Aug. 2006).

9. A. Catlin, C. Cowan, S. Heffler, B. Washington, and the National Health Expenditure Accounts Team, "National Health Spending in 2005: The Slowdown Continues," *Health Affairs,* Jan./Feb. 2007 26(1):142–153.

10. B. Frogner and G. Anderson, *Multinational Comparisons of Health Systems Data, 2005* (New York: The Commonwealth Fund, Apr. 2006).

11. G. F. Anderson, D. G. Shea, P. S. Hussey et al., "Doughnut Holes and Price Controls," *Health Affairs* Web Exclusive (July 21, 2004):W4-396–W4-404; G. Anderson, U. E. Reinhardt, P. S. Hussey et al., "It's the Prices, Stupid: Why the United States Is So Different from Other Countries," *Health Affairs,* May/June 2003 22(3):89–105.

12. B. Frogner and G. Anderson, *Multinational Comparisons of Health Systems Data, 2005* (New York: The Commonwealth Fund, Apr. 2006).

13. G. F. Anderson, B. K. Frogner, R. A. Johns et al., "Health Care Spending and Use of Information Technology in OECD Countries," *Health Affairs,* May/June 2006 25(3):819–831.

14. J. S. Skinner, D. O. Staiger, and E. S. Fisher, "Is Technological Change in Medicine Always Worth It? The Case of Acute Myocardial Infarction," *Health Affairs* Web Exclusive (Feb. 7, 2006):w34–w47; B. Starfield, L. Shi, and J. Macinko, "Contribution of Primary Care to Health Systems and Health," *The Milbank Quarterly,* 2005 83(3):457–502.

15. C. Schoen, R. Osborn, P. T. Huynh, M. Doty, K. Zapert, J. Peugh, and K. Davis, "Taking the Pulse of Health Care Systems: Experiences of Patients with Health Problems in Six Countries," *Health Affairs* Web Exclusive (Nov. 3, 2005):w509–w525.

16. C. Schoen, S. K. H. How, I. Weinbaum, J. E. Craig, Jr., and K. Davis, *Public Views on Shaping the Future of the U.S. Health System* (New York: The Commonwealth Fund, Aug. 2006).

17. P. S. Hussey, G. F. Anderson, R. Osborn et al., "How Does the Quality of Care Compare in Five Countries?" *Health Affairs,* May/June 2004 23(3):89–99.

18. C. Schoen, R. Osborn, P. T. Huynh, M. Doty, K. Zapert, J. Peugh, and K. Davis, "Taking the Pulse of Health Care Systems: Experiences of Patients with Health Problems in Six Countries," *Health Affairs* Web Exclusive (Nov. 3, 2005):w509–w525; C. Schoen, R. Osborn, P. T. Huynh, M. Doty, J. Peugh, and K. Zapert, "On the Front Lines of Care: Primary Care Doctors' Office Systems, Experiences, and Views in Seven Countries," *Health Affairs* Web Exclusive (Nov. 2, 2006):w555–w571.

19. A. M. J. Audet, M. M. Doty, J. Shamasdin, and S. C. Schoenbaum, *Physicians' Views on Quality of Care: Findings from The Commonwealth Fund National Survey of Physicians and Quality of Care* (New York: The Commonwealth Fund, May 2005).

20. K. Davis, *Time for Change: The Hidden Costs of a Fragmented Health Insurance System.* Invited Testimony, Senate Special Committee on Aging, March 10, 2003.

21. A. Catlin, C. Cowan, S. Heffler, B. Washington, and the National Health Expenditure Accounts Team, "National Health Spending in 2005: The Slowdown Continues," *Health Affairs,* Jan./Feb. 2007 26(1):142–153.

22. C. Schoen, K. Davis, S. K. H. How, and S. C. Schoenbaum, "U.S. Health System Performance: A National Scorecard," *Health Affairs* Web Exclusive (Sept. 20, 2006):w457–w47.

23. K. Davis, "The Danish Health System Through an American Lens," *Health Policy,* Jan. 2002 59(2):119–132.

24. E. Mossialos, "Citizens' Views on Health Care Systems in the 15 Member States of the European Union," *Health Economics,* 1997 6:109–16.

25. B. Starfield, "Why More Primary Care: Better Outcomes, Lower Costs, Greater Equity," Presentation to the Primary Care Roundtable: Strengthening Adult Primary Care: Models and Policy Options, October 3, 2006.

26. I. Johansen, "What Makes a High Performance Health Care System and How Do We Get It? Denmark," Presentation to the Commonwealth Fund International Symposium, November 3, 2006.

27. D. Protti, "A Comparison of Information Technology in General Practice in Ten Countries," Presentation to the Commonwealth Fund International Symposium, November 3, 2006.

28. M. Hallek, "Typical Problems and Recent Reform Strategies in German Health Care—with Emphasis on the Treatment of Cancer," Presentation to the Commonwealth Fund International Symposium, November 2, 2006.

29. T. Doran, C. Fullwood, H. Gravelle et al., "Pay-for-Performance Programs in Family Practices in the United Kingdom." *New England Journal of Medicine,* 2006 355(4):375–384.

30. K. Davis, S. C. Schoenbaum, K. S. Collins, K. Tenney, D. L. Hughes, and A.-M. J. Audet, *Room for Improvement: Patients Report on the Quality of Their Health Care* (New York: The Commonwealth Fund, Apr. 2002); K. Davis, C. Schoen, S. C. Schoenbaum, A.-M. J. Audet, M. M. Doty, A. L. Holmgren, and J. L. Kriss, "Mirror, Mirror on the Wall: The Quality of American Health Care" (New York: The Commonwealth Fund, forthcoming).

31. K. Davis, C. Schoen, and S. C. Schoenbaum, "A 2020 Vision for American Health Care." *Archives of Internal Medicine,* Dec. 2000 160(22):3357–62.

32. The Commonwealth Fund Commission on a High Performance Health System, *Framework for a High Performance Health System for the United States* (New York: The Commonwealth Fund, Aug. 2006).

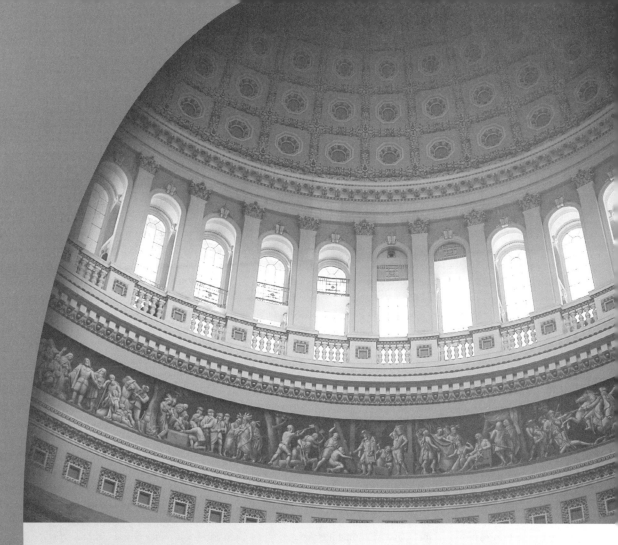

PART V

Tools for Health Policy Analysis

When researching health policy options and developing policy proposals, analysts rely on journal articles, textbooks, and other resources that are familiar to many students and professionals. As they hone their craft, policy analysts also turn to resources that may be less obvious to the casual observer of the policymaking process. In this section, we provide one background article and a selection of less familiar resources generated by both public and private sources that are nonetheless emblematic of the practical tools that policy analysts frequently use.

The opening article by Gail Wilensky, entitled "Framing the Public Policy Questions: Financial Incentives for Efficiency and Effectiveness," illustrates the value of the policy analysis tools that are provided in this section by discussing how and why research should inform the policymaking process. We then turn to examples of policy documents developed by the federal government: administrative regulations, memoranda, and budgets. Federal administrative agencies are responsible for implementing many programs created by Congress. When implementing a program, these agencies promulgate regulations detailing background information, definitions of terms, and specific requirements that regulated individuals and entities must adhere to when participating in a program (these regulations are published in what is called the *Federal Register* and can be accessed on-line in their entirety at http://www.gpoaccess.gov/fr/index.html.) To provide a sense of how federal regulations shape policy, we include portions of the regulations developed by the Office for Civil Rights (OCR; an agency of the Department of Health and Human Services) that detail standards for privacy of individual health information as required by the Health Information Portability and Accountability Act.

Federal agencies also issue less formal documents to clarify a specific aspect of a program. For example, the Centers for Medicare and Medicaid Services (CMS) issues State Medicaid Director Letters (SMDL) to assist states and help staff implement the Medicaid program consistently throughout the country (a list of recent SMDLs is available on the CMS website at http://www.cms.hhs.gov/SMDL/01_overview.asp#TopOfPage). We include an example of one such letter, which provides information explaining certain sections of the Deficit Reduction Act of 2005.

Budget-related documents also can form the basis for policy-making and policy analysis. At the federal level, the budget process begins with agencies (such as OCR and CMS) submitting budget proposals to department officials. Departments then submit budget requests to the president's staff. The president, in turn, submits a budget for the Executive Branch to Congress, which is the only branch able to appropriate money for the purpose of keeping the federal government operating. All of these various proposals are more than a collection of charts with revenue and expenditure estimates. They also function as policy documents that explain and justify program decisions made in the past and highlight priority items for the upcoming year. As an example of the type of policy information available in budget documents, we include part of the fiscal year 2008 budget request from CMS to fund the Medicaid and the State Children's Health Insurance programs. (For access to all of the public documents and charts related to the president's budget proposal, go to www.whitehouse.gov.)

When assessing legislative proposals, Congress considers various types of policy documents. The Congressional Budget Office (CBO), which provides Congress with nonpartisan analysis of economic and budgetary issues to assist Congress in crafting legislation, formulates one policy tool that is particularly helpful for policy analysts: the cost estimate. Through cost estimates, CBO presents Congress with the potential impact on federal spending and revenue for every bill reported by congressional committees; because the financial impact of a policy option is likely to be a key factor in whether the option is adopted or rejected, these nonpartisan estimates are critical. Included in this section is the estimate for the Improving Head Start Act of 2007, one of the many health-related cost estimates produced by CBO each year.

State governments are another important source of information for policy analysts. Because many important policies are made on the state level and policies and laws vary from state to state, it is essential that analysts are familiar with actions taken by the state or states involved in their analysis. By way of example, we include a regulatory amendment to the New York City Health Code that bans the use of trans fat in New York City food services establishments.

Finally, the private sector also develops useful tools for health policy analysts. Think tanks and advocacy organizations often take complex information provided by federal and state governments and other sources and distill it into forms that are easy to understand and use. These groups produce reports, fact sheets, side-by-side analyses, and chart packs that can be helpful to policy analysts—though bear in mind when reading them that many private organizations advocate a particular policy position that is reflected in their work. To give you a sense of the type of resources generated by private organizations, we include a report published by the Center on Budget and Policy Priorities (CBPP) analyzing proposed changes to the State Children's Health Insurance Program by distilling information provided in both the president's budget proposal and CBO's cost estimate.

IN THIS SECTION

Gail Wilensky, "Framing the Public Policy Questions: Financial Incentives for Efficiency and Effectiveness"

Selections from Department of Health and Human Services Regulations on Standards for Privacy of Individually Identifiable Health Information as required by the Health Information Portability and Accountability Act

State Medicaid Director Letter Concerning the Deficit Reduction Act of 2005

Department of Health and Human Services 2008 Budget in Brief concerning Medicaid and SCHIP

Congressional Budget Office Cost Estimate Concerning the Improving Head Start Act of 2007

New York City Department of Health and Mental Hygiene Board of Health, Amendment to the New York City Health Code, Concerning Phasing out Artificial Trans-Fat in New York City Food Services establishments

Edwin Park and Matt Broaddus, "SCHIP Reauthorization: President's Budget Would Provide Less than Half the Funds That States Need to Maintain SCHIP Enrollment."

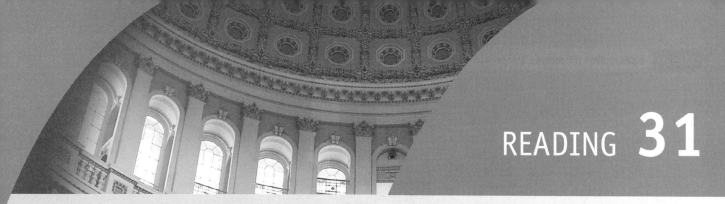

Framing the Public Policy Questions: Financial Incentives for Efficiency and Effectiveness

Gail R. Wilensky

Source: Framing the Public Policy Questions: Financial Incentives for Efficiency and Effectiveness, Gail R. Wilensky, Center for Health Affairs, Project HOPE, *Medical Care Research and Review* 2004; 61; 31, DOI: 10.1177/1077558704266769.

Despite the efforts of many policy researchers, there is a growing sense that we do not yet have or understand the policy levers needed to produce quality health care efficiently and effectively. In part, this reflects the relatively late recognition that much of what is done in health care is based on "art" rather than science and occurs without the underlying clinical rigor of scientific testing. In part, it is also the recognition that too often research and analysis have not kept pace with the changing organizational structures involved in the delivery of health care. Creating the understanding needed to develop such policy tools will require the efforts of individuals with a variety of disciplines and policy experiences.

In this article, I try and set the stage for some of the more detailed discussions of the types of research needed to better understand how physicians respond to differing financial incentives and to differing relationships with health plans that themselves bear risk differentially. First, I briefly consider how research and researchers can and should inform the policy process. Second, I review some of the policy levers available in Medicare and ways to make use of these policy levers to produce and/or monitor change in the delivery of health care.

INFORMING THE POLICY PROCESS

For policy research to be useful in helping decision makers make better-informed decisions, the implications of implementing a policy need to be clearly articulated. Obviously, the cost of developing and initiating policies needs to be clear and known, and the consequences of implementing the policy also need to be clear and known. Volumes have been written about ways to estimate the direct and indirect costs and benefits associated with various projects as well as about the more esoteric issues of appropriate discount rates to be used in discounting to present values. My interest here is to discuss the role of the researcher in communicating the results of well-done policy research to the decision maker rather than focusing on how that research itself should be done.

All policy options will have intended and unintended consequences. To inform the policy process, researchers need to be as clear about any unintended consequences of a particular policy as they are about the intended consequences. Obviously, a policy should be judged in large part as to whether and how well it carries out its intended goals and objectives. Less obvious but equally important is an assessment of what else is likely to result from a policy, whether or not it is the intended goal of the policy. In the 1980s, for example, serious consideration was being given to making subsidized health insurance available to individuals who had recently become unemployed. However, it was discovered that many of the people who had lost their jobs in the early 1980s did not have insurance when they were employed, and it was realized that if highly subsidized insurance were only available when an individual was unemployed, it would reduce the incentive for an unemployed individual to reenter the labor market. As a result, legislation to subsidize insurance for unemployed individuals was put on hold.

The unintended consequences of a policy are more likely to be known with the increasing use of sophisticated statistical models than was the case before the use of such models. What is less clear is whether the unintended consequences will always be conveyed to the policy maker with the same sense of urgency or commitment as the intended consequences of a policy. Unfortunately for the policy maker, individuals and institutions respond as well to unintended incentives as they do to intended incentives.

Since all policies are likely to have some unintended consequences, it is especially useful if the policy analyst can formulate several alternative strategies that can accomplish a particular goal or objective. The presumption should be that each of the strategies will accomplish the intended objective more or less well and that each will also have some number of unintended consequences. By considering the alternatives available to accomplish a given objective and the likely consequences associated with each, the decision maker is best able to make the trade-offs inherently present in any choice set. What most decision makers are less likely to be able to do is identify the relevant choice set and unintended consequences associated with each choice.

To be helpful in developing sets of alternative policies, the researcher needs to understand the questions that are likely to be asked and also the data that will be needed to answer the questions being addressed by alternative policies. In some cases, the most important questions are likely to be the most obvious ones (i.e., how can spending be reduced without reducing quality or changing outcomes, or how will changing demographics affect health care utilization) but in other cases, questions that will be important to answer at one point in time will not have been obvious at an earlier period (identifying cost-effective strategies for implementing smallpox immunization in the event of bioterrorism). In helping to make data needs known and available, it is also important for researchers to understand the trade-offs between having data that are accurate and data that are timely, that is, trade-offs that match precision needs with relevancy. Because the kinds of data that will be needed will be partly determined by the types of analyses that are likely to be done, an understanding of these analyses are key to being responsive to such issues as timeliness and relevance in the data collection process.

As important as timeliness is for relevance, it is not the only requirement that researchers will need to respond to in order to inform the policy process. Equally important is the ability to use language that allows the presentation of data and the implications of research to be understood by individuals outside the research community. Perhaps most important of all is the need for analysts to maintain high levels of credibility, both in their roles as objective analysts and in the credibility of the data they present. This does not mean than an individual who is a researcher cannot ever act as an advocate but it does mean that these roles have to be kept clearly separate and dis-

tinct. Taken together, these steps will allow researchers to effectively help decision makers understand the likely consequences of alternative policies prior to making a decision.

MEDICARE'S POLICY LEVERS

Understanding how research can and does inform the policy process, the implications for data, the implications for researchers and ultimately, the implications for the research agenda are important but no more so than understanding the incentives available in Medicare to affect the delivery of efficient and effective health care. This is a very large topic that has been the subject of many academic articles and dissertations. I am going to consider these issues in terms of a broad overview of the strategies Medicare has used to affect cost and quality of health care and then focus on the current attempts to influence the quantity and quality of services delivered by physicians.

The goal of Medicare has been clear: timely access to high-quality, clinically appropriate health care at the lowest cost to the taxpayer. The problem is that this goal contains inherent tensions and conflicts in addition to not always knowing what is the most clinically appropriate health care or how to get it delivered at high levels of quality.

The focus of Medicare in its early years was more limited—expanding access to the millions of seniors who had been unable to access health care and health insurance prior to the passage of Medicare. The legislation modeled Medicare after the Blue Cross/Blue Shield plans of the 1960s, the dominant insurance carrier of the time, in an effort to provide health care to seniors that was comparable to the health care provided to the rest of the American population. Hospitals and physicians were reimbursed using usual, customary, and reasonable fees (UCR) and per diem reimbursement, the most frequently used reimbursement strategies of the time. As has been well documented, these reimbursement strategies are inherently inflationary. Thus, while UCR and per diem reimbursement supported increased access to care, a stated goal of Medicare, they also helped produce the intolerable increases in Medicare spending that also characterized that period.

Following its first decade, Medicare's focus increasingly turned to ways of restraining spending with periodic concerns raised about both access and quality. The most dramatic change in payment strategy that affected not only Medicare spending but potentially quality as well was the introduction of prospective payment for inpatient hospital reimbursement in 1983. Rather than reimburse hospitals on a per diem basis, Medicare began reimbursing hospitals according to the diagnosis at discharge. This change fundamentally changed the incentives facing hospitals, producing a significant shock to the way health care was delivered (and billed) in hospitals. Rather than encouraging patients to spend an extra day in the hospital, hospitals were incited to discharge patients as quickly as possible. While prospective payment has been credited with slowing down inpatient spending, it has also led to concerns about whether patients may have been discharged sooner than was medically appropriate ("quicker but sicker") and also whether it led to moving patients to other settings that were less regulated, whether or not the other setting was more clinically appropriate. Studies attempting to answer these questions continue 20 years after the introduction of prospective payment in hospitals.

The trend since the introduction of prospective payment for inpatient hospital reimbursement has been to expand prospective payment to other areas of reimbursement. The first expansion was to capital expenditures by hospitals. The *Balanced Budget Act of 1997* expanded prospective payment to the outpatient portion of hospital spending as well as to home health care and skilled nursing homes. The introduction of prospective payment in these areas not only reflected the success experienced on the inpatient side but also responded to the unexpected rapid spending growth in these other areas, in part induced by the use of prospective payment in the inpatient sector—again a reminder that incentives produce changes not only where they are intended but also in other areas.

The one area that has moved in an entirely different direction has been Medicare's reimbursement for physicians. Rather than move to bundled services with preset prices, physician reimbursement continues to use a disaggregated fee schedule with an aggregate spending control that feeds back to the fee schedule. The expansion of prospective payment to areas other than inpatient hospital spending and the development of a resource-based relative value scale fee schedule tied to a spending target for physicians have increased the interest in understanding what has happened to access, cost, and quality as a result of these changes. The use of a disaggregated fee schedule for physicians and an aggregated reimbursement strategy for other parts of Medicare has led to a second set of questions as to what happens to access and quality when the incentives associated with reimbursement for hospitals, home care, and nursing homes are fundamentally different from the incentives associated with physicians' services.

In trying to respond to these questions, it is important to understand the various policy levers contained within the Medicare program. The primary policy levers are the payment structure and the payment level. But there are a variety of other levers that pertain to the way the prospective payment is structured and/or updated and the rules regarding participation in Medicare. Some of these levers include the medical classifica-

tions system, the updating mechanism, the risk adjusters, the conditions of participation, and the rules regarding private contracting. Each of these will need to be assessed to understand the ways in which different institutional providers and physician groups respond to financial risk and how that response may affect access and quality. In assessing the effects of these policy levers, it is important to understand the ongoing tension within Medicare to develop policies that can maintain access and quality while restraining spending and to establish the "right" price while rewarding quality.

The effects of the policy levers and incentives in Medicare are particularly complex when it comes to understanding physician behavior. First, because the reimbursement for physicians is fundamentally out of sync with the reimbursement for other areas of spending, the behavior that will be observable will represent the net effect of the institutional providers they interact with and the incentives they face directly. Second, much of the earlier research has been directed to how an individual physician would respond to different reimbursement strategies, such as fee for service, salary, or capitation. Because many physicians now practice in groups, the focus needs to be on how physician groups bear financial risk, whether the individual physician faces financial risk in the same way as does the group, and the way in which physician groups interact with insurance plans. This substantially increases the complexity of the analysis since it requires an understanding of the incentives facing the organizational structure, the individual physicians, and the interaction between these incentives. Although it could be argued that as long as the organization faces the right incentives and is held accountable, it might not matter whether the incentives facing the individual physician were consistent with the incentives of the organization. The concern is that if there is enough internal dissonance between the incentives facing the group and those facing the individual physician, the effects of the incentives facing the larger organization may begin to unravel.

To bring this back to where I started, there is a need for further work to better understand the policy levers available to Medicare that can change physician behavior in ways that will improve both quality and health care efficiency. That will require an understanding of the likely response of physicians to current incentives and to any changes in incentives that might be introduced. It will be especially important to carry out these analyses with an understanding of how physicians in groups bear risk that may not be the same as the risk faced by the group. Finally, there needs to be a better understanding of how research informs the policy process and the kind of evidence that is needed to influence policy and policy decision makers.

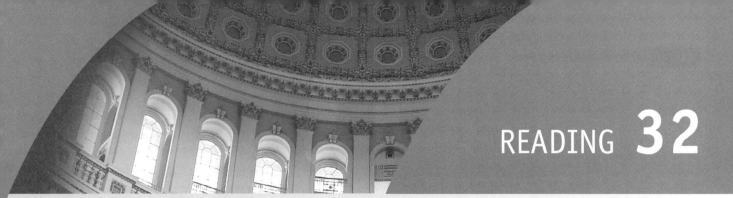

READING 32

Selections from Department of Health and Human Services Regulations on Standards for Privacy of Individually Identifiable Health Information as Required by the Health Information Portability and Accountability Act

Federal Register

Wednesday, August 14, 2002

[Note: Portions of this rule have been omitted]

Part V
Department of Health and Human Services
Office of the Secretary
45 CFR Parts 160 and 164
Standards for Privacy of Individually Identifiable Health Information; Final Rule
Department of Health and Human Services
Office of the Secretary

SUMMARY

The Department of Health and Human Services ("HHS" or "Department") modifies certain standards in the Rule entitled "Standards for Privacy of Individually Identifiable Health Information" ("Privacy Rule"). The Privacy Rule implements the privacy requirements of the Administrative Simplification subtitle of the Health Insurance Portability and Accountability Act of 1996.

The purpose of these modifications is to maintain strong protections for the privacy of individually identifiable health information while clarifying certain of the Privacy Rule's provisions, addressing the unintended negative effects of the Privacy Rule on health care quality or access to health care, and relieving unintended administrative burdens created by the Privacy Rule.

Dates

This final rule is effective on October 15, 2002.
For Further Information Contact:
Felicia Farmer, 1-866-OCR-PRIV (1-866-627-7748) or TTY 1-866-788-4989.
Supplementary Information:
Availability of copies, and electronic access.

Copies: To order copies of the *Federal Register* containing this document, send your request to: New Orders, Superintendent of Documents, P.O. Box 371954, Pittsburgh, PA 15250-7954. Specify the date of the issue requested and enclose a check or money order payable to the Superintendent of Documents, or enclose your Visa or Master Card number and expiration date. Credit card orders can also be placed by calling the order desk at (202) 512-1800 (or toll-free at 1-866-512-1800) or by fax to (202) 512-2250. The cost for each copy is $10.00. Alternatively, you may view and photocopy the *Federal Register* document at most libraries designated as Federal Depository Libraries and at many other public and academic libraries throughout the country that receive the *Federal Register*.

Electronic Access: This document is available electronically at the HHS Office for Civil Rights (OCR) Privacy Web site at http://www.hhs.gov/ocr/hipaa/, as well as at the web site of the Government Printing Office at http://www.access.gpo.gov/su_docs/aces/aces140.html.

I. BACKGROUND

A. Statutory Background

Congress recognized the importance of protecting the privacy of health information given the rapid evolution of health information systems in the Health Insurance Portability and Accountability Act of 1996 (HIPAA), Public Law 104-191, which became law on August 21, 1996. HIPAA's Administrative Simplification provisions, sections 261 through 264 of the statute, were designed to improve the efficiency and effectiveness of the health care system by facilitating the electronic exchange of information with respect to certain financial and administrative transactions carried out by health plans, health care clearinghouses, and health care providers who transmit information electronically in connection with such transactions. To implement these provisions, the statute directed HHS to adopt a suite of uniform, national standards for transactions, unique health identifiers, code sets for the data elements of the transactions, security of health information, and electronic signature.

At the same time, Congress recognized the challenges to the confidentiality of health information presented by the increasing complexity of the health care industry, and by advances in the health information systems technology and communications. Thus, the Administrative Simplification provisions of HIPAA authorized the Secretary to promulgate standards for the privacy of individually identifiable health information if Congress did not enact health care privacy legislation by August 21, 1999. HIPAA also required the Secretary of HHS to provide Congress with recommendations for legislating to protect the confidentiality of health care information. The Secretary submitted such recommendations to Congress on September 11, 1997, but Congress did not pass such legislation within its self-imposed deadline.

With respect to these regulations, HIPAA provided that the standards, implementation specifications, and requirements established by the Secretary not supersede any contrary State law that imposes more stringent privacy protections. Additionally, Congress required that HHS consult with the National Committee on Vital and Health Statistics, a Federal advisory committee established pursuant to section 306(k) of the Public Health Service Act (42 U.S.C. 242k(k)), and the Attorney General in the development of HIPAA privacy standards.

After a set of HIPAA Administrative Simplification standards is adopted by the Department, HIPAA provides HHS with authority to modify the standards as deemed appropriate, but not more frequently than once every 12 months. However, modifications are permitted during the first year after adoption of the standards if the changes are necessary to permit compliance with the standards. HIPAA also provides that compliance with modifications to standards or implementation specifications must be accomplished by a date designated by the Secretary, which may not be earlier than 180 days after the adoption of the modification.

B. Regulatory and Other Actions to Date

HHS published a proposed Rule setting forth privacy standards for individually identifiable health information on November 3, 1999 (64 FR 59918). The Department received more than 52,000 public comments in response to the proposal. After reviewing and considering the public comments, HHS issued a final Rule (65 FR 82462) on December 28, 2000, establishing "Standards for Privacy of Individually Identifiable Health Information" ("Privacy Rule").

In an era where consumers are increasingly concerned about the privacy of their personal information, the Privacy Rule creates, for the first time, a floor of national protections for the privacy of their most sensitive information—health information. Congress has passed other laws to protect consumers' personal information contained in bank, credit card, other financial records, and even video rentals. These health privacy protections are intended to provide consumers with similar assurances that their health information, including genetic information, will be properly protected. Under the Privacy Rule, health plans, health care clearinghouses, and certain health care providers must guard against misuse of individuals' identifiable health information and limit the sharing of such information, and consumers are afforded significant new rights to enable them to understand and control how their health information is used and disclosed.

After publication of the Privacy Rule, HHS received many inquiries and unsolicited comments through telephone calls, e-mails, letters, and other contacts about the impact and operation of the Privacy Rule on numerous sectors of the health care industry. Many of these commenters exhibited substantial confusion and misunderstanding about how the Privacy Rule will operate; others expressed great concern over the complexity of the Privacy Rule. In response to these communications and to ensure that the provisions of the Privacy Rule would protect patients' privacy without creating unanticipated consequences that might harm patients' access to health care or quality of health care, the Secretary of HHS opened the Privacy Rule for additional public comment in March 2001 (66 FR 12738).

After an expedited review of the comments by the Department, the Secretary decided that it was appropriate for the Privacy Rule to become effective on April 14, 2001, as scheduled (65 FR 12433). At the same time, the Secretary directed the Department immediately to begin the process of developing guidelines on how the Privacy Rule should be implemented and to clarify the impact of the Privacy Rule on health care activities. In addition, the Secretary charged the Department with proposing appropriate changes to the Privacy Rule during the next year to clarify the requirements and correct potential problems that could threaten access to, or quality of, health care. The comments received during the comment period, as well as other communications from the public and all sectors of the health care industry, including letters, testimony at public hearings, and meetings requested by these parties, have helped to inform the Department's efforts to develop proposed modifications and guidance on the Privacy Rule.

On July 6, 2001, the Department issued its first guidance to answer common questions and clarify certain of the Privacy Rule's provisions. In the guidance, the Department also committed to proposing modifications to the Privacy Rule to address problems arising from unintended effects of the Privacy Rule on health care delivery and access. The guidance will soon be updated to reflect the modifications adopted in this final Rule. The revised guidance will be available on the HHS Office for Civil Rights (OCR) Privacy Web site at http://www.hhs.gov/ ocr/ hipaa/.

In addition, the National Committee for Vital and Health Statistics (NCVHS), Subcommittee on Privacy and Confidentiality, held public hearings on the implementation of the Privacy Rule on August 21–23, 2001, and January 24–25, 2002, and provided recommendations to the Department based on these hearings. The NCVHS serves as the statutory advisory body to the Secretary of HHS with respect to the development and implementation of the Rules required by the Administrative Simplification provisions of HIPAA, including the privacy standards. Through the hearings, the NCVHS specifically solicited public input on issues related to certain key standards in the Privacy Rule: consent, minimum necessary, marketing, fundraising, and research. The resultant public testimony and subsequent recommendations submitted to the Department by the NCVHS also served to inform the development of these proposed modifications.

II. OVERVIEW OF THE MARCH 2002 NOTICE OF PROPOSED RULEMAKING (NPRM)

As described above, through public comments, testimony at public hearings, meetings at the request of industry and other stakeholders, as well as other communications, the Department learned of a number of concerns about the potential unintended effects certain provisions would have on health care quality and access. On March 27, 2002, in response to these concerns, and pursuant to HIPAA's provisions for modifications to the standards, the Department proposed modifications to the Privacy Rule (67 FR 14776).

The Department proposed to modify the following areas or provisions of the Privacy Rule: consent; uses and disclosures for treatment, payment, and health care operations; notice of privacy practices; minimum necessary uses and disclosures, and oral communications; business associates; uses and disclosures for marketing; parents as the personal representatives of unemancipated minors; uses and disclosures for research purposes; uses and disclosures for which authorizations are required; and deidentification. In addition to these key areas, the proposal included changes to other provisions where necessary to clarify the Privacy Rule. The Department also included in the proposed Rule a list of technical corrections intended as editorial or typographical corrections to the Privacy Rule.

The proposed modifications collectively were designed to ensure that protections for patient privacy are implemented in a manner that maximizes the effectiveness of such protections while not compromising either the availability or the quality of medical care. They reflected a continuing commitment on the part of the Department to strong privacy protections for medical records and the belief that privacy is most effectively protected by requirements that are not exceptionally difficult to implement. The Department welcomed comments and suggestions for alternative ways effectively to protect patient privacy without adversely affecting access to, or the quality of, health care.

Given that the compliance date of the Privacy Rule for most covered entities is April 14, 2003, and the Department's interest in having the compliance date for these revisions also be no later than April 14, 2003, the Department solicited public comment on the proposed modifications for only 30 days. As stated above, the proposed modifications addressed public concerns already communicated to the Department through a wide variety of sources since publication of the Privacy Rule in December 2000. For these reasons, the Department believed that 30 days should be sufficient for the public to state its views fully to the Department on the proposed modifications to the Privacy Rule. During the 30-day comment period, the Department received in excess of 11,400 comments.

III. SECTION-BY-SECTION DESCRIPTION OF FINAL MODIFICATIONS AND RESPONSE TO COMMENTS

A. Section 164.501—Definitions

1. Marketing

December 2000 Privacy Rule

The Privacy Rule defined "marketing" at § 164.501 as a communication about a product or service, a purpose of which is to encourage recipients of the communication to purchase or use the product or service, subject to certain limited exceptions.

To avoid interfering with, or unnecessarily burdening communications about, treatment or about the benefits and services of health plans and health care providers, the Privacy Rule explicitly excluded two types of communications from the definition of "marketing": (1) communications made by a covered entity for the purpose of describing the participating providers and health plans in a network, or describing the services offered by a provider or the benefits covered by a health plan; and (2) communications made by a health care provider as part of the treatment of a patient and for the purpose of furthering that treatment, or made by a provider or health plan in the course of managing an individual's treatment or recommending an alternative treatment. Thus, a health plan could send its enrollees a listing of network providers, and a health care provider could refer a patient to a specialist without either an authorization under § 164,508 or having to meet the other special requirements in § 164.514(e) that attach to marketing communications. However, these communications qualified for the exception to the definition of "marketing" only if they were made orally or, if in writing, were made without remuneration from a third party. For example, it would not have been marketing for a pharmacy to call a patient about the need to refill a prescription, even if that refill reminder was subsidized by a third party; but it would have been marketing for that same, subsidized refill reminder to be sent to the patient in the mail.

Generally, if a communication was marketing, the Privacy Rule required the covered entity to obtain the individual's authorization to use or disclose protected health information to make the communication. However, the Privacy Rule, at § 164.514(e), permitted the covered entity to make health-related marketing communications without such authorization, provided it complied with certain conditions on the manner in which the communications were made. Specifically, the Privacy Rule permitted a covered entity to use or disclose protected health information to communicate to individuals about the health-related products or services of the covered entity or of a third party, without first obtaining an authorization for that use or disclosure of protected health information, if the communication: (1) Identified the covered entity as the party making the communication; (2) identified, if applicable, that the covered entity received direct or indirect remuneration from a third party for making the communication; (3) with the exception of general circulation materials, contained instructions describing how the individual could opt-out of receiving future marketing communications; and (4) where protected health information was used to target the communication about a product or service to individuals based on their health status or health condition, explained why the individual had been targeted and how the product or service related to the health of the individual.

For certain permissible marketing communications, however, the Department did not believe these conditions to be practicable. Therefore, § 164.514(e) also permitted a covered entity to make a marketing communication that occurred in a face-to-face encounter with the individual, or that involved products or services of only nominal value, without meeting the above conditions or requiring an authorization. These provisions, for example, permitted a covered entity to provide sample products during a face-to-face communication, or to distribute calendars, pens, and the like, that displayed the name of a product or provider.

March 2002 NPRM
The Department received many complaints concerning the complexity and unworkability of the Privacy Rule's marketing requirements. Many entities expressed confusion over the Privacy Rule's distinction between health care communications that are excepted from the definition of "marketing" versus those that are marketing but permitted subject to the special conditions in § 164.514(e). For example, questions were raised as to whether disease management communications or refill reminders were "marketing" communications subject to the special disclosure and opt-out conditions in § 164.514(e). Others stated that it was unclear whether various health care operations activities, such as general health-related educational and wellness promotional activities, were to be treated as marketing under the Privacy Rule.

The Department also learned that consumers were generally dissatisfied with the conditions required by § 164.514(e). Many questioned the general effectiveness of the conditions and whether the conditions would properly protect consumers from unwanted disclosure of protected health information to commercial entities, and from the intrusion of unwanted solicitations. They expressed specific dissatisfaction with the provision at § 164.514(e)(3)(iii) for individuals to opt-out of future marketing communications. Many argued for the opportunity to opt-out of marketing communications before any marketing occurred. Others requested that the Department limit marketing communications to only those consumers who affirmatively chose to receive such communications.

In response to these concerns, the Department proposed to modify the Privacy Rule to make the marketing provisions clearer and simpler. First, the Department proposed to simplify the Privacy Rule by eliminating the special provisions for marketing health-related products and services at § 164.514(e). Instead, any use or disclosure of protected health information for a communication defined as "marketing" in § 164.501 would require an authorization by the individual. Thus, covered entities would no longer be able to make any type of marketing communications that involved the use or disclosure of protected health information without authorization simply by meeting the disclosure and opt-out conditions in the Privacy Rule. The Department intended to effectuate greater consumer privacy protection by requiring authorization for all uses or disclosures of protected health information for marketing communications, as compared to the disclosure and opt-out conditions of § 164.514(e).

Second, the Department proposed minor clarifications to the Privacy Rule's definition of "marketing" at § 164.501. Specifically, the Department proposed to define "marketing" as "to make a communication about a product or service to encourage recipients of the communication to purchase or use the product or service." The proposed modification retained the substance of the "marketing" definition, but changed the language slightly to avoid the implication that in order for a communication to be marketing, the purpose or intent of the covered entity in making such a communication would have to be determined. The simplified language permits the Department to make the determination based on the communication itself.

Third, with respect to the exclusions from the definition of "marketing" in § 164.501, the Department proposed to simplify the language to avoid confusion and better conform to other sections of the regulation, particularly in the area of treatment communications. The proposal retained the exclusions for communications about a covered entity's own products and services and about the treatment of the individual. With respect to the exclusion for a communication made "in the course of managing the treatment of that individual," the Department proposed to modify the language to use the terms "case management" and "care coordination" for that individual. These terms are more consistent with the terms used in the definition of "health care operations," and were intended to clarify the Department's intent.

One substantive change to the definition proposed by the Department was to eliminate the condition on the above exclusions from the definition of "marketing" that the covered entity could not receive remuneration from a third party for any written communication. This limitation was not well understood and treated similar communications differently. For example, a prescription refill reminder was marketing if it was in writing and paid for by a third party, while a refill reminder that was not subsidized, or was made orally, was not marketing. With the proposed elimination of the health-related marketing requirements in § 164.514(e) and the proposed requirement that any marketing communication require an individual's prior written authorization, retention of this condition would have adversely affected a health care provider's

ability to make many common health-related communications. Therefore, the Department proposed to eliminate the remuneration prohibition to the exceptions to the definition so as not to interfere with necessary and important treatment and health-related communications between a health care provider and patient.

To reinforce the policy requiring an authorization for most marketing communications, the Department proposed to add a new marketing provision at § 164.508(a)(3) explicitly requiring an authorization for a use or disclosure of protected health information for marketing purposes. Additionally, if the marketing was expected to result in direct or indirect remuneration to the covered entity from a third party, the Department proposed that the authorization state this fact. As noted above, because a use or disclosure of protected health information for marketing communications required an authorization, the disclosure and opt-out provisions in § 164.514(e) no longer would be necessary and the Department proposed to eliminate them. As in the December 2000 Privacy Rule at § 164.514(e)(2), the proposed modifications at § 164.508(a)(3) excluded from the marketing authorization requirements face-to-face communications made by a covered entity to an individual. The Department proposed to retain this exception so that the marketing provisions would not interfere with the relationship and dialogue between health care providers and individuals. Similarly, the Department proposed to retain the exception to the authorization requirement for a marketing communication that involved products or services of nominal value, but proposed to replace the language with the common business term "promotional gift of nominal value."

As noted above, because some of the proposed simplifications were a substitute for § 164.514(e), the Department proposed to eliminate that section, and to make conforming changes to remove references to § 164.514(e) at § 164.502(a)(1)(vi) and in paragraph (6)(v) of the definition of "health care operations" in § 164.501.

Overview of Public Comments

The following discussion provides an overview of the public comment received on this proposal. Additional comments received on this issue are discussed below in the section entitled, "Response to Other Public Comments."

The Department received generally favorable comment on its proposal to simplify the marketing provisions by requiring authorizations for uses or disclosures of protected health information for marketing communications, instead of the special provisions for health-related products and services at § 164.514(e). Many also supported the requirement that authorizations notify the individual of marketing that results in direct or indirect remuneration to the covered entity from a third party. They argued that for patients to make informed decisions, they must be notified of potential financial conflicts of interest. However, some commenters opposed the authorization requirement for marketing, arguing instead for the disclosure and opt-out requirements at § 164.514(e) or for a one-time, blanket authorization from an individual for their marketing activities.

Commenters were sharply divided on whether the Department had properly defined what is and what is not marketing. Most of those opposed to the Department's proposed definitions objected to the elimination of health-related communications for which the covered entity received remuneration from the definition of "marketing." They argued that these communications would have been subject to the consumer protections in § 164.514(e) but, under the proposal, could be made without any protections at all. The mere presence of remuneration raised conflict of interest concerns for these commenters, who feared patients would be misled into thinking the covered entity was acting solely in the patients' best interest when recommending an alternative medication or treatment. Of particular concern to these commenters was the possibility, of a third party, such as a pharmaceutical company, obtaining a health care provider's patient list to market its own products or services directly to the patients under the guise of recommending an "alternative treatment" on behalf of the provider. Commenters argued that, even if the parties attempted to cloak the transaction in the trappings of a business associate relationship, when the remuneration flowed from the third party to the covered entity, the transaction was tantamount to selling the patient lists and ought to be considered marketing.

On the other hand, many commenters urged the Department to broaden the categories of communications that are not marketing. Several expressed concern that, under the proposal, they would be unable to send newsletters and other general circulation materials with information about health-promoting activities (e.g., screenings for certain diseases) to their patients or members without an authorization. Health plans were concerned that they would be unable to send information regarding enhancements to health insurance coverage to their members and beneficiaries. They argued, among other things, that they should be excluded from the definition of "marketing" because these communications would be based on limited, non-clinical protected health information, and because policyholders benefit and use such information to fully evaluate the mix of coverage most appropriate to their needs. They stated that providing such information is especially important given that individual and market-wide needs, as well as benefit offerings, change over time and by statute. For exam-

ple, commenters informed the Department that some States now require long-term care insurers to offer new products to existing policyholders as they are brought to market and to allow policyholders to purchase the new benefits through a formal upgrade process. These health plans were concerned that an authorization requirement for routine communications about options and enhancements would take significant time and expense. Some insurers also urged that they be allowed to market other lines of insurance to their health plan enrollees.

A number of commenters urged the Department to exclude any activity that met the definitions of "treatment," "payment," or "health care operations" from the definition of "marketing" so that they could freely inform customers about prescription discount card and price subsidy programs. Still others wanted the Department to broaden the treatment exception to include all health-related communications between providers and patients.

Final Modifications. The Department adopts the modifications to marketing substantially as proposed in the NPRM, but makes changes to the proposed definition of "marketing" and further clarifies one of the exclusions from the definition of "marketing" in response to comments on the proposal. The definition of "marketing" is modified to close what commenters characterized as a loophole, that is, the possibility that covered entities, for remuneration, could disclose protected health information to a third party that would then be able to market its own products and services directly to individuals. Also, in response to comments, the Department clarifies the language in the marketing exclusion for communications about a covered entity's own products and services.

As it proposed to do, the Department eliminates the special provisions for marketing health-related products and services at § 164.514(e). Except as provided for at § 164.508(a)(3), a covered entity must have the individual's prior written authorization to use or disclose protected health information for marketing communications and will no longer be able to do so simply by meeting the disclosure and opt-out provisions, previously set forth in § 164,514(e). The Department agrees with commenters that the authorization provides individuals with more control over whether they receive marketing communications and better privacy protections for such uses and disclosures of their health information. In response to commenters who opposed this proposal, the Department does not believe that an opt-out requirement for marketing communications would provide a sufficient level of control for patients regarding their health information. Nor does the Department believe that a blanket authorization provides sufficient privacy protections for individuals. Section 164.508(c) sets forth the core elements of an authorization necessary to give individuals control of their protected health information. Those requirements give individuals sufficient information and notice regarding the type of use or disclosure of their protected health information that they are authorizing. Without such specificity, an authorization would not have meaning. Indeed, blanket marketing authorizations would be considered defective under § 164.508(b)(2).

The Department adopts the general definition of "marketing" with one clarification. Thus, "marketing" means "to make a communication about a product or service that encourages the recipients of the communication to purchase or use the product or service." In removing the language referencing the purpose of the communication and substituting the term "that encourages" for the term "to encourage", the Department intends to simplify the determination of whether a communication is marketing. If, on its face, the communication encourages recipients of the communication to purchase or use the product or service, the communication is marketing. A few commenters argued for retaining the purpose of the communication as part of the definition of "marketing" based on their belief that the intent of the communication was a clearer and more definitive standard than the effect of the communication. The Department disagrees with these commenters. Tying the definition of "marketing" to the purpose of the communication creates a subjective standard that would be difficult to enforce because the intent of the communicator rarely would be documented in advance. The definition adopted by the Secretary allows the communication to speak for itself.

The Department further adopts the three categories of communications that were proposed as exclusions from the definition of "marketing." Thus, the covered entity is not engaged in marketing when it communicates to individuals about: (1) The participating providers and health plans in a network, the services offered by a provider, or the benefits covered by a health plan; (2) the individual's treatment; or (3) case management or care coordination for that individual, or directions or recommendations for alternative treatments, therapies, health care providers, or settings of care to that individual. For example, a doctor that writes a prescription or refers an individual to a specialist for follow-up tests is engaging in a treatment communication and is not marketing a product or service. The Department continues to exempt from the "marketing" definition the same types of communications that were not marketing under the Privacy Rule as published in December 2000, but has modified some of the language to better track the terminology used in the definition of "health care operations." The commenters generally supported this clarification of the language.

The Department, however, does not agree with commenters that sought to expand the exceptions from marketing for all communications that fall within the definitions of "treatment," "payment," or "health care operations." The purpose of the exclusions from the definition of marketing is to facilitate those communications that enhance the individual's access to quality health care. Beyond these important communications, the public strongly objected to any commercial use of protected health information to attempt to sell products or services, even when the product or service is arguably health related. In light of these strong public objections, ease of administration is an insufficient justification to categorically exempt all communications about payment and health care operations from the definition of "marketing."

However, in response to comments, the Department is clarifying the language that excludes from the definition of "marketing" those communications that describe network participants and the services or benefits of the covered entity. Several commenters, particularly insurers, were concerned that the reference to a "plan of benefits" was too limiting and would prevent them from sending information to their enrollees regarding enhancements or upgrades to their health insurance coverage. They inquired whether the following types of communications would be permissible: enhancements to existing products; changes in deductibles/co-pays and types of coverage (e.g., prescription drug); continuation products for students reaching the age of majority on parental policies; special programs such as guaranteed issue products and other conversion policies; and prescription drug card programs. Some health plans also inquired if they could communicate with beneficiaries about "one-stop shopping" with their companies to obtain long-term care, property, casualty, and life insurance products.

The Department understands the need for covered health care providers and health plans to be able to communicate freely to their patients or enrollees about their own products, services, or benefits. The Department also understands that some of these communications are required by State or other law. To ensure that such communications may continue, the Department is broadening its policy, both of the December 2000 Privacy Rule as well as proposed in the March 2002 NPRM, to allow covered entities to use protected health information to convey information to beneficiaries and members about health insurance products offered by the covered entity that could enhance or substitute for existing health plan coverage. Specifically, the Department modifies the relevant exemption from the definition of "marketing" to include communications that describe "a health-related product or service (or payment for such product or service) that is provided by, or included in a plan of benefits of, the covered entity making the communication, including communications about: the entities participating in a health care provider network or health plan network; replacement of, or enhancements to, a health plan; and health-related products or services available only to a health plan enrollee that add value to, but are not part of, a plan of benefits." Thus, under this exemption, a health plan is not engaging in marketing when it advises its enrollees about other available health plan coverages that could enhance or substitute for existing health plan coverage. For example, if a child is about to age out of coverage under a family's policy, this provision will allow the plan to send the family information about continuation coverage for the child. This exception, however, does not extend to excepted benefits (described in section 2791(c)(1) of the Public Health Service Act, 42 U.S.C. 300gg-91(c)(1)), such as accident-only policies), nor to other lines of insurance (e.g., it is marketing for a multi-line insurer to promote its life insurance policies using protected health information).

Moreover, the expanded language makes clear that it is not marketing when a health plan communicates about health-related products and services available only to plan enrollees or members that add value to, but are not part of, a plan of benefits. The provision of value-added items or services (VAIS) is a common practice, particularly for managed care organizations. Communications about VAIS may qualify as a communication that is about a health plan's own products or services, even if VAIS are not considered plan benefits for the Adjusted Community Rate purposes. To qualify for this exclusion, however, the VAIS must meet two conditions. First, they must be health-related. Therefore, discounts offered by Medicare+ Choice or other managed care organizations for eyeglasses may be considered part of the plan's benefits, whereas discounts to attend movie theaters will not. Second, such items and services must demonstrably "add value" to the plan's membership and not merely be a pass-through of a discount or item available to the public at large. Therefore, a Medicare+Choice or other managed care organization could, for example, offer its members a special discount opportunity for a health/fitness club without obtaining authorizations, but could not pass along to its members discounts to a health fitness club that the members would be able to obtain directly from the health/fitness clubs.

In further response to comments, the Department has added new language to the definition of "marketing" to close what commenters perceived as a loophole that a covered entity could sell protected health information to another company for the marketing of that company's products or services. For example, many were concerned that a pharmaceutical company could pay a provider for a list of patients with a particular con-

dition or taking a particular medication and then use that list to market its own drug products directly to those patients. The commenters believed the proposal would permit this to happen under the guise of the pharmaceutical company acting as a business associate of the covered entity for the purpose of recommending an alternative treatment or therapy to the individual. The Department agrees with commenters that the potential for manipulating the business associate relationship in this fashion should be expressly prohibited. Therefore, the Department is adding language that would make clear that business associate transactions of this nature are marketing. Marketing is defined expressly to include "an arrangement between a covered entity and any other entity whereby the covered entity discloses protected health information to the other entity, in exchange for direct or indirect remuneration, for the other entity or its affiliate to make a communication about its own product or service that encourages recipients of the communication to purchase or use that product or service." These communications are marketing and can only occur if the covered entity obtains the individual's authorization pursuant to § 164.508. The Department believes that this provision will make express the fundamental prohibition against covered entities selling lists of patients or enrollees to third parties, or from disclosing protected health information to a third party for the marketing activities of the third party, without the written authorization of the individual. The Department further notes that manufacturers that receive identifiable health information and misuse it may be subject to action taken under other consumer protection statutes by other Federal agencies, such as the Federal Trade Commission.

The Department does not, however, agree with commenters who argued for retention of the provisions that would condition the exclusions from the "marketing" definition on the absence of remuneration. Except for the arrangements that are now expressly defined as "marketing," the Department eliminates the conditions that communications are excluded from the definition of "marketing" only if they are made orally, or, if in writing, are made without any direct or indirect remuneration. The Department does not agree that the simple receipt of remuneration should transform a treatment communication into a commercial promotion of a product or service. For example, health care providers should be able to, and can, send patients prescription refill reminders regardless of whether a third party pays or subsidizes the communication. The covered entity also is able to engage a legitimate business associate to assist it in making these permissible communications. It is only in situations where, in the guise of a business associate, an entity other than the covered entity is promoting its own products using protected health information it has received from, and for which it has paid, the covered entity, that the remuneration will place the activity within the definition of "marketing."

In addition, the Department adopts the proposed marketing authorization provision at § 164.508(a)(3), with minor language changes to conform to the revised "marketing" definition. The Rule expressly requires an authorization for uses or disclosures of protected health information for marketing communications, except in two circumstances: (1) When the communication occurs in a face-to-face encounter between the covered entity and the individual; or (2) the communication involves a promotional gift of nominal value. A marketing authorization must include a statement about remuneration, if any. For ease of administration, the Department has changed the regulatory provision to require a statement on the authorization whenever the marketing "involves" direct or indirect remuneration to the covered entity from a third party, rather than requiring the covered entity to identify those situations where "the marketing is expected to result in" remuneration.

Finally, the Department clarifies that nothing in the marketing provisions of the Privacy Rule are to be construed as amending, modifying, or changing any rule or requirement related to any other Federal or State statutes or regulations, including specifically anti-kickback, fraud and abuse, or self-referral statutes or regulations, or to authorize or permit any activity or transaction currently proscribed by such statutes and regulations. Examples of such laws include the anti-kickback statute (section 1128B (b) of the Social Security Act), safe harbor regulations (42 CFR part 1001), Stark law (section 1877 of the Social Security Act) and regulations (42 CFR parts 411 and 424), and HIPAA statute on self-referral (section 1128C of the Social Security Act). The definition of "marketing" is solely applicable to the Privacy Rule and the permissions granted by the Rule are only for a covered entity's use or disclosure of protected health information. In particular, although this regulation defines the term "marketing" to exclude communications to an individual to recommend, purchase, or use a product or service as part of the treatment of the individual or for case management or care coordination of that individual, such communication by a "white coat" health care professional may violate the anti-kickback statute. Similar examples for pharmacist communications with patients relating to the marketing of products on behalf of pharmaceutical companies were identified by the OIG as problematic in a 1994 Special Fraud Alert (December 19, 1994, 59 FR 65372). Other violations have involved home health nurses and physical therapists acting as marketers for durable medical equipment companies. Although a particular communication under the

Privacy Rule may not require patient authorization because it is not marketing, or may require patient authorization because it is "marketing" as the Rule defines it, the arrangement may nevertheless violate other statutes and regulations administered by HHS, the Department of Justice, or other Federal or State agency.

Response to Other Public Comments
Comment: Some commenters recommended that the definition of "marketing" be broadened to read as follows: "any communication about a product or service to encourage recipients of the communication to purchase or use the product or service or that will make the recipient aware of the product or service available for purchase or use by the recipient." According to these commenters, the additional language would capture marketing campaign activities to establish "brand recognition."

Response: The Department believes that marketing campaigns to establish brand name recognition of products are already encompassed within the general definition of "marketing" and that it is not necessary to add language to accomplish this purpose.

Comment: Some commenters opposed the proposed deletion of references to the covered entity as the source of the communications, in the definition of those communications that were excluded from the "marketing" definition. They objected to these nonmarketing communications being made by unrelated third parties based on protected health information disclosed to these third parties by the covered entity, without the individual's knowledge or authorization.

Response: These commenters appear to have misinterpreted the proposal as allowing third parties to obtain protected health information from covered entities for marketing or other purposes for which the Rule requires an individual's authorization. The deletion of the specific reference to the covered entity does not permit disclosures to a third party beyond the disclosures already permitted by the Rule. The change is intended to be purely editorial: since the Rule applies only to covered entities, the only entities whose communications can be governed by the Rule are covered entities, and thus the reference to covered entities there was redundant. Covered entities may not disclose protected health information to third parties for marketing purposes without authorization from the individual, even if the third party is acting as the business associate of the disclosing covered entity. Covered entities may, however, use protected health information to communicate with individuals about the covered entity's own health-related products or services, the individual's treatment, or case management or care coordination for the individual. The covered entity does not need an authorization for these types of communications and may make the communication itself or use a business associate to do so.

Comment: Some commenters advocated for reversion to the provision in § 164.514(e) that the marketing communication identify the covered entity responsible for the communication, and argued that the covered entity should be required to identify itself as the source of the protected health information.

Response: As modified, the Privacy Rule requires the individual's written authorization for the covered entity to use or disclose protected health information for marketing purposes, with limited exceptions. The Department believes that the authorization process itself will put the individual sufficiently on notice that the covered entity is the source of the protected health information. To the extent that the commenter suggests that these disclosures are necessary for communications that are not "marketing" as defined by the Rule, the Department disagrees because such a requirement would place an undue burden on necessary health-related communications.

Comment: Many commenters opposed the proposed elimination of the provision that would have transformed a communication exempted from marketing into a marketing communication if it was in writing and paid for by a third party. They argued that marketing should include any activity in which a covered entity receives compensation, directly or indirectly, through such things as discounts from another provider, manufacturer, or service provider in exchange for providing information about the manufacturer or service provider's products to consumers, and that consumers should be advised whenever such remuneration is involved and allowed to opt-out of future communications.

Response: The Department considered whether remuneration should determine whether a given activity is marketing, but ultimately concluded that remuneration should not define whether a given activity is marketing or falls under an exception to marketing. In fact, the Department believes that the provision in the December 2000 Rule that transformed a treatment communication into a marketing communication if it was in writing and paid for by a third party blurred the line between treatment and marketing in ways that would have made the Privacy Rule difficult to implement. The Department believes that certain health care communications, such as refill reminders or informing patients about existing or new health care products or services, are appropriate, whether or not the covered entity receives remuneration from third parties to pay for them. The fact that remuneration is received for a marketing communication does not mean the communication is biased or inaccurate. For the same reasons, the Department does not believe that the communications that are exempt from the

definition of "marketing" require any special conditions, based solely on direct or indirect remuneration received by the covered entity. Requiring disclosure and opt-out conditions on these communications, as § 164.514(e) had formerly imposed on health-related marketing communications, would add a layer of complexity to the Privacy Rule that the Department intended to eliminate. Individuals, of course, are free to negotiate with covered entities for limitations on such uses and disclosures, to which the entity may, but is not required to, agree.

The Department does agree with commenters that, in limited circumstances, abuses can occur. The Privacy Rule, both as published in December 2000 and as proposed to be modified in March 2002, has always prohibited covered entities from selling protected health information to a third party for the marketing activities of the third party, without authorization. Nonetheless, in response to continued public concern, the Department has added a new provision to the definition of "marketing" to prevent situations in which a covered entity could take advantage of the business associate relationship to sell protected health information to another entity for that entity's commercial marketing purposes. The Department intends this prohibition to address the potential financial conflict of interest that would lead a covered entity to disclose protected health information to another entity under the guise of a treatment exemption.

Comment: Commenters argued that written authorizations (opt-ins) should be required for the use of clinical information in marketing. They stated that many consumers do not want covered entities to use information about specific clinical conditions that an individual has, such as AIDS or diabetes, to target them for marketing of services for such conditions.

Response: The Department does not intend to interfere with the ability of health care providers or health plans to deliver quality health care to individuals. The "marketing" definition excludes communications for the individual's treatment and for case management, care coordination or the recommendation of alternative therapies. Clinical information is critical for these communications and, hence, cannot be used to distinguish between communications that are or are not marketing. The covered entity needs the individual's authorization to use or disclose protected health information for marketing communications, regardless of whether clinical information is to be used.

Comment: The proposed modification eliminated the § 164.514 requirements that permitted the use of protected health information to market health-related products and services without an authorization. In response to that proposed modification, many commenters asked whether covered entities would be allowed to make communications about "health ed-ucation" or "health promoting" materials or services without an authorization under the modified Rule. Examples included communications about health improvement or disease preven-tion, new developments in the diagnosis or treatment of disease, health fairs, health/wellness-oriented classes or support groups.

Response: The Department clarifies that a communica-tion that merely promotes health in a general manner and does not promote a specific product or service from a particular provider does not meet the general definition of "marketing." Such communications may include population-based activities to improve health or reduce health care costs as set forth in the definition of "health care operations" at § 164.501. There-fore, communications, such as mailings reminding women to get an annual mammogram, and mailings providing informa-tion about how to lower cholesterol, about new developments in health care (e.g., new diagnostic tools), about health or "wellness" classes, about support groups, and about health fairs are permitted, and are not considered marketing.

Comment: Some commenters asked whether they could communicate with beneficiaries about government programs or government-sponsored programs such as information about SCHIP; eligibility for Medicare/Medigap (e.g., eligibil-ity for limited, six-month open enrollment period for Medicare supplemental benefits).

Response: The Department clarifies that communications about government and government-sponsored programs do not fall within the definition of "marketing." There is no com-mercial component to communications about benefits avail-able through public programs. Therefore, a covered entity is permitted to use and disclose protected health information to communicate about eligibility for Medicare supplemental ben-efits, or SCHIP. As in our response above, these communica-tions may reflect population-based activities to improve health or reduce health care costs as set forth in the definition of "health care operations" at § 164.501.

Comment: The proposed modification eliminated the § 164.514 requirements that allowed protected health informa-tion to be used and disclosed without authorization or the op-portunity to opt-out, for communications contained in newsletters or similar general communication devices widely distributed to patients, enrollees, or other broad groups of indi-viduals. Many commenters requested clarification as to whether various types of general circulation materials would be permit-ted under the proposed modification. Commenters argued that newsletters or similar general communication devices widely distributed to patients, enrollees, or other broad groups of indi-viduals should be permitted without authorizations because they are "common" and "serve appropriate information distri-bution purposes" and, based on their general circulation, are less intrusive than other forms of communication.

Response: Covered entities may make communications in newsletter format without authorization so long as the content of such communications is not "marketing," as defined by the Rule. The Department is not creating any special exemption for newsletters.

Comment: One commenter suggested that, even when au-thorizations are granted to disclose protected health informa-tion for a particular marketing purpose to a non-covered entity, there should also be an agreement by the third party not to re-disclose the protected health information. This same commenter also recommended that the Privacy Rule place re-strictions on nonsecure modes of making communications pursuant to an authorization. This commenter argued that protected health information should not be disclosed on the outside of mailings or through voice mail, unattended FAX, or other modes of communication that are not secure.

Response: Under the final Rule, a covered entity must ob-tain an individual's authorization to use or disclose protected health information for a marketing communication, with some exceptions. If an individual wanted an authorization to limit the use of the information by the covered entity, the individ-ual could negotiate with the covered entity to make that clear in the authorization. Similarly, individuals can request confi-dential forms of communication, even with respect to author-ized disclosures. See § 164.522(b).

Comment: Commenters requested that HHS provide clear guidance on what types of activities constitute a use or disclo-sure for marketing, and, therefore, require an authorization.

Response: The Department has modified the "marketing" definition to clarify the types of uses or disclosures of protected health information that are marketing, and, therefore, require prior authorization and those that are not marketing. The Department intends to update its guidance on this topic and ad-dress specific examples raised by commenters at that time.

Comment: A number of commenters wanted the Depart-ment to amend the face-to-face authorization exception. Some urged that it be broadened to include telephone, mail and other common carriers, fax machines, or the Internet so that the ex-ception would cover communications between providers and patients that are not in person. For example, it was pointed out that some providers, such as home delivery pharmacies, may have a direct treatment relationship, but communicate with patients through other channels. Some raised specific concerns about communicating with "shut-ins" and "persons living in rural areas." Other commenters asked the Department to make the exception more narrow to cover only those mar-keting communications made by a health care provider, as opposed to by a business associate, or to cover only those marketing communications of a provider that arise from a treatment or other essential health care communication.

Response: The Department believes that expanding the face-to-face authorization exception to include telephone, mail, and other common carriers, fax machines or the Internet would create an exception essentially for all types of marketing communications. All providers potentially use a variety of means to communicate with their patients. The authorization exclusion, however, is narrowly crafted to permit only face-to-face encounters between the covered entity and the individual.

The Department believes that further narrowing the exception to place conditions on such communications, other than that it be face-to-face, would neither be practical nor better serve the privacy interests of the individual. The Department does not intend to police communications between doctors and patients that take place in the doctor's office. Further limiting the exception would add a layer of complexity to the Rule, encumbering physicians and potentially causing them to second-guess themselves when making treatment or other essential health care communications. In this context, the individual can readily stop any unwanted communications, including any communications that may otherwise meet the definition of "marketing."

2. Health Care Operations: Changes of Legal Ownership

December 2000 Privacy Rule. The Rule's definition of "health care operations" included the disclosure of protected health information for the purposes of due diligence with respect to the contemplated sale or transfer of all or part of a covered entity's assets to a potential successor in interest who is a covered entity, or would become a covered entity as a result of the transaction.

The Department indicated in the December 2000 preamble of the Privacy Rule its intent to include in the definition of health care operations the actual transfer of protected health information to a successor in interest upon a sale or transfer of its assets. (65 FR 82609.) However, the regulation itself did not expressly provide for the transfer of protected health information upon the sale or transfer of assets to a successor in interest. Instead, the definition of "health care operations" included uses or disclosures of protected health information only for due diligence purposes when a sale or transfer to a successor in interest is contemplated.

March 2002 NPRM. A number of entities expressed concern about the discrepancy between the intent as expressed in the preamble to the December 2000 Privacy Rule and the actual regulatory language. To address these concerns, the Department proposed to add language to paragraph (6) of the definition of

"health care operations" to clarify its intent to permit the transfer of records to a covered entity upon a sale, transfer, merger, or consolidation. This proposed change would prevent the Privacy Rule from interfering with necessary treatment or payment activities upon the sale of a covered entity or its assets.

The Department also proposed to use the terms "sale, transfer, consolidation or merger" and to eliminate the term "successor in interest" from this paragraph. The Department intended this provision to apply to any sale, transfer, merger or consolidation and believed the current language may not accomplish this goal.

The Department proposed to retain the limitation that such disclosures are health care operations only to the extent the entity receiving the protected health information is a covered entity or would become a covered entity as a result of the transaction. The Department clarified that the proposed modification would not affect a covered entity's other legal or ethical obligation to notify individuals of a sale, transfer, merger, or consolidation.

Overview of Public Comments. The following discussion provides an overview of the public comment received on this proposal. Additional comments received on this issue are discussed below in the section entitled, "Response to Other Public Comments."

Numerous commenters supported the proposed modifications. Generally, these commenters claimed the modifications would prevent inconvenience to consumers, and facilitate timely access to health care. Specifically, these commenters indicated that health care would be delayed and consumers would be inconvenienced if covered entities were required to obtain individual consent or authorization before they could access health records that are newly acquired assets resulting from the sale, transfer, merger, or consolidation of all or part of a covered entity. Commenters further claimed that the administrative burden of acquiring individual permission and culling records of consumers who do not give consent would be too great, and would cause some entities to simply store or destroy the records instead. Consequently, health information would be inaccessible, causing consumers to be inconvenienced and health care to be delayed. Some commenters noted that the proposed modifications recognize the realities of business without compromising the availability or quality of health care or diminishing privacy protections one would expect in the handling of protected health information during the course of such business transactions.

Opposition to the proposed modifications was limited, with commenters generally asserting that the transfer of records in such circumstances would not be in the best interests of individuals.

Final Modifications. The Department agrees with the commenters that supported the proposed modifications and, therefore, adopts the modifications to the definition of health care operations. Thus, "health care operations" includes the sale, transfer, merger, or consolidation of all or part of the covered entity to or with another covered entity, or an entity that will become a covered entity as a result of the transaction, as well as the due diligence activities in connection with such transaction. In response to a comment, the final Rule modifies the phrase "all or part of a covered entity" to read "all or part of the covered entity" to clarify that any disclosure for such activity must be by the covered entity that is a party to the transaction.

Under the final definition of "health care operations," a covered entity may use or disclose protected health information in connection with a sale or transfer of assets to, or a consolidation or merger with, an entity that is or will be a covered entity upon completion of the transaction; and to conduct due diligence in connection with such transaction. The modification makes clear it is also a health care operation to transfer records containing protected health information as part of the transaction. For example, if a pharmacy which is a covered entity buys another pharmacy which is also a covered entity, protected health information can be exchanged between the two entities for purposes of conducting due diligence, and the selling entity may transfer any records containing protected health information to the new owner upon completion of the transaction. The new owner may then immediately use and disclose those records to provide health care services to the individuals, as well as for payment and health care operations purposes. Since the information would continue to be protected by the Privacy Rule, any other use or disclosure of the information would require an authorization unless otherwise permitted without authorization by the Rule, and the new owner would be obligated to observe the individual's rights of access, amendment, and accounting. The Privacy Rule would not interfere with other legal or ethical obligations of an entity that may arise out of the nature of its business or relationship with its customers or patients to provide such persons with notice of the transaction or an opportunity to agree to the transfer of records containing personal information to the new owner.

Response to Other Public Comments

Comment: One commenter was concerned about what obligations the parties to a transaction have regarding protected health information that was exchanged as part of a transaction if the transaction does not go through.

Response: The Department believes that other laws and standard business practices are adequate to address these situations and accordingly does not impose additional requirements of this type. It is standard practice for parties contemplating such transactions to enter into confidentiality agreements. In addition to exchanging protected health information, the parties to such transactions commonly exchange confidential proprietary information. It is a standard practice for the parties to these transaction to agree that the handling of all confidential information, such as proprietary information, will include ensuring that, in the event that the proposed transaction is not consummated, the information is either returned to its original owner or destroyed as appropriate. They may include protected health information in any such agreement, as they determine appropriate to the circumstances and applicable law.

3. Protected Health Information: Exclusion for Employment Records

December 2000 Privacy Rule. The Privacy Rule broadly defines "protected health information" as individually identifiable health information maintained or transmitted by a covered entity in any form or medium. The December 2000 Privacy Rule expressly excluded from the definition of "protected health information" only educational and other records that are covered by the Family Education Rights and Privacy Act of 1974, as amended, 20 U.S.C. 1232g. In addition, throughout the December 2000 preamble to the Privacy Rule, the Department repeatedly stated that the Privacy Rule does not apply to employers, nor does it apply to the employment functions of covered entities, that is, when they are acting in their role as employers. For example, the Department stated:

> Covered entities must comply with this regulation in their health care capacity, not in their capacity as employers. For example, information in hospital personnel files about a nurses' (sic) sick leave is not protected health information under this rule.

65 FR 82612. However, the definition of protected health information did not expressly exclude personnel or employment records of covered entities.

March 2002 NPRM. The Department understands that covered entities are also employers, and that this creates two potential sources of confusion about the status of health information. First, some employers are required or elect to obtain health information about their employees, as part of their routine employment activities [e.g., hiring, compliance with the Occupational Safety and Health Administration (OSHA) requirements]. Second, employees of covered health care providers or health plans sometimes seek treatment or reimbursement from that provider or health plan, unrelated to the employment relationship.

To avoid any confusion on the part of covered entities as to application of the Privacy Rule to the records they maintain as employers, the Department proposed to modify the definition of "protected health information" in § 164.501 to expressly exclude employment records held by a covered entity in its role as employer. The proposed modification also would alleviate the situation where a covered entity would feel compelled to elect to designate itself as a hybrid entity solely to carve out its employment functions. Individually identifiable health information maintained or transmitted by a covered entity in its health care capacity would, under the proposed modification, continue to be treated as protected health information.

The Department specifically solicited comments on whether the term "employment records" is clear and what types of records would be covered by the term.

In addition, as discussed in section III.C.1. below, the Department proposed to modify the definition of a hybrid entity to permit any covered entity that engaged in both covered and noncovered functions to elect to operate as a hybrid entity. Under the proposed modification, a covered entity that primarily engaged in covered functions, such as a hospital, would be allowed to elect hybrid entity status even if its only noncovered functions were those related to its capacity as an employer. Indeed, because of the absence of an express exclusion for employment records in the definition of protected health information, some covered entities may have elected hybrid entity status under the misconception that this was the only way to prevent their personnel information from being treated as protected health information under the Rule.

Overview of Public Comments. The following discussion provides an overview of the public comment received on this proposal. Additional comments received on this issue are discussed below in the section entitled, "Response to Other Public Comments."

The Department received comments both supporting and opposing the proposal to add an exemption for employment records to the definition of protected health information. Support for the proposal was based primarily on the need for clarity and certainty in this important area. Moreover, commenters supported the proposed exemption for employment records because it reinforced and clarified that the Privacy Rule does not conflict with an employer's obligation under numerous other laws, including OSHA, Family and Medical Leave Act (FMLA), workers' compensation, and alcohol and drug free workplace laws.

Those opposed to the modification were concerned that a covered entity may abuse its access to the individually identifiable health information in its employment records by using that information for discriminatory purposes. Many com-

menters expressed concern that an employee's health information created, maintained, or transmitted by the covered entity in its health care capacity would be considered an employment record and, therefore, would not be considered protected health information. Some of these commenters argued for the inclusion of special provisions, similar to the "adequate separation" requirements for disclosure of protected health information from group health plan to plan sponsor functions (§ 164.504(f)), to heighten the protection for an employee's individually identifiable health information when moving between a covered entity's health care functions and its employer functions.

A number of commenters also suggested types of records that the Department should consider to be "employment records" and, therefore, excluded from the definition of "protected health information." The suggested records included records maintained under the FMLA or the Americans with Disabilities Act (ADA), as well as records relating to occupational injury, disability insurance eligibility, sick leave requests and justifications, drug screening results, workplace medical surveillance, and fitness-for-duty test results. One commenter suggested that health information related to professional athletes should qualify as an employment record.

Final Modifications. The Department adopts as final the proposed language excluding employment records maintained by a covered entity in its capacity as an employer from the definition of "protected health information." The Department agrees with commenters that the regulation should be explicit that it does not apply to a covered entity's employer functions and that the most effective means of accomplishing this is through the definition of "protected health information."

The Department is sensitive to the concerns of commenters that a covered entity not abuse its access to an employee's individually identifiable health information which it has created or maintains in its health care, not its employer, capacity. In responding to these concerns, the Department must remain within the boundaries set by the statute, which does not include employers per se as covered entities. Thus, we cannot regulate employers, even when it is a covered entity acting as an employer.

To address these concerns, the Department clarifies that a covered entity must remain cognizant of its dual roles as an employer and as a health care provider, health plan, or health care clearinghouse. Individually identifiable health information created, received, or maintained by a covered entity in its health care capacity is protected health information. It does not matter if the individual is a member of the covered entity's workforce or not. Thus, the medical record of a hospital employee who is receiving treatment at the hospital is protected health information and is covered by the Rule, just as the medical record of any other patient of that hospital is protected health information and covered by the Rule. The hospital may use that information only as permitted by the Privacy Rule, and in most cases will need the employee's authorization to access or use the medical information for employment purposes. When the individual gives his or her medical information to the covered entity as the employer, such as when submitting a doctor's statement to document sick leave, or when the covered entity as employer obtains the employee's written authorization for disclosure of protected health information, such as an authorization to disclose the results of a fitness for duty examination, that medical information becomes part of the employment record, and, as such, is no longer protected health information. The covered entity as employer, however, may be subject to other laws and regulations applicable to the use or disclosure of information in an employee's employment record.

The Department has decided not to add a definition of the term "employment records" to the Rule. The comments indicate that the same individually identifiable health information about an individual may be maintained by the covered entity in both its employment records and the medical records it maintains as a health care provider or enrollment or claims records it maintains as a health plan. The Department therefore is concerned that a definition of "employment record" may lead to the misconception that certain types of information are never protected health information, and will put the focus incorrectly on the nature of the information rather than the reasons for which the covered entity obtained the information. For example, drug screening test results will be protected health information when the provider administers the test to the employee, but will not be protected health information when, pursuant to the employee's authorization, the test results are provided to the provider acting as employer and placed in the employee's employment record. Similarly, the results of a fitness for duty exam will be protected health information when the provider administers the test to one of its employees, but will not be protected health information when the results of the fitness for duty exam are turned over to the provider as employer pursuant to the employee's authorization.

Furthermore, while the examples provided by commenters represent typical files or records that may be maintained by employers, the Department does not believe that it has sufficient information to provide a complete definition of employment record. Therefore, the Department does not adopt as part of this rulemaking a definition of employment record, but does clarify that medical information needed for an employer to carry out its obligations under FMLA, ADA, and similar laws, as well as files or records related to occupational injury, disability insurance eligibility, sick leave requests and justifications, drug screening results, workplace medical surveillance, and fitness-for-duty tests of employees, may be part of the employment records maintained by the covered entity in its role as an employer.

Response to Other Public Comments

Comment: One commenter requested clarification as to whether the term "employment record" included the following information that is either maintained or transmitted by a fully insured group health plan to an insurer or HMO for enrollment and/or disenrollment purposes: (a) the identity of an individual including name, address, birth date, marital status, dependent information and SSN; (b) the individual's choice of plan; (c) the amount of premiums/contributions for coverage of the individual; (d) whether the individual is an active employee or retired; (e) whether the individual is enrolled in Medicare.

Response: All of this information is protected health information when held by a fully insured group health plan and transmitted to an issuer or HMO, and the Privacy Rule applies when the group health plan discloses such information to any entity, including the plan sponsor. There are special rules in § 164.504(f) which describe the conditions for disclosure of protected health information to the plan sponsor. If the group health plan received the information from the plan sponsor, it becomes protected health information when received by the group health plan. The plan sponsor is not the covered entity, so this information will not be protected when held by a plan sponsor, whether or not it is part of the plan sponsor's "employment record."

Comment: One commenter asked for clarification as to how the Department would characterize the following items that a covered entity may have: (1) medical file kept separate from the rest of an employment record containing (a) doctor's notes; (b) leave requests; (c) physician certifications; and (d) positive hepatitis test results; (2) FMLA documentation including: (a) physician certification form; and (b) leave requests; (3) occupational injury files containing (a) drug screening; (b) exposure test results; (c) doctor's notes; and (d) medical director's notes.

Response: As explained above, the nature of the information does not determine whether it is an employment record. Rather, it depends on whether the covered entity obtains or creates the information in its capacity as employer or in its capacity as covered entity. An employment record may well contain some or all of the items mentioned by the commenter;

but so too might a treatment record. The Department also recognizes that the employer may be required by law or sound business practice to treat such medical information as confidential and maintain it separate from other employment records. It is the function being performed by the covered entity and the purpose for which the covered entity has the medical information, not its record keeping practices, that determines whether the health information is part of an employment record or whether it is protected health information.

Comment: One commenter suggested that the health records of professional athletes should qualify as "employment records." As such, the records would not be subject to the protections of the Privacy Rule.

Response: Professional sports teams are unlikely to be covered entities. Even if a sports team were to be a covered entity, employment records of a covered entity are not covered by this Rule. If this comment is suggesting that the records of professional athletes should be deemed "employment records" even when created or maintained by health care providers and health plans, the Department disagrees. No class of individuals should be singled out for reduced privacy protections. As noted in the preamble to the December 2000 Rule, nothing in this Rule prevents an employer, such as a professional sports team, from making an employee's agreement to disclose health records a condition of employment. A covered entity, therefore, could disclose this information to an employer pursuant to an authorization.

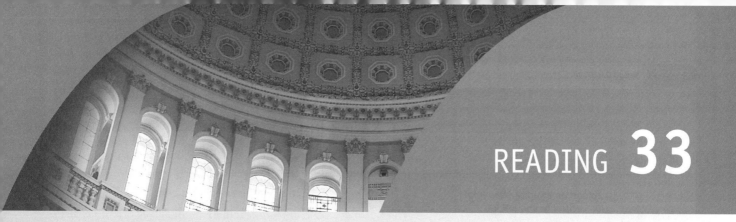

Department of Health & Human Services, Centers for Medicare & Medicaid Services, State Medicaid Director Letter

Centers for Medicare & Medicaid Services

7500 Security Boulevard, Mail Stop S2-26-12 Baltimore, Maryland 21244-1850

Centers for Medicaid and State Operations

August 15, 2007 SMDL #07-010

Dear State Medicaid Director:

The purpose of this letter is to provide you with additional information about sections 6041, 6042, and 6043 of the Deficit Reduction Act (DRA) of 2005, Public Law No.109-171, and to provide guidance on changes enacted by the Tax Relief and Health Care Act (TRHC) of 2006, Public Law No.109-432. We are also providing specific guidance about Section 6043 of the DRA, "Emergency Room Co-payments for Non-Emergency Care." This provision added a new subsection 1916A(e) of the Social Security Act (the Act), which provides a State option to impose higher cost sharing for non-emergency care furnished in a hospital emergency department without a waiver, and also added a new subsection 1903(y) of the Act providing $50,000,000 in Federal grant funds over 4 years for States to use for the establishment of alternate non-emergency service providers, or networks of such providers.

The addition of sections 1916A(e) and 1903(y) of the Act provides new opportunities for States to work with the Federal Government to implement effective reforms to slow spending growth while maintaining needed coverage. These sections also will help people to get the kind of care they prefer in non-emergency settings. These provisions are effective as of January 1, 2007.

On June 16, 2006, we issued a State Medicaid Director's letter to provide guidance on the alternate cost-sharing provisions of DRA sections 6041 and 6042. The TRHC, enacted on December 20, 2006, made some technical changes to those provisions. Those changes are described below and are effective as if originally enacted in the DRA.

Technical Changes to Sections 6041 and 6042 of the DRA Related to Individuals With Family Incomes At or Below 100 Percent of the Federal Poverty Level (FPL)

The TRHC clarified that, in the case of individuals at or below 100 percent of the FPL, cost sharing for non-emergency services furnished in a hospital emergency room may be imposed as long as no cost sharing is imposed to receive such care through an outpatient department or other alternative health care provider in the geographic area of the hospital emergency room. Such cost sharing may not exceed nominal cost sharing levels, and is subject to the aggregate cost sharing cap of 5 percent of family income.

The cost sharing limitations under section 1916 shall continue to apply with the exception of cost sharing for pharmacy or non-emergency use of an emergency room which the State elects under section 1916A(c) or (e).

The amount, scope, and duration of benefit requirements of section 1902(a)(10)(B) shall continue to apply to cost sharing.

The enforceability provisions of section 1916A(d) do not apply.

The total aggregate cost sharing cap of 5 percent of family income (as determined by the State on a quarterly or monthly basis) would apply to the extent that cost sharing is permitted under sections 1916, 1916A(c) (pharmacy), and 1916A(e) (non-emergency use of the emergency room).

Subsection 1916A(e) – Emergency Room Co-Payments for Non-emergency Services

Section 1916A(e) of the Act allows States to amend their State plans to allow hospitals to impose cost sharing on an individual (within one or more groups of individuals specified by the State) who receives non-emergency care furnished in the hospital emergency department. In order for the hospital to impose cost sharing:

- The individual must actually have available and accessible an alternate non-emergency services provider with respect to the necessary services.
- The hospital must inform the beneficiary (after the beneficiary has received an appropriate medical screening examination under section 1867—the Emergency Medical Treatment and Active Labor Act, or EMTALA provision of the Act, and after a determination has been made that the individual does not have an emergency medical condition) before providing the non-emergency services that:
- The hospital may require the payment of the State-specified cost sharing before the service can be provided;
- The hospital provides the name and location of an alternate non-emergency services provider that is actually available and accessible;
- An alternate provider can provide the services without the imposition of the State-specified higher cost sharing for the inappropriate use of the emergency room (nothing under this language should be construed as preventing a State from applying (or waiving) cost sharing otherwise permissible under section 1916A of the Act); and
- The hospital provides a referral to coordinate scheduling of this treatment.

Under this provision, the term "non-emergency services" means care or services furnished in an emergency department of a hospital that do not constitute an appropriate medical screening examination, or stabilizing examination, and treatment required to be provided by the hospital under section 1867 of the Act.

Also, the term "alternative non-emergency services provider" means, with respect to non-emergency services for the diagnosis or treatment of a condition, a health care provider—such as a physician's office, health care clinic, community health center, hospital outpatient department, or similar health care provider that:

- can provide clinically appropriate services for the diagnosis or treatment of a condition concurrently with the provision of the non-emergency services that would be provided in an emergency department of a hospital for the diagnosis or treatment of a condition; and
- is participating in the Medicaid program.

LIMITATIONS RELATING TO COST SHARING FOR OTHER INDIVIDUALS

Individuals with Family Incomes between 100 and 150 percent of the FPL

For an individual with a family income between 100 and 150 percent of the FPL, the co-payments imposed under section 1916A(e) may not exceed twice the amount determined to be nominal under section 1916 of the Act. Such cost sharing is also subject to the aggregate cost sharing cap of 5 percent of family income under section 1916A(b)(2)(A).

Individuals Exempt under Section 1916A of the Act

In the case of an individual who is identified as otherwise exempt from alternative cost sharing under section 1916A(b)(3) of the Act, a State may impose emergency room co-payments for non-emergency care in an amount that does not exceed a nominal amount (as determined under section 1916) as long as no cost sharing would be imposed in order to receive the care through an outpatient department or other alternative non-emergency health care provider in the geographic area of the hospital emergency department involved. States may not impose cost-sharing on individuals receiving emergency services (as defined by the Secretary and consistent with current law outlined in Section 1916(a)(2)(D) of the Act) in an emergency room. Below is a list of exempt populations and services not subject to cost sharing under section 1916A(b)(3) of the Act:

- Individuals under 18 years of age who are required to be provided Medicaid under section 1902(a)(10)(A)(i) of the Act, and including services furnished to individuals to whom child welfare services are made available under part B of title IV on the basis of being a child in foster care or individuals with respect to whom adoption or foster care assistance is made available under part E of title IV, without regard to age;
- Pregnant women, if such services relate to the pregnancy or to any other medical condition which may complicate the pregnancy;
- Any terminally ill individual who is receiving hospice care;

- Any individual who is an inpatient in a hospital, nursing facility, intermediate care facility for the mentally retarded, or other medical institution, if such individual is required, as a condition of receiving services in such institution under the State plan, to spend for costs for medical care all but a minimal amount of the individual's income required for personal needs;
- Women who are receiving medical assistance by virtue of the application of breast or cervical cancer provisions;
- Preventive services (such as well baby and well child care and immunizations) provided to children under 18 years of age regardless of family income;
- Family planning services and supplies, and
- Services furnished to disabled children who are receiving medical assistance by virtue of the application of sections 1902(a)(10)(A)(ii)(XIX) and 1902(cc). (This group was added by the TRHC).

APPLICATION OF AGGREGATE CAP AND RELATIONSHIP TO OTHER COST SHARING

Cost sharing applied under this provision is subject to the 5 percent maximum aggregate cap for cost sharing as specified under 1916A of the Act, as applied on a monthly or quarterly basis (as specified by the State). This total aggregate cost sharing cap of 5 percent of family income applies to any cost-sharing amounts under sections 1916, 1916A(a), 1916A(c) (pharmacy), and 1916A(e) (non-emergency use of the emergency room).

If co-payments are imposed under this provision, no other co-payments or co-insurance may otherwise be imposed for the emergency room services under sections 1916A(a), 1916(a)(3), or 1916(b)(3) of the Act.

EMTALA and Prudent Layperson Requirements

Nothing in this provision limits a hospital's obligations with respect to screening and stabilizing treatment of an emergency medical condition under section 1867 of the Act, or modifies any obligations under either State or Federal standards relating to the application of a prudent-layperson standard with respect to payment or coverage of emergency services by any managed care organization.

State Plan Submission

States may use the enclosed State plan preprint page (Enclosure A) to adopt cost sharing pursuant to this provision, States must include it in their approved State plan. For your convenience we have enclosed a template for a State plan amendment. Please submit your State plan amendment electronically in a "PDF" file format to your Centers for Medicare & Medicaid Services (CMS) regional office in order to implement this provision.

Subsection 1903(y) – Grant Funds for Establishment of Alternate Non-emergency Services Providers

Subsection 1903(y) of the Act authorizes the payment of $50,000,000 during the 4-year period beginning in 2007 in order to provide payment to States for the establishment of alternate non-emergency service providers or networks of providers. (See page 2 for the definition of an alternate non-emergency services provider.)

In providing for payments to States under subsection 1903(y) of the Act, the Secretary shall provide preference to States that establish, or provide for, alternate non-emergency services providers or networks of providers that:

- serve rural or underserved areas where Medicaid beneficiaries may not have regular access to providers of primary care services; or
- are in partnership with local community hospitals.

Additionally, in reviewing applications, CMS will consider as a special circumstance whether the grant funding is necessary to further the implementation of a pending or approved State plan amendment for section 1916A(e) of the Act for hospitals to impose cost sharing for non-emergency services provided in a hospital emergency department.

The Funding Opportunity Number is HHS-2007-CMS-ANESP-0005. To apply, go to www.grants.gov. You must "Get Registered" before you apply. On the left of the screen, select "Get Registered" and follow the directions. When that is completed, select "Apply for Grants" and follow the directions. Please do not wait until the application deadline date to begin the application process through the Web site www.grants.gov. We recommend you visit the Web site at least 30 days prior to filing your application to fully understand the process and requirements. Also, submit your application well in advance of the closing date in order to allow time to submit a hard copy by overnight mail if difficulties are encountered. For questions on the application process select "Contact Us" at the www.grants.gov Web site and you will be given the option to telephone or e-mail your questions to the support center.

We strongly encourage you to consider these grant opportunities to develop proposals to enhance your Medicaid program. The CMS contact for this new legislation is Ms. Jean Sheil, Director, Family and Children's Health Programs, who may be reached at (410) 786-5647. If you have any additional questions, please let us know.

Sincerely,
Dennis G. Smith, Director
Enclosure
cc:

CMS REGIONAL ADMINISTRATORS

CMS Associate Regional Administrators Division of Medicaid and Children's Health

Martha Roherty Director, Health Policy Unit American Public Human Services Association Joy Wilson Director, Health Committee National Conference of State Legislatures

Matt Salo Director of Health Legislation National Governors Association

Jacalyn Bryan Carden Director of Policy and Programs Association of State and Territorial Health Officials

Christie Raniszweski Herrera Director, Health and Human Services Task Force American Legislative Exchange Council

Debra Miller Director for Health Policy Council of State Governments

Department of Health and Human Services 2008 Budget in Brief Concerning Medicaid and SCHIP

Department of Health and Human Services

United States Department of Health and Human Services, Budget in Brief Fiscal Year 2008

MEDICAID

| | (Dollars in millions) | | | |
| | **2006** | **2007** | **2008** | |
	Actual	**Continuing Resolution**	**President's Budget**	**+/− 2007 Cont. Res.**
Current Law:				
Benefits[1]	171,485	181,959	193,871	+11,912
State Administration	9,141	9,882	10,015	+133
Total Outlays, Current Law	180,625	191,841	203,886	+12,045

[1]Includes Vaccines for Children Outlays.

Federal and State Governments jointly fund Medicaid, a program that provides medical assistance to certain low-income groups. The Federal Government's share of a State's expenditures is called the Federal Medical Assistance Percentage (FMAP). The FMAP has a floor rate of 50 percent and for FY 2008, the highest FMAP is 76.29 percent. Overall, the Federal Government will pay for approximately 57 percent of medical assistance payments.

In FY 2008, HHS estimates that approximately 50 million individuals in States and Territories will be covered by Medicaid. This includes children, the aged, blind, and/or disabled, and people who meet eligibility criteria under the old Aid to Families with Dependent Children (AFDC) program. Additionally, Medicaid will cover many other individuals who are eligible for benefits through waivers and amended State plans with somewhat higher income eligibility limits. The Medicaid current law baseline assumes passage of a full-year Continuing Resolution. In FY 2008, the Federal share of current law Medicaid outlays is expected to be $204 billion. This is a $12 billion (6.3 percent) increase over projected FY 2007 spending.

How Medicaid Works

States are required to cover individuals who meet categorical and financial eligibility levels. This includes individuals who qualified under the 1996 AFDC rules; most Supplemental Security Income (SSI) recipients; pregnant women and children under age 6 whose family income is at or below 133 percent of the Federal poverty level (FPL); children ages 6 to 19 whose family income, is below the FPL, all of whom are commonly referred to as "the categorically eligible." States may also cover "medically needy" individuals. These individuals meet the categorical eligibility criteria, but have too much income or too many resources to meet the financial criteria. This includes pregnant women through a 60-day postpartum period, children under age 18, newborns and certain protected blind individuals. In FY 2007, the FPL for a family of three was $17,170 in the continental United States. For more information, see www.aspe.hhs.gov/poverty/07poverty.shtml.

| | Medicaid Enrollment (enrollees in millions) | | |
	2006	**2007**	**2008**
Aged 65 and Over	4.9	5.0	5.1
Blind and Disabled	8.3	8.5	8.6
Needy Adults	10.8	11.1	11.3
Needy Children	22.9	23.5	24.0
Territories	1.0	1.0	1.0
Total	**47.9**	**49.1**	**50.0**

FIGURE 34-1 Estimated State and Federal Medicaid Outlays FY 2008-2017 (dollars in billions)

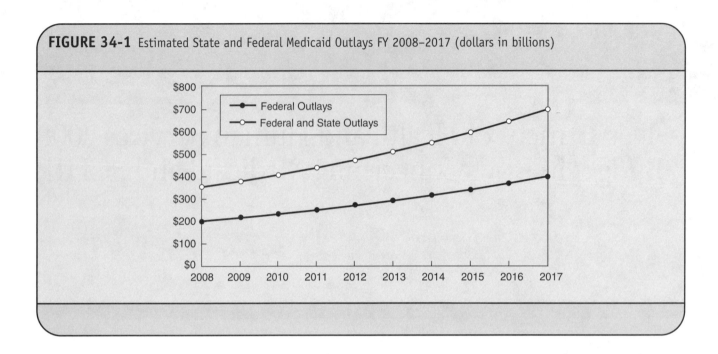

On February 8, 2006, President Bush signed the Deficit Reduction Act (DRA) of 2005 (P.L. 109-171). The DRA was an important step in bringing mandatory spending under control and reforming Medicaid. In the long run, the biggest challenge to the budget is mandatory spending—or entitlement programs—like Medicare, Medicaid, and Social Security. Together, these programs are now growing faster than the economy and the population—and nearly three times the rate of inflation. By 2030, projected spending for Medicare, Medicaid, and Social Security alone will be almost 60 percent of the entire Federal budget. The annual growth of entitlement programs needs to be slowed to affordable levels.

The DRA reduces Medicaid spending for prescription drugs so that taxpayers do not have to pay inflated prices. The law gives governors more flexibility to design Medicaid benefits that efficiently and affordably meet State needs, and it closes loopholes that allowed higher income people to game the system by transferring assets in order to qualify for Medicaid benefits.

The President's Budget continues to exercise fiscal discipline in Medicaid. It proposes $1.9 billion in Medicaid savings in FY 2008 and approximately $13.0 billion in savings over five years. The President's proposals slow the average annual growth in Medicaid over the next five years from 7.3 percent a year to 7.1 percent a year.

FY 2008 PROPOSED LEGISLATION

Last year the DRA made important strides in modernizing the financing, benefit structure, and infrastructure of Medicaid. The FY 2008 President's Budget continues these efforts to restrain unsustainable growth rates in this vital program.

Medicaid Administrative Services Reforms

Streamline Administrative Match Rates: Creates consistency in the administrative matching structure across Medicaid, by proposing to align all administrative reimbursement rates in Medicaid at 50 percent.

Implement Cost Allocation: Recoups Medicaid administrative costs included in the Temporary Assistance for Needy Families (TANF) block grant.

Medicaid Reimbursement Reforms

Require State Reporting and Link Performance to Reimbursement: Requires States to report on Medicaid performance measures and link performance to Federal Medicaid grant awards.

Reimburse Targeted Case Management (TCM) at 50 percent: Aligns reimbursement for TCM services with the standard administrative matching rate of 50 percent.

Medicaid Pharmacy Reforms

Rationalize Pharmacy Reimbursement: Builds on changes to pharmacy reimbursement in the DRA by reducing the Federal upper limit reimbursement for multiple source drugs to 150 percent of the average manufacturer price of the lowest priced drug in the group.

Allow Optional Managed Formulary: Allows States to use private sector management techniques to leverage greater discounts through negotiations with drug manufacturers.

Require Tamper-Resistant Prescription Pads: Requires all States where providers use handwritten prescription pads to use "tamper-resistant" pads.

Replace Best Price with Budget Neutral Rebate: Replaces the "best price" component of the Medicaid drug rebate formula with a budget neutral flat rebate. Medicaid best-price currently deters manufacturers from offering lower prices to other drug purchasers.

Program Integrity Reforms

Expand Asset Verification Demonstration: Expands a Social Security Administration (SSA) pilot using electronic financial records for verifying an applicant's assets to appropriate HHS programs. State Medicaid agencies would be required to establish pilots in locations where SSA is operating such a pilot.

Enhance Third Party Liability: Enhances current law by allowing States to avoid costs for prenatal and preventive pediatric claims where a third party is responsible; collect for medical child support where health insurance is derived from a noncustodial parent's obligation to provide coverage; and recover Medicaid expenditures from beneficiary liability settlements.

Extend 1915(b) Waiver Period: Extends the renewal period for 1915(b) "freedom of choice" waivers from two to three years.

Long-Term Care Reform

Define Home Equity Definition at $500,000: Removes the State option to increase the $500,000 home equity limit to $750,000 by proposing to codify the substantial home equity definition at $500,000.

Authorization Extensions and Modifications

Modify Health Insurance Portability and Accountability Act (HIPAA): Includes two legislative changes to ensure that Medicaid and State Children's Health Insurance Program (SCHIP) beneficiaries receive the benefits of HIPAA-related coverage, which increases the continuity, portability, and accessibility of health insurance.

Extend Transitional Medical Assistance (TMA): Extends TMA which allows families to remain eligible for Medicaid for up to 12 months after they lose welfare cash benefits due to increased earnings. The Tax Relief and Health Care Act of 2006 (P.L. 109432) extends TMA through June 30, 2007. This legislative proposal extends TMA through September 30, 2008.

Extend Qualified Individuals (QI) Program: Extends premium assistance for QIs, Medicare beneficiaries with incomes of at least 120 percent and less than 135 percent FPL and who have limited financial resources, through September 30, 2008. The QI extension will continue Federal coverage of Medicare Part B premiums.

Other

Extend Refugee Exemption: This SSA proposal, which has a Medicaid impact, extends the seven-year exemption to eight years so that refugees and asylees will have one additional year to complete the citizenship application process without penalty.

ADMINISTRATIVE PROPOSALS

The President's Budget also announces plans for several administrative initiatives that achieve additional Medicaid savings. The Administration believes it can implement the following initiatives through either regulatory or sub-regulatory guidance.

Revise Payments for Government Providers: Builds on past CMS efforts to curb questionable financing practices by recovering Federal funds that are diverted from government providers and retained by the State. In addition, this proposal caps payments to government providers to no more than the cost of furnishing services to Medicaid beneficiaries.

School-Based Services: Announces planned administrative actions to phase out Medicaid reimbursement for some services, including transportation and administrative claiming related to Medicaid services provided in schools.

Eliminate Medicaid Graduate Medical Education (GME): Clarifies that Medicaid will no longer be available as a source of funding for GME. Paying for GME is outside of Medicaid's primary purpose, which is to provide medical care to low-income populations.

Clarify Rehabilitation Services: Proposes a regulation clearly defining allowable services that may be claimed as rehabilitation services, which are optional Medicaid services typically offered to individuals with special needs or disabilities to help improve their health and quality of life.

Issue Guidance Defining 1915(b)(3) Services: Announces regulation clarifying which services provided under section 1915(b)(3) of the Social Security Act will be allowed.

Third Party Liability—Eliminate "Pay & Chase" for Pharmacy: Requires States to uphold the cost avoidance standard for pharmacy claims, and eliminates waivers that permit "pay and chase."

Payment Reform: Clarify Provider Tax Policy: Clarifies the mechanism by which Congress originally intended the provider tax limitations to operate.

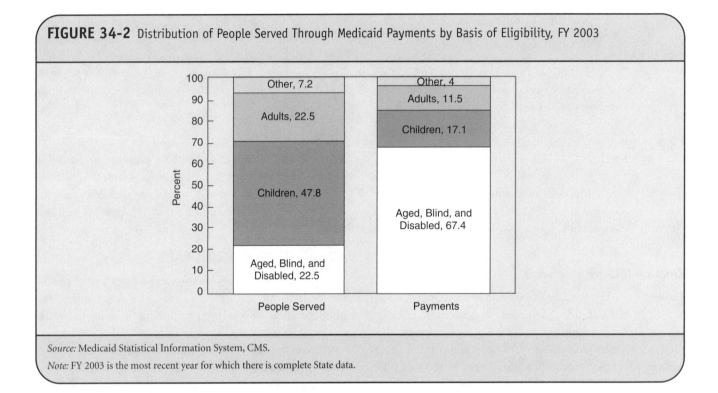

FIGURE 34-2 Distribution of People Served Through Medicaid Payments by Basis of Eligibility, FY 2003

Source: Medicaid Statistical Information System, CMS.

Note: FY 2003 is the most recent year for which there is complete State data.

Codify Disproportionate Share Hospital (DSH) Provisions in Regulation: Provides further clarification of allowable DSH costs that may be claimed for Federal reimbursement.

MEDICAID COMMISSION

The Secretary established the Medicaid Commission in May 2005 to provide recommendations on ways to modernize the Medicaid program. Many of the Commission's preliminary recommendations, released in September 2005, were incorporated into the DRA. This past December, the Commission released its final report detailing recommendations to ensure the long-term sustainability of Medicaid.

Some of the Commission's recommendations include:

- Promote individual responsibility and planning for long-term care needs.
- Give States greater flexibility to design Medicaid benefits packages.
- Aggressively promote and support the implementation of health IT.

The full Medicaid Commission report is available at www.aspe.hhs.gov/medicaid/.

RECENT PROGRAM DEVELOPMENTS

Tax Relief and Health Care Act of 2006, (RL. 109-432)

In addition to tax provisions that address Medical Savings Accounts and Health Savings Accounts, this law included provisions related to Medicaid, including:

Extension of Transitional Medical Assistance (TMA) and Abstinence Education Program: Extends TMA and Abstinence education programs through June 30, 2007.

Provider Taxes: Codifies the maximum rate at which a State can tax its health care providers at six percent, in effect on November 1, 2006. Beginning January 1, 2008 through FY 2011, the rate will be temporarily reduced to 5.5 percent.

DSH Allotments: Provides FY 2007 DSH allotments for Tennessee and Hawaii.

Medicaid DRA Technical Corrections: Clarifies that Medicaid beneficiaries at less than 100 percent of the FPL continue to pay no more than nominal cost sharing and sets an aggregate cap for their cost sharing at five percent of family income, and expands exemption from DRA citizenship documentation requirements to beneficiaries of Medicare, SSI, SSDI, old-age and survivors insurance benefits as a result of disability, and Titles IV-B or IV-E foster children.

Key DRA Implementation Issues

The DRA enables Medicaid to better respond to the health care needs of 21st century Americans. For example, when the program was established in the 1960s, institutional care was the norm for long-term care services. Provisions in the DRA represent the most important reforms in 15 years to end the longstanding Medicaid bias toward institutional care. Institutional care may still be the best choice for many, but the DRA helped make home- and. community-based care a real option for Medicaid beneficiaries. The law created strong financial incentives and opportunities for States through options like Money Follows the Person and Cash and Counseling, which give disabled Medicaid beneficiaries, their caregivers, and families the ability to choose the optimal setting for long-term care needs.

The DRA also permits Medicaid to cover more people at lower cost, with care that is portable and has greater continuity. This approach has already seen promise through demonstrations in States where innovative programs enable Medicaid to work better with mainstream insurance to increase access to affordable health coverage.

Medicaid Flexibility: The Administration has maintained its focus on providing States with options to expand the use of Medicaid with a focus on flexibility. States can apply limited premiums and cost sharing for certain groups of Medicaid beneficiaries and services, as well as provide Medicaid coverage to certain groups of individuals through enrollment in benchmark benefit packages, similar to those offered in the SCHIP.

Medicaid Transformation Grants: This program provides new grant funds to States for the adoption of innovative methods to improve the effectiveness and efficiency in providing medical assistance under Medicaid. Congress authorized and appropriated $75 million in each FY 2007 and FY 2008. Grants to 27 States were awarded in January 2007.

Reforming Long-Term Care and Services for the Disabled: Beginning January 1, 2007, both home- and community-based services (HCBS) for the elderly and self-directed personal assistance services for the elderly and disabled became optional benefits for States.

Money Follows the Person Demonstration: This demonstration supports State efforts to "rebalance" their long-term support systems by offering $1.75 billion over five years in competitive grants to States.

The Family Opportunity Act (FOA): The FOA was included as part of the DRA and includes a provision that allows States to offer middle-income families with disabled children the option of buying into Medicaid. FOA includes a demonstration that provides States with the opportunity to offer home and community based alternatives to psychiatric residential treatment facilities for children as part of the New Freedom Initiative first proposed by the President. The FOA also restores Medicaid eligibility for certain SSI beneficiaries.

Medicaid Integrity Program: The Medicaid Integrity Program was implemented in FY 2006. The Secretary is promoting Medicaid integrity by entering into contracts with eligible entities to carry out certain specified activities including reviews, audits, identification of over-payments, education, and technical support to States.

Medicaid Growth: The slowdown in Medicaid growth has resulted from many actions, including the shift in drug costs for the dually-eligible to the new Medicare drug benefit. While nursing home care, community-based long-term care costs, and payments to health plans are significant contributors to the growth in Medicaid outlays, the Administration's continued focus on eliminating fraud and abuse will assist in reducing outlays in the future.

PERFORMANCE HIGHLIGHT

Medicaid received a rating of Adequate in its 2006 Program Assessment Rating Tool (PART) review. As a result of the PART process, CMS developed a range of new performance measures, including:

- Increase the number of States that demonstrate improvement related to access and quality health care through the Medicaid Quality Improvement Program;
- Track return on investment resulting from implementation of the Medicaid Integrity Program; and
- Increase percentage of beneficiaries who receive home and community based services.

MEDICAID AND SCHIP PROPOSALS

	(Outlays in millions)	
	2008 President's Budget	Five Year 2008–2012
Medicaid Legislative Proposals		
Streamline Administrative Match Rates	−945	−5,315
Implement Cost Allocation	−280	−1,770
Require State Reporting and Link Performance to Reimbursement	—	−330
Reimburse Targeted Case Management at 50 Percent	−200	−1,160
Rationalize Pharmacy Reimbursement	−160	−1,200
Allow Optional Managed Formulary	−160	−870
Require Tamper Resistant Prescription Pads	−35	−210

	(Outlays in millions)	
	2008 President's Budget	Five Year 2008–2012
Medicaid Legislative Proposals		
Replace Best Price with Budget Neutral Rebate	—	—
Expand Asset Verification Demonstration	−65	−640
Enhance Third Party Liability	−10	−85
Define Home Equity Definition at $500,000	−70	−430
Extend Section 1915(b) Waiver Period	—	—
Modify HIPAA	—	—
Extend Transitional Medical Assistance (TMA)	460	665
Extend Qualified Individual (QI) Program[1]	425	425
Adjustment for QI Transfer from Medicare[1]	−425	−425
Subtotal, Medicaid Legislative Proposals	−1,465	−11,345
Other Proposals with Impact on Medicaid		
Refugee Exemption Extension	33	99
SCHIP Reauthorization (Medicaid Impact)	−510	−1,770
Total, Medicaid Legislative Proposals	−1,942	−13,016
Medicaid Administrative Proposals		
Revise Payments for Government Providers	−530	−5,000
School Based Services: Eliminate Admin./ Transportation	−615	−3,645
Eliminate Medicaid Graduate Medical Education	−140	−1,780
Clarify Rehabilitation Services	−230	−2,290
Issue Guidance Defining 1915(b)(3) Services	—	—
Third Party Liability: Eliminate Pay and Chase for Pharmacy	—	—
Payment Reform: Clarify Provider Tax Policy	—	—
Codify DSH Provisions in Regulation	—	—
Total, Medicaid Administrative Proposals	−1,515	−12,715
Total, Medicaid Budget Proposals	−3,457	−25,731
SCHIP Legislative Proposals		
SCHIP Reauthorization	1,220	5,930
Total, SCHIP Legislative Proposals	1,220	5,930
Total, Medicaid and SCHIP Budget Proposals	−2,237	−19,801

[1] States pay the Medicare Part B premium costs for QIs, which are in turn offset by a reimbursement from Medicare Part B.

STATE CHILDREN'S HEALTH INSURANCE PROGRAM

	(Dollars in millions)			
	2006	2007	2008	
	Actual	Continuing Resolution	President's Budget	+/− 2007 Cont. Res.
Current Law:				
Total Outlays	5,451	5,647	5,424	−223

The Balanced Budget Act of 1997 (BBA) created the State Children's Health Insurance Program (SCHIP) under Title XXI of the Social Security Act.

SCHIP is a partnership between Federal and State Governments that helps provide children with the health insurance coverage they need. The program improves access to health care and quality of life for millions of vulnerable children under 19 years of age. SCHIP reaches children whose families have incomes too high to qualify for Medicaid, but too low to afford private health insurance.

The BBA appropriated almost $40 billion to the program over 10 years (FY 1998 through FY 2007). States with an approved SCHIP plan are eligible to receive an enhanced Federal matching rate, which ranges from 65 to 85 percent, drawn from a capped allotment.

States have a high degree of flexibility in designing their programs. They can implement SCHIP by:

- Expanding Medicaid;
- Creating a new, non-Medicaid Title XXI separate State program; or
- A combination of both approaches.

Generally, SCHIP targets Medicaid-ineligible uninsured children who are under 19 years old from families with incomes at or below 200 percent of the Federal poverty level (FPL).

Implementation and Enrollment

Every State, the District of Columbia, and all five Territories have had approved SCHIP plans since September 1999. As of January 2007, States have received approval for 16 Medicaid expansion programs, 18 separate programs, 22 combination programs, and 275 State plan amendments.

As of January 18, 2007, 27 States and the District of Columbia cover children in families with incomes up to and including 200 percent of the FPL. Sixteen States cover children above that level. Of the 16, eight States cover children up to and including 300 percent of the FPL. One State, New Jersey, covers children up to 350 percent of the FPL.

During FY 2006, 6.6 million children were enrolled in SCHIP. This represents an increase of approximately 473,000 children, or 7.7 percent, over FY 2005 enrollment.

Proposed Legislation

SCHIP Reauthorization: The authorization for SCHIP expires at the end of FY 2007. The Administration proposes to reauthorize SCHIP for five years, consistent with submission of a five-year Budget to the Congress, and focuses each of the program elements on SCHIP's original objectives to provide health insurance coverage for uninsured, low-income children

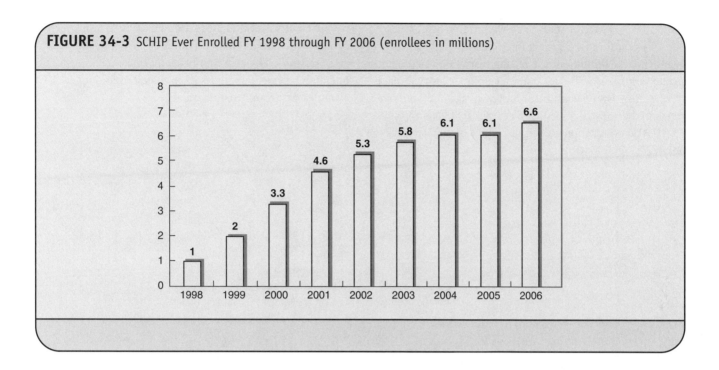

FIGURE 34-3 SCHIP Ever Enrolled FY 1998 through FY 2006 (enrollees in millions)

at or below 200 percent of the FPL. Toward this end, the Budget provides approximately $5 billion over five years for additional allotment funds.

Recent Programs Development

National Institutes of Health Reform Act of 2006 (P.L. 109-482) FY 2007 Funding Shortfalls: Requires the Secretary to redistribute unspent FY 2004 and FY 2005 State SCHIP allotments to some of the 14 States experiencing shortfalls in FY 2007. Funding is to be redistributed on a monthly basis, in the order by which States realize monthly funding shortfalls. Redistributed funds can only be used for populations eligible for SCHIP under the State plan on October 1, 2006. Regular Federal matching for coverage of populations other than children or pregnant women (instead of enhanced Federal matching normally available) will apply using redistributed funds.

Use of certain SCHIP funds for Medicaid Expenditures: Extends the ability of certain "qualifying States" to use up to 20 percent of available SCHIP allotment amounts for FY 2006 and FY 2007 as Federal matching funds to provide medical assistance under Medicaid for individuals under age 19 who are not eligible for SCHIP and whose family income exceeds 150 percent of the FPL. "Qualifying States" are those States that, prior to the implementation of SCHIP, were providing medical assistance to this population under Medicaid.

SCHIP Performance

When SCHIP began in FY 1998, CMS adopted a goal of enrolling five million children by FY 2005. CMS exceeded this enrollment goal by 1.1 million children in FY 2005. For FY 2008, CMS is focusing on a goal to improve health care quality across the SCHIP program. States will collect measures related to access to care, asthma medications, and child wellness visits. These performance measures involve improving health care quality across the SCHIP program and support HHS Strategic Goal three: Increase the percentage of the Nation's children and adults who have access to health care services, and expand consumer choices.

SCHIP Waivers

The requirements of Federal law and regulations can be waived by the Secretary to give States programmatic flexibility to increase health insurance coverage, improve quality of services, and encourage innovation in their SCHIP programs. Using section 1115 of the Social Security Act, States can more effectively tailor their programs to meet local needs and experiment with new approaches to providing health care services. In the past, section 1115 waivers have provided health insurance to uninsured children, parents, caretaker guardians, pregnant women, and childless adults.

The Administration has promoted the Health Insurance Flexibility and Accountability (HIFA) waiver, one type of section 1115 waiver, for States to develop comprehensive insurance coverage for individuals at twice the FPL and below, using SCHIP and Medicaid funds. The Administration places a particular emphasis on broad, statewide approaches that maximize both private health insurance coverage and employer sponsored insurance. As of January 2007, CMS has approved 15 HIFA demonstration waivers that could expand coverage to nearly one million people.

The DRA prohibited the use of Title XXI funds for the coverage of non-pregnant childless adults, other than caretaker relatives. The provision, effective October 1, 2005, did not apply to existing waivers or to the extension, renewal, or amendments of any existing waivers.

Congressional Budget Office Cost Estimate Concerning the Improving Head Start Act of 2007

Congressional Budget Office Cost Estimate

March 22, 2007
H.R. 1429
Improving Head Start Act of 2007
—As ordered reported by the House Committee
on Education and Labor on March 14, 2007

SUMMARY

H.R. 1429 would reauthorize the Head Start program through 2012. Head Start was authorized through 2003 by the Coats Human Services Reauthorization Act of 1998 (Public Law 105-285) and has since been extended through annual appropriation acts.

CBO estimates that the bill would authorize additional appropriations of $6.0 billion in 2008 and $36.8 billion over the 2008–2012 period, assuming that annual authorizations are adjusted for inflation when specific annual appropriation levels are not provided. (Without such inflation adjustments, the authorizations would total about $35.4 billion over the 2008–2012 period.) CBO estimates that appropriation of the authorized levels would result in additional outlays of $33.1 billion over the 2008–2012 period, assuming annual adjustments for inflation. (Outlays would total about $31.9 billion without adjustments for inflation.) Enacting H.R. 1429 would not affect direct spending or receipts.

H.R. 1429 contains no intergovernmental or private-sector mandates as defined by the Unfunded Mandates Reform Act (UMRA). Any costs to state, local, or tribal governments would result from complying with conditions for receiving federal assistance.

ESTIMATED COST TO THE FEDERAL GOVERNMENT

The estimated budgetary impact of H.R. 1429 is shown in the following table. The costs of this legislation fall within budget function 500 (education, training, employment, and social services).

	By Fiscal Year, in Millions of Dollars					
	2007	2008	2009	2010	2011	2012
Spending Subject to Appropriation						
Head Start Spending Under Current Law						
Budget Authority[a]	6,889	1,389	0	0	0	0
Estimated Outlays	6,846	3,751	761	97	14	0
Proposed Changes						
Estimated Authorization Level	0	5,961	7,490	7,629	7,769	7,916
Estimated Outlays	0	3,398	6,654	7,464	7,689	7,847
Total Spending Under H.R. 1429						
Estimated Authorization Level	6,889	7,350	7,490	7,629	7,769	7,916
Estimated Outlays	6,846	7,149	7,415	7,560	7,703	7,847

Notes: Components may not sum to totals because of rounding.

[a] The 2007 level is the amount appropriated for the Head Start program, including an advance of $1.389 billion. The 2008 level is the amount provided in an advance appropriation.

BASIS OF ESTIMATE

H.R. 1429 would reauthorize the Head Start program through 2012. The program is currently authorized through September 30, 2007, by the Revised Continuing Appropriations Resolution, 2007 (Public Law 110-5). For this estimate, CBO assumes that the bill will be enacted before the start of fiscal year 2008, that the estimated amounts shown in the table will be appropriated for each year, and that outlays will follow historical spending patterns.

The Head Start program provides comprehensive child development services to low-income children. Services include education, health, nutrition, and social services with the goal of increasing the school readiness of young children in low-income families.

The bill would authorize the appropriation of $7.350 billion in 2008 (including the $1.389 billion advance already appropriated for fiscal year 2008), and such sums as may be necessary in 2009 through 2012. CBO estimates that the total authorizations of additional appropriations for the 2008–2012 period would be $36.8 billion, assuming adjustments for inflation from 2009 through 2012, with resulting additional outlays of $33.1 billion over those five years.

Funding for this program for a given fiscal year is provided by both a regular appropriation for that fiscal year and an advance appropriation provided earlier. Although the program has been funded by two separate appropriations since 2001, funding does not need to be authorized separately because all of the funds for a fiscal year could be provided in one appropriation.

INTERGOVERNMENTAL AND PRIVATE-SECTOR IMPACT

H.R. 1429 contains no intergovernmental or private-sector mandates as defined in UMRA. Grant funds authorized by the bill would benefit state, local, and tribal governments that participate in the Head Start program. Any costs they incur from complying with increased management and oversight responsibilities would result from complying with conditions for receiving federal assistance.

PREVIOUS CBO ESTIMATE

On March 20, 2007, CBO transmitted a cost estimate for S. 556 as ordered reported by the Senate Committee on Health, Education, Labor, and Pensions on February 14, 2007. That bill would authorize the overall Head Start program from 2008 through 2012. S. 556 would authorize slightly more funding than H.R. 1429, including two new grant programs that are not in the House bill. It also would establish a specific authorization level for Head Start for 2009 and 2010, whereas H.R. 1429 would authorize such sums as necessary for those years.

Estimate Prepared By:
Federal Costs: Jonathan Morancy
Impact on State, Local, and Tribal Governments: Lisa Ramirez-Branum
Impact on the Private Sector: Paige Shevlin

Estimate Approved By:
Robert A. Sunshine
Assistant Director for Budget Analysis

New York City Department of Health and Mental Hygiene Board of Health, Amendment to the New York City Health Code, Concerning Phasing out Artificial Trans-Fat in New York City Food Services Establishments

Department of Health and Mental Hygiene Board of Health

Notice of Adoption of an Amendment (§81.08) to Article 81 of the New York City Health Code

In compliance with §1043(b) of the New York City Charter (the "Charter") and pursuant to the authority granted to the Board of Health by §558 of said Charter, a notice of intention to amend Article 81 of the New York City Health Code (the "Health Code"), adding a new §81.08, was published in the City Record on September 29, 2006, and a public hearing was held on October 30, 2006. Approximately 2,200 written and oral comments were received in support of the proposal and 70 comments in opposition to the proposal. At its meeting on December 5, 2006 the Board adopted the following resolution.

STATUTORY AUTHORITY

This amendment to the Health Code is promulgated pursuant to §§558 and 1043 of the Charter. Section 558(b) and (c) of the Charter empowers the Board of Health to amend the Health Code and to include in the Health Code all matters to which the Department's authority extends. Section 1043 grants the Department rule-making authority.

STATEMENT OF BASIS AND PURPOSE

The Department of Health and Mental Hygiene (the "Department") enforces provisions of the New York City Health Code ("Health Code") and other applicable law relating to food served directly to the consumer throughout the City, including food that is commercially prepared, and sold or distributed for free, by food service establishments, a broad category which includes restaurants, caterers and mobile food vending units. The Department also regulates non-retail food processing establishments, such as mobile food vending commissaries, as defined in Health Code §89.01, which supply food for mobile vending units.

Background

Restaurants (the term is being used interchangeably with "food service establishments" or "FSEs") are an important source of daily food intake for New York City residents: an estimated one third of daily caloric intake comes from foods purchased in restaurants.[1] Assuring safe and healthy dining options is a public health priority. The Department issues permits and inspects all New York City FSEs and non-retail food processing establishments, as defined in §81.03(j) and (p) of the Health Code. The public health concern addressed by this amendment is the presence of trans fat in foods served in restaurants, which represents a dangerous and entirely preventable health risk to restaurant goers. Yet New York City restaurant patrons currently have no practical way to avoid this harmful substance.

Accordingly, the Board of Health has amended Article 81 of the New York City Health Code to restrict the service of products containing artificial trans fats at all FSEs.

The Department is charged with preventing and controlling diseases, including chronic disease, through approaches that may address individual behavior or the community environment. By restricting FSEs from serving food that contains artificial trans fat, except for food served in the manufacturer's original sealed package, we can reduce New Yorkers' exposure

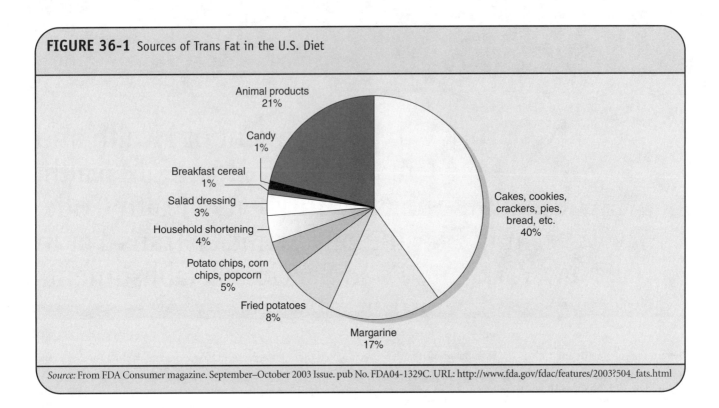

FIGURE 36-1 Sources of Trans Fat in the U.S. Diet

Source: From FDA Consumer magazine. September–October 2003 Issue. pub No. FDA04-1329C. URL: http://www.fda.gov/fdac/features/2003?504_fats.html

to an avoidable hazard in the food environment that is associated with increased heart disease risk.

Basis for Restricting Service of Products Containing Artificial Trans Fat

Heart disease is New York City's leading cause of death. In 2004, 23,000 New York City residents died from heart disease and nearly one-third of these individuals died before the age of 75.[2] Scientific evidence demonstrates a clear association between increased trans fat intake and the risk of coronary heart disease. Most dietary trans fat is found in partially hydrogenated vegetable oil ("PHVO")—oil that has been chemically modified. Scientific studies which examine the change in cholesterol levels when trans fat is replaced with currently available heart healthy alternatives conservatively estimate a reduction of 6% in coronary heart disease events such as heart attacks.[3] Even in the most conservative estimates, based on replacing trans fat primarily by saturated fat—an unlikely outcome given the widespread trend to healthier fats by food producers—a significant although smaller reduction in coronary heart disease events is still expected. Other scientific studies, based upon observing large groups of people over time estimate that up to 23%, of coronary heart disease events could be avoided by replacing trans fat with healthy alternatives. Because an estimated one third

of dietary trans fat comes from foods purchased in restaurants, the continued presence of PHVO in restaurant foods represents an important contribution to cardiovascular risk for New York City diners.[4]

Dietary trans fat increases the risk of heart disease by elevating LDL ("bad") cholesterol, and lowering HDL ("good") cholesterol.[5] Because of its negative effect on "good cholesterol," trans fat appears to be even worse than saturated fat. The Institute of Medicine ("IOM") reviewed the scientific evidence and concluded that there is "a positive linear trend between trans fatty acid intake and total and LDL concentration, and therefore increased risk of coronary heart disease."[6] The 2005 Dietary Guidelines for Americans, issued by the United States Department of Agriculture ("USDA"), recommends that dietary intake of trans fat be "as low as possible"[7] and the American Heart Association guidelines issued in June 2006 recommend that trans fat intake be kept below 1% of total energy intake.[8] In January of 2006, the FDA's mandatory listing of trans fat content on the nutrition facts labels of packaged foods came into effect.[9]

Approximately 80% of dietary trans fat is found in industrially-produced PHVO, which is used for frying and baking and is present in many processed foods.[10] Approximately 20% is naturally occurring and is found in small amounts in dairy and meat products from ruminant animals.

The artificial trans fat found in PHVO is produced when hydrogen is added to vegetable oil in a process called hydrogenation. Common FSE sources of artificial trans fat include: foods fried in partially hydrogenated vegetable oils; margarine and vegetable shortening; prepared foods such as pre-fried French fries, fried chicken, taco shells and donuts; baked goods such as hamburger buns, pizza dough, crackers, cookies, and pies; and pre-mixed ingredients such as pancake and hot chocolate mix.

The major source of dietary trans fat, found in PHVO, can be replaced with currently available heart healthy alternatives. Denmark has recently successfully removed artificial trans fat by limiting industrially produced trans fat content in food to 2% of total calories from fat. In addition, in June 2006 the Canadian Trans Fat Task Force issued a report recommending that Canada limit trans fat in food service establishments to 2% of total fat content in margarines and vegetable oils and 5% of total fat content in all other food ingredients.[12] "Zero grams" trans fat packaged foods in the US, both new products and those already in production, have been extensively marketed since the labeling requirement for packaged foods became effective in January of 2006. Many manufacturers have reformulated a number of their existing products that are now widely available as "zero grams" trans fat (defined by the FDA as <0.5 grams per serving) on supermarket shelves. A recent *New England Journal of Medicine* article reports that industry and government representatives agreed that the restriction of trans fat in Denmark "did not appreciably affect the quality, cost or availability of food."[13] This experience demonstrates that artificial trans fat can be replaced without consumers noticing an effect.[14] Acceptable healthier alternatives to PHVOs include traditional mono and poly unsaturated vegetable oils (e.g., canola, corn, olive, etc.) that have not been hydrogenated, as well as newly developed oils such as those made from specially cultivated varieties of soybeans, safflowers, and sunflowers. Further, many of the newer trans fat-free oils have long "fry lives" and other favored characteristics of PHVOs. Educational and enforcement efforts will seek to promote a shift to healthier fats. In response to increased demand, US companies are expanding production of products that will increase the market supply of alternatives to hydrogenated oils.[15,16]

Consumer Trans Fat Consumption and the Contribution of FSEs

National surveys show that Americans spend almost half (47%) of their food dollars eating out.[17] One third of daily caloric intake comes from foods purchased in restaurants.[18] The continued presence of artificial trans fat in restaurant foods needlessly increases the risk for heart disease for all of our city's residents.

Consumer concern about trans fat in food is evidenced by the increase in national sales of products labeled "no trans fat" by 12% to $6.4 billion for the 52 weeks ended October 2, 2004, compared with the previous 52-week period.[19] Nutrition ranks second after taste as the factor most frequently influencing food purchases.[20] Moreover, artificial trans fat can be replaced with heart-healthier oils and fats without changing the taste of foods.

Prevalence of Use of Partially Hydrogenated Vegetable Oil in NYC FSEs

In June 2005, the Department launched the Trans Fat Education Campaign. The campaign called on all NYC FSEs to voluntarily remove PHVO from the foods they were serving. This was supported by extensive educational outreach to food suppliers, consumers and to every licensed restaurant in New York City.

To assess use of PHVO-containing products by FSEs, the Department conducted two surveys: one prior to the campaign (May 9 through June 10, 2005) and another nine months after the campaign (April 3 through May 5, 2006).

In both the 2005 and 2006 survey findings, the prevalence of PHVO-containing oils used for frying, baking or spreads was approximately 50% at FSEs where product content could be determined. While a lack of labeling or product identification of some products precludes a precise, estimate of the prevalence of use, the data show that PHVO use remained common and has not declined substantially despite the Trans Fat Education Campaign.

Why Focus on Trans Fat over Other Fats?

The IOM conclusion that there is no safe level of artificial trans fat consumption[21] is in contrast to other dietary fats which, when consumed in moderation, are a natural part of a healthy diet. Artificially produced trans fat is relatively new to our food supply and confers no known health benefit. Because healthy, inexpensive alternatives exist for the most common source of trans fat, PHVO, their continued use by FSEs poses an unnecessary public health threat.

Why use 0.5 Grams per Serving of Trans Fat as a Threshold?

Current FDA labeling regulations allow manufacturers of foods packaged for direct sale to consumers in retail markets to list trans fat content as "0 grams" if the product contains less than 0.5 grams per serving.[22] This allows for the presence of naturally occurring trans fat in meat and dairy foods as well as newer "low trans fat" foods, which may have PHVO listed as an ingredient. The proposed provision intentionally allows for products that have less than 0.5 grams per serving (evidenced either on a Nutrition Facts label or in information provided by the manufacturer) in order to accommodate most of the newly formulated low trans fat margarines on the market, and allows for substitute spreads.

Response to Comments

The Department received more than 2,200 written and oral comments in favor of the amendment, and 70 comments opposed to the proposed amendment. It was brought to the Department's attention that the term "margarine" is found in some ingredients lists on labels of products, and that margarines may contain artificial trans fat. While only subdivision (d) of the original proposal included the term "margarine," the proposal has been amended to clarify that it is intended to restrict use of margarine that contains artificial trans fat. In addition, since some comments stated that in practice it could take longer to reformulate recipes to accommodate the restriction on artificial trans fat in baked goods and deep fried yeast dough and cake batter, the proposal has been amended. Accordingly, the effective date of the restriction on use of oils, margarines and vegetable shortenings containing artificial trans fats that are used for frying and as spreads will remain July 1, 2007, but the effective date for oils and shortenings used for deep frying yeast dough and cake batter and for all other foods containing artificial trans fat has been extended to July 1, 2008.

STATEMENT PURSUANT TO SECTION 1042— REGULATORY AGENDA

The proposed amendment was not included in the Department's Regulatory Agenda because it resulted from a recent analysis by the Department.

The proposal is as follows:

Note-matter in brackets [ ] to be deleted

Matter <u>underlined</u> is new.

RESOLVED, that Article 81 of the New York City Health Code, set forth in title 24 of the Rules of the City of New York, as amended by resolution adopted on the seventh of June, two thousand five, be and the same hereby is further amended by adding a new §81.08, to be printed together with explanatory notes, as follows:

§81.08 Foods containing artificial trans fat.

(a) *Artificial trans fat restricted.* No foods containing artificial trans fat, as defined in this section, shall be stored, distributed, held for service, used in preparation of any menu item or served in any food service establishment or by any mobile food unit commissary, as defined in §89.01 of this Code or successor provision, except food that is being served directly to patrons in a manufacturer's original sealed package.

(b) *Definition.* For the purposes of this section, a food shall be deemed to contain artificial trans fat if the food is labeled as, lists as an ingredient, or has vegetable shortening, margarine or any kind of partially hydrogenated vegetable oil. However, a food whose nutrition facts label or other documentation from the manufacturer lists the trans fat content of the food as less than 0.5 grams per serving, shall not be deemed to contain artificial trans fat.

(c) Labels required.

  (1) *Original labels.* Food service establishments and mobile food unit commissaries shall maintain on site the original labels for all food products:

    (i) that are, or that contain, fats, oils or shortenings, and

    (ii) that are, when purchased by such food service establishments or mobile food unit commissaries, required by applicable federal and state law to have labels, and

    (iii) that are currently being stored, distributed, held for service, used in preparation of any menu items, or served by the food service establishment or by the mobile food unit commissary.

  (2) *Documentation instead of labels.* Documentation acceptable to the Department from the manufacturers of such food products, indicating whether the food products contain vegetable shortening, margarine or any kind of partially hydrogenated vegetable oil, or indicating trans fat content, may be maintained instead of original labels.

  (3) *Documentation required when food products are not labeled.* If baked goods, or other food products restricted pursuant to subdivision (a) of this section, that are or that contain fats, oils or shortenings, are not required to be labeled when purchased, food service establishments and mobile food commissaries shall obtain and maintain documentation acceptable to the Department from the manufacturers of the food products, indicating whether the food products contain vegetable shortening. margarine or any kind of partially hydrogenated vegetable oil, or indicating trans fat content.

(d) *Effective date.* This section shall take effect on July 1, 2007 with respect to oils, shortenings and margarines containing artificial trans fat that are used for frying or in spreads: except that the effective date of this section with regard to oils on shortenings used for deep frying of yeast dough or cake batter, and all other foods containing artificial trans fat, shall be July 1, 2008.

Notes: Section 81.08 was added by resolution adopted on December 5, 2006 to restrict use of artificial trans fat in food service establishments in New York City in an effort to decrease the well-documented risk of ischemic heart and other disease conditions associated with consumption of such products.

RESOLVED, that the list of Section Headings in Article 81 of the New York City Health Code, set forth in title 24 of the Rules of the City of New York, as amended by resolution adopted on the seventh of June, two thousand five, be, and the same hereby is, further amended, to be printed together with explanatory notes, as follows:

ARTICLE 81
FOOD PREPARATION AND FOOD ESTABLISHMENTS
* * *
§81.07 Food; sanitary preparation, protection against contamination.
§81.08 Foods containing artificial trans fat.
§81.09 Food; temperature requirements
* * *

Notes: Section 81.08 was added by resolution adopted on December 5, 2006 to restrict service of unhealthful artificial trans fat by food service establishments.

REFERENCES

1. Guthrie JF. et al. Role of Food Prepared Away from Home in the American Diet, 1977–78 Versus 1994–96: Changes and Consequences. *Society for Nutrition Education* 2002; 34: 140–150.
2. NYC DOHMH, Office of Vital Statistics. NYC Vital Statistics 2004, Accessed on EpiQuery. 2006.
3. Mozaffarian D. Katan MB. Ascherio A. Stampfer MJ. Willett WC. Trans Fatty Acids and Cardiovascular Disease. *New England Journal of Medicine.* April 13, 2006. 354;15:1601–13.
4. Guthrie JF. et al. Role of Food Prepared Away from Home in the American Diet, 1977–78 Versus 1994–96: Changes and Consequences. *Society for Nutrition Education* 2002; 34:140–150.
5. Ascherio A. Katan MB. Zock PL. Stampfer MJ. Willett WC. Trans fatty acids and coronary heart disease. *New England Journal of Medicine.* 1999; 340:1994–1998.
6. Panel on Macronutrients, Institute of Medicine. Letter report on dietary reference intakes for trans fatty acids drawn from the Report on dietary reference intakes for energy, carbohydrate, fiber, fat, fatty acids, cholesterol, protein, and amino acids. 2002. Washington, DC, Institute of Medicine. Page 14.
7. Dietary Guidelines Advisory Committee. King J, et al. Dietary Guidelines for Americans 2005. January 12, 2005. http://www.health.gov/dietaryguidelines/dga2005/document/pdf/ExecutiveSummary.pdf.
8. American Heart Association Nutrition Committee. Lichtenstein, A. et al. Diet and lifestyle recommendations revision 2006: a scientific statement from the American Heart Association Nutrition Committee. *Circulation.* 2006 July 4;114(1)e27.
9. US Food and Drug Administration. Trans Fatty Acids in Nutrition Labeling, Nutrient Content Claims, and Health Claims. Published July 11, 2003 Accessed October 15, 2004 a 5 A.D. October 20; URL: http://www.cfsan.fda.gov/~dms/qatrans2.html#s2q1.
10. *FDA Consumer magazine.* September–October 2003 Issue. Pub No. FDA04-1329C. URL: http://www.fda.gov/fdac/features/2003/503_fats.html.
11. *FDA Consumer magazine.* September–October 2003 Issue. Pub No. FDA04-1329C. URL: http://www.fda.gov/fdac/features/2003/503_fats.html.
12. Report of the Trans Fat Task Force submitted to the Minister of Health. TRANSforming the Food Supply. June 2006. URL: http://www.hc-sc.gc.ca/fn-an/alt_formats/hpfb-dgpsa/pdf/nutrition/tf-gt_rep-rap_e.pdf.
13. Mozaffarian D. Katan MB. Ascherio A. Stampfer MJ. Willett WC. Trans Fatty Acids and Cardiovascular Disease. *New England Journal of Medicine.* April 13, 2006. 354; 15:1601–13.
14. Stender S. et al. *A Trans World Journey.* Atherosclerosis Supplements 7 (2006) 47–52.
15. Staff Reporter. Cargill Expands Trans-fat Lowering Soyoil Production. FoodNavigator-USA.com. February 2, 2006. URL: http://www.foodnavigator-usa.com/news/ng.asp?id=65561-cargill-monsanto-vistive.
16. Monsanto Press Release. *Monsanto Research Platform Focuses on Reducing Unhealthy Fats in Soybean Oil.* URL: http://www.monsanto.com/monsanto/layout/media/03/10-27-03.asp.
17. National Restaurant Association (NRA). "Industry at a Glance." 2005.
18. Guthrie JF. et al. Role of Food Prepared Away from Home in the American Diet, 1977–78 Versus 1994–96: Changes and Consequences. *Society for Nutrition Education* 2002; 34: 140–150.
19. Staff Reporter. Cargill Expands Trans-fat Lowering Soyoil Production. FoodNavigator-USA.com. February 2, 2006. URL: http://www.foodnavigator-usa.com/news/ng.asp?id=65561-cargill-monsanto-vistive.
20. Guthrie JF, Derby BM, Levy AS. What people know and do not know about nutrition. In: Frazao E, ed. *America's Eating Habits: Changes and Consequences.* Washington, DC: Economic Research Service, United States Dept of Agriculture; 1999. Agriculture Information Bulletin No. 750:243–280.
21. Panel on Macronutrients, Institute of Medicine. Letter report on dietary reference intakes for trans fatty acids drawn from the Report on dietary reference intakes for energy, carbohydrate, fiber, fat, fatty acids, cholesterol, protein, and amino acids. 2002. Washington, DC, Institute of Medicine.
22. US Food and Drug Administration. Trans Fatty Acids in Nutrition Labeling, Nutrient content Claims, and Health Claims (68 Fed. Reg. 41443 (July 11, 2003)) accessed on October 15 at http://www.cfsan.fda.gov/~lrd/fr03711a.html.

S: HC 81.08 adopt

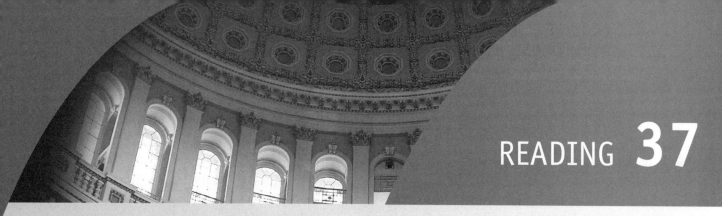

SCHIP Reauthorization: President's Budget Would Provide Less Than Half the Funds That States Need to Maintain SCHIP Enrollment

Edwin Park and Matt Broaddus

Source: **Courtesy of the Center on Budget and Policy Priorities. SCHIP Reauthorization: President's Budget Would Provide Less Than Half the Funds That States Need to Maintain SCHIP Enrollment. Edwin Park and Matt Broaddus, Center on Budget and Policy Priorities, Washington, DC, March 2007.**

The President's fiscal year 2008 budget proposes to reauthorize the State Children's Health Insurance Program (SCHIP) for five years but provides less than half of the funding needed for states to maintain their existing SCHIP caseloads, let alone to make progress in covering more uninsured low-income children. Under the President's budget, we estimate that states would experience a total federal funding shortfall of $7 billion over the next five years. (In other words, federal SCHIP funds would fall a total of $7 billion short of what will be needed to sustain states' current programs.)

The SCHIP program, which provides comprehensive health insurance coverage to more than four million children and is financed jointly by the federal government and the states, is in the final year of its original 10-year authorization and must be extended this year. If SCHIP is reauthorized but funding remains frozen at the current annual funding level of $5.04 billion per year (as is assumed in the OMB and CBO budget baselines), states will not have sufficient federal funding to sustain their programs. According to CBPP estimates based on the most recent SCHIP data, the total federal funding shortfall will equal as much as $13.4 billion over the next five years under the baseline funding levels.[1] (The Congressional Research Service estimates the shortfall at $12.1 billion over this period.[2]) The proposals in the President's budget would close a little less than half of this shortfall.

Unless the shortfalls are closed, states will have to scale back their SCHIP programs by reducing eligibility, capping enrollment, eliminating benefits, increasing beneficiary cost-sharing or cutting payments to providers, unless states are able to come up with sufficient additional state funds to plug the federal funding shortfalls.[3] In states that cut back their programs, significant numbers of SCHIP beneficiaries would be at risk.

The President's budget proposes to reauthorize the SCHIP program and to provide some additional funding. The President's budget would:

- Reauthorize the SCHIP program for five years at baseline levels of $5.04 billion per year.
- Provide an additional $4.8 billion to states, above the baseline funding levels, starting in fiscal year 2009. The President's budget would presumably distribute these funds to states that face federal funding shortfalls.
- Accelerate the redistribution of unspent SCHIP funds from prior years. Under current law, the Secretary recaptures and redistributes any SCHIP funds allocated to states that remain unspent after *three* years; the funds are then reallocated to states that need them. The President's budget would require the Secretary to recapture and redistribute SCHIP funds that remain unspent after *one* year.
- Reduce the federal matching rate for certain SCHIP beneficiaries. Under current law, the federal government pays, on average, 70 percent of the cost of covering SCHIP beneficiaries. The President's budget would reduce the SCHIP matching rate to the Medicaid matching rate (on average, 57 percent) for children in families with incomes above 200 percent of the poverty line (just

over $34,000 for a family of three in 2007). The President's budget also would substitute the lower Medicaid matching rate for the SCHIP matching rate for SCHIP coverage of adults, the large majority of whom are working-poor parents of low-income children enrolled in Medicaid or SCHIP. About 11 states cover some parents through SCHIP, under waivers granted by the federal government. (In the typical, or median, state, the income eligibility limit for working parents under Medicaid is only 65 percent of the poverty line, or about $11,200 for a family of three. Working-poor parents with incomes above that level are ineligible for Medicaid in the typical state.) Five states also cover poor adults other than parents.

While some details of the Administration's SCHIP reauthorization proposal have not yet been made public, the President's budget—along with additional detail provided by Administration officials to Congressional staff—provides sufficient information to estimate the likely effects of the President's proposals. Using the Center on Budget and Policy Priorities' SCHIP financing model, which is based on a financing model originally developed by the Office of the Actuary at the Centers for Medicare and Medicaid Services and is similar to the model used by the Congressional Research Service, we estimate that the President's SCHIP proposals would have the following effects.

1. States would face a total federal SCHIP funding short-fall estimated at $7 billion over the next five years. Under the President's budget, the total federal funding shortfall would be approximately $7 billion over a five-year period (2008–2012). This is a little more than half of the $13.4 billion total shortfall that states otherwise would incur (i.e., that states would incur under the baseline funding levels).[4] The shortfall would remain this large because the President's proposal provides a little more than $6.3 billion in federal SCHIP funds to avert shortfalls among the states, of which only $4.8 billion would represent additional funds above the levels already assumed in the baseline. (See Figure 1 for a year-by-year comparison between the President's budget and the budget baseline.)

The other $1.5 billion of the $6.3 billion that the President's budget would provide to address shortfalls consists of *existing* SCHIP funds that already are expected to be spent in the future. The Administration's proposal to hasten the redistribution of unspent funds—by reducing the period of time for which states may retain SCHIP funds from three years to one—would accelerate the spending of such funds, with more of these funds being spent in fiscal years 2008 and 2009 than would otherwise be the case. But fewer of these funds then would remain to be used in the latter part of the five-year period. As discussed below, using these funds to address shortfalls in 2008 and 2009 would help to eliminate or greatly reduce the shortfalls in those years but would increase the number of states that face shortfalls in later years.

2. By 2012, some 46 states would face a total shortfall of $2.9 billion, which is equal to the average annual cost of covering 1.4 million children through SCHIP. Our analysis indi-

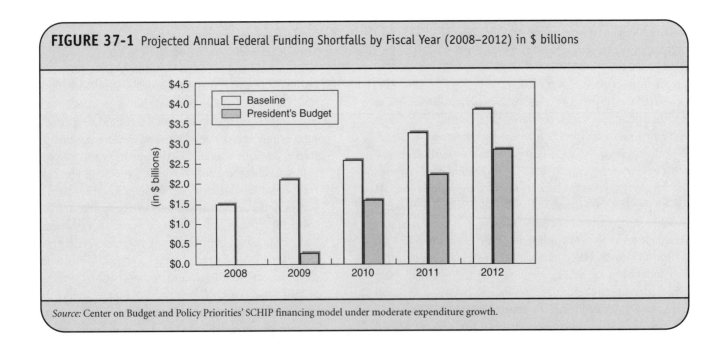

FIGURE 37-1 Projected Annual Federal Funding Shortfalls by Fiscal Year (2008–2012) in $ billions

Source: Center on Budget and Policy Priorities' SCHIP financing model under moderate expenditure growth.

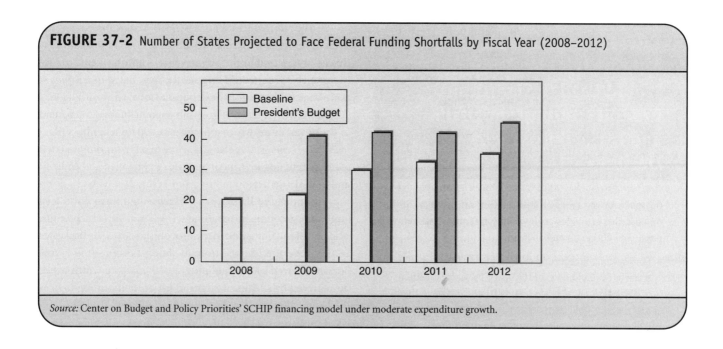

FIGURE 37-2 Number of States Projected to Face Federal Funding Shortfalls by Fiscal Year (2008–2012)

Source: Center on Budget and Policy Priorities' SCHIP financing model under moderate expenditure growth.

cates that the President's budget would provide sufficient funding in fiscal year 2008 to avert shortfalls. In 2009, an estimated 41 states would face shortfalls, but the shortfalls would be relatively small, totaling $331 million. (See Figures 1 and 2.) The 2009 shortfall is equivalent to the cost of covering 196,000 chil-

dren; see Figure 3 for a year-by-year comparison of the number of children potentially at risk.) In the years after 2009, however, the shortfalls would become progressively larger, and the number of SCHIP beneficiaries at risk of losing their health insurance coverage would rise.[5] Indeed, under the President's

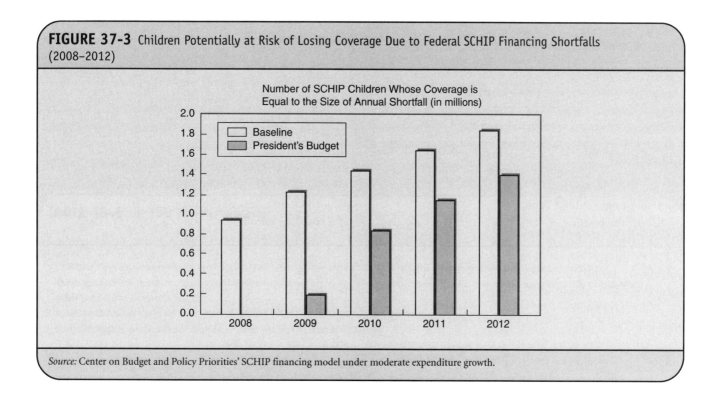

FIGURE 37-3 Children Potentially at Risk of Losing Coverage Due to Federal SCHIP Financing Shortfalls (2008–2012)

Source: Center on Budget and Policy Priorities' SCHIP financing model under moderate expenditure growth.

CBO Estimates that the Administration's Proposal Would Lead to Significant Federal Funding Shortfalls and Large Enrollment Declines

On March 9, the Congressional Budget Office issued its own detailed estimates of the Administration's SCHIP proposal. The CBO estimates indicate:*

- States would face a total federal funding shortfall of as much as $7.6 billion over the next five years (if current SCHIP matching rates are retained), which is more than half the $13.4 billion shortfall that CBO estimates states will experience under baseline funding levels. The Administration's proposal to reduce the federal SCHIP matching rate for certain beneficiaries would, if adopted, reduce the shortfall to $4.6 billion by shifting up to $3 billion in costs to states.

- SCHIP enrollment of children and pregnant women over the course of a year would decline from 7.6 million in 2007 (assuming Congress closes the current-year shortfalls) to 6.2 million by 2012, a reduction of 1.4 million. Total SCHIP enrollment would fall by 1.6 million.

---

* Congressional Budget Office, "Additional Information on CBO's Estimate of the Administration's SCHIP Proposals," March 9, 2007. See also Edwin Park and Matt Broaddus, "CBO Estimates President's SCHIP Proposal Would Lead to Large Enrollment Declines and Funding Shortfalls," March 13, 2007.

proposals, the number of states experiencing shortfalls in these years would exceed the number of states that would face shortfalls under the budget baseline (although the total size of the shortfalls would not be as large; see Figures 1 and 2).

Under the baseline, 36 states are estimated to have insufficient federal funding in 2012 to maintain their existing SCHIP programs. Under the President's budget, the number of states facing shortfalls in 2012 would increase to 46. This would occur because the provision accelerating the redistribution of unspent SCHIP funds would shift to states facing shortfalls in 2008 and 2009 funds that otherwise would be spent by other states in subsequent years. The states that would give up these unspent funds would have fewer SCHIP funds at their disposal and be more likely eventually to face shortfalls. (See Figure 2.)

3. **Shortfall states whose SCHIP programs cover children in families with incomes above $34,000 for a family of three (200 percent of the poverty line) and/or parents of low-income children would encounter new fiscal incentives to scale back coverage for these populations.** Currently, at least 16 states cover children with family incomes above 200 percent of the poverty line, which is about $34,000 for a family of three in 2007.[6] Eleven states also use some SCHIP funding to cover some parents of low-income children enrolled in Medicaid and SCHIP.[7]

As noted, the President's budget would leave states with large and growing shortfalls starting in 2009, which would place substantial financial pressures on states to scale back their SCHIP coverage.[8] In addition, the budget proposes $24.7 billion in cuts to the Medicaid program, the bulk of which would be achieved by shifting a larger share of Medicaid costs from the federal government to the states. That would place added fiscal pressures on the states.[9]

As a result of the proposed reduction in the federal matching rates for these populations, SCHIP children over 200 percent of the poverty line and low-income working parents would be at particular risk of losing coverage. Indeed, such a result is explicitly intended under the President's budget, in order to "refocus" SCHIP on children in families below 200 percent of the poverty line.[10] To continue to cover these populations, states would have to increase state funding enough *both* to offset the overall federal funding shortfalls they still would face *and* to offset the reduction in the federal matching rate for covering these children and parents.

Furthermore, not only would children over 200 percent of the poverty line who lose SCHIP likely end up uninsured, but many children *below* 200 percent of the poverty line who live in states that currently cover parents could end up uninsured as well. A large body of research has found that public-program coverage of *parents* of low-income who are children eligible for Medicaid and SCHIP markedly increases the enrollment of their *children* in the programs, as well.[11] States that face funding shortfalls and a lower federal matching rate and respond by scaling back or eliminating SCHIP coverage for parents could see enrollment among children fall as well.

The fiscal incentives for states to scale back coverage for these populations would be even greater if the President's budget also restricts the availability of its $4.8 billion in new funding and the unspent funds that would be recovered and redistributed. (The Administration has not yet specified whether its proposal contains these restrictions, although it seems likely its proposal would contain these restrictions in some form.) If the President's budget limits the provision of these funds to shortfall states that do *not* cover such populations, or allows the use of these funds only to plug shortfalls attributable to children with incomes below 200 percent of the poverty line, that would place still greater pressure on states to cease covering these populations.

4. The President's budget would do nothing to help states cover more uninsured children, since it does not even eliminate the shortfalls that states would experience under their existing programs. Many health care providers, insurers, low-income advocates, and state governments, as well as a number of members of Congress of both parties, have voiced support for making further significant progress toward the goal of covering all uninsured children, and for utilizing SCHIP reauthorization as a vehicle for that effort. However, since the President's budget would provide fewer funds than are needed just to ensure that states can sustain their existing SCHIP programs, no progress in covering more uninsured children would be made.

Research indicates that 74 percent of the nearly nine million U.S. children who are uninsured are already eligible for Medicaid or SCHIP but are not enrolled.[12] Enrolling and covering these children would require a significantly larger increase in federal funding for SCHIP (and Medicaid) than the President's budget includes. Sufficient funding would be needed both to fully close the SCHIP shortfalls and to cover a large portion of the uninsured low-income children who are eligible for Medicaid or SCHIP but are not participating.

CONCLUSION

The President's budget for SCHIP reauthorization falls short on two counts. First, while it acknowledges the need for additional SCHIP funding above the levels assumed in the budget baseline, it does not provide sufficient funding for states simply to sustain their existing programs, and it erects fiscal incentives for states to cease providing SCHIP coverage to children with modest incomes and low-income parents. The likely result of the large federal funding shortfalls that would remain would be fewer individuals covered through SCHIP and more people who are uninsured.

Second, the budget does not encourage states to continue making progress toward covering more uninsured children, despite the growing consensus that SCHIP reauthorization should serve as a vehicle for reaching the several million low-income children who are eligible for Medicaid or SCHIP but remain unenrolled and uninsured.

NOTES

1. See Matt Broaddus and Edwin Park, "Freezing SCHIP Funding in Coming Years Would Reverse Recent Gains in Children's Health Coverage," Center on Budget and Policy Priorities, Revised February 22, 2007. This analysis estimates a five-year shortfall of $12.3 billion to $13.4 billion, assuming that SCHIP is reauthorized but funding is frozen at current levels. The $12.3 billion estimate is the result of the low-growth version of the CBPP SCHIP financing model. The $13.4 billion estimate is the result of the moderate-growth version of the CBPP SCHIP financing model. For purposes of analyzing the President's budget, we estimate its effects relative to the estimated shortfall under the moderate-growth scenario. For an explanation of the differences between the two cost growth scenarios, see Broaddus and Park.

2. Chris Peterson, "Funding Projections and State Redistribution Issues", Congressional Research Service, Updated January 30, 2007.

3. States could address part of the shortfalls they face by expanding their Medicaid programs to cover some of their current SCHIP beneficiaries. However, this would require states to bear a significantly higher share of the cost of covering these beneficiaries, because the federal Medicaid matching rate is, on average, 13 percentage points lower than the average federal SCHIP matching rate.

4. Under the low-expenditure growth version of the CBPP SCHIP financing model, we estimate that the President's budget would leave a remaining shortfall of $5.7 billion over five years.

5. Under the low-expenditure growth version of the CBPP SCHIP financing model, we estimate that 43 states would face a total shortfall of $2.2 billion in 2012, equal to the cost of covering 1.1 million children.

6. The 16 states are California, Connecticut, Georgia, Hawaii, Maryland, Massachusetts, Minnesota, Missouri, New Hampshire, New Jersey, New Mexico, New York, Rhode Island, Vermont, Washington and West Virginia. In addition, both Pennsylvania and the District of Columbia are scheduled to implement SCHIP expansions to children above 200 percent of the poverty line.

7. Arizona, Illinois, Minnesota, New Jersey, Rhode Island and Wisconsin cover parents through their SCHIP programs. In addition, Arkansas, Idaho, Nevada, New Mexico, and Oregon cover a very limited number of parents through their SCHIP-funded premium assistance programs, which generally use SCHIP funds to subsidize the purchase of employer-based coverage.

8. In calculating the aggregate shortfall that states will experience over the five-year period (2008–2012), we do not take into account the effect of the lower matching rate that the President's proposal would institute for certain SCHIP beneficiaries. The lower matching rate would artificially reduce the need for federal SCHIP funds among the states that cover those beneficiaries and hence would reduce the overall shortfall. We did not include this effect in our estimates of the shortfall because our estimates are intended to reflect the funding gap between how much states will need to sustain their current programs under current rules (including the current rules governing federal matching rates) and how much federal funding states will have available under the President's proposal. Taking into account the lower matching rate would reduce our estimate of the size of the five-year shortfall from $7.0 billion to $5.1 billion.

9. See Leighton Ku, Andy Schneider and Judy Solomon, "The Administration Again Proposes to Shift Federal Medicaid Costs to States," Center on Budget and Policy Priorities, February 14, 2007.

10. Office of Management and Budget, "Budget of the United States Government, Fiscal Year 2008," February 5, 2007.

11. See Leighton Ku and Matthew Broaddus, "Coverage of Parents Helps Children Too," Center on Budget and Policy Priorities, October 20, 2006.

12. See, for example, Kaiser Commission on Medicaid and the Uninsured, "Enrolling Low-Income Uninsured Children in Medicaid and SCHIP," January 2007.

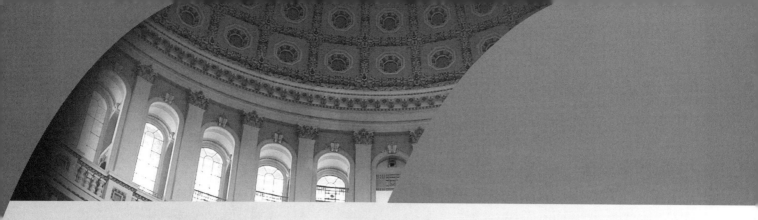

Index